EXOTIC
ANIMAL MEDICINE

Dedicated to my parents, Edna and Gordon, who have suffered fish, snakes, and escaping frogs, as well as childhood holidays dictated by zoo locations, and to my sons Charlton, Quaid, and Lloyd, who over the years have been enthusiastic but frequently bemused spectators of the animal antics in both my professional and home life.

EXOTIC
ANIMAL MEDICINE
A QUICK REFERENCE GUIDE

Lance Jepson MA, VetMB, CBiol, MIBiol, MRCVS
Origin Vets Veterinary Referral & Consultancy
Service for Zoo, Avian, Aquatic and Unusual Pets, Wales, UK

ELSEVIER

ELSEVIER

3251 Riverport Lane
St. Louis, Missouri 63043

EXOTIC ANIMAL MEDICINE: A QUICK REFERENCE GUIDE,   ISBN: 978-0-323-32849-4
SECOND EDITION

Library of Congress Cataloging-in-Publication Data
Jepson, Lance, author.
 Exotic animal medicine : a quick reference guide / Lance Jepson.—2.
    p. ; cm.
 Includes bibliographical references and index.
 ISBN 978-0-323-32849-4 (pbk. : alk. paper)   1. Exotic animals–Diseases–Handbooks, manuals, etc.   I. Title.
 [DNLM: 1. Animal Diseases–Handbooks.   2. Pets–Handbooks. SF 997.5.E95]
 SF997.5.E95J47 2016
 591.6′2–dc23
                                                                    2015022319

Content Strategy Director: Penny Rudolph
Associate Content Development Specialist: Laura Klein
Publishing Services Manager: Hemamalini Rajendrababu
Project Manager: Manchu Mohan
Designer: Miles Hitchen

Printed in the United States of America.

Last digit is the print number: 13 12 11 10 9

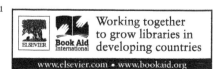

Working together
to grow libraries in
developing countries

www.elsevier.com • www.bookaid.org

Acknowledgments

· ·

Exotic pets are more popular than ever. In some cases they provide companionship, in others they are a fascination and a hobby, and in still others, a cause. I am privileged to be a veterinary surgeon who works solely with exotic species. A great many people have influenced and inspired my professional life in both its course and its content. Many of these are colleagues, students, or clients who have become more friends than "customers." To single them out would be to put one above the other and I cannot do that, but thank you all.

Introduction to the Second Edition

How to use this book

During their training, veterinarians are trained to apply the same core set of clinical skills and thought processes to the health problems and management of several different domestic species. Often due to time constraints and outmoded perceptions, exotic pets fall off the radar. The practicing veterinarian often therefore feels at a disadvantage when presented with the more unusual species, yet those same core skills, backed by relevant information, can be applied as easily to a bearded dragon as they can to a bearded collie.

The Quick Reference Guide to Exotic Pet Medicine was conceived to aid the veterinary clinician to professionally and quickly deal with a wide array of exotic pets and their problems. It allows the veterinarian to create a diagnostic and treatment plan in a short space of time for a wide range of exotic pets, some of which he or she may not be familiar with. This second edition has been updated to include advances in our knowledge of exotic animal diseases and also includes three new chapters covering hedgehogs, common marmosets, and sugar gliders.

The approach is hoped to be a practical one, combining both clinical signs and/or an organ system perspective. Thus a parrot may present with a loss of flight (clinical sign) or have a liver disorder diagnosed on blood sampling (organ system). Where relevant, there is cross-referencing between the different sections.

Lists of differential diagnoses

These provide the clinician with a rapid overview of the likely conditions to be encountered in a given animal group. Where no examples are listed but the heading is still included, these should still be considered even though no examples have been reported in the literature. As an example, neoplasia should occur on most lists of differential diagnoses.

Findings on clinical examination

These list the most common signs seen within the given group of disorders. Not every clinical sign will be seen in every case, and because of this some may appear contradictory. They are given as an aid to diagnosis. Some diseases may present as a syndrome of typical signs; where this occurs, an indication of that disease is given in brackets at the end of the description. I have tried to make these complete and accurate wherever possible, but the huge range of individual and species-related responses to a multitude of diseases and challenges means that variations outside those listed are possible.

Investigations

A list of the basic types of investigative procedures is offered to stimulate ideas on how to approach a given case. In some cases useful general tips are given; in others normal values (or expected abnormalities) that may be difficult to find in the literature are given where it may aid a diagnosis. In some cases, specific tests for certain diseases (e.g., polymerase chain reaction) are listed to aid the clinician with what tests are potentially available (although this may vary from country to country). The basic list of investigations is as follows and is included in every section to act as a reminder:

- Radiography
- Routine hematology and biochemistry
- Culture and sensitivity
- Endoscopy
- Biopsy/necropsy
- Ultrasonography

It is hoped that by the consideration and undertaking of appropriate tests, diagnoses can be achieved even if these fall outside of the potential differential lists. Other more advanced, potential investigative techniques, such as magnetic resonance imaging and computed tomography scans, are not to be ruled out or discounted. Where practical their use can make a significant contribution to the diagnostic procedure, but it is assumed that most practicing clinicians will not have ready access to these facilities.

Management

In most cases the clinician is referred to the section on general nursing care at the beginning of each chapter. In some conditions more specific recommendations are given.

Treatment/specific therapy

For each condition, suggested treatment options are given. Not every drug variation is listed, as there are some excellent resources, such as *Carpenter's Exotic Animal Formulary* (Saunders) and *The Veterinary Formulary* (Pharmaceutical Press), that amply cover this information and to which the clinician may already have access. However, an extensive index is provided to aid the rapid recovery of drug dosage regimens cited in the species covered. The majority of the drugs mentioned are not licensed for use in the species described, and where applicable, consent should be gained from the owner before their use. Due consideration should be given to mandatory drug selection procedures where such systems exist—for example, the cascade system in the UK.

Contents

Ferrets

Ferrets *(Mustela putorius furo)* are thought to be a domesticated form of the European polecat *(M. putorius)* and, not surprisingly, have a history extending back alongside the domestic rabbit. Originally kept as working animals, selective breeding for color varieties and temperament has resulted in a significant rise in their being kept as pets and show animals.

Table 1-1 The ferret: Key facts	
Average life span	5-8+ years
Weight	Male: 1.0-2.0 kg
	Female: 0.5-1.0 kg
Body temperature (°C)	37.8-40
Respiratory rate (per min)	33-36
Heart rate (beats per min)	180-250
Gestation (days)	41-42
Age at weaning	6-8 weeks
Sexual maturity	4-8 months (in the first spring following birth—typically March)

Consultation and handling

Ferrets vary markedly in their temperament; working ferrets are perhaps slightly more unpredictable, whereas pet ferrets are usually well handled and unlikely to bite unless provoked. When handling a ferret, it can be easily restrained around the neck; a towel can be used—draped over the body—before grasping the neck to protect from scratching. For those ferrets determined to bite, scruffing and holding with all four legs off the table will usually relax them to allow a reasonable examination.

Many ferrets intensely enjoy certain commercially available dietary supplements (e.g., 8 in 1 FerreTone) to the extent that they will readily tolerate some procedures such as electrocardiography as long as they are supplied with a steady stream of product to lick.

Always weigh the ferret whenever examined to monitor weight trends. A healthy ferret aboveground walks with a dorsal flexure in its back. Hind-leg paresis can be a nonspecific sign of ill health in the ferret due to weakness of the muscle groups needed to maintain this position.

Odor is a feature of ferret life and is likely to be used for transmitting and receiving information about individuals, such as identification, age, sex, and sexual readiness. Most of this smell comes from the sebaceous skin glands, which regress following routine castration, ovariohysterectomy or deslorelin implantation. The anal sacs can produce a strong-smelling liquid, but this tends only to occur if the ferret is frightened. Therefore, routine anal gland removal ("descenting") of ferrets is largely pointless and could constitute unnecessary surgery.

Blood sampling

Suitable sites for venipuncture are the jugular, cephalic, and saphenous veins. Alternatively the ventral tail artery and veins can be used.

Blood collection from the tail in the ferret

1. The ferret is held on its back with ventral tail shaved.
2. Use a 21- or 23- gauge 25-mm needle.
3. There is a flattened area on the ventral side for the proximal 4 to 5 cm overlying the ventral concavity of the caudal vertebrae.
4. The artery there is flanked by two veins.
5. The needle is inserted at a shallow angle toward the body around 3 to 4 cm from the base of the tail.

If blood sampling is done under isoflurane anesthetic, note that isoflurane has been linked with a reduction in packed cell volume (PCV), hemoglobin level, and RBC count. In addition, one may need to centrifuge the blood for 20% longer than for other species and collect 3× plasma volume required. This may be due to increased erythropoiesis from the spleen.

The typical WBC count is neutrophilic with <30% lymphocytes. Absolute and relative increases in lymphocyte counts may indicate lymphosarcoma.

It is not uncommon for ferrets to have two or more pathologic conditions ongoing at the same time. Combinations include variations on insulinomas, hyperadrenocortism, lymphoma, and cardiomyopathy. The clinician should always be aware that the situation may be more complicated than it initially appears and be prepared to investigate several possible clinical problems simultaneously.

Avoid gentamicin as it has been associated with nephrotoxicity and ototoxicity (deafness) in ferrets.

Nursing care

• •

Thermoregulation

For general principles, see "Thermoregulation" under *Nursing Care* in Chapter 2.

Fluid therapy

The normal maintenance water intake for ferrets is 75 to 100 mL/kg/day. In ferrets, the choice of fluid used is indicated as with other mammals. Fluid replacement calculations are as for other species. All fluids should be warmed to 38° C.

Recommended fluid replacement rates for ferrets

1. Subcutaneous: 30 to 60 mL
2. Intraperitoneal: 30 to 60 mL
3. Ferrets in shock or suffering from profound losses from vomiting and diarrhea may need up to 180 to 240 mL/kg over a 24-hour period.
4. Crystalloids: For ferrets the maintenance fluid rate is 75 to 100 mL/kg/24 hours. Shock rate is up to 100 mL/kg over 1 hour.
5. Colloids: A bolus of 10 to 15 mL/kg over 30 minutes can be given up to four times daily.

Blood transfusions

Blood volume is 40 to 60 mL per ferret. Blood groups have not been demonstrated (Manning and Bell 1990), so there is thought to be no need for cross matching.

Estimation of blood volume requirement

Based upon an assumption of 70 mL/kg/hr maintenance fluid requirement (Orcutt 1998):

$$\text{Anticoagulated blood volume (mL)} = \text{body weight (kg)} \times 70 \times \frac{\text{PCV desired} - \text{PCV recipient}}{\text{PCV of donor in anticoagulant}}$$

Nutritional support

- Ferrets are prone to hypoglycemia, so nutritional support is imperative. If anorexic for even a comparatively short time, a ferret may be hypoglycemic, so test with a commercial glucometer on a small sample of blood. IV or IP glucose can be given to these cases once identified (see *Pancreatic Disorders* in this chapter for normal blood glucose values).
- Commercially available high-energy dog and cat recovery foods (e.g., Prescription Diet a/d Canine/Feline Critical Care by Hills Pet Products) are suitable.
- Force-feeding is possible with these supplements at 2 to 5 mL, 3 to 4 times daily.

Analgesia

Table 1-2   The ferret: Analgesic doses

Analgesic	Dose
Buprenorphine	0.01-0.03 mg/kg SC, IM, or IV every 8-12 hours
Butorphanol	0.1-0.5 mg/kg SC, IM, or IV every 2-4 hours
Carprofen	1.0-2.0 mg/kg SC or IM every 12-24 hours
Ketoprofen	1.0 mg/kg SC or IM every 12-24 hours
Meloxicam	0.1-0.3 mg/kg SC or PO every 24 hours
Morphine	0.5-5.0 mg/kg SC or IM every 2-6 hours
Meperidine/pethidine	5-10 mg/kg SC, IM, IV every 2-4 hours
Nalbuphine	0.5-1.5 mg/kg IM or IV every 2-3 hours
Tramadol	5-10 mg/kg PO every 24 hours

Table 1-3   The ferret: Gastroprotectants

Cimetidine	10 mg/kg PO, SC, IM, or IV (slow) q.i.d.
Ranitidine	3.5 mg /kg PO b.i.d.
Famotidine	2.5 mg/ferret PO, SC, or IV s.i.d.
Omeprazole	4 mg/kg s.i.d. PO
Sucralfate	25 mg/kg PO q.i.d.

Anesthesia

Ferrets have a very short gut transit time of around 3 hours; therefore, if starved overnight there is a high risk of hypoglycemia. Do not starve preoperatively.

There are many anesthetic protocols written up in the literature. The author has found the following protocols useful

---

Anesthetic protocol

1. Premedication
   a. Midazolam 0.25 to 0.3/kg IM or IV
   b. Diazepam at 2 mg/kg IM or SC
2. Ferrets are easily induced with 5% isoflurane, head held in a mask.
3. Intubate

Parenteral anesthesia

1. Propofol at 2 to 10 mg/kg IV *or*
2. Ketamine at 5 mg/kg; medetomidine at 80 µg/kg; butorphanol at 0.1 mg/kg, all given simultaneously IM
3. Intubate and maintain with isoflurane as necessary.
4. Reverse with atipamezole SC, IV, IP, or IM at same volume of administered medetomidine.

- Intraoperative care
  - Keep warm (see "Thermoregulation").
  - Replace fluids (see "Fluid Therapy").
- Postoperative aftercare
  - Reverse medetomidine (if used) with atipamezole at same volume as administered medetomidine IM.
  - Supply analgesia—as for other small mammals.
  - Must be offered food as soon as animal recovers.
  - Keep warm.

Cardiopulmonary resuscitation

1. Intubate and ventilate at 20 to 30 breaths/min.
2. Reverse medetomidine (if used) with atipamezole at same volume as administered medetomidine IM.
3. If cardiac arrest, external cardiac massage at around 100 compressions/min.
4. Epinephrine at
   a. 0.2 to 0.4 mg/kg diluted in sterile saline intratracheal.
   b. 0.2 mg/kg intracardiac, IV or IO
5. Fluid therapy (see above)
6. If bradycardic, atropine at 0.05 mg/kg IV or 0.05 to 0.1 mg/kg intratracheal.

Skin disorders

Ferrets undergo a seasonal cycle of hair thinning that occurs during the summer months. There are multiple sebaceous glands in the skin that impart both a greasy feel to the coat and the typical musky ferret smell. These glands are more numerous in males, and in some albino males they can produce a dirty, yellow appearance. Neutering and deslorelin implantation causes some atrophy of these glands, reducing the odor.

Pruritus

- Ectoparasites
  - Note that *Sarcoptes scabiei* presents in two clinical patterns—generalized and localized to the feet.

- Hyperadrenocorticism (see *Endocrine Disorders*)
- Pyoderma
  - Staphylococci
  - Streptococci
  - *Corynebacterium*
  - *Pasteurella*
  - *Actinomyces*
  - *Escherichia coli*
- Dermatophytosis

Alopecia

- Self-mutilation
- Hormonal
- Hyperadrenocorticism (see *Endocrine Disorders*, Fig. 1-1)
- Ovarian pedicle neoplasia (Patterson et al 2003)
- Alopecia at tail base (hyperestrogenism—see *Reproductive Disorders*)
- Seasonal alopecia
- Pregnancy toxemia/ketosis (see *Reproductive Disorders*)
- Dermatophytosis
- Mucormycosis *(Absidia corymbifera)*
- Biotin deficiency (feeding raw eggs)

Scaling and crusting

- Canine distemper virus (CDV—see *Systemic Disorders*)
- Pyoderma
- Dermatophytosis

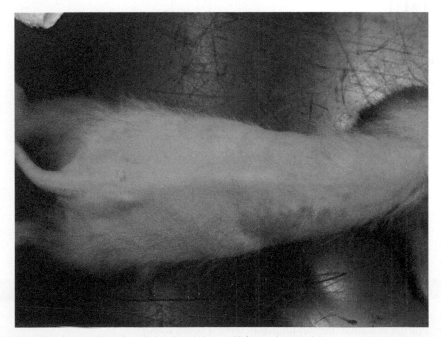

Fig 1-1. Bilateral symmetrical alopecia in a female ferret with hyperadrenocorticism.

Erosions and ulceration

- Excoriation from self-inflicted trauma if pruritic
- Bite wound
- *Blastomyces dermatitidis*
- *Cryptococcus bacillisporus*

Nodules and nonhealing wounds

- Abscess
- Hematoma
- Granuloma
- Swollen mammary glands
  - Painful, discolored (acute mastitis, neoplasia—see *Reproductive Disorders*)
  - Nonpainful, normal color (chronic mastitis, neoplasia—see *Reproductive Disorders*)
- Swollen, discharging swellings around neck (actinomycosis)

Changes in pigmentation

- Dry, dull coat (poor diet)
- CDV (see *Systemic Disorders*)
- Swollen, painful mammary glands; may turn black (gangrenous) (acute mastitis—see *Reproductive Disorders*)
- Ectoparasites
  - Fleas (*Ctenocephalides* spp.)
  - Ear mites *(Otodectes cynotis)*
  - Ticks
  - *Sarcoptes scabiei*
  - *Demodex* spp.
  - *Lynxacarus mustelae* (fur mite)
  - Myiasis
  - *Cuterebra* spp.
  - *Hypoderma bovis*

Neoplasia

- Mast cell tumor
- Sebaceous gland adenoma
- Hemangioma
- Squamous cell carcinoma
- Benign cystic adenoma
- Preputial adenocarcinoma
- Dermatofibroma
- Carcinoma
- Fibroma
- Fibrosarcoma
- Histiocytoma
- Sarcoma
- Lymphoma (rarely presents as a skin lesion)

Findings on clinical examination

- Thick brown, waxy exudate from ears (ear mites)
- Pruritis and inflammation limited to feet *(Sarcoptes scabiei)*

- Hyperkeratosis of the footpads and erythematous cutaneous rashes in the inguinal area and under the chin. Oculonasal discharge (CDV)
- Swellings with discharging sinuses in the cervical area (bite wounds, actinomycosis)

Investigations

1. Microscopy: examine fur pluck, acetate strips, or skin scrapes to affected area and examine for ectoparasites.
2. Examine material from ear canals for *Otodectes cynotis*.
3. Bacteriology and mycology: hair pluck or swab lesions for routine culture and sensitivity
4. Fine-needle aspirate followed by staining with rapid Romanowsky stains
5. Biopsy obvious lesions.
6. Ultraviolet (Wood's) lamp—positive for *Microsporum canis* only (not all strains fluoresce)
7. Radiography
8. Routine hematology and biochemistry
9. Culture and sensitivity
10. Endoscopy
11. Biopsy
12. Ultrasonography

Treatment/specific therapy

- Fleas
  - Commercial flea treatments at cat dose rates
  - Lufenuron at 10 mg/kg SC or 30 mg/kg PO in food
  - Topical spot-on preparations of 10% (w/v) imidacloprid (Advantage, Bayer) at 10 mg/kg and 10% (W/V) imidacloprid/50% (w/v) permethrin (Advantix, Bayer) at 10 mg/kg have proven efficacious at flea control on the mink (Larsen et al 2005) and should be safe on the ferret. Environmental flea control will be required.
- Sarcoptic mange
  - Ivermectin at 0.2 to 0.4 mg/kg SC every 7 to 14 days to resolution
  - Selamectin at dose for ear mites (see *Ear Mites* below)
  - Moxidectin at dose for ear mites (see *Ear Mites* below)
- Ear mites
  - Topical antiparasitic ear preparations, although the small size of the ear canal may prevent effective treatment.
  - Selamectin spot-on at 6 mg/kg as a topical spot-on preparation; has proven safe at 45 mg/adult ferret (Stronghold Cat, Pfizer) (Revolution , Zoetis) (Miller et al 2006)
  - 10% imidacloprid/1% moxidectin (Advocate (UK) Revolution, Zoetis (USA), Bayer) at 1 drop per 100 g body weight (Beck 2007)
  - Cross-infection with dogs and cats in the same household may occur.
- Demodex
  - Amitraz (0.05%) topically every 7 days
- Myiasis
  - Remove larvae.
  - Clean and debride wounds.
  - Systemic parasiticide (e.g., ivermectin, selamectin, imidacloprid)
  - Covering antibiosis
  - Supportive therapy if necessary

- Pyoderma, bacterial dermatitis, and cellulitis
  - Shave any badly infected areas.
  - Apply topical and parenteral antibiotics.
  - Cleaning with chlorhexidine solution may be beneficial.
- Surgical removal of abscesses
- Bites and lacerations
  - Clean and debride well.
  - Covering broad-spectrum antibiosis
- Actinomycosis
  - Debride and clean lesion.
  - Appropriate antibiosis
- Dermatophytosis, *Blastomyces,* and mucormycosis
  - Miconazole/chlorhexidine (Malaseb, Leo) shampoo—bath once daily
  - Griseofulvin at 25 mg/kg PO s.i.d. for 21 to 30 days
  - Itraconazole at 25 to 33 mg/kg PO s.i.d. for 30 days
  - Ketoconazole at 10 to 30 mg/kg PO s.i.d. for 60 days
- *Cryptococcus*
  - Amphotericin B, at 150 µg/kg i.v. 3 times weekly for 2-4 months
- Seasonal alopecia
  - In breeding season (March to August); will regrow
  - Hair loss occurring in winter and early spring may be an early indicator of hyperadrenocorticism (see *Endocrine Disorders*).
- Self-mutilation
  - Lack of suitable hiding places or other stressors
  - Females plucking hair for nesting
- Biotin deficiency
  - Associated with diets >10% raw egg
  - Reduce egg intake and supplement with proprietary vitamin formula.
- Neoplasia
  - Aggressive surgical resection
  - Chemotherapy may be attempted. Accessible cutaneous tumors can be treated by injecting cisplatin directly into the tissue mass on a weekly basis as a debulking exercise.

Respiratory tract disorders

Ferrets constantly investigate and monitor their environment by sniffing all available surfaces; hence sneezing is not uncommon.

Viral

- CDV (see *Systemic Disorders*)
- Influenza virus (orthomyxovirus)

Bacterial

- Bacterial pneumonias
- *Streptococcus zooepidemicus, S. pneumoniae,* group C and G streptococci
- *E. coli*
- *Klebsiella pneumoniae*
- *Pseudomonas aeruginosa*

- *Bordetella bronchiseptica*
- *Listeria monocytogenes*
- Mycobacteriosis: *M. bovis, M. abscessus*

Fungal

- Fungal mycoses (e.g., *Aspergillus*—rare)

Protozoal

- *Pneumocystis jiroveci*

Parasitic

- *Angiostrongylus vasorum* (lungworm)

Neoplasia

- Lymphoma/lymphosarcoma (see *Systemic Disorders*)
- Lung metastases

Other noninfectious problems

- Cardiac disorders
- Hyperestrogenism (see *Reproductive Disorders*)
- Gastric bloat (see *Gastrointestinal Tract Disorders*)

Findings on clinical examination

- Sneezing
- Coughing
- Dyspnea and tachypnea
- Air hunger
- Cyanosis
- Respiratory signs varying from a catarrhal rhinitis to pneumonia, plus oculonasal discharge, hyperkeratosis, and gastrointestinal signs (CDV)
- Pale mucous membranes (anemia—see *Cardiac and Hematologic Disorders*)
- Ocular and/or nasal discharges (CDV, influenza)
- Lethargy, dullness, depression, and pyrexia in addition to upper respiratory signs (influenza)
- Coughing, dyspnea, exercise intolerance, anorexia, and weight loss (interstitial pneumonia and hemorrhage); pulmonary hypertension and congestive heart failure; coagulopathy can result in anemia, melena, subcutaneous hematomas, and CNS signs (*Angiostrongylus vasorum*).

Investigations

1. Tracheal wash/bronchoalveolar lavage
2. Culture and sensitivity
3. Cytology
4. Pleural tap and cytology
5. Radiography
   a. Mediastinal lymphoma with pleural effusions occurs more commonly in younger ferrets.
6. Routine hematology and biochemistry
   a. Anemia; eosinophilia: *Angiostrongylus vasorum*

9

7. Serology for CDV, *Mycobacterium bovis*, influenza (hemagglutination inhibition tests and enzyme-linked immunosorbent assays [ELISAs] may be of benefit in detecting influenza A)
   a. Serology, polymerase chain reaction (PCR) fecal examination for *Angiostrongylus vasorum*
8. Endoscopy
9. Biopsy
10. Ultrasonography

Management

1. Provide supportive treatment (e.g., fluids), covering antibiosis.
2. Reduce stress levels. Hospitalize away from dogs and noisy cats; keep in darkened position.
3. Supply oxygen, preferably via an oxygen tent.
4. Mucolytics (e.g., bromhexine, *N*-acetylcysteine) may be useful.
5. Pleural effusion—consider tube thoracostomy.

Treatment/specific therapy

- CDV (see *Systemic Disorders*)
- Influenza
  - Ferrets are very susceptible to the human influenza virus as well as the H5N1 strain (Govorkova et al 2005), showing pyrexia, anorexia, weight loss, lethargy, diarrhea, and death.
  - It can be transmitted from ferret to ferret and, more important, from human to ferret.
  - It may also be a potential zoonosis.
  - Usually transient and self-limiting—most ferrets will recover without treatment, although the H5N1 strain is potentially fatal.
  - Supportive care, including fluids and nutritional support, can be given if necessary.
  - Diphenhydramine at 1 mg/kg PO b.i.d.
  - Amantadine at 6.0 mg/kg PO b.i.d. or by nebulizer
  - Covering antibiosis to prevent secondary infections (mucopurulent oculonasal discharges)
- Bacterial pneumonia
  - Appropriate antibiosis
  - Otherwise care as described under *Management*
- Mycobacteriosis
  - Potential zoonosis, so consider euthanasia.
  - *M. abscessus* has been successfully treated with clarithromycin (Lunn et al 2005).
- Fungal mycoses
  - Ketoconazole at 10 to 30 mg/kg PO s.i.d. for 60 days
  - plain Amphotericin B
    - 0.25 to 1.0 mg/kg IV s.i.d. or every other day until a total dose of 7 to 25 mg has been given
    - For *Cryptococcus*, 150 µg/kg i.v. 3 times weekly for 2-4 months
  - Itraconazole at 25 to 33 mg/kg PO s.i.d. long term

- *Pneumocystis jiroveci*
  - Pentamidine isethionate at 3 to 4 mg/kg on alternate days for a maximum of 10 treatments
  - Co-trimoxazole at 30 mg/kg PO or SC b.i.d.
- *Angiostrongylus vasorum*
  - Uncommon but is an emerging disease of dogs in Europe; has been recorded in ferrets (Helm et al 2010)
  - Adult worms in pulmonary artery and right ventricle. Low burdens may be asymptomatic.
  - Moxidectin 1.0 to 4.0 mg/kg as Advocate (UK), Advantage Multi (USA) (Europe) or Advantage Multi for Cats (USA) 40 mg imidacloprid + 4 mg moxidectin spot-on solution for small cats and ferrets (Bayer). May need to be repeated monthly.
  - Avoid access to intermediate hosts, such as terrestrial mollusks like slugs, and paratenic hosts.

Gastrointestinal tract disorders

Permanent dental formula of the ferret

$$I:\frac{3}{3}, \quad C:\frac{1}{1}, \quad PM:\frac{3}{3}, \quad M:\frac{1}{2}$$

The permanent incisors erupt at around 6 to 8 weeks while the other permanents are usually through by 10 weeks.

Deciduous dental formula of the ferret

$$I:\frac{4}{3}, \quad C:\frac{1}{1}, \quad PM:\frac{0}{0}, \quad M:\frac{3}{3}$$

Disorders of the oral cavity

- Dental disease
  - Periodontal disease, gingivitis, and dental tartar not uncommon
  - May be associated with moist or semi-moist foods
  - Fractured canines are commonly found but are rarely painful unless the pulp is exposed.
  - If pulp/dentin is red/pink (recently exposed) or tan colored and the tooth color has been retained, these teeth can potentially be saved with an amalgam filling (Johnson-Delaney and Nelson 1992).
  - If pulp/dentin is dull gray, it is likely to be devitalized; if black, it is necrotic.
  - Manage as for dog and cat dental disease.
- Salivary mucocele
  - Facial swellings.
  - Aspirate sample for analysis, including cytology (differentiate from abscess, neoplasia, hematoma).
  - Surgical resection of the affected gland is the best option to prevent recurrence. Zygomatic and buccal glands are commonly affected—may require removal of zygomatic arch to aid surgical resection (Mullen 1997).

- Neoplasia
  - Salivary gland adenocarcinoma
  - Investigate as for salivary mucocele.
  - Oral fibrosarcoma
    - Solid mass from oral mucosa that gradually grows over the teeth, eventually interfering with feeding
    - Surgical resection, although it often becomes a debulking exercise as complete resection is difficult

Differential diagnoses for gastrointestinal disorders

Viral

- CDV (see *Systemic Disorders*)
- Rotavirus
- Influenza virus (transient diarrhea)
- Coronavirus (epizootic catarrhal enteritis, green slime disease)

Bacterial

- *Lawsonia intracellularis* (proliferative bowel disease, PBD)
- *Helicobacter mustelae*
- Salmonellosis, esp. *S. typhimurium, S. newport,* and *S. choleraesuis*
- *Campylobacter jejuni*
- *Clostridium perfringens* (possible cause of gastric bloat)
- Mycobacteriosis, esp. *M. bovis* and *M. avium*
- Anal gland abscess

Fungal

- *Cryptococcus neoformans* var. *grubii* (Malik et al 2002)

Protozoal

- *Isospora*
- *Giardia*
- *Cryptosporidium*

Parasitic

- *Toxascaris* (uncommon)
- *Toxocara* (uncommon)
- *Ancylostoma* (uncommon)
- Cestodes (uncommon)

Neoplasia

- Lymphoma/lymphosarcoma (see *Systemic Disorders*)
- Polyps
- Adenocarcinoma
- Anal gland neoplasia

Other noninfectious problems

- Eosinophilic gastroenteritis (EGE)
- Megaesophagus
- Foreign body
- Trichobezoar (hairball)
- Gastric ulceration (may be iatrogenic, e.g., NSAID overdose)

- Gastric bloat
- Rectal prolapse
- Anal sac impaction

Findings on clinical examination

- Diarrhea (with or without blood/melena; for melena, see also *Urinary Disorders*)
- Green diarrhea (epizootic catarrhal enteritis—see *Hepatic Disorders*)
- Vomiting/gagging
- Dehydration
- Anorexia
- Dysphagia
- Hypersalivation
- Teeth grinding and abdominal pain
- Weight loss
- Gastric distension, dyspnea, cyanosis
- Hemorrhagic diarrhea in young ferrets; occasional rectal prolapse *(Isospora)*
- Fecal tenesmus (especially in ferrets under 1 year of age) (PBD)
- Thickened bowel palpable (PBD, EGE)
- Colitis-like signs—increased amount of mucus and frank blood in the stool (PBD, EGE)
- Vomiting (± blood from erosions or ulcers), black tarry diarrhea (small intestine), watery diarrhea with frank blood (large intestine), and weight loss (EGE)
- Enlarged mesenteric lymph nodes may be palpable (EGE).
- Palpable foreign body
- Gastrointestinal signs are rare with CDV, but it should be considered if accompanied by oculonasal discharge, hyperkeratosis, and respiratory signs.

Investigations

1. Fecal examination
   a. *Isospora* oocysts
   b. Modified Ziehl-Neelsen (MZN) staining for *Cryptosporidium*
   c. Nematode eggs
2. Radiography
   a. Megaesophagus (contrast study with barium at 10 mL/kg PO)
   b. Foreign body
3. Routine hematology and biochemistry
   a. Eosinophilia—10% to 35% (normal range 3% to 5%) (EGE [eosinophilia not always present], parasitism)
   b. Anemia (severe gastric ulceration—see also *Cardiovascular and Hematologic Disorders*)
   c. Hypoalbuminemia (severe intestinal disease, including PBD, EGE, and *Helicobacter*)
4. Serology for CDV, *Helicobacter mustelae*
5. PCR for *Lawsonia*, ferret coronavirus
6. Culture and sensitivity
7. Endoscopy
   a. Gastric ulceration (also biopsy)

8. Biopsy
   a. Lymphoma
   b. *Helicobacter*
9. Ultrasonography
   a. Enlarged mesenteric lymph node (EGE)

Management

1. Fluid therapy (see *Nursing Care*)
2. If vomiting:
   a. Do not feed for 6 to 12 hours and use antiemetics (e.g., metoclopramide at 0.2 to 1.0 mg/kg SC t.i.d.).
   b. Monitor blood glucose—consider dextrose/saline fluids.

Treatment/specific therapy

1. Rotavirus
   a. Supportive treatment only
   b. Usually in young ferrets 2 to 6 weeks old
2. Influenza virus (see *Respiratory Tract Disorders*)
3. Epizootic catarrhal enteritis
   a. Supportive treatment plus covering antibiotics
4. Bacterial diseases, including salmonellosis
   a. See *Management* above.
   b. Appropriate antibiosis
5. PBD
   a. Chloramphenicol at 50 mg/kg IM, SC, or PO b.i.d.
   b. Metronidazole at 20 mg/kg PO b.i.d. for 3 weeks
6. *Helicobacter mustelae*
   a. A common isolate from gastric ulcers, its significance is uncertain.
   b. Combination therapy of:
      i. Amoxicillin at 10 to 20 mg/kg PO or SC b.i.d.
      ii. Metronidazole at 20 mg/kg PO b.i.d.
      iii. Bismuth subsalicylate at 0.25 to 1.0 mL/kg PO q.i.d.
7. Mycobacteriosis
   a. Potential zoonosis
   b. Consider euthanasia.
8. *Cryptococcus*
   a. Amphotericin B at 150 µg/kg i.v. 3 times weekly for 2-4 months
9. *Isospora*
   a. Sulfadimethoxine at 30 mg/kg PO b.i.d.
   b. Amprolium at 119 mg/kg PO in food or water daily for 7 to 10 days
10. *Giardia*
    a. Metronidazole at 10 to 20 mg/kg PO b.i.d. for 10 days
11. *Cryptosporidium*
    a. Often subclinical
    b. No effective treatment recognized
    c. Potentiated sulfonamides may be of use, as may nitazoxanide at 5 mg/kg PO s.i.d.
    d. Potential zoonosis, so consider euthanasia.

12. Nematodes
    a. Fenbendazole at 20 mg/kg PO s.i.d. for 5 days or 100 mg/kg as a single dose
    b. Mebendazole at 50 mg/kg PO b.i.d. for 2 days
    c. Ivermectin at 0.2-0.4 mg/kg sc, PO repeated after 14 days. Repeat after 1 week.
13. Cestodes
    a. Praziquantel at 5 to 10 mg/kg SC. Repeat after 2 weeks.
14. Eosinophilic gastroenteritis
    a. May be an allergic or immune-mediated response
    b. Prednisolone at 1.25 to 2.5 mg/kg PO s.i.d., continuing for 3 to 4 weeks after clinical resolution
    c. Ivermectin at 0.4 mg/kg SC once only. Repeat after 2 weeks.
15. Megaesophagus
    a. Feed from a raised platform.
    b. Gut motility enhancers (e.g., metoclopramide at 0.2 to 1.0 mg/kg PO or SC every 6 to 8 hours; cisapride at 0.5 mg/kg PO every 8 to 24 hours
    c. If esophagitis, cimetidine at 5 to 10 mg/kg PO or IV t.i.d.
16. Gastric ulceration
    a. Investigate possible underlying etiologies.
    b. Cimetidine at above dose
    c. Bismuth subsalicylate at 0.25 to 1.0 mL/kg PO q.i.d.
    d. Sucralfate at 25 to 30 mg PO q.i.d.
    e. For *Helicobacter*—see above.
17. Foreign body
    a. Surgical removal
18. Trichobezoars
    a. Likely to require surgical removal
    b. Attempt prevention by regular use of cat laxatives.
    c. May be linked to abnormal gut motility arising from underlying gastrointestinal disease (e.g., lymphoma—see *Systemic Disorders*)
19. Gastric bloat
    a. May be related to foreign body or *Clostridium perfringens* overgrowth
    b. Decompress either by passing esophageal tube or trocharization.
    c. Fluid therapy
    d. Treat as for gastric ulceration.
20. Solid neoplasms and polyps
    a. Surgical resection
21. Rectal prolapse
    a. Moisten prolapse, clean up; if necessary apply osmotic solution (e.g., concentrated sugar water) to shrink prolapse prior to reinsertion.
    b. Replace and insert rectal pursestring suture.
    c. Address possible underlying causes.
22. Anal sac impaction
    a. Express and treat as for other small animals.

Nutritional disorders

Ferrets have a rapid gut transit time of around 5 hours. They should be fed a diet high in protein and fat and low in fiber.

Ferret nutrition

1. Protein requirement is around 30% to 40% and the quality must be good—in the region of 85% to 90% digestable. Diets high in plant proteins predispose to urinary calculi (see *Urinary Disorders*).
2. Fat levels should be 15% to 30%.
3. Carbohydrate levels should be below 40%. The rapid gut transit time and low brush border enzyme levels present in ferrets result in a poor ability to utilize carbohydrates, and the animal will fail to thrive if the carbohydrate concentration exceeds 40%. Note that the only carbohydrates that ferrets would normally have access to are in the gut contents of their prey.

It can be normal for ferrets to undergo seasonal weight increases, under the influence of photoperiod. This is normal and should not be a cause of concern.

- Hypoglycemia from starvation (see *Pancreatic Disorders* for management)
- Nutritional osteodystrophy
  - Young kits fed on a low-calcium diet (day-old chicks)
  - Deformities of the long bones, soft jaw
  - Supplement with dietary calcium and vitamin D_3 supplement.
- Hepatic lipidosis
  - Linked to long-term anorexia
  - Aggressive fluid therapy
  - Parenteral nutrition with glucose and vitamins
  - Assisted feeding by syringe (see *Nursing Care*)
  - Calcium gluconate PO or propylene glycol PO may be of use.
  - Dexamethasone at 0.2 mg/kg IV, SC, or PO

Hepatic disorders

Nutritional
- Hepatic lipidosis
- Copper toxicosis
- Ketosis (see *Reproductive Disorders*)

Neoplasia
- Lymphoma/lymphosarcoma (see *Systemic Disorders*)
- Metastases (e.g., insulinoma)
- Hemangiosarcoma
- Adenocarcinoma
- Hepatocellular adenoma
- Bile duct cyst adenoma
- Biliary carcinoma

Other noninfectious problems
- Lymphocytic hepatitis
- Cholangiohepatitis

Findings on clinical examination

- Reduced or loss of appetite
- Vague signs of ill health

- Abnormal feces
- Hepatomegaly
- Jaundice (rare)
- Ascites
- Bile-tinged (green) diarrhea
- Lethargy, hypothermia, hyperthermia, jaundice (copper toxicosis)
- Seizures

Investigations

1. Radiography
2. Routine hematology and biochemistry
   a. Raised liver enzymes; alanine transaminase (ALT) usually >275 IU/L (normal 78 to 289 IU/L); alkaline phosphatase (ALP) may be raised; total bilirubin levels often normal
3. Culture and sensitivity
4. Endoscopy
5. Biopsy
6. Ultrasonography

Management

1. Fluid therapy (see *Nursing Care*)
2. Lactulose at 150 to 750 mg/kg PO b.i.d. or t.i.d.
3. Milk thistle *(Silybum marianum)* is hepatoprotectant. Dose at 4 to 15 mg/kg PO b.i.d. or t.i.d.

Treatment/specific therapy

- Hepatic lipidosis (see *Nutritional Disorders*)
- Copper toxicosis
  - Penicillamine at 10 mg/kg PO s.i.d.—offer as divided dose if vomiting occurs.
  - Trientine at 10 mg/kg PO b.i.d.
  - Supportive therapy
  - Possibly inherited susceptibility
  - Poor prognosis

Splenic disorders

- Splenomegaly can be a normal finding in ferrets; however, it is also found in a range of disorders, the most significant of which are:
  - Hemangiosarcoma and hemangioma
  - Cardiac disease (see *Cardiovascular and Hematologic Disorders*)
  - Lymphoma/lymphosarcoma (see *Systemic Disorders*)
  - Insulinoma (see *Pancreatic Disorders*)
  - Aleutian disease (see *Systemic Disorders*)
  - Idiopathic splenomegaly

Treatment

- Address underlying cause.
- Splenectomy
  - Hypersplenism
  - Splenic rupture
  - Splenic torsion
  - Neoplasia
  - Splenitis

Pancreatic disorders

Neoplasia

- Insulinoma (pancreatic beta cell tumor)
- Exocrine pancreatic adenocarcinoma

Other noninfectious problems

- Diabetes mellitus

Findings on clinical examination

- Signs of an insulinoma include transient episodes of inactivity during which the ferret is unresponsive to external stimuli, hind-limb weakness, and eventually seizures, coma, and death.
- Ataxia and hind-limb paresis
- Lethargy
- Hypersalivation
- "Glazed-eye" appearance
- Abdominal distension
- Pain
- Abdominal mass palpable

Investigations

1. Radiography
2. Routine hematology and biochemistry (Table 1-4)
   a. Provisional diagnosis of an insulinoma is based on a low fasting blood glucose sample (a 4-hour fast will suffice). Insulinomas often also show

Table 1-4 The ferret: Routine hematology and biochemistry

	Normal range	Insulinoma	Diabetes mellitus
Blood glucose *normal resting* (mmol/L)	5.22-11.49	<3.89 (commonly 1.12-2.24)	>16.65
Blood glucose *normal fasting* (mmol/L)	5.0-6.94		
Normal insulin (pmol/L)	35-250	772.7-12470	
Mean fasting insulin (pmol/L)	58		
Normal insulin/glucose ratio (pmol/mmol)	4.6-44.2		

neutrophilia, leukocytosis, and monocytosis plus raised ALT and aspartate transaminase (AST).
   b. Blood insulin levels
3. Culture and sensitivity
4. Urinalysis
   a. Glycosuria/ketonuria
5. Endoscopy
6. Exploratory surgery and biopsy
7. Ultrasonography

Management

1. Treatment of hypoglycemia

Hypoglycemia
1. Rub honey or sugared water onto the gingiva, taking care not to get bitten.
2. Give 0.5- to 2.0-mL bolus IV of 50% dextrose solution slowly (so as not to overstimulate a possible insulinoma).
3. Provide fluid therapy (see *Nursing Care*) with 5% dextrose infusion.
4. If ferret fails to respond, can give shock dose of dexamethasone at 4 to 8 mg/kg IV or IM once only.
5. Diazepam at 1 to 2 mg IV as needed to control if are seizures persistent.

Treatment/specific therapy

- Diabetes mellitus
  - Neutral protamine Hagedorn (NPH) insulin at a starting dose of 0.1 IU/ferret SC b.i.d. until stabilized. Monitor blood glucose levels.
  - Maintain on ultralente insulin s.i.d.
- Insulinoma
  - Surgical resection
    - Fluid therapy with 5% dextrose saline
    - Partial resection or nodulectomy
    - Metastasis is very common.
  - Medical management
    - Prednisolone 0.5 to 2.0 mg/kg PO b.i.d., raising until clinical signs subside
    - Diazoxide at 5 to 10 mg/kg PO b.i.d. (may induce vomiting and anorexia)
  - Medical management may give 6 to 18 months of control of clinical signs, although it will not prevent further growth and spread of the insulinoma.
  - Hyperglycemia following pancreatic surgery will usually resolve within 2 weeks and requires no action.
- Pancreatic exocrine adenocarcinoma
  - Readily metastasize. Surgery is a possible option, but metastasis is highly likely before diagnosis is confirmed.

Cardiovascular and hematologic disorders

Viral
- Aleutian disease (see *Systemic Disorders*)

Bacterial

- Bacteremia/septicemia
- Endocarditis

Protozoal

- *Toxoplasma gondii* (myocarditis—see *Neurologic Disorders*)

Parasitic

- *Dirofilaria immitis* (heartworm)
- *Angiostrongylus vasorum* (lungworm—see *Respiratory Tract Disorders*)

Neoplasia

- Lymphoma (see *Systemic Disorders*)

Other noninfectious problems

- Cardiomyopathy
- Dilative
- Hypertrophic
- Valvular heart disease
- Hyperestrogenism (see *Reproductive Disorders*)
- Gastric ulceration (see *Gastrointestinal Tract Disorders*)
- Congenital disorders

Findings on clinical examination

- Cyanosis or pallor of the mucous membranes
- Anemia (hyperestrogenism, gastric ulceration)
- Slow capillary refill time
- Dyspnea
- Precordial thrill
- Abormalities of femoral arterial pulse, including weakness, irregularities, pulse deficits
- Arrhythmia
- Lack of thoracic percussion with auscultation
- Abnormal lung sounds
- Abnormal heart sounds
- Exercise intolerance
- Ascites
- Hepatomegaly, splenomegaly
- Weight loss
- Sudden death

Investigations

1. Auscultation
2. Blood pressure: systole: 140 ± 35 mm Hg; diastole: 110 ± 31 mm Hg
3. ECG
   a. Use adhesive ECG contacts designed for children; metal clips and needles are poorly tolerated in the conscious ferret.
   b. Distract the ferret by offering a favored food or food supplement (e.g., 8 in 1 FerreTone).

Table 1-5 The ferret: Normal lead II ECGs

Parameter	Ketamine-xylazine anesthesia[a]	Ketamine-diazepam anesthesia[b]	
		Right lateral recumbency	Sternal recumbency
Heart rate (beats/min)	233 ± 22	250-430	
Frontal plane MEA (°)	+77.22 ± 12	+75-+100	+65-+90
Lead II			
P amplitude (mV)	0.122 ± 0.007	≤0.2	≤0.3
P duration (s)	0.024 ± 0.004	0.01-0.03	
PR interval (s)	0.047 ± 0.003	0.03-0.06	
QRS duration (s)	0.043 ± 0.003	0.02-0.05	
Q wave amplitude (mV)		−0.05-0	
R amplitude (mV)	1.46 ± 0.84	1.0-2.8	1.0-3.1
QT interval (s)	0.12 ± 0.04	0.06-0.16	
S wave amplitude		0	
T amplitude (mV)		−0.4-+0.4	
		Most often > 0	>0 or <0
Lead I			
Q(S) wave amplitude (mV)		−0.4-0.0	0
R amplitude (mV)		≤+0.9	≤+1.25
Lead aVF			
R amplitude (mV)		1.0-3.1	

[a]Stamoulis et al 1997.
[b]Bublot et al 2006.

    c. Normal ferret lead II ECGs:
      i. The P waves are small.
      ii. The R waves are large.
      iii. Short QT interval
      iv. Elevated ST segment (Table 1-5)
4. Radiography
    a. Vertebral heart score:
      i. Thoracic radiograph taken in right lateral recumbency.
      ii. Measure the long axis (LA) and short axis or width of the heart (SA) in cm.
      iii. Measure the combined length of thoracic vertebrae T5-T8 in cm.
      iv. Divide the sum of the axes by the thoracic vertebral measurement:
        (LA + SA) cm/T5-T8 (cm)
        Males: Ratio = 1.35 (SD 0.07); Females: Ratio = 1.34 (SD 0.06)
        After Stepien et al (1999)
    b. Pleural effusions and cardiomegaly are common findings with cardiomyopathy and dirofilariasis.

Table 1-6 The ferret: Normal echocardiographic values

Parameter	Mean value
Left ventricle, end-diastolic (mm)	11.0
Left ventricle, end-systolic (mm)	6.4
Left ventricular posterior or free wall (mm)	3.3
Fractional shortening (%)	42
End point septal separation	

    c. A globoid heart shape is often indicative of cardiac disease, usually with increased cardiosternal contact.

    d. Anterior mediastinal masses (lymphoma)

5. Ultrasonography/echocardiography

    a. Normal echocardiographic values for ferrets (from Stamoulis et al 1997) (Table 1-6)

    b. Detection of dirofilariasis (Sasai et al 2000)

6. Routine hematology and biochemistry

    a. Microfilaria in peripheral bloodstream (uncommon) *(Dirofilaria)*

    b. Anemia (hyperestrogenism, high ectoparasite count, Aleutian disease, gastrointestinal hemorrhage due to, e.g., gastric ulceration or gastroenteritis)

7. Serology for *Dirofilaria* antigen, *Toxoplasma*

8. Culture and sensitivity

9. Endoscopy

10. Biopsy

Management

- Reduce stress (e.g., keep in a cool, shaded or darkened area away from potential stressors such as dogs).
- Provide a high oxygen environment.
- For pleural effusion, consider tube thoracostomy.

Treatment/specific therapy

- *Dirofilaria immitis*
  - Due to the small size of the ferret, even only a few worms may cause serious problems, with clinical signs ranging from heart failure to pulmonary edema.
  - Treatment is also difficult because the worms may cause thromboembolisms, resulting in acute death.
  - Treatment protocol
    - Thiacetarsemide at 2.2 mg/kg IV b.i.d. for 2 days.
    - Start heparin at 100 units/ferret SC every 24 hrs for 21 days.
    - After 3 weeks stop heparin and start on aspirin at 22 mg/kg PO s.i.d. for 3 months.
    - Treat concurrently for cardiac disease if appropriate.
    - Alternatively try topical 10% imidacloprid/1.0% moxidectin (Advocate (UK) Advantage Multi (USA), Bayer) at 0.4 mL per ferret.
    - Prevention is with ivermectin at 0.2-0.4 mg/kg SC, PO repeated after 14 days once monthly in areas where heartworm is endemic.

- Cardiomyopathies
  - Dilated (congestive) cardiomyopathy
    - Furosemide at 1 to 4 mg/kg b.i.d.
    - Enalapril at 0.5 mg/kg PO every 48 hours. Ferrets appear very sensitive to the hypotensive effects of ACE inhibitors.
    - Benazepril 0.25 to 0.5 mg/kg s.i.d. Less nephrotoxic than enalapril
    - Digoxin at 0.01 mg/kg PO s.i.d.
    - Nitroglycerin at 3 mm of 2% ointment applied to skin s.i.d. or b.i.d.
    - Pimobendan at 0.2-1.25 mg/kg PO b.i.d.
  - Hypertrophic cardiomyopathy
    - Atenolol at 3.125-6.25 mg/kg PO s.i.d.
    - Diltiazem at 1.5-7.5 mg/kg PO b.i.d.
- Valvular heart disease
  - Treat as for dilated cardiomyopathy
- Hyperestrogenism (see *Reproductive Disorders*)

Systemic disorders

Viral
- Coronavirus
- CDV (see also *Neurologic Disorders*)
- Aleutian disease (parvovirus)
- Rabies

Bacterial
- Bacteremia/septicemia

Nutritional
- Copper toxicosis (see *Hepatic Disorders*)
- Ketosis (see *Reproductive Disorders*)

Neoplasia
- Insulinoma (see *Pancreatic Disorders*)
- Hyperadrenocorticism (see *Endocrine Disorders*)
- Lymphoma/lymphosarcoma (see also *Respiratory Tract Disorders* and *Cardiovascular and Hematologic Disorders*)
- Mesothelioma

Other noninfectious problems
- Hyperestrogenism (see *Reproductive Disorders*)

Findings on clinical examination

- Weight loss, dyspnea, hind-leg weakness, ascites (coronavirus, Aleutian disease, lymphoma)
- Bilateral mucopurulent ocular and/or nasal discharges—the ocular discharge dries to a crust at the eyelid margins, sealing the eyes shut (CDV)
- Hyperkeratosis of the footpads and erythematous cutaneous rashes in the inguinal area and under the chin (CDV)

- Chronic upper respiratory infections, dyspnea, general lethargy, wasting, and lymphadenopathy (lymphoma). Peripheral lymphadenopathy is more common in older animals.
- Palpable abdominal masses (splenomegaly, mesenteric and/or gastric lymph nodes) (lymphoma)
- Distended abdomen (mesothelioma)

Investigations

1. Radiography
   a. Renomegaly, splenomegaly, lymphadenopathy (coronavirus)
   b. Mediastinal masses, pleural effusions, abdominal masses (lymphoma) (Table 1-7)
2. Routine hematology and biochemistry
   a. Persistent high WBC counts (10×10^9/L or above) with a high lymphocyte count (lymphoma). Consider lymphoma if lymphocytosis (3.5×10^9/L or greater) or 60% lymphocytes. Immature ferrets (<6 months old) can have a natural lymphocytosis. In older ferrets with chronic lymphoma there may be a lymphopenia.
   b. Bacterial infections tend to cause a smaller rise in WBC count with a relative neutrophilia of >85% with the presence of bands.
   c. Hyperglobulinemia (coronavirus, Aleutian disease); note that not all ferrets with Aleutian disease are hypergammaglobulinemic (Une et al 2000).
   d. Aleutian disease produces immune complexes that trigger renal disease, including glomerulonephritis, so renal parameters are likely to be high.
3. Bone marrow aspirate/lymph node cytology (lymphoma)

Technique for bone marrow aspirate (performed under GA)

1. Prepare at least four slides.
2. Draw some EDTA (can mix from EDTA blood tube with sterile saline).
3. Use a 5- or 10-mL syringe with around 1 mL of EDTA solution present.
4. Use an 18G or 21G 25-mm needle.
5. Identify the trochanteric fossa.
6. Grind into bone so that needle is parallel to long axis of femur.
7. Perform several aspirates—marrow appears as thick blood.
8. Apply the collected marrow to each of the slides.
9. Leave for approximately 30 seconds for bone spicules to settle onto slide.
10. With half of the slides, tip and drain away excess, including the spicules.
11. For the other half, place a clean slide across at right angles and draw across to create a "squash" preparation (but without squashing!).
12. Air dry and submit to lab.

Table 1-7 The ferret: Grading of lymphoma

Grading of lymphoma	
Stage 1	Single focus
Stage 2	Two foci on same side of diaphragm
Stage 3	Involving the spleen and lymph node(s)
Stage 4	Multiple sites

4. Abdominal centesis and cytology
5. Serology for CDV, Aleutian disease, rabies
6. PCR for ferret coronavirus
7. Culture and sensitivity
8. Endoscopy
9. Biopsy/necropsy
   a. Pyogranulomatous enteritis (coronavirus)
   b. Lymphoma (especially mesenteric lymph node, peripheral lymph nodes, spleen, liver, and any abnormal organs); see Table 1-7.
   c. CDV
10. Ultrasonography

Management

- See *Nursing Care.*

Treatment/specific therapy

- Coronavirus
  - Symptomatic treatment only
- CDV
  - The incubation period described for CDV in ferrets is from 7 to 10 days. The usual course of disease, from exposure to death, is 12 to 25 days.
  - There is no treatment—consider supportive therapy including covering antibiosis. The mortality rate is close to 100%. Those that do recover are likely to die later from CNS disturbances (see *Neurologic Disorders*).
  - Prevent by vaccination. Consult manufacturers first as some CDV vaccines derived from ferret tissue cultures may increase the risk of vaccine-induced disease. Where possible, do not use multivalent vaccines. Where CDV is endemic, an initial vaccination course of 3 injections is recommended at 6 to 8 weeks of age, 10 to 12 weeks, and 13 to 14 weeks with annual boosters to follow. If CDV is not endemic, give a single dose at 12 weeks of age with annual boosters.
  - Adverse reactions to vaccination are vomiting and diarrhea (Moore et al 2005).
  - CDV is readily destroyed by normal cleaning and disinfection routines.
- Rabies
  - Significant zoonosis. Euthanize.
  - Prevent by vaccination given at 12 weeks of age with an annual booster.
- Aleutian disease
  - Many ferrets can be serologically positive for Aleutian disease but show no clinical signs.
  - Supportive therapy
  - Steroids may prove useful in reducing the formation and effect of the immune complexes.
- Bacteremia/septicemia
  - Appropriate antibiosis
  - Supportive therapy as necessary (see *Nursing Care*)
- Lymphoma/lymphosarcoma
  - Chemotherapy protocols for small animals are regularly altered and updated, so if in doubt, consult a veterinary oncologist. The following two protocols (from Brown 1997) have been found to be useful.

Table 1-8 The ferret: Chemotherapy protocol 1

Week	Day	Drug	Dose
1	1	Prednisolone	1 mg/kg PO b.i.d. Continue throughout treatment.
	1	Vincristine	0.12 mg/kg IV
	3	Cyclophosphamide	10 mg/kg PO
2	8	Vincristine	0.12 mg/kg IV
3	15	Vincristine	0.12 mg/kg IV
4	22	Vincristine	0.12 mg/kg IV
	24	Cyclophosphamide	10 mg/kg PO
7	46	Cyclophosphamide	10 mg/kg PO
9		Prednisolone	Start reducing dose to end by 4 weeks.

- The author finds it useful to give the owner a modified copy of the above protocol adjusted to specific days/dates for administration of the different medications.
- Weekly PCV should be performed before administration of next dose of vincristine to assess degree of anemia; consider halting treatment at values below 20%.

Table 1-9 The ferret: Chemotherapy protocol 2

Week	Drug	Dose
1	Vincristine	0.07 mg/kg IV
	Asparaginase	400 IU/kg IP
	Prednisolone	1 mg/kg PO s.i.d. Continue throughout treatment.
2	Cyclophosphamide	10 mg/kg PO
3	Doxorubicin	1 mg/kg IV
4-6	Discontinue asparaginase, otherwise as for weeks 1-3	
8	Vincristine	0.07 mg/kg IV
10	Cyclophosphamide	10 mg/kg PO
12	Vincristine	0.07 mg/kg IV
14	Methotrexate	0.5 mg/kg IV

- Palliative treatment for lymphoma
  - Prednisolone at 0.5 mg/kg PO b.i.d., increasing to control signs. Note that prednisolone treatment alone is likely to make the lymphoma refractory to chemotherapy.
  - Vitamin C (ascorbic acid) at 50 to 100 mg/kg PO b.i.d
  - Regular annual CBC to screen for lymphoma.
- Clusters of outbreaks have occurred and in some cases may be due to a retrovirus-like agent (Erdman et al 1995), although attempted detection using feline leukemia virus (FeLV) serology, PCR, or ELISA all proved negative (Erdman et al 1996).

- Mesothelioma
  - Surgical resection and chemotherapy may be worth attempting, but the prognosis is poor.

Musculoskeletal disorders

Viral
- Aleutian disease (see *Systemic Disorders*)

Neoplasia
- Multiple myeloma
- Chondroma
- Chondrosarcoma
- Fibrosarcoma
- Osteoma
- Chordoma

Other noninfectious problems
- Traumatic fractures
- Any causes of weakness
  - See *Neurologic Disorders*
  - See *Cardiovascular and Hematologic Disorders*
  - See *Systemic Disorders*
  - See *Pancreatic Disorders*

Findings on clinical examination

- Pain
- Lameness
- Swelling
- Hind-leg paresis/paralysis
- Small rounded mass at tip of tail (chordoma)

Investigations

1. Radiography
2. Osteolysis, pathological fractures (multiple myeloma)
3. Traumatic fractures
4. Routine hematology and biochemistry
5. Culture and sensitivity
6. Endoscopy
7. Biopsy
8. Ultrasonography

Treatment/specific therapy

- Multiple myeloma
  - No treatment recorded.

- Traumatic fractures
  - Repair using standard small animal techniques.
- Neoplasia
  - Surgical resection, amputation, chemotherapy, or radiation therapy as for other small animals
  - Note that chordomas may metastasize (Munday et al 2004).

Neurologic disorders

Viral

- CDV (see *Systemic Disorders*)
- Rabies
- Coronavirus

Bacterial

- Bacterial meningitis or other CNS infection
- Otitis media/interna

Fungal

- Cryptococcal meningitis
- Blastomycosis

Protozoal

- Toxoplasmosis

Nutritional

- Hypoglycemia
- Ketosis (see *Reproductive Disorders*)

Neoplasia

- Schwannoma
- Insulinoma (hypoglycemia—see *Pancreatic Disorders*)
- Lymphoma (see *Systemic Disorders*)
- T-cell lymphoma (Hanley et al 2004)

Other noninfectious problems

- Toxins
- Spinal lesions (e.g., intervertebral disc prolapse—see Lu et al 2004; fractures)
- Eosinophilic granulomatous infiltrate (as part of eosinophilic gastroenteritis—see *Gastrointestinal Tract Disorders*)

Findings on clinical examination

- Apparent weakness
- Posterior paralysis/paresis
- Anxiety, lethargy, constipation, bladder atony, posterior paresis, aggression (rabies)
- Seizures (uncommon except with chronic neurotrophic form of CDV)
- Salivation, muscle tremors, seizures, and coma (CDV)
- Otitis externa (see also "Ear Mites" in *Skin Disorders*)

Investigations

1. Full neurologic examination
2. Radiography
   a. Myelography—access as for cerebrospinal fluid (CSF) tap (see below)
   b. 0.25 to 0.5 mL/kg iohexol
3. Routine hematology and biochemistry
4. Serology for toxoplasmosis
5. Culture and sensitivity

Cerebrospinal fluid tap in the ferret

1. Collect as from dog or cat.
2. Sites for CSF tap are the atlantooccipital joint and lumbar (L5-L6) region.
3. 21G or 22G needle
4. Endoscopy
5. Biopsy
6. Ultrasonography

Management

- Important to differentiate from other causes of weakness (insulinoma, lymphoma etc.)

Treatment/specific therapy

- Rabies (see *Systemic Disorders*)
- Bacterial CNS infection
  - Appropriate antibiosis
  - Supportive care
- Fungal infections
  - Ketoconazole at 10 to 30 mg/kg PO s.i.d. for 60 days
  - Amphotericin B
    - 0.25 to 1.0 mg/kg IV s.i.d. or every other day until a total dose of 7 to 25 mg has been given
    - For *Cryptococcus*, 150 µg/kg i.v. 3 times weekly for 2-4 months
  - Itraconazole at 25 to 33 mg/kg PO s.i.d. long term
- Toxoplasmosis
  - Clindamycin at 12.5 mg/kg PO b.i.d. for at least 2 weeks
  - Combination therapy consisting of:
    - Co-trimoxazole at 30 mg/kg PO b.i.d.
    - Pyrimethamine at 0.5 mg/kg PO b.i.d.
    - Folic acid at 3.0 to 5.0 mg/kg PO s.i.d.
- Hypoglycemia
  - For management of hypoglycemic episodes, see *Pancreatic Disorders*.
- Orthopedic conditions
  - Treat as for other small animals.

Ophthalmic disorders

The ferret eye is similar to the canine eye except that the pupil is horizontal rather than vertical.

Viral

- CDV (see *Systemic Disorders*)
- Influenza A (see *Respiratory Tract Disorders*)

Bacterial

- *Salmonella* spp.
- *Mycobacterium* spp.

Protozoal

- Toxoplasmosis (see *Neurological Disorders*)

Nutritional

- Hypovitaminosis A

Neoplasia

- Carcinoma of the ocular globe

Other noninfectious problems

- Salivary mucocele (see *Gastrointestinal Tract Disorders*)
- Hereditary cataracts
- Idiopathic cataract
- Retinal degeneration (may be hereditary)
- Foreign body

Findings on clinical examination

- Corneal ulceration
- Conjunctivitis (influenza, CDV, hypovitaminosis A)
- Nasal discharge
- Uveitis
- Corneal edema, hypopyon, and synechiae
- Cataracts
- Exophthalmos
- Megaglobus/glaucoma
- Night blindness (hypovitaminosis A, retinal degeneration)
- Periocular swelling (salivary mucocele)
- Cataracts (hereditary, hypovitaminosis A, idiopathic)
- Bilateral mucopurulent ocular and/or nasal discharges—the ocular discharge dries to a crust at the eyelid margins, sealing the eyes shut; accompanied by hyperkeratosis of the footpads and skin rashes (CDV)

Investigations

1. Ophthalmic examination
   a. Schirmer tear test 5.31 ± 1.32 mm/min (Montiani-Ferreira et al 2006)
   b. Central corneal thickness 0.337 ± 0.020 mm

2. Topical fluorescein to assess extent of ulceration
3. Tonometry
   a. Intraocular pressure 14.5 ± 3.27 mm Hg
4. Skull radiography
5. Routine hematology and biochemistry
6. Serology for CDV, toxoplasmosis
7. Culture and sensitivity
8. Biopsy
9. Ultrasonography

Treatment/specific therapy

- Corneal ulceration
  - Topical and systemic antibiosis
  - Once infection is cleared, treat as for other small animals (e.g., scarification to encourage healing, conjunctival grafts).
- Uveitis
  - Topical ophthalmic steroid or NSAID preparations
  - Topical ophthalmic antibiotic preparations plus systemic antibiosis if appropriate
  - Enucleation if severe
- Cataracts
  - Treat for any uveitis as above.
  - Cataract removal either surgically or by phacoemulsification
- Neoplasia
  - Enucleation
- Toxoplasmosis (see *Neurologic Disorders*)
- Mycobacteriosis
  - Topical chloramphenicol b.i.d. for 60 to 90 days
  - Systemic antimycobacterial drugs such as rifampin, clofazimine, and clarithromycin
  - Guarded prognosis; potential zoonosis so consider euthanasia

Endocrine disorders

Neoplasia
- Adrenal neoplasia
- Adrenal hyperplasia
- Adrenal adenoma/carcinoma
- Pituitary gonadotrophic adenomas (Schoemaker et al 2004)
- Insulinoma (see *Pancreatic Disorders*)

Other noninfectious problems
- Hyperestrogenism (see *Reproductive Disorders*)

Findings on clinical examination

- Hyperadrenocorticism
  - Symmetrical alopecia
  - Over 30% may be pruritic.

- Vulval swelling (also in spayed females)
- Male behavior in castrated males
- Dysuria in males (urethral obstruction secondary to prostatic hyperplasia)
- Splenomegaly
- Enlarged adrenal glands may be palpable (not consistent).

Investigations

1. Radiography
2. Routine hematology and biochemistry
   a. Hyperadrenocorticism
      i. Blood hormone levels. Which are elevated varies among individuals; cortisol is the least likely to be raised and a diagnosis is more likely if androstenedione, estradiol, and hydroxyprogesterone are measured (Table 1-10).
      ii. Ideally blood samples for hyperadrenocorticism should be taken under anesthesia because manual restraint increases plasma cortisol and ACTH but decreases α-melanocyte-stimulating hormone (α-MSH) production (Schoemaker et al 2003). However, it should be noted that isoflurane (but not medetomidine) anesthesia increases the α-MSH from the pituitary gland, which may subsequently affect the concentrations of adrenal hormones.
      iii. Pancytopenia (severe cases)
      iv. Raised AST
      v. For suspect female ferrets, differentiate from ovarian remnant (or estrus if entire) by giving 2 injections of 100 IU hCG 7 days apart. This should cause regression of vulval swelling unless the ferret has hyperadrenocorticism.
   b. Thyroid levels (Table 1-11)

Thyroid stimulation test (Keeble 2001)

1. Thyroid-stimulating hormone (TSH) at 1.0 IU given IV
2. Blood for T_4 taken at 120 minutes

Table 1-10 The ferret: Blood hormone levels

Parameter	Normal range	Hyperadrenocorticism (mean values)
Androstenedione (nmol/L)	0-15	67
Dehydroepiandrosterone sulfate (μmol/L)	0.01 (mean)	0.03
Estradiol (pmol/L)	30-180	167
17-hydroxyprogesterone (nmol/L)	0-0.8	3.2
Cortisol (nmol/L)	0-140	
ACTH (adrenocorticotropic hormone) (ng/L)	13-98	
α-MSH (melanocyte-stimulating hormone) (ng/L)	16-74	
Sodium (mmol/L)	137-162	
Potassium (mmol/L)	4.3-7.7	

Table 1-11 The ferret: Thyroid levels

	Male	Female
Thyroxine (T$_4$) (nmol/L)	13.0-106.9	9.14-32.69
Triiodothyronine (T$_3$) (nmol/L)	0.007-0.012	0.004-0.011

3. Culture and sensitivity
4. Endoscopy
5. Biopsy
6. Ultrasonography
   a. Enlarged adrenal gland
   b. Normal values: left adrenal gland normally 6 to 8 mm length; right adrenal gland 8 to 11 mm length. Accessory nodules of adrenal tissue occur in some individuals.

Treatment/specific therapy

- Hyperadrenocorticism
  - The disease is linked to luteinizing hormone (LH) effects on the sex steroid-producing cells of the adrenal cortex (Schoemaker et al 2002), which in turn may explain the predisposing factor of early age of neutering.
  - Treatment of choice is deslorelin implant: 4.7 mg lasts up to 12 months while 9.4 mg implant lasts from 16 months up to 4 years (NOAH Suprelorin datasheet).
  - The protective effects of deslorelin implants and their ease of use mean that where they are available, castration and ovariohysterectomy are no longer recommended for ferrets.
- Other medical management
  - Mitotane
  - Trilostane at 2 mg/kg PO s.i.d.
  - Leuprolide acetate at 100 µg/kg SC every 21 to 30 days
  - Ketoconazole ineffective at 15 mg/kg b.i.d. (cited in Keeble 2001)
  - Temporary cessation of clinical signs due to reduced hormone levels can be achieved with deslorelin, given as a single, slow-release 3-mg implant, with an average of 13.7 ± 3.5 months to recurrence of signs (Wagner et al 2005).
- Surgical management (adrenalectomy)
  - Surgery is no longer the treatment of choice.
  - In cases of bilateral adrenal disease, then either completely remove one (the left is easiest) and perform a subtotal adrenalectomy on the other (right) with subsequent medical management, or consider medical management only.
  - If bilateral adrenalectomy, consider the use of supplementary glucocorticoids (prednisolone at 0.1 mg/kg PO s.i.d.) [Martorell et al 2005] for several days post surgery to prevent hypoadrenocorticism. Monitor serum electrolyte ranges and titrate to effect; partial adrenalectomy or presence of accessory nodules may result in continued normal electrolyte levels without treatment.
  - Temporary tube cystotomy may be beneficial in those cases with urinary obstruction from prostatic hyperplasia/prostatic cysts (Nolte et al 2002). Removal is after 5 to 10 days.
- Gonadotrophic adenomas
  - Unknown significance

Urinary disorders

Viral

- Aleutian disease (see *Systemic Disorders*)

Bacterial

- Cystitis

Nutritional

- Urolithiasis (males > females) (see also *Reproductive Disorders*)

Neoplasia

- Lymphoma (see *Systemic Disorders*)
- Transitional cell carcinoma
- Renal carcinoma

Other noninfectious problems

- Chronic interstitial nephritis
- Hydronephrosis
- Renal cysts
- Prostatic hyperplasia (see "Hyperadrenocorticism" in *Endocrine Disorders*)
- Gentamicin toxicity

Findings on clinical examination

- Depression
- Anorexia/weight loss
- Polydipsia/polyuria
- Oral ulceration
- Hematuria (urolithiasis, cystitis, neoplasia)
- Hind-leg weakness
- Melena
- Dysuria/polyuria
- Urine dribbling, wet perineum, constant licking at genitalia (urolithiasis)
- Painful urination, stranguria (urolithiasis, cystitis)
- Death
- Palpable abnormalities
  - Distended bladder (urethral obstruction)
  - Cystic calculi/sand

Investigations

1. Urinalysis (normal urine parameters) (Table 1-12)
   a. Magnesium ammonium phosphate (struvite) crystals (urolithiasis)
   b. Ketonuria (ketosis—see *Reproductive Disorders*)
2. Radiography
   a. Useful to differentiate uncomplicated cystitis from urolithiasis
   b. Contrast studies (pyelography, double contrast bladder studies, pneumocystographies)

Table 1-12 The ferret: Normal urine parameters

Volume	8-140 mL/kg/hr
pH	6.0-7.5
Protein	7-33 mg/dL
Ketones	Trace
Glucose	Negative
Crystals	Negative

Table 1-13 The ferret: GFR evaluation

Parameter	Normal mean ± SD
Exogenous creatinine clearance (mL/min/kg)	3.32 ± 2.16
Inulin clearance (mL/min/kg)	3.02 ± 1.78
Endogenous creatinine clearance (mL/min/kg)	2.5 ± 0.93

3. Routine hematology and biochemistry
   a. With renal disease, urea can be >42.5 mmol/L in renal disease (normal 10 to 15 mmol/L), but creatinine is rarely raised unless renal disease is severe and long-standing.
   b. Phosphorus often raised with renal disease
   c. Nonregenerative anemia (advanced renal disease)
   d. GFR evaluation (from Hillyer 1997) (Table 1-13)
4. Cytology
   a. Renal casts, neoplastic cells
5. Culture and sensitivity
6. Endoscopy
7. Biopsy
8. Ultrasonography

Management

1. Fluid therapy (see *Nursing Care*)
2. Appropriate antibiosis

Treatment/specific therapy

- Renal cysts
  - No treatment
  - If large, painful, and unilateral, consider nephrectomy.
- Hydronephrosis
  - Nephrectomy
  - Some cases may be linked to accidental ureteral occlusion during routine ovariohysterectomy.

- Urolithiasis
  - If urethral obstruction:
    - Attempt catheterization (can be difficult in males due to J-shaped os penis).
    - Cystocentesis
    - Surgical cystotomy
    - If unable to clear urethra, create a perineal urethrostomy.
- Cystic calculi
  - Cystotomy
  - Submit any stones/sand for analysis.
  - Administer antibiosis (usually has accompanying cystitis) and other supportive care.
  - Note that diets high in plant protein (especially dog food or poor-quality cat food) may predispose ferrets to urinary calculi formation as well as urinary bacterial infections.
  - Change diet to commercial ferret food or high-quality cat food.
- Neoplasia
  - Transitional cell carcinoma of the bladder: surgery is difficult because cancer is often diffuse. Chemotherapy may prove useful.
- Renal carcinoma
  - Nephrectomy

Reproductive disorders

Ferrets are induced ovulators; ovulation occurs 30 to 40 hours after copulation. Failure to mate can result in a prolonged estrus (up to 6 months) and a resultant aplastic anemia (see "Hyperestrogenism" below). Estrus is indicated by a pronounced swollen vulva (Fig. 1-2); any female in season for longer than 1 month is considered at risk of hyperestrogenism.

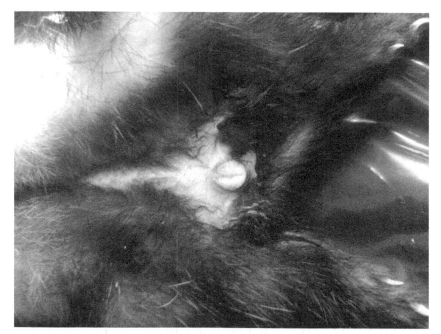

Fig 1-2. Swollen vulva of a ferret in estrus.

Males have a J-shaped os penis.

Where available, the routine use of deslorelin implants has superseded routine castration and ovariohysterectomy of ferrets due to its ease of administration and its protective effects against hyperadrenocorticism (see *Endocrine Disorders*).

Bacterial

- Prostatitis
- Metritis/pyometra
- Mastitis (*Staphylococcus* spp., coliforms)
- *Staphylococcus intermedius* (chronic mastitis)

Nutritional

- Ketosis/pregnancy toxemia (in pregnant jills)

Neoplasia

- Hyperadrenocorticism (see *Endocrine Disorders*)
- Prostatic hyperplasia and prostatic cysts
- Testicular neoplasia
- Sertoli cell tumors
- Interstitial cell tumors
- Prostatic carcinoma
- Ovarian stump neoplasia
- Undifferentiated carcinoma
- Leiomyoma
- Fibrosarcoma
- Ovarian teratoma
- Mammary cystic carcinoma
- Uterine adenoma

Other noninfectious problems

- Hyperestrogenism
- Failure to mate
- Adrenal neoplasia (see *Endocrine Disorders*)
- Ovarian remnant following ovariohysterectomy
- Urolithiasis (in pregnant jills)
- Dystocia
  - Low litter size (unborn kits will die after 43 days' gestation)
  - Physical abnormalities
  - Large kits
  - Deformed/anasarca kits
  - Maternal pelvic abnormalities

Findings on clinical examination

- Vulval hyperplasia (hyperestrogenism, hyperadrenocorticism, estrus, ovarian remnant/ neoplasia)
- Other signs of hyperestrogenism include tachypnea, anemia (pale mucous membranes), ecchymotic and petechial hemorrhages, melena, weakness, hind-limb paresis, secondary infections, and alopecia at tail base.
- Vaginal prolapse (may accompany rectal prolapse) (urolithiasis)
- Swollen uterus palpable; vaginal discharge may, but not always, be present (pyometra, metritis)

- Dysuria/stranguria (prostatic hyperplasia)
- Alopecia and pruritis in entire male ferret (Sertoli cell tumor)
- Swollen, painful, discolored mammary glands (acute mastitis, neoplasia)
- Swollen but otherwise normal mammary glands (chronic mastitis)
- Lethargy dehydration in pregnant female (jill); melena may be present; hair loss (pregnancy toxemia)

Investigations

1. Radiography
   a. Prostatic hyperplasia (will also help differentiate from urolithiasis)
2. Routine hematology and biochemistry
   a. PCV (normal 46% to 61%). For hyperestrogenism, PCV can be used as a prognostic indicator (from Keeble 2001) (Table 1-14).
   b. Other blood values consistent with hyperestrogenism reflect a pancytopenia and include a normocytic normochromic or macrocytic hypochromic anemia plus a thrombocytopenia, neutropenia, eosinopenia.
   c. Pregnancy toxemia/ketosis
   d. In additon to low blood glucose (<2.8 mmol/L) and high blood urea, Batchelder et al (1999) report anemia, hypoproteinemia, hypocalcemia, hyperbilirubinemia, and raised liver enzymes.
3. Urinalysis
   a. Ketonuria (ketosis)
4. Culture and sensitivity
5. Endoscopy
6. Biopsy
7. Ultrasonography
   a. Prostatic hyperplasia/cysts

Table 1-14   The ferret: PCV

PVC (%)	Prognosis	Treatment options
>25	Good	Ovariohysterectomy hCG or GnRH injection
15-25	Guarded	hCG or GnRH injection Supportive care before surgery
<15	Poor	hCG or GnRH injection IV fluids Vitamin B Iron Prophylactic antibiotics Blood transfusion(s), then consider surgery

Management

1. Fluid therapy, including blood transfusions (see *Nursing Care*)
2. Vitamin B complex at 1 to 2 mg/kg thiamine content as needed, IM.
3. Iron dextran at 10 mg/kg IM every 7 days.
4. Prophylactic antibiotics

Treatment/specific therapy

- Hyperestrogenism
  - Ovarohysterectomy
  - hCG at 100 IU/ferret SC IM. Repeat after 7 days if necessary.
  - GnRH at 20 µg/ferret IM or SC. Repeat after 7 to 14 days if necessary.
  - Prevention
    - Routine ovariohysterectomy
    - Routine proligestone injections at 50 mg/kg IM once only before breeding season
    - Mate with vasectomized male.
    - Altering and maintaining the photoperiod at 14 hours light : 10 hours dark may prevent estrus.
- Prostatic hyperplasia
  - Often resolves following treatment of hyperadrenocorticism.
  - Surgical debulking or marsupialization
  - Appropriate antibiosis if prostatitis suspected
- Testicular neoplasia
  - Castration
- Metritis
  - Induce uterine contractions with 0.5 mg prostaglandin $F_{2\alpha}$ SC.
  - Antibiosis
- Pyometra
  - Ovariohysterectomy
  - Antibiosis
- Stump pyometra (following ovariohysterectomy) may occur in some ferrets with hyperadrenocorticism. These will require surgical removal of the stump as well as treatment for adrenal disease.
- Mastitis
  - Acute mastitis
    - Antibiosis and fluids
    - NSAIDs may have anti-endotoxin effects (see "Analgesia" in *Nursing Care*).
    - Debride or surgically resect affected mammary tissue.
    - Fostering kits may spread pathogens to other females.
  - Chronic mastitis
    - Often nonresponsive to therapy
  - Kits may need supplemental feeding (see *Neonatal Disorders*).
- Urolithiasis in pregnant jills
  - If possible, undertake cesarean with 24 hours of parturition date.
  - At the same time perform cystotomy.
  - For management of urolithiasis, see *Urinary Disorders*.
- Ketosis
  - Usually linked to period of anorexia/starvation during pregnancy. This can be as little as 12 to 24 hours.
  - In some cases linked to large litters (15+).
  - Supportive treatment, including fluids, warmth, and IV glucose/force-feeding (see *Nursing Care*)
  - Perform cesarean as soon as possible.
  - Foster or euthanize young (<40 days) as ferret young are hard to hand-rear and the recovering female is unlikely to lactate.

- Dystocia
  - Small litter size
  - Induce parturition at day 41 with 0.5 mg prostaglandin $F_{2\alpha}$ SC, followed by 0.2 to 3.0 units oxytocin SC, IM 1 to 4 hours later. Birth should be 2 to 12 hours later. If not, either repeat treatment or undertake cesarean.
  - Large or deformed kits, pelvic abnormalities, and other anomalies
  - Cesarean

Neonatal disorders

- Some normal parameters of neonatal kits (from Bell 1997)

Table 1-15 The ferret: Neonatal kits normal parameters

Approximate weight at birth (g)	8-10
Approximate weight at 7 days (g)	30
Approximate weight at 14 days (g)	60-70
Approximate weight at 21 days (g)	100
Age of eyes opening	30-35 days
Age of weaning	6-8 weeks

Viral
- Rotavirus

Bacterial
- Eye infections prior to 35 days

Other noninfectious problems
- Hypothermia (especially in first 2 weeks as kits are unable to thermoregulate)
- Lack of maternal milk
- Mastitis (see *Reproductive Disorders*)
- Maternal metritis (see *Reproductive Disorders*)
- Maternal systemic illness
- Tangled umbilical cords

Findings on clinical examination

- Lethargy
- Failure to feed
- History of lack of maternal care
- Failure to grow
- Diarrhea (may not be apparent as female continually licks clean)
- Swelling of the unopened eyes in kits less than 3 weeks old

Investigations

1. Weigh kits
2. Radiography

3. Routine hematology and biochemistry
4. Culture and sensitivity
5. Endoscopy
6. Biopsy
7. Ultrasonography

Management

- Nursing care, especially provision of warmth and fluids, is extremely important with neonates.

Treatment/specific therapy

- Rotavirus
  - Kits over 7 days old may not require treatment.
  - Fluids as 0.5 to 1.0 mL saline SC repeated several times daily
  - Covering antibiosis
- Tangled umbilical cords
  - Gently disentangle from each other and associated nesting material, resecting umbilical cords where appropriate.
- Lack of maternal milk production
  - Supplement with commercial puppy or kitten milk replacer enhanced with cream to give a fat content of around 20%, q.i.d.
  - Foster only if appropriate to do so (may transfer pathogens between females).
  - Investigate underlying problem in the dam.
- Eye infections
  - Incise along the eyelid suture line.
  - Flush out any debris or pus.
  - Apply a topical ophthalmic antibiotic preparation b.i.d.

Rabbits

Table 2-1 The rabbit: Key facts

Average life span (years)	5-10
Weight (kg)	1.0 kg (Netherland Dwarf) to 10 kg (giant breeds)
Body temperature (°C)	38-39.6
Respiratory rate (breaths/min)	30-60
Heart rate (beats/min)	120-325
Gestation (days)	28-35
Age at weaning (weeks)	4-6
Sexual maturity (months)	4.5-9

Rabbits are prey animals and, therefore, may exhibit extreme antipredator behavior, such as jumping from the examination table. During a clinical examination, movements should be moderated and deliberate with loud noises avoided as these may startle the rabbit. The scent of potential predators such as dogs, cats, and ferrets may be stressful to some rabbits, so these should be removed by cleaning your hands, examination table, and equipment as best as possible prior to examination.

Always weigh the rabbit at every consultation; weight loss may be the first occult sign of chronic disease such as dental disease. Most rabbits can be examined on a table with minimal restraint. If lifted, one hand is placed beneath the chest while the other supports the back end and legs. Many rabbits can have their perineum and ventral surface examined by gently turning them on their backs, such that the rabbit is held and supported upside-down between the examiner's chest and arm. The oral cavity can be examined with the use of an auroscope, although in the conscious rabbit this can never be regarded as a full oral examination.

Use of glucose and sodium as prognostic indicators in the rabbit

Stressed and ill rabbits commonly show hyperglycemia with a compensatory hyponatremia. However, the hyponatremia may be either a true sodium deficiency or an apparent, but not actual, pseudohyponatremia. Pseudohyponatremia (which can occur with congestive heart failure, severe liver disease, and hyperlipidemia) does not require treatment, whereas true hyponatremia does. These are distinguished by comparing the sodium levels with the calculated tonicity. Calculated osmolarity has less diagnostic significance.

Calculated tonicity:

$$\text{Ton (mOsm/L)} = 2 \times (\text{mEq/L}) + \text{Glucose (mg/dL)}/18$$

Calculated osmolarity:

$$P_{osm} \text{ (mOsm/L)} = 2 \times \text{Na (mEq/L)} + \text{Glucose (mg/dL)}/18 + \text{BUN (mg/dL)}/2.8$$

Table 2-2 The rabbit: glucose and sodium values as prognostic indicators.

Physiologic state	Blood glucose	Sodium	Osmolarity	Tonicity
	mmol/L	mEq/L	mOsm/L	mOsm/L
Normal	4.2-8.2	136-147	284-312	278-302
Stress (e.g., handling)	8.0-10.0			
Severe disease (e.g., enterotoxemia, mucoid enteropathy, hepatic lipidosis, bladder obstruction, ureteral stones, intestinal obstruction)	20.0-30.0	<129 carries a 2.3 times mortality risk.		
Diabetes mellitus	30-33.4			

Adapted from Bonvehi et al 2014 and Harcourt-Brown and Harcourt-Brown 2012.

Nursing care

Thermoregulation

This is one of the most crucial homeostatic mechanisms for rabbits (and other small mammals). They are susceptible to both hyperthermia and hypothermia (which acts as a general depressant and is also immunosuppressive). Body temperature is achieved and maintained at some cost to the rabbit, which must generate and maintain a high metabolic rate. However, their small size means that they have a large surface area compared with body mass, with a consequent high potential for conductive, convective, and radiative heat loss. In the conscious rabbit, heat loss is countered by a variety of mechanisms such as dense coats and subcutaneous fat (insulative layers) plus physiologic methods—peripheral vasoconstriction/dilatation, piloerection, and shivering. Behavior also alters to either enhance or reduce heat loss. High respiratory rates secondary to stress can mean a significant evaporative heat loss.

Management of hyperthermia

See *Systemic Disorders.*

Management of hypothermia

1. Assess the rectal temperature of the rabbit. If in doubt, assume that the animal is hypothermic and that this should be corrected as soon as possible.
2. Applying insulation such as bubble wrap is often insufficient—collapsed or otherwise inactive rabbits are not generating heat, and this may insulate it from a higher ambient temperature.
3. Place these animals onto a heat mat, onto which is placed an absorptive towel or other material to reduce the risk of localized burns.
4. Alternatives include heated operating tables, commercial warm air generators, or incubators; "hot hands" (gloves filled with warm water) carry too high a risk of burns and cool too quickly.
5. Place insulative material over the animal and heat source.
6. Areas of the body where there is a high risk of radiative heat loss such as the pinnae or feet can be covered with aluminum foil to further conserve heat.

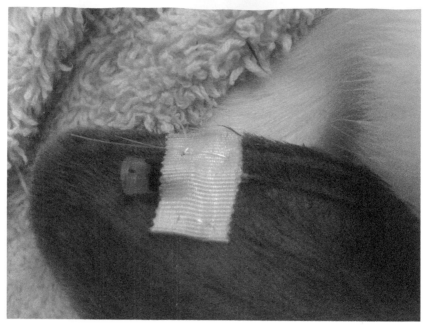

Fig 2-1. Correct placement of a catheter into the marginal auricular vein.

7. By either quickly raising the body temperature or allowing the rabbit to maintain its core temperature with ease, we remove the need for costly hyperthermic physiologic processes, such as shivering.
8. Treat high risk of enterotoxemia following die-off of gut bacteria according to general principles outlined in *Management* in *Gastrointestinal Tract Disorders.*

Fluids

In small mammals the choice of fluid used is as indicated with other mammals. Venous access in the rabbit is via the cephalic, lateral saphenous, and marginal ear veins (Fig. 2-1). Jugular cutdown can be undertaken under general anesthesia (GA) but may result in respiratory embarrassment. Fluids can be given IV either by bolus or by infusion.

In hypovolemic patients, vascular access may be impossible and it may be better to consider either IP or IO administration. For IO it is relatively simple under GA to insert either an intraosseous catheter or a hypodermic needle into the marrow of either the femur (via the greater trochanter) or tibia (through the tibial crest). Fluids, colloids, and even blood can be given IO if necessary.

Fluid administration

- All fluids should be warmed to 38°C.
- Daily fluid maintenance requirement for a rabbit is 100 mL/kg per day.
- Fluid replacement calculations are as for other species. Recommendations for rabbits are:
  - Crystalloids: For rabbits the maintenance fluid rate is 75 to 100 mL/kg per 24 hours. Shock rate is up to 100 mL/kg over 1 hour.
  - Colloids: A bolus of 10 to 15 mL/kg over 30 minutes can be given up to four times daily.
- Whole blood: Transfusions from other rabbits can be done, usually over a period of 20 to 30 minutes. Transfusion reactions are rare, but a major and minor cross-match are recommended.

Nutritional support

Many rabbits are presented as emergencies after a prolonged period of ill health that will have affected their food intake (e.g., suffering from undiagnosed chronic dental disease). These animals are often hypoglycemic, so testing beforehand (a commercial glucometer is suitable) is beneficial, followed by IV or IP glucose to those cases identified.

Longer-term support can be given by syringe feeding commercially available food supplements, e.g., Oxbow Critical Care and Science Recovery Diet. The following caveats apply:
- Use a relatively wide-bore syringe, as blockage at the correct concentration is common. Feeding a dilute mixture may be counterproductive.
- Nasogastric tubes can be fitted, but these are prone to blockage.
- If the rabbit is very debilitated, then choking/failure to swallow may occur; in these cases concentrate on parenteral fluids, dextrose, and vitamin B therapy.

Analgesia

Table 2-3   The rabbit: Analgesic doses

Analgesic	Dose
Buprenorphine	0.01-0.05 mg/kg SC, IM, or IV every 6-12 h
Butorphanol	0.1-1.0 mg/kg SC, IM, or IV every 2-4 h
Carprofen	1.0-2.0 mg/kg SC or PO b.i.d.
Ketoprofen	1-3 mg/kg IM, SC s.i.d.
Meloxicam	0.1-0.3 mg/kg SC or PO s.i.d.
Morphine	2.0-5.0 mg/kg SC or IM every 4 h
Meperidine/pethidine	5.0-10 mg/kg SC or IM every 2-4 h
Nalbuphine	1.0-2.0 mg/kg IM or IV every 2-4 h
Tramadol	2-4 mg/kg PO b.i.d.

Table 2-4   Continuous rate infusions delivered via syringe driver

Ketamine	Loading dose 0.25-0.5 mg/kg; maintenance dose 0.02-0.2 mg/kg/hr
Morphine	Loading dose 0.5 mg/kg; maintenance dose 0.1-0.4 mg/kg/hr
Dexmedetomidine	Loading dose 0.005 mg/kg; maintenance 0.001 mg/kg/hr

Anesthesia

There are many safe anesthetic techniques described for rabbits despite the persistent myth that rabbits do not survive anesthesia. The author finds the following protocols of use:

Preanesthetic protocol

1. Rabbits rarely vomit, so starving is not only unnecessary but should be avoided due to their high metabolic rate.
2. Administering metoclopramide (0.5 mg/kg SC or PO every 6 to 8 hours) postoperatively will help to prevent a postsurgical ileus, especially following painful or abdominal surgery.
3. Monitor feeding and fecal output for 24 hours following surgery.

Anesthesia of high-risk cases

Typically these are rabbits that have chronic dental disease, have not been able to eat normally for some time, and have marked weight loss. Clinical assessment is vital and if necessary correction of fluid deficit and stabilization should be attempted prior to anesthesia. Such rabbits should ideally have a rapid induction and a rapid recovery from anesthesia to regain temperature homeostasis and imitate feeding. Masking with volatile anesthetics alone can achieve the latter although induction can be prolonged. Alternatively the author has found induction with IV propofol to be generally safe.

The advantage of gaseous anesthetic induction is rapid recovery without the need to metabolize large amounts of drug. Isoflurane appears to be less stressful for induction than halothane, based on lower corticosterone levels (González-Gil et al 2006).

Gaseous anesthetic induction protocol

1. Preoxygenate rabbits before induction.
2. When masking down rabbits, breath holding is very common. This can lead to hypoxia, hypercapnia, and bradycardia.
3. Monitor breathing closely and only increase anesthetic concentration when rabbit is seen breathing.
4. If the concentration is increased rapidly, there is increased risk of inhalation of high concentrations of anesthetic gas quickly and increased risk of cardiovascular consequences once rabbit starts to breathe.
5. Once sufficiently anesthetized, intubate—use an uncuffed endotracheal tube. Rabbits can exhibit laryngeal spasm, so beware excessive trauma. Use local anesthetic spray.

Propofol induction

- Following the application of local anesthetic cream a catheter is placed into the marginal auricular vein (see Fig. 2-1).
- Propofol is administered at 10 mg/kg IV.
- Intubate (see below) and maintain on gaseous anesthetics.
- Anesthesia can be maintained for very short periods by repeated boluses of propofol, but the cardiac and respiratory depressant effects mean that it should not be used for longer procedures.

Blind intubation of rabbits

1. Spray glottis with local anesthetic spray.
2. Place rabbit in sternal recumbency.
3. Run endotracheal (usually 2.0, 2.5, or 3.0 mm uncuffed) tube along midline of palate to back of pharynx.
4. Look for gagging reflex.
5. Listen for breaths.
6. Feel for exhalations.
7. Feel for sensation of tube passing over tracheal rings.
8. *Or* use laryngoscope with long blade.
9. Having an assistant hold the mouth open with pieces of bandage gauze behind the upper and lower incisors may be of some use.

Pre-medication protocol

1. Alternatively sedate with diazepam (0.2 mg/kg IM or IV) or midazolam (2.0 mg/kg IM or IP) or a combination of butorphanol (1.5 mg/kg) and medetomidine (0.1 mg/kg) IV. These may still not prevent breath-holding.
2. Once sleepy, mask with isoflurane.
3. Spray glottis with local anesthetic spray.
4. Intubate once able to and maintain with isoflurane.

- Oxygen can also be delivered via the nasal cavities—a small-diameter catheter or tube is inserted into the ventral nasal meatus. Even moderate flow rates risk an explosive exit of such a tube! If necessary, a tracheotomy may need to be performed.
- Premedication with doxapram at 10 mg/kg IP, IV, or sublingually (SL) 5 to 10 minutes beforehand is occasionally recommended, but this will increase oxygen demand and the author finds it usually unnecessary.

Parenteral anesthesia

- Ketamine/medetomidine/butorphanol given IM simultaneously:
  - Ketamine at 10 mg/kg
  - Medetomidine at 0.1 mg/kg
  - Butorphanol at 1.5 mg/kg
- At end of procedure reverse medetomidine with atipamezole at 0.75 mg/kg IM.

Cardiopulmonary resuscitation

Respiratory arrest

1. Administer 100% oxygen.
2. Assist ventilation—compress thorax at around 60x/minute.
3. Doxapram SL or at 10 mg/kg IV or IP. *Note:* This will increase the animal's oxygen demand.
4. If appropriate, give atipamezole.

Cardiac arrest

As for respiratory arrest but also:
1. Compress thorax at around 90x/minute.
2. If asystole—give epinephrine at 0.1 mg/kg of 1:10,000 IV.
3. If ventricular fibrillation—lidocaine (lignocaine) at 1 to 2 mg/kg IV.

Skin disorders

Normally rabbits have a soft, short undercoat covered with larger guard hairs. Rex breeds have short guard hairs that do not exceed the undercoat, while Angoran breeds have very long guard and undercoat hairs. Lionhead rabbits retain the long hair around the head, neck, and rump area. Satin breeds have altered hair fiber structure.

Findings on clinical examination

Signs of skin disease:
- Pruritus
  - Typically hairs will be damaged. There may be areas of reddened and inflamed skin.
  - Edema may accompany a cellulitis.
  - Ectoparasites, especially *Cheyletiella*, *Leporacarus*, and *Psoroptes*. Occasionally fleas (rabbit flea—*Spilopsyllus cuniculi* [Pinter 1999], cat and dog fleas—*Ctenocephalides* spp.), lice, sarcoptic and *Demodex* mites, and blowfly maggots. *Cheyletiella* may act as a vector for myxomatosis.
  - Ear mites *(Psoroptes cuniculi):* inflammation and pruritus of the pinnae (Fig. 2-2). Can spread onto surrounding face and neck.
  - Bacterial disease, typically *Staphylococcus* and *Pasteurella* species (Fig. 2-3). *Pseudomonas* is typically linked to moist dermatitis under the chin (blue fur disease).
  - Occasionally due to *Trichophyton*

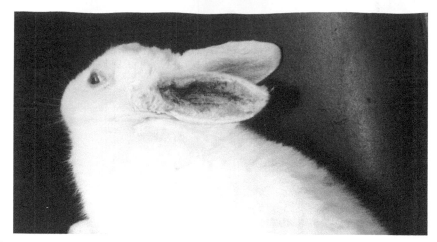

Fig 2-2. Ear mite *(Psoroptes cuniculi)* infestation.

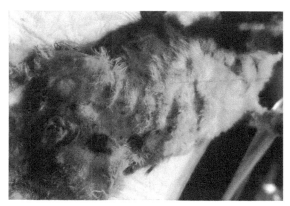

Fig 2-3. Severe bacterial dermatitis in a rabbit.

- Alopecia
  - Self-mutilation secondary to pruritus
  - Sebaceous adenitis (Whitbread et al 2002)
  - Lack of dietary fiber can lead to "barbering" if two or more rabbits present
  - Endocrinologic
  - Cystic ovaries and other ovarian diseases
  - Suckling does will remove hair from around teats
  - Atypical myxomatosis
- Scaling and crusting
  - Ectoparasitic infestations, especially *Cheyletiella*
  - Thickened crustlike material on pinnae and in ear canal strongly suggestive of *Psoroptes cuniculi*
  - Sebaceous adenitis
  - *Trichophyton mentagrophytes, Scopulariopsis brevicaulis* (Vangeel et al 2000), and rarely *Microsporum*
  - Myxomatosis lesions

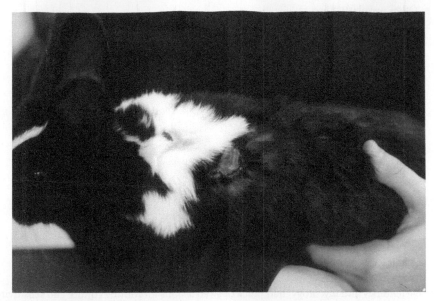

Fig 2-4. Skin lacerations and subsequent dermal necrosis from fighting.

- Rabbit syphilis *Treponema cuniculi*, especially at mucocutaneous junctions. Vesicles may be present.
  - Atypical myxomatosis
- Erosions and ulceration
  - Bacterial disease, especially *Staphylococcus* and *Pseudomonas*
  - Myiasis
  - Cutaneous lymphosarcoma
  - Bites and lacerations (Fig. 2-4)
  - Pododermatitis
  - Atypical myxomatosis
  - Rabbit syphilis
  - Vaccine reactions; can happen with oil adjuvant vaccines or if part of vaccine given intradermally (as manufacturer may recommend)
- Nodules, swellings, and nonhealing wounds
  - Abscess. If these are around the mouth, strongly suspect underlying dental disease.
  - Salivary mucocele (soft fluctuant swelling on jaw—see *Gastrointestinal Disorders*)
  - Herpesvirus (circular, reddened skin lesions)
  - Poxvirus—initial nasal discharge and fever, followed by generalized formation of papules and nodules; edema of the face and perineum
  - *Cuterebra* larvae
  - Mycobacteriosis
  - Myxomatosis (may see concurrent palpebral edema, swollen pinnae, swelling of external genitalia and perineum)
  - Shope papilloma virus (papovavirus)
  - Shope fibroma virus (poxvirus)
  - Acrochordon
  - Lymphoma/lymphosarcoma

- Other neoplastic diseases
  - Fibrosarcoma
  - Squamous cell carcinoma
  - Trichoepithelioma
  - Basal cell tumor
  - Lipoma
  - Apocrine adenocarcinoma (Miwa et al 2006)
- Excessively pronounced dewlap
  - Some breeds selected for this
  - More prominent in females
  - May be site of recurrent moist dermatitis, especially *Pseudomonas,* where the dewlap is consistently moist, as from water bowls

Investigations

1. Microscopy: examine fur pluck, acetate strips, or skin scrapes to affected area and examine for ectoparasite.
2. Examine material from ear canals for *Psoroptes cuniculi.*
3. Examine teeth. Rabbits with dental disease may have difficulty grooming normally.
4. Bacteriology and mycology: hair pluck or swab lesions for routine culture and sensitivity.
5. Fine-needle aspirate followed by staining with rapid Romanowsky stains
6. Biopsy obvious lesions.
7. Ultraviolet (Wood's) lamp—positive for *Microsporium canis* only (not all strains fluoresce)
8. Routine hematology and biochemistry
9. Serology for *Treponema cuniculi* titer
10. Endocrine analysis (see *Endocrine Disorders*)
11. Normal plasma thyroid level: 22 nM/L (Hulbert 2000)
12. If barbering suspected, examine hair under microscope to see if chewed; separate from other rabbit; supply extra hay.

Management

1. Rabbits with dental disease or those that have had incisor extractions are unable to groom and will require regular grooming by their owner.
2. Routine and regular examination of the perineum of pet rabbits is essential. The presence of caecotrophs adhered to the perineum will encourage myiasis (see *Failure to Caecotroph*).

Treatment/specific therapy

- Treat for any ectoparasites.
  - Ivermectin at 200 µg/kg SC, topically or as topical application (Beaphar Anti-Parasite Spot-On for Small Animals, USA, Genitrix Xeno 450, UK) works well for mites such as *Cheyletiella,* although treatment should be continued for longer than 6 weeks (life cycle = 5 weeks). Also for myiasis.
  - Imidacloprid (Advantage, Bayer) applied as a 40-mg spot-on. Can be applied weekly for lice and myiasis
  - Permethrin applied as either a dusting powder or shampoo
- Ear mites *(Psoroptes cuniculi)*
  - Ivermectin at 200 µg/kg SC, topically or as topical application (Beaphar Anti-Parasite Spot-On for Small Animals, USA, Genitrix Xeno 450, UK)

- Topical selamectin at 6 to 18 mg/kg (Hack et al 2002)
- Topical 10% imidacloprid/1.0% moxidectin (Advocate (UK), Advantage Multi, Bayer (USA)) at 10 mg/kg (imidacloprid) and 1 mg/kg (moxidectin) every 4 weeks for 3 treatments (Beck 2007)
- Soften material in ear canal using either acaricidal eardrops or nonacaricidal products.
- After 5 to 7 days the crusty exudate should have softened sufficiently to allow atraumatic removal.
- Myiasis
  - Initial treatment involves clipping of the fur and cleaning the affected area, with manual removal of maggots plus flushing with a dilute chlorhexidine or povidone-iodine cleanser. Supportive treatment should be aggressive with therapy for toxic shock plus ivermectin or imidacloprid to kill any maggots or emergent larvae that cannot be removed.
  - The underlying cause of the caecotroph accumulation must be addressed (see *Failure to Caecotroph*) and regular perineal inspection and cleaning, plus protection from exposure to flies, is crucial in preventing the condition.
  - Topical cyromazine (Rearguard (UK) Larvadex (US), Novartis) applied as a 6% solution topically every 6 to 10 weeks as a preventative for myiasis
  - *Cuterebra* larvae: Either remove via the breathing hole, surgically, or by using ivermectin at 200 µg/kg SC, topical or as topical application (Beaphar Anti-Parasite Spot-On for Small Animals, USA, Genitrix Xeno 450, UK).
- Pododermatitis
  - Risk factors (in part from Mancinelli et al 2014)
    - Large breeds
    - Older rabbits
    - Females > Males
    - Neutered > entire (<100% neutered females)
    - Obesity
    - Substrate. Hay bedding appeared to be preventative.
  - Typically on hocks. A pet rabbit pododermatitis scoring system (PRPSS) has been developed (Mancinelli et al 2014)

Table 2-5 The rabbit: Pet Rabbit Pododermatitis Scoring System

Grading scale	Macroscopic description
Grade 0	No lesions
Grade 1	A small, circular area on the plantar aspect of the metatarsal bone-calcaneus (mono or bilateral lesions), with minimal alopecia, minimal epidermal hyperemia and/or hyperkeratosis of the skin, but with no evidence of infection or bleeding of underlying tissues
Grade 2	Circumscribed area of varying size localized at the caudal plantar aspect of the metatarsal-calcaneal area or extending linearly along the plantar aspect of the cranial metatarsal area with alopecia, erythema, and scaling of surrounding tissues
Grade 3	Area of varying size focally ulcerated and with varying degree of keratinization abnormalities. Infection of subcutaneous tissue present
Grade 4	Full-thickness skin loss with swelling and necrotic debris may be present with infection of underlying tissues. Purulent exudates may be adherent to the lesions.
Grade 5	Severe infections with involvement of deep structures, including bones and tendons with tenosynovitis, osteomyelitis, and arthritis
Grade 6	End-stage disease with loss of pedal function

- Once established, difficult to resolve
- Appropriate antibiosis and analgesia
- May need repeated dressing (some rabbits may not tolerate such bandages)
- IntraSite Gel applied several times per day is beneficial.
- Maintain on hay substrate.
- Bacterial dermatitis and cellulitis
  - Topical and parenteral antibiotics
  - Cleaning with chlorhexidine solution may be beneficial.
- Surgical removal of abscesses. Draining and flushing of rabbit abscesses rarely work.
- Bites and lacerations
  - Clean and debride well. These are prone to infection, so it may be better to surgically excise the lesion and heal by first intention.
  - Covering broad-spectrum antibiosis
- Poxvirus, Shope fibroma virus
  - Supportive treatment only; usually spontaneously regress
- Shope papilloma virus
  - Can trigger warts, especially on eyelids and ears
  - Consider surgical resection as may eventually become carcinomas
  - Spread by insect vector so antiectoparasiticidal treatment important adjunct
- Myxomatosis
  - Supportive therapy is required. Fluids, assisted feeding, and covering antibiosis are essential if the rabbit is to stand any chance of survival.
  - Spread by insect vectors so antiectoparasiticidal treatment important adjunct
  - Atypical myxomatosis. Three atypical forms have been described:
    - Partially immune (vaccinated) rabbits may develop a papillomatous form that progresses to crusting lesions, especially on the eyelids and other mucocutaneous junctions. These usually resolve with appropriate care.
    - Papules and plaques appear in recently depilated areas. These progress to hemorrhagic and necrotic lesions. Recovery is spontaneous.
    - Respiratory form
  - Vaccines are available.
- Dermatophytosis
  - Griseofulvin at 25 mg/kg PO once daily for 4 weeks
  - Miconazole/chlorhexidine (Malaseb, Leo) shampoo—bathe once daily
  - Itraconazole at 5.0 mg/kg PO s.i.d. for 30 days
- *Treponema* (rabbit syphilis)
  - Responds well to penicillin at 50,000 IU/kg SC given once weekly for 3 weeks. In view of slight risk of inducing an enterotoxemia, where possible always have serologic test done first.
  - Tetracyclines and chloramphenicol can also be effective.
- Lymphoma/lymphosarcoma
  - See *Systemic Disorders.*
- Neoplasia
  - Surgical debulking, resection, or euthanasia
  - Accessible cutaneous tumors can be treated by injecting cisplatin directly into the tissue mass on a weekly basis as a debulking exercise.
- Dewlap dermatitis
  - Clean with chlorhexidine solution.
  - Antibiosis
  - Dewlap resection

Respiratory tract disorders

Rabbits are obligate nasal breathers. The back of the pharynx is comparatively small and is occupied by the main body of the tongue, preventing easy visualization of the caudal pharynx.

Disorders of the upper respiratory tract

- Dental disease
- Pasteurellosis (includes atrophic rhinitis-like condition)
- Other bacterial infections
- Poxvirus
- *Treponema cuniculi*
- Toxoplasmosis (see *Neuromuscular Disorders*)
- Allergy

Findings on clinical examination

- Nasal discharge
- Conjunctivitis (see *Ophthalmic Disorders*)
- Dacryocystitis (see *Ophthalmic Disorders*)
- Vesicles, erosions, and crusty lesions *(Treponema cuniculi)*
- Fever (>40° C), oculonasal discharge, increased respiratory rate, CNS signs (toxoplasmosis)

Investigations and management

- See *Differential Diagnoses for Respiratory Disorders*.

Treatment

- Poxvirus—initial nasal discharge and fever; followed by generalized formation of papules and nodules; edema of the face and perineum; self-limiting
- See also *Differential Diagnoses for Respiratory Disorders*.

Differential diagnoses for respiratory disorders

Viral

- Myxomatosis (see *Skin Disorders*)
- Viral hemorrhagic disease (VHD) (calicivirus)
- Herpesvirus
- Paramyxovirus (Sendai virus)

Bacterial

- Pasteurellosis (including *P. multocida*)
- *Bordetella bronchiseptica*
- *Staphylococcus aureus*
- Streptococci
- *Moraxella* spp.
- *Pseudomonas aeruginosa*

- Mycobacteriosis
- Cilia-associated respiratory bacillus
- *Mycoplasma pulmonis*
- *Chlamydophila*

Protozoal

- Toxoplasmosis (see *Neuromuscular Disorders*)

Neoplasia

- Lung metastases from uterine adenocarcinoma
- Thymomas

Other noninfectious problems

- Allergic
- Congestive heart failure
- Traumatic tracheitis (secondary to endotracheal intubation)
- Heatstroke

Findings on clinical examination

- Rhinitis
- Sinusitis
- Conjunctivitis
- Dacryocystitis (see *Ophthalmic Disorders*)
- Otitis
- Abscessation (can involve skin and variety of organs or joints due to bacteremic spread)
- Increased respiratory noise
- Dyspnea/tachypnea
- Fever
- Bilateral exophthalmia (thymomas)
- Anorexia and weight loss
- Loss of exercise tolerance
- Associated cardiovascular disease (e.g., pericarditis with *Pasteurella* bacteremia—see *Cardiovascular Disorders*)

Investigations

1. Auscultation
   a. Rales and rattles: Differentiate between upper respiratory tract disease and lower respiratory tract disease (pneumonia).
   b. Areas of consolidation may be silent.
2. Radiography
   a. Skull (dental disease, bulla abscessation, turbinate atrophy)
   b. Contrast studies on nasolacrimal ducts
   c. Spine (discospondylitis)
   d. Thorax (lung metastases, cardiac disease, consolidated lung tissue, effusion lines)
3. Routine hematology and biochemistry
   a. Look for alterations in heterophil/lymphocyte ratios.
4. Serology for *Pasteurella*, *Mycoplasma pulmonis*, *Chlamydophila*, myxomatosis

5. Culture and sensitivity (including from tracheal wash)
   a. Always have anaerobic culture performed as well as aerobic.
6. *Chlamydophila* polymerase chain reaction (PCR)
7. Cytology from tracheal wash
8. Pleural tap and cytology
9. Endoscopy
10. Ultrasonography
    a. Thymoma
11. Biopsy

Management

1. Give supportive treatment (e.g., covering antibiosis).
2. Reduce stress levels. Hospitalize away from dogs and noisy cats; keep in darkened position.
3. Supply oxygen, preferably via an "oxygen tent."
4. Mucolytics may be useful (e.g., bromhexine, *N*-acetylcysteine).

Treatment/specific therapy

- VHD
  - No treatment; supportive treatment only
- Pasteurellosis and other bacterial infections: broad-spectrum antibiotics plus anaerobic cover (e.g., metronidazole at 20 mg/kg PO b.i.d.)
  - Surgical removal or debridement of abscesses often necessary
  - If surgery is not practical, then some abscesses may be allowed to heal by second intention. Daily topical applications of IntraSite Gel (Smith and Nephew Health) are helpful. Topical Manuka honey is also said to be useful.
- Heatstroke (see *Systemic Diseases*)
- Thymoma
  - Radiation therapy; 24 Gy given in 3 fractions of 8 Gy on days 0, 7, and 21 (Sanchez-Migallon et al 2006)

Dental disorders

- The permanent dental formula of the rabbit (Fig. 2-5) is:

Permanent dental formula of the rabbit

$$I : \frac{2}{1}, \quad C : \frac{0}{0}, \quad PM : \frac{3}{2}, \quad M : \frac{3}{3}$$

Protozoal

- *E. cuniculi* (meningitis may produce abnormal chewing muscle movements; partial paralysis of tongue secondary to hypoglossal nerve damage)

Nutritional

- Lack of long fiber (e.g., hay) in diet
- Inappropriate nutrition

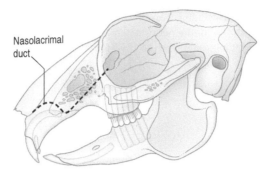

Fig 2-5. A diagram of a rabbit skull showing position of teeth and track of nasolacrimal duct.

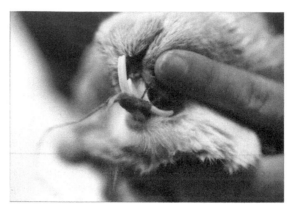

Fig 2-6. Overgrown maxillary and mandibular incisors, with hair matted around the lower teeth.

Neoplasia

- Osteosarcoma of the mandible

Other noninfectious problems

- Congenital incisor malocclusion (esp. brachycephalic breeds such as Netherland Dwarf, Lionhead, and Mini-Lops)

Findings on clinical examination

- Incisor malocclusion (Fig. 2-6)
- Mandibular swelling (unilateral or bilateral) due to bone remodeling to accommodate tooth root overgrowth
- Gross swelling, typically in the mandibular area (Fig. 2-7), but can be at maxilla, secondary to tooth root abscess
- Excessive salivation/moist fur on chin and ventral neck
- Weight loss
- Anorexia (may be intermittent)
- Perineal accumulations of caecotrophs
- Ectoparasitic disease
- Dacryocystitis

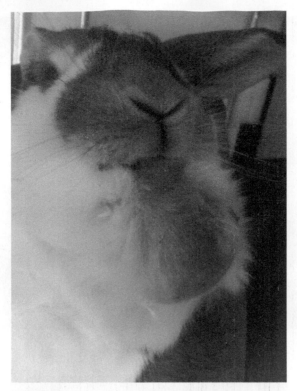

Fig 2-7. Mandibular tooth root abscess.

- Conjunctivitis
- Exophthalmos (secondary to retrobulbar abscess) (see *Ophthalmic Disorders*)

Investigations

1. Otoscopic examination
   a. Spurs on cheek teeth (tend to be lingual on the mandibular cheek teeth and buccal on the maxillary)
   b. Lingual tilting of mandibular cheek teeth and buccal tilting of maxillary cheek teeth (Fig. 2-8)
   c. Ulceration of tongue and cheeks
   d. Purulent material in mouth
   e. Otoscopic examination does not constitute a complete examination of the oral cavity as structures at the back of the pharynx can be difficult to see due to its depth and the large size of the tongue.
2. Radiography
   a. Lateral, dorsoventral (DV) views of skull. *Note:* Skulls often appear osteoporotic, probably due to an atrophy of disuse but has been linked to hypocalcemia.
   b. Left and right lateral oblique views of skull allow assessment of individual tooth roots. Any divergence of maxillary or mandibular tooth roots away from each other suggests abnormal root elongation (Figs. 2-9, 2-10).
   c. Contrast study on nasolacrimal ducts

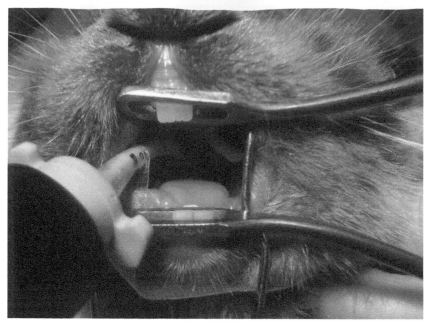

Fig 2-8. Buccal tilting and overgrowth of the upper first premolar.

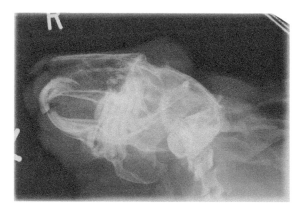

Fig 2-9. Right lateral oblique view of skull showing osteolysis around the root of the left first mandibular premolar associated with a tooth root abscess; there is also overgrowth of the second premolar, first molar, and incisor roots.

3. Check patency of nasolacrimal ducts (Fig. 2-11).
4. Routine hematology and biochemistry
   a. Concerns that rabbits with dental disease are hypocalcemic are ill-founded. Calcium levels are readily responsive to dietary levels, and calcium status is monitored with ionized calcium (total calcium 3.0 to 4.0 mmol/L; ionized 1.57 to 1.83 mmol/L).
5. Culture and sensitivity
   a. Aerobic and anaerobic culture of abscesses
6. Endoscopy

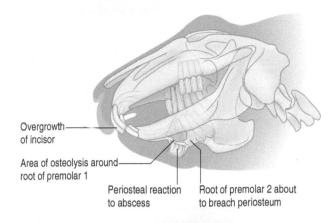

Overgrowth of incisor

Area of osteolysis around root of premolar 1

Periosteal reaction to abscess

Root of premolar 2 about to breach periosteum

Fig 2-10. Explanatory diagram of Fig. 2-9.

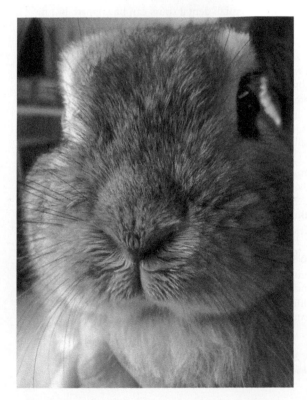

Fig 2-11. Fluorescein can be used to check nasolacrimal duct patency.

7. Examination of oral cavity under GA
8. Biopsy (osteosarcoma)

Management

1. Chronic cases often cachexic—may need parenteral fluid support. Check blood glucose levels (normal range 4.2 to 8.2 mmol/L).

2. Syringe feeding with commercial feed suspensions (e.g., Oxbow Critical Care or Science Recovery Diet); may require nasogastric tube
3. Flushing of nasolacrimal ducts and antibiosis.

Treatment/specific therapy

- Regular coronal reduction
  - Always burr overgrown incisors in preference to clipping due to risk of fracture, pulpal hemorrhage, and infection.
  - For cheek teeth, this will likely necessitate heavy sedation or GA. "Conscious" dental work on the cheek teeth is stressful to the rabbit and risks serious traumatic back injuries, including fracture of lumbar vertebrae (see *Neuromuscular Disorders*).
  - Often coronal reduction alone is insufficient; often by the time of presentation, dental disease has progressed to a quite advanced stage.
  - Use of a dental drill or equivalent is essential; dental spurs can be clipped, but the teeth must be burred down and clipping is likely to fracture the tooth.
- Incisor extraction
- Cheek teeth extraction
- Surgical debridement of tooth root abscesses, including removal of infected bone and affected tooth roots, followed by:
  - Packing with antibiotic-impregnated methyl-methacrylate (bone cement or similar) *and/or*
  - Marsupialization, leaving ostium for recurrent povidone-iodine/antibiotic application during second intention healing
  - Antibiosis
    - Usually a broad-spectrum antibiotic such as enrofloxacin at 5 mg/kg PO s.i.d. or co-trimoxazole at 30 mg/kg PO b.i.d. *plus*
    - Anaerobic antibiosis, e.g., metronidazole at 10 to 20 mg/kg PO s.i.d. or b.i.d. or procaine G benzylpenicillin at 20,000 to 60,000 IU/kg IM or SC s.i.d.
- Drilling out of tooth root apices to initiate tooth root death where extraction is not viable
- Analgesia (e.g., meloxicam at 0.3 mg/kg PO s.i.d.) can be given for many weeks.
- Where possible, wean rabbit onto a diet high in long fiber (i.e., grass and hay), as this encourages normal chewing and dental wear on the back teeth.
- Osteosarcoma: Treatment is difficult even with surgical debridement and chemotherapy—consider euthanasia.

Gastrointestinal tract disorders

Viral

- Rotavirus
- Papillomatosis
- VHD

Bacterial

- The normal gut flora of the rabbit is predominantly gram-positive. Typical inhabitants include *Bacteroides* spp., *Propionibacterium* spp., and *Butyrivibrio* spp. *plus* gram-negative oval and fusiform rods. Also present are large ciliated protozoa

(Isotricha) and yeasts *(Cyniclomyces guttulatus)*. Coliforms are not present in healthy animals.

- *Escherichia coli*
- *Staphylococcus* (enteritis in newborn/suckling rabbits)
- *Clostridium spiroforme*
- *Clostridium piliforme* (Tyzzei disease)
- Salmonellosis
- *Klebsiella pneumoniae* (Coletti et al 2001)
- *Pseudomonas*
- *Mycobacterium avium paratuberculosis* (Greig et al 1997)

Protozoal
- Intestinal coccidiosis (especially *Eimeria perforans, E. magna, E. media,* and *E. irresidua*)
- Hepatic coccidiosis *(Eimeria stiedae)*
- *Cryptosporidium* (young rabbits)
- *Giardia duodenalis* (nonpathogenic)
- *Monocercomonas cuniculi* (nonpathogenic)
- *Retortamonas cuniculi* (nonpathogenic)
- *Entamoeba cuniculi* (nonpathogenic)
- The commensal yeast *(Cyniclomyces guttulatus)* should not be mistaken for *Eimeria* oocysts.

Parasitic
- Nematodes
  - Pinworms *(Passalurus ambiguus)*
  - *Trichostrongylus*
  - *Obeliscoides cuniculi*
- Cestodes
  - *Cittotaenia variablis*
  - *Mosgovoyia pectinata americana, M. perplexa*
  - *Monoecocestus americana*
  - *Ctenotaenia ctenoids*
- Trematodes
  - *Hasstilesia tricolor*
  - *Fasciola hepatica*
  - Cysticercosis (see *Liver Disease*)

Nutritional
- Insufficient fiber in diet, especially long fiber (grass and hay)
- Excessive carbohydrate intake (predisposes to *Clostridium* overgrowth)
- Selective feeding out of mixed pellet and grain diets is an unsubstantiated but possible problem.

Neoplasia
- Adenocarcinomas
- Leiomyomas
- Leiomyosarcoma
- Metastases from uterine adenocarcinoma
- Rectal papillomas
- Inflammatory fibroid polyps

Other noninfectious problems

- Salivary mucocele
- Gastric trichobezoars (usually secondary to gut motility problems, lack of dietary fiber, or dehydration)
- Caecoliths
- Mucoid enteropathy
- Dysautonomia
- Dental disease (see *Dental Disease*)
- Iatrogenic enterotoxemia secondary to antibiotic use. Problem antibiotics include clindamycin, erythromycin, lincomycin, ampicillin, and amoxicillin. Less likely, but capable of causing problems, is the cephalosporin family of antibiotics. Antibiotics that rarely if ever cause problems include the fluoroquinolones such as enrofloxacin and marbofloxacin, the potentiated sulfonamide drugs, and the aminoglycosides.
- Failure to caecotroph
- Gastric stasis and bloat
- Foreign body
- Ingestion of toxin
- Intussusception (can be secondary to severe coccidiosis, cecal polyp)
- Liver lobe torsion (see *Hepatic Disorders*)

Findings on clinical examination

- Diarrhea (may be hemorrhagic, e.g., due to coccidiosis or *Klebsiella*, or green, e.g., due to rotavirus)
- Abnormal feces (jelly-like mucus with mucoid enteropathy, dysautonomia)
- Lack of feces (gut stasis, occasionally mucoid enteropathy, dysautonomia)
- Depression
- Dehydration
- Perineal accumulations of caecotrophs (see *Failure to Caecotroph*)
- Anorexia, weight loss
- Abdominal distension (gastric bloat, ileus, gut stasis)
- Collapse, hypothermia
- Hepatomegaly, ascites, jaundice (*E. stiedae*, liver neoplasia, cysticercosis)
- Fever, diarrhea, abortions, sudden death (salmonellosis)
- Small white growths on ventral tongue (papillomatosis)
- Gut stasis, raised liver enzymes, abdominal pain (liver lobe torsion—see *Hepatic Disorders*)
- Soft fluctuant mass on jaw (salivary mucocele)

Investigations

1. Radiography
   a. Lateral and DV. Normal rabbit abdomen very variable in appearance
   b. Contrast studies. Can be complicated by reingestion of caecotrophs
2. Microscopy
3. Parasitology
4. Gram stain
5. Staining/cytology

6. Routine hematology and biochemistry
   a. Slightly raised liver enzymes (cysticercosis)
7. Serologil test for rotavirus, VHD, *Clostridium piliforme*
8. Culture and sensitivity
9. Endoscopy
   a. Gastroscopy
10. Laparoscopy
11. Ultrasonography
12. Exploratory laparotomy and biopsy
13. Postmortem

Management

1. Fluid therapy (see *Nursing Care*)
2. High-fiber diet
3. May need to syringe feed
4. Probiotics
   a. May be of benefit—the natural low pH of the rabbit stomach may reduce the amount of probiotics gaining access to the large intestine/cecum.
   b. Transfaunation, using caecotrophs from a healthy rabbit, may help natural gut flora to reestablish.
5. Only use antibiotics if indicated. Many cases do not require their use, which can be counterproductive.
6. Gut motility modifiers
   a. Metoclopramide at 0.5 mg/kg SC or PO every 6 to 8 hours
   b. Cisapride 0.5 mg/kg PO s.i.d. or b.i.d.
7. Analgesics can be necessary but avoid those likely to exacerbate gastrointestinal tract ulceration (e.g., flunixin).

Treatment/specific therapy

1. Salivary mucocele
   a. Drain aseptically as required.
   b. Should heal spontaneously
   c. Likely to be due to trauma, but radiograph skull to assess for underlying pathologies such as dental disease.
2. Rotavirus
   a. Usually just in young rabbits
   b. Supportive treatment
3. Papillomatosis
   a. Covering antibiotics and analgesia if required. Usually self-limiting (<145 days)
4. VHD
   a. Supportive treatment only (see *Systemic Disorders*)
5. Bacterial enteritis
   a. Appropriate antibiosis based upon culture and sensitivity
   b. Cholestyramine at 2 g/20 mL water PO s.i.d. for 14 days for *C. spiroforme* infections
6. Enterotoxemia
   a. Treat according to general principles as outlined in *Management* above.

7. Coccidiosis
   a. Usually seen in rabbits younger than age 12 to 14 weeks
   b. Co-trimoxazole at 30 mg/kg PO b.i.d.
   c. Sulfamethazine in drinking water 0.2% 100 to 233 mg/L over 3 days
   d. Improve hygiene to prevent ingestion of contaminated feces.
8. *Cryptosporidium*
   a. Potentiated sulfonamides at 30 mg/kg PO b.i.d. may be of use.
   b. Nitazoxanide may prove useful.
9. Pinworms and *Obeliscoides*
   a. Ivermectin at 200 µg/kg or as topical (450 µg/tube) spot-on (Beaphar Anti-Parasite Spot-On for Small Animals, USA, Genitrix Xeno 450, UK)
   b. Fenbendazole (Panacur) at 10 to 20 mg/kg; repeat after 2 weeks
10. Cestodes, including cysticercosis
    a. Praziquantel at 5 to 10 mg/kg PO as a single dose
11. Trematodes
    a. *Hasstilesia tricolor:* Usually nonpathogenic. Intermediate host is snails
    b. *Fasciola hepatica:* Intermediate host is aquatic snails; infected from foods collected from wet meadows and streamsides
    c. Praziquantel at 5 to 10 mg/kg PO as a single dose
12. Trichobezoars—usually symptomatic of gut motility problem or dehydration
    a. Aggressive fluid therapy
    b. Analgesia
    c. Gut motility modifiers (e.g., metoclopramide at 0.2 to 1.0 mg/kg PO SC and cisapride at 0.5 to 1.0 mg/kg PO)
    d. The use of enzyme papain, bromelain, or pineapple juice (10 mL PO t.i.d.) to break down hair accretions often unsuccessful
    e. Avoid surgery unless absolutely necessary.
13. Mucoid enteropathy and dysautonomia
    a. Usually seen in young rabbits 4 to 14 weeks old
    b. Fluid therapy, high-fiber diet, gut motility modifiers, and analgesics
14. Intussusception
    a. Surgical correction
    b. May be secondary due to cecal fibroid polyp (Pizzi et al 2007)
15. Gastric stasis and bloat
    a. Decompress by passing stomach tube (insert and maintain in diastema as may bite through tube with incisors).
    b. Cimetidine at 5 to 10 mg/kg PO, SC, IV, or IM b.i.d. or t.i.d.
    c. Nursing care as under *General Management* above
    d. Investigate underlying etiology (e.g., foreign body).

Failure to caecotroph

Nutritional

- High plane of nutrition
- Obesity
- Excess caecotroph production (low-fiber, high-protein, and high-carbohydrate diet)
- Unpalatable caecotrophs (diet high in protein and carbohydrate) (Richardson 2001)

Other noninfectious problems

- Dental disease
- Incisor extraction
- Spondylosis
- Spondylitis
- Other illness

Findings on clinical examination

- Fecal accumulation or impaction around the perineum, especially in the skinfolds either side of the genitalia
- Underlying skin is sore—liable to tear under mild traction to remove overlying feces
- Maggots (see "Myiasis" in *Skin Disorders*)
- Overt dental disease (e.g., incisor malocclusion, bilateral mandibular swelling) (see *Dental Disease*)
- The rabbit may appear overtly overweight.

Investigations

1. Radiography
   a. Include full spinal radiography lateral and DV
   b. Skull radiography for dental disease
2. Routine hematology and biochemistry
3. Culture and sensitivity
4. Cytology
5. Endoscopy
6. Ultrasonography
7. Exploratory laparotomy
8. Biopsy

Management

1. Gentle removal of impacted fecal material. May require anesthetic as skin is very friable around perineum
2. Cleaning of underlying skin with dilute chlorhexidine or povidone-iodine solution. Topical antibiotics may be used if there is an underlying dermatitis.
3. Reevaluation of diet—consider switching to a lower energy diet with high-fiber intake to encourage normal caecotrophy.

Treatment/specific therapy

- Spondylosis/spondylitis: NSAIDs (e.g., meloxicam at 0.3 mg/kg PO s.i.d.) plus appropriate antibiosis if necessary. Spondylitis may be present as part of a bacteremic spread.
- Weight reduction; see "Reevaluation of Diet" under *Management* above)
- Dental disease (see *Dental Disease*)

Nutritional disorders

- Hypovitaminosis A
  - Reproductive disorders, including infertility, fetal resorptions, and abortion
  - High neonatal mortality and morbidity
  - CNS abnormalities, including hydrocephalus
  - Supplement with commercial vitamin A preparations.
- Hypovitaminosis E
  - Reproductive disorders, including infertility, fetal resorptions, and abortion
  - High neonatal mortality and morbidity
  - Muscular dystrophies
  - Supplement with commercial vitamin E preparations.
- Hepatic lipidosis
  - Linked to obesity
  - Can predispose to diabetes mellitus and ketosis
  - Ketones in blood and urine (ketonuria)
  - Treatment: See *Systemic Disorders*
- Lack of dietary fiber
  - Increased risk of gastrointestinal disease secondary to altered gut motility and gut environment/commensal flora
  - Barbering of conspecifics
  - Supplement with long fiber (grass and hay)
- Copper deficiency
  - Anemia in weanlings, decreased growth, hair loss, dry scaly skin, and graying of black hairs
  - Recommended daily intake is 2.7 mg, and foods should have an absolute minimum of around 8 mg copper/kg
- Excess calcium intake
  - Calcium levels are readily responsive to dietary levels, and there is a theoretical risk of hypercalcemia. This has been linked to urolithiasis and arteriosclerosis.
  - Total calcium 3.0 to 4.0 mmol/L; ionized 1.57 to 1.83 mmol/L

Hepatic disorders

Viral
- VHD (calicivirus—see *Systemic Disorders*)

Bacterial
- Bacterial hepatitis

Protozoal
- *Eimeria stiedae*

Parasitic
- Cysticercosis

Nutritional
- Hepatic lipidosis
- Aflatoxicosis

Neoplasia
- Bile duct adenoma
- Bile duct adenocarcinoma
- Metastatic spread of uterine adenocarcinoma

Other noninfectious problems
- Heart disease (see *Cardiovascular Disorders*)
- Liver lobe torsion

Findings on clinical examination

- Reduced or loss of appetite
- Vague signs of ill health
- Abnormal feces
- Hepatomegaly
- Jaundice
- Ascites

Investigations

1. Radiography
   a. Hepatomegaly
   b. Ascitic fluid
2. Routine hematology and biochemistry
   a. Raised liver enzymes
   b. Raised alkaline phosphatase, aspartate transaminase, and alanine transaminase associated with painful anterior abdomen, and occasional borborygmi (liver lobe torsion); pallor of mucous membranes
3. Culture and sensitivity
4. Cytology
5. Peritoneal tap
6. Endoscopy
7. Laparoscopy
8. Ultrasonography
9. Biopsy
10. Postmortem
    a. Demonstration of *E. stiedae* oocysts from characteristic yellow-colored liver lesions or distended bile ducts
11. Feed analysis—food concentrations of aflatoxin B_1 >100 ppm are toxic.

Management

1. Fluid therapy (see *Nursing Care*)
2. Lactulose at 0.5 mL/kg PO b.i.d.
3. Milk thistle *(Silybum marianum)* is a hepatoprotectant. Dose at 4 to 15 mg/kg PO b.i.d. or t.i.d.

Treatment/specific therapy

- Bacterial hepatitis
  - Appropriate antibiosis
- *E. stiedae*
  - Usually seen in rabbits younger than age 12 to 14 weeks
  - Toltrazuril at 7.0 mg/kg PO daily for 2 days. Repeat after 12 days.
  - Co-trimoxazole at 30 mg/kg PO b.i.d.
  - Often have concurrent gastric bloat and gut stasis, so treat as in *Gastrointestinal Tract Disorders*.
  - Improve hygiene to prevent ingestion of contaminated feces.
- Cysticercosis
  - Praziquantel at 5 mg/kg SC or PO one off treatment
  - Regular worming of in-contact dogs and cats
- Neoplasia
  - No treatment
- Liver lobe torsion
  - Stabilization and lobectomy

Pancreatic disorders

Noninfectious problems

- Diabetes mellitus (see *Endocrine Disorders*)

Cardiovascular disorders

Viral

- Coronavirus (pleural effusion/dilated cardiomyopathy [DCM])

Bacterial

- Pericarditis and endocarditis (especially *Pasteurella, Staphylococcus* spp., *Salmonella* spp., and *Streptococcus viridans*)

Protozoal

- *Encephalitozoon cuniculi* (myocarditis)
- *Trypanosoma cruzi* (ventricular hypertrophy and dilatation)

Nutritional

- Hypovitaminosis E (myocardial muscular dystrophy)

Neoplasia

- Thymomas (exophthalmos)

Other noninfectious problems

- Congenital
  - Ventricular septal defects
  - Atrial septal defects
  - Valvular cysts
- Hypertrophic cardiomyopathy

- DCM
- Bicuspid valve insufficiency
- Mitral valve insufficiency
- Coronary atherosclerosis
- Doxorubicin administration (DCM)
- Alpha agonist drugs (myocardial fibrosis)
- Catecholamines (coronary vasoconstriction with resultant myocardial fibrosis)
- Arteriosclerosis (possibly linked to hypercalcemia)
- Atherosclerosis (possibly linked to hyperlipidemia)

Findings on clinical examination

- Cyanosis or pallor of the mucous membranes
- Slow capillary refill time
- Exophthalmos (venous congestion of retrobulbar venous plexus)
- Dyspnea (normal respiratory rate = 30 to 60/min)
- Precordial thrill
- Arrhythmia (normal rate = 180 to 250 beats/min; excited healthy rabbits increase to 330 beats/min)
- Lack of thoracic percussion with auscultation
- Abnormal lung sounds
- Abnormal heart sounds
- Exercise intolerance
- Ascites
- Weight loss

Investigations

1. Routine hematology and biochemistry
   a. Renal and hepatic parameters may be raised due to congestion and/or poor perfusion.
   b. Raised cholesterol (0.1 to 2.0 mmol/L) and triglycerides (2.67 to 4.29 mmol/L)
2. E. cuniculi serology
3. Blood plasma K-tocopherol (vitamin E). Should be >0.5 µg/mL
4. Blood calcium (total calcium 3.0 to 4.0 mmol/L; ionized 1.57 to 1.83 mmol/L)
5. Serology for coronavirus
6. Pleural tap
   a. Cytology of effusions
7. ECG
   a. P waves are positive in standard limb leads
   b. Normal ECG values (from Reusch and Boswood 2003, see Table 2-6)
8. Radiography
   a. Lateral and DV views
   b. Note that thymus is persistent into adulthood
   c. Lateral view: normal heart around two rib spaces; 2.5 to 3 rib spaces suggests cardiomegaly (Fig. 2-12)
9. Echocardiography
   a. Normal values for echocardiographic parameters in rabbits (from Marini et al 1999, see Table 2-7)

Table 2-6 The rabbit: Normal lead II ECGs

ECG parameter (lead II)	Value
Heart rate (beats/min)	198-330
P-wave duration (s)	0.01-0.05
P-wave amplitude (mV)	0.04-0.12
P-R interval (s)	0.04-0.08
QRS duration (s)	0.02-0.06
R-wave amplitude (mV)	0.03-0.39
Q-T interval (s)	0.08-0.16
T-wave amplitude (mV)	0.05-0.17
Mean electrical axis (degrees)	−43 to +80

Table 2-7 The rabbit: Normal echocardiographic values

Measurement	Cardiac timing	Mean ± SD
Left ventricular internal diameter (cm)	Diastole	1.17 ± 0.19
	Systole	0.70 ± 0.09
Left ventricular free wall (cm)	Diastole	0.31 ± 0.08
Interventricular septum (cm)	Diastole	0.25 ± 0.05
Fractional shortening (%)		39.5 ± 5.39
E-point septal separation (cm)	Diastole	0.05 ± 0.05
Aorta (cm)	Diastole	0.67 ± 0.10
Left atrial dimension (cm)	Systole	0.17 ± 0.41
Right ventricular outflow tract velocity (m/s)		0.83 ± 0.10
Left ventricular outflow tract velocity (m/s)		0.65 ± 0.14
Body weight (kg)		2.32 ± 0.36

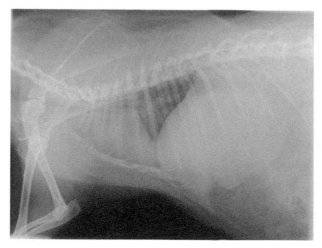

Fig 2-12. Cardiomegaly.

Table 2-8 Echocardiographic variables in male New Zealand white rabbits anesthetized with a combination of ketamine and medetomidine

Variable	Mean ± SD	Range
Body weight (kg)	2.59 ± 0.25	2.2-3.2
Thickness of the interventricular septum (IVS) in diastole (mm)	2.03 ± 0.37	1.43-3.10
Thickness of the IVS in systole (mm)	3.05 ± 0.45	2.17-4.03
Left ventricular internal diameter (LVID) in diastole (mm)	14.37 ± 1.49	11.87-19.06
LVID in systole (mm)	10.05 ± 1.22	7.83-13.53
Thickness of the left ventricular free wall (LVFW) in diastole (mm)	2.16 ± 0.25	1.60-2.80
Thickness of the LVFW in systole (mm)	3.48 ± 0.55	2.43-4.55
Fractional shortening (%)	30.13 ± 2.98	22.60-36.83
Ejection fraction (%)	61.29 ± 4.66	49.07-70.0
Aortic diameter (mm)	8.26 ± 0.76	6.73-9.80
Left atrial appendage diameter (mm)	9.66 ± 1.14	7.53-12.0
Left atrium: Aortic diameter	1.17 ± 0.14	0.94-1.54
Mitral valve E-point–septal separation interval (mm)	1.71 ± 0.29	1.20-2.33
Doppler heart rate (beats/min)	155 ± 29	115-234
Maximal aortic outflow velocity (m/s)	0.85 ± 0.11	0.56-1.06
Maximal pulmonary artery outflow velocity (m/s)	0.59 ± 0.10	0.34-0.84
Maximal mitral E-wave velocity (m/s)	0.59 ± 0.10	0.41-0.83
Maximal mitral A-wave velocity (m/s)	0.28 ± 0.07	0.19-0.44
Mitral E:A	2.19 ± 0.46	1.34-3.55

Table 2-9 The rabbit: Blood pressure

	Normal range (mm Hg)
Mean arterial pressure	80-91
Systolic pressure	92.7-135
Diastolic pressure	64-75

10. Table 2-8 (Fontes-Sousa et al 2006) gives these values for 2-dimensional, M-mode, and Doppler echocardiographic variables in male New Zealand white rabbits anesthetized with a combination of ketamine and medetomidine.
11. Blood pressure (cited in Reusch 2005, Table 2-9)

Management

1. Reduce stress (e.g., keep in a cool, shaded or darkened area away from dogs, cats, ferrets, and other "predators").
2. Monitor closely—diuretics can produce dehydration, which in rabbits can present as a gastric or cecal impaction.
3. Supply oxygen.

Treatment/specific therapy

- Cardiomyopathy
  - Taurine at 100 mg/kg s.i.d. PO for 8 weeks
- Arrhythmias
  - Digoxin at 0.003 to 0.03 mg/kg PO every 12 to 48 hours
  - Lidocaine 1 to 2 mg/kg IV or 2 to 4 mg/kg IT
- Congestive heart failure
  - Furosemide 0.3 to 4 mg/kg PO, SC, IM, or IV s.i.d. or b.i.d.
  - Enalapril 0.1 to 0.5 mg/kg PO every 24 to 48 hours. Beware hypotensive side effects.
  - Nitroglycerin ointment (2%) at 3 mm applied topically to the inner pinna every 6 to 12 hours
- Other medications
  - Atenolol 0.5 to 2 mg/kg PO s.i.d.
  - Verapamil 0.2 mg/kg PO, SC, or IV t.i.d.
  - Diltiazem 0.5 to 1 mg/kg PO b.i.d. or s.i.d.
  - Atropine 0.05 to 0.5 mg/kg SC or IM. Note that rabbits have high tissue and serum atropinase levels.
  - Glycopyrronium (glycopyrrolate) 0.01 to 0.1 mg/kg SC, IM, or IV
  - Pimobendan at 0.2 mg/kg PO s.i.d.
  - Benazepril at 0.1 to 0.5 mg/kg PO s.i.d. Note that rabbits appear very susceptible to the hypotensive side effects of benazepril.
  - Enalapril 0.25 to 0.5 mg/kg PO every 24 to 48 hours

Systemic disorders

Viral
- VHD, calicivirus.

Bacterial
- Salmonellosis

Neoplasia
- Lymphosarcoma/lymphoma (Gómez et al 2002)

Other noninfectious problems
- Hypoglycemia (especially with chronic dental disease)
- Heatstroke
- Pregnancy toxemia/ketosis
- Severe cardiovascular disease

Findings on clinical examination

- Anorexia: A recent history of anorexia (e.g., with dental disease or other ill health) suggests hypoglycemia or ketosis.
- Weight loss/poor physical condition
- Marked dental disease
- Lethargy

- Ataxia, convulsions (ketosis)
- Collapse
- Pale mucous membranes (lymphosarcoma)
- Hyperthermia (>40.5° C) (heatstroke)
- Lymphadenopathy (lymphosarcoma)
- Tachypnea/dyspnea (heatstroke, lymphosarcoma)
- Obesity (ketosis)
- Late pregnancy (pregnancy toxemia)
- Acute onset epistaxis and/or respiratory signs and/or diarrhea (VHD)
- High mortalities (VHD)
- Fever, diarrhea, abortion, sudden death (salmonellosis, VHD)
- Dyspnea

Investigations

1. Radiography
2. Routine hematology and biochemistry
   a. WBC count and differential
   b. Blood glucose levels (normal glucose 4.2 to 8.2 mmol/L)
   c. Ketosis
3. Serology for VHD
4. Urinalysis
   a. Ketonuria (ketosis/pregnancy toxemia)
   b. Aciduria (pH 5 to 6—ketosis)
5. Culture and sensitivity
6. Cytology
7. Bone marrow aspirate/biopsy
8. Laparoscopic endoscopy
9. Ultrasonography
10. Biopsy
    a. Multiorgan biopsies for lymphosarcoma
11. Necropsy
    a. Hepatic necrosis, hemorrhagic viscera (VHD)
    b. Hepatomegaly, splenomegaly, mesenteric lymphadenopathy (lymphosarcoma)

Management

1. Supportive therapy—parenteral fluids, assisted feeding
2. May require additional heat if recumbent

Treatment/specific therapy

- Lymphosarcoma
  - The author has found that a chemotherapy regimen, modified from that used for ferrets (Brown 1997), can be beneficial (Table 2-10).
- Hypoglycemia
  - IV glucose by bolus and infusion
  - Assisted feeding

Table 2-10 The rabbit: Chemotherapy protocol

Week	Day	Drug	Dose
1	1	Vincristine	0.1 mg/kg IV
		Prednisolone	1 mg/kg PO b.i.d. throughout therapy
1	3	Cyclophosphamide	10 mg/kg PO
2	8	Vincristine	0.1 mg/kg IV
3	15	Vincristine	0.1 mg/kg IV
4	22	Vincristine	0.1 mg/kg IV
4	24	Cyclophosphamide	10 mg/kg PO
7	46	Cyclophosphamide	10 mg/kg PO
9		Prednisolone	Begin to wean off prednisolone over the next 4 weeks

- Hepatic lipidosis/ketosis/pregnancy toxemia
  - Aggressive fluid therapy
  - Parenteral nutrition with glucose and vitamins
  - Assisted feeding either by syringe or nasogastric tube. Calcium gluconate PO or propylene glycol PO may be of use.
  - Dexamethasone at 0.2 mg/kg IV, SC, or PO once only. Repeat doses may immune compromise.
- Heatstroke
  - Monitor core body temperature.
  - Cool (not cold) body (e.g., damp towels, water bath)
  - Dexamethasone at 2 to 4 mg/kg IV once only
  - Supportive treatment such as cool IV fluids; heatstroke may have unforeseen sequelae (e.g., gut stasis).
- VHD: Supportive treatment only
  - Environmental cleaning with 0.5% sodium hypochlorite will inactivate virus.
  - Virus can survive for some time in the environment and can be carried on fomites.
  - Vaccine available; recommended annual vaccination. Vaccinated rabbits can develop a subclinical infection.

Neuromuscular disorders

Viral

- Herpes simplex
- Rabies

Bacterial

- Pasteurellosis (otitis media/interna, encephalitis)
- Other bacteria frequently isolated from otitis media are *Staphylococcus aureus* and *Bordetella bronchiseptica*.
- Discospondylitis
- Osteomyelitis
- *Listeria monocytogenes*

Protozoal

- *E. cuniculi*
- *Toxoplasma gondii*
- *Sarcocystis* (myositis)

Parasitic

- *Baylisascaris procyonis*
- Other aberrant migrant parasites (e.g., *Ascaris* spp.)
- *Psoroptes cuniculi* (predisposes to otitis media)

Nutritional

- Hypovitaminosis A (hydrocephalus and other CNS defects)
- Hypovitaminosis E (muscular dystrophy)

Neoplasia

- Osteosarcomas
- Osteochondromas
- CNS metastases

Other noninfectious problems

- Trauma
  - Vertebral fracture—typically L6 or L7
  - Other fractures
  - Electrocution (lumbar or pelvic fractures following spasm of lumbar musculature)
  - Intervertebral disc disease
  - Metastatic calcification of cerebral vasculature/arteriosclerosis
- Atherosclerosis
- Splay leg—autosomal recessive defect (unable to adduct one or more limbs, accompanies distortion of joints and long bones)
- Idiopathic epilepsy
- Intoxication
  - Heavy metals
  - Fertilizers, herbicides, insecticides
  - Fipronil application

Findings on clinical examination

- Otitis media/externa (see also "Ear Mites" in *Skin Disorders*)
- Mild head tilt or torticollis
- Nystagmus (only in acute disease)
- Extreme twisting of the body along the longitudinal axis.
- Hind-limb paresis or paralysis
- Paresis or paralysis of one or more legs
- Seizures
- Anorexia
- Fever (>40° C), oculonasal discharge, increased respiratory rate (toxoplasmosis)
- Ophthalmic disease (see *Ophthalmic Disorders*)

Investigations

1. Neurologic examination
2. Radiography
   a. Skull—check tympanic bullae
   b. Lateral and DV spinal radiographs
   c. Myelography
   d. Ingested metal in gut
3. Routine hematology and biochemistry
   a. Triglycerides and cholesterol for atherosclerosis
   b. Blood lead levels; basophilic stippling of RBCs
4. Serology for *E. cuniculi, T. gondii, Pasteurella, Sarcocystis,* and rabies
5. Culture and sensitivity
   a. Swab if perform bulla osteotomy
6. Cytology from CSF tap (Table 2-11)

Collection of CSF

- Collect as from the cat.
- Undertake ventral flexion of neck.
- Collect from the atlantooccipital joint, using a 22G needle, and direct toward nose.

---

7. Toxicology
8. Endoscopy of ear canal
9. Ultrasonography
10. Exploratory laparotomy
11. Biopsy

Table 2-11 The rabbit: CSF parameters (adapted from Weisbroth and Manning 1974 and Jass et al 2008)

Parameter	Value	*E. cuniculi* infected (Jass et al 2008)
WBC (per µL)	0-4	5-78
Glucose (mmol/L)	4.2	
Urea nitrogen (mmol/L)	10.8	
Creatinine (mmol/L)	1.5	
Cholesterol (mmol/L)	0.858	
Total protein (g/L)	0.13-0.31	0.31-1.54
ALP (U/L)	50.0	
CO_2 (mL%)	41.2-48.5	
Na (mmol/L)	149	
K (mmol/L)	3.0	
Cl (mmol/L)	127	
Ca (mmol/L)	1.35	
Mg (mmol/L)	1.1	
PO_4 (mmol/L)	0.74	
Lactic acid (mmol/L)	0.16-0.44	
Nonprotein nitrogen (mmol/L)	4.0-12	

Management

1. May require food and fluid support if unable to feed. Consider fluid therapy, syringe feeding, or nasogastric tube.
2. Supportive harnesses may be useful where there is hind-limb paresis/paralysis.
3. Nursing care to prevent pressure sores, urine scalding, and perineal caecotroph accumulation

Treatment/specific therapy

- Otitis media: Treat with appropriate antibiotics, both topical and systemic. Ensure eardrum is intact before treatment.
- Otitis interna
  - Covering antibiotics
  - May require bulla osteotomy. Swab for culture and sensitivity if so.
- *E. cuniculi*
  - Co-trimoxazole at 30 mg/kg b.i.d. PO for at least 3 weeks
  - Albendazole at 10 mg/kg PO s.i.d. for 6 weeks
  - Fenbendazole at 10 to 20 mg/kg PO s.i.d. for 1 month
  - Also treatment protocol for *Toxoplasma* effective (see "*T. gondii*")
- *T. gondii*
  - Combination therapy consisting of:
    - Co-trimoxazole at 30 mg/kg PO b.i.d.
    - Pyrimethamine at 0.5 mg/kg PO b.i.d.
    - Folic acid at 3.0 to 5.0 mg/kg PO s.i.d.
  - Rabbits with acute toxoplasmosis have congested tissues and marked splenomegaly.
  - Avoid access to soil/food contaminated with *Toxoplasma* oocysts.
- *Sarcocystis*
  - Treat with co-trimoxazole and pyrimethamine at *Toxoplasma* dose rates.
  - The Virginia opossum is the primary host; cockroaches can act as paratenic hosts.
- *Baylisascaris procyonis*
  - Adults found in raccoon *(Procyon lotor)*
  - Attempt treatment with fenbendazole at 20 mg/kg PO daily for 5 days, plus supportive therapy. Consider euthanasia.
- Vertebral fracture usually requires euthanasia.
- Other fractures, especially long-bone fractures, usually respond well to orthopedic procedures. Because they are relatively light, external fixation techniques are especially useful providing chewing can be avoided.
- Intervertebral disc disease
  - Spondylitis—antibiotics and NSAIDs (e.g., meloxicam at 0.3 mg/kg PO s.i.d.)
  - Intervertebral disc prolapse—may require surgery (e.g., disc fenestration); guarded prognosis
- Metastatic calcification of cerebral vasculature/arteriosclerosis
  - Guarded prognosis. Consider cerebral vasodilators such as nicergoline and propentofylline
- Atherosclerosis
  - Switch to a lower fat/carbohydrate diet.

- Toxin ingestion
  - Supportive therapy. Antidote if applicable (e.g., calcium EDTA for lead poisoning at 27.5 mg/kg q.i.d. IM for 5 days; repeat after week if required)
- Fipronil application
  - Supportive therapy only
- Rabies: euthanasia
- Idiopathic epilepsy/control of seizures
  - Phenobarbital at 1 to 4 mg/kg PO every 8-12 hours

Ophthalmic disorders

The rabbit eye differs from that of carnivores in several respects. A tapetum is absent, and there is a merangiotic retina with a horizontal band of myelinated nerve fibers and blood vessels. These provide a horizontal, photoreceptor-rich, macula-like region. It may be that, combined with lateral positioning of eyes, a band of high-resolution vision across the whole horizon is produced. There is a large ventral retrobulbar venous sinus, which can cause serious intraoperative complications during enucleation.

Differential diagnoses of ocular disorders

Viral

- Myxomatosis

Bacterial

- Retrobulbar abscess (often secondary to dental disease)
- *Staphylococcus* spp., *Pasteurella, Haemophilus*
- *Treponema cuniculi*

Protozoal

- *E. cuniculi* (uveitis)

Neoplasia

- Thymoma

Other noninfectious problems

- Glaucoma in New Zealand white rabbits (autosomal recessive disorder)
- Corneal occlusion syndrome—aberrant covering of cornea by conjunctiva
- Entropion
- Foreign bodies
- Diabetes mellitus (cataracts)

Findings on clinical examination

- Ulceration
- Severe blepharitis and whitish ocular discharge (myxomatosis). Look for other signs of myxomatosis (see *Skin Disorders*).
- Conjunctivitis (distinguish from dacryocystitis)
- Dacryocystitis is common in rabbits (often secondary to dental disease as the nasolacrimal duct runs close to roots of incisor teeth and premolars).
- Microabscesses in eyelid margins—often a sequel to severe or chronic periocular infection
- Nasal discharge

- Uveitis
- Corneal edema, hypopyon, and synechiae; may see large iridial abscesses; occasionally secondary cataracts
- Exophthalmos
- Third eyelid may be prolapsed and swollen
- Megaglobus/glaucoma
- Cataracts

Investigations

1. Ophthalmic examination
   a. Conjunctivitis is common in rabbits, often associated with dacryocystitis. Differentiate from dacryocystitis by cannulation of nasolacrimal duct (single ventral nasolacrimal punctum at medial canthus) (Fig. 2-13).
   b. Topical fluorescein to assess extent of ulceration (Fig. 2-14)
2. Schirmer tear test 2.0 to 11.0 mm/min (Biricik et al 2005)
3. Phenol red thread test 15 to 27 mm/15 seconds
4. Tonometry
   a. Normal intraocular pressure is 15 to 23 mm Hg. With hereditary glaucoma in New Zealand white rabbits it is 26 to 48 mm Hg.
5. Radiography
   a. Assess tooth roots for underlying dental disease.
   b. Contrast studies of nasolacrimal duct to determine if occluded
6. Cannulate and flush the nasolacrimal duct to collect sterile samples for culture, sensitivity, and cytology if appropriate.
7. Ultrasonography

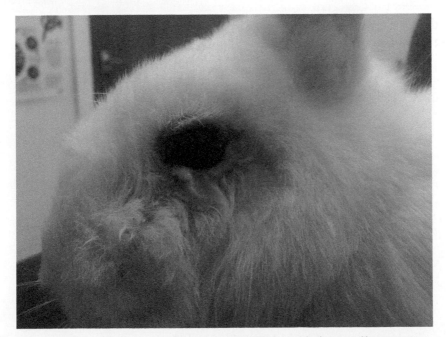

Fig 2-13. Proliferative lymphatic tissue response of the conjunctiva in chronic dacryocystitis.

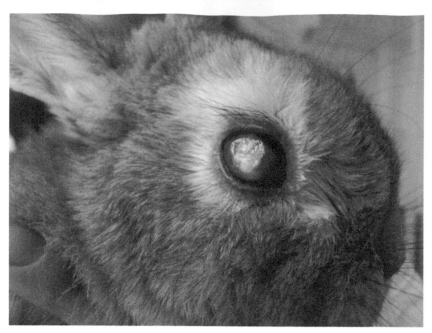

Fig 2-14. Fluorescein-positive corneal ulcer in a rabbit with keratitis.

Treatment/specific therapy

- Corneal ulceration
  - Topical and systemic antibiosis
  - Once infection cleared, treat as for other small animals (e.g., scarification to encourage healing, conjunctival grafts). Note that third eyelid may not cover whole cornea if attempt a third eyelid flap
- Dacryocystitis
  - Topical ophthalmic antibiotic preparations. Conjunctival bacterial flora can be both gram-positive and gram-negative, so select antibiotic according to sensitivity results.
  - Regularly cannulate and flush the nasolacrimal ducts.
  - Incisor or premolar extraction if linked to nasolacrimal disease
- *Encephalitozoon cuniculi*
  - Can cause cataracts or even lens capsule rupture, producing a phacoclastic uveitis
  - Co-trimoxazole at 30 mg/kg b.i.d. PO for at least 3 weeks
  - Albendazole at 10 mg/kg PO s.i.d. for 6 weeks
  - Fenbendazole 10 to 20 mg/kg PO s.i.d. for 1 month
  - Combination therapy consisting of:
    - Co-trimoxazole at 30 mg/kg PO b.i.d.
    - Pyrimethamine at 0.5 mg/kg PO b.i.d.
    - Folic acid at 3.0 to 5.0 mg/kg PO s.i.d.
  - Consider lens removal, preferably by phacoemulsification

- Retrobulbar abscess
  - Start on antibiotics—treat for anaerobic as well as aerobic (see under "Treatment/ specific therapy" in *Dental Disorders*).
  - Remove affected teeth.
  - May require enucleation. Hemorrhage is likely to be a significant complication due to the large retrobulbar abscess.
  - Dental disease: Treat as under *Dental Disorders*.
- Corneal occlusion syndrome: Surgery and topical cyclosporine
- Diabetes mellitus (see *Endocrine Disorders*)

Endocrine disorders

- Diabetes mellitus
- Adrenal disease
- Hypertestosteronism in castrated males secondary to adrenal hyperplasia/neoplasia

Findings on clinical examination

- Sudden-onset cataracts
- Polydipsia
- Polyuria
- Weight loss despite good appetite
- Increased aggression and sexual behavior in castrated male rabbits (hypertestosteronism)

Investigations

1. Radiography
2. Routine hematology and biochemistry
   a. High blood glucose usually associated with stress (see *Use of Glucose and Sodium as Prognostic Indicators in the Rabbit*); for diabetes mellitus, correlate with glycosuria, polydipsia, and polyuria. Normal glucose is 4.2 to 8.2 mmol/L.
   b. Normal rabbit fructosamine is 289 to 399 µmol/L.

ACTH stimulation test
- Cortisol (resting) 1.0 to 2.04 µg/dL
- Give ACTH at 6.0 µg/dL IM.
- Resample after 30 minutes; cortisol 12.0 to 27.8.
- Note that corticosterone is the principal adrenocortical hormone in rabbits, with an approximate ratio of 20:1 corticosterone:cortisol.

---

3. Blood testosterone levels
   a. Normal intact New Zealand white rabbits (reported in Lennox and Chitty 2006) = 0.51 to 9.16 ng/mL. Castrated males have significantly lower testosterone levels >0.1 ng/mL.
4. Urinalysis—should be glucose negative, but glycosuria can also occur after periods of stress and certain diseases (e.g., ketosis)
5. Cytology

6. Endoscopy
7. Ultrasonography
8. Biopsy

Treatment/specific therapy

- Diabetes mellitus
  - Insulin is not usually required.
  - Maintain on a high-fiber, low-carbohydrate diet.
- Hypertestosteronism secondary to adrenal hyperplasia/neoplasia
  - Adrenalectomy
  - Trilostane
  - The poor result of trial treatment with leuprolide acetate described in Lennox and Chitty (2006) suggests that hormonal antagonism as a treatment is likely to be of limited value.

Urinary disorders

Bacterial

- Pyelonephritis *(Staphylococcus aureus, Pasteurella multocida)*
- Cystitis *(S. aureus, P. multocida)*

Protozoal

- *E. cuniculi*

Nutritional

- Urolithiasis (usually combined with a cystitis)
- Renal calcinosis (hypercalemia, hypervitaminosis D)
- Fatty degeneration

Neoplasia

- Embryonal nephroma
- Renal carcinoma
- Renal leiomyoma

Other noninfectious problems

- Congenital abnormalities
- Renal
- Inguinal hernias
- Poor mobility (e.g., discospondylitis) contributes to calciuria/urolithiasis
- Hemolytic anemias
- Nephrotoxic drugs (gentamicin, zolazepam)

Findings on clinical examination

- Polydipsia, polyuria
- Urinary tenesmus
- Apparent hematuria (uterine adenocarcinoma, endometrial venous aneurysms, porphyrinuria). Differentiate from porphyrinuria by either urinalysis dipstick test or expose to ultraviolet light: porphyrins fluoresce a purple-like color.

- Anorexia
- Depression
- Urolithiasis
- Sandlike material in the urine
- Small stones present in the urine or lodged in the penis

Investigations

1. Urinalysis (Table 2-12)
   a. Culture and sensitivity
   b. Sediment examination/cytology
2. Urolith analysis
3. Radiography
   a. Uroliths or calciuria in the renal pelvices, ureters, bladder, or urethra
   b. Radiodense lesions in the kidney *(E. cuniculi)*
   c. Intravenous urograms
4. Routine hematology and biochemistry
   a. Renal parameters may be raised (i.e., raised urea, creatinine, calcium, phosphate, and potassium)
5. Serology for *E. cuniculi, Pasteurella*
6. Endoscopic laparotomy
7. Ultrasonography
8. Exploratory laparotomy
9. Biopsy

Table 2-12   The rabbit: Typical urinalysis values

Volume	20-350 mL/kg per 24 hr
Specific gravity	1.003-1.036, but can be difficult to measure due to crystals
pH	≈ 8.2. Can fall to 6.0 in anorectic or fasted animals
Color	Cloudy, pale to dark yellow BUT may be pink/rust/red due to porphyrins (see "Findings on Clinical Examination" under *Urinary Disorders*)
Protein	Negative to trace
Casts	None
Crystals	Triple phosphate, $CaCO_3$
Epithelial cells	None or rare
Bacteria	None or rare
Glucose	Negative
Ketones	Negative
WBC	Rare
RBC	Rare

Management

1. Fluid therapy if appropriate
2. Consider whether diet is too high in calcium; dietary modification alone unlikely to resolve or prevent recurrence of excess sand/urolithiasis.

Treatment/specific therapy

- Acute and chronic renal failure
  - Fluid therapy
  - Daily fluid maintenance requirement for a rabbit is 100 mL/kg per day.
  - Recommended approximate volumes for fluid replacement therapy (mL) are 10 to 15 mL/kg SC in divided sites or 15 mL/kg IP. Fluids can also be given IV either by bolus or by infusion.
- Pyelonephritis
  - Appropriate antibiosis (avoid aminoglycosides and other known nephrotoxic drugs)
  - Fluid therapy
- Calciuria
  - Catheterization and flushing of the bladder under anesthetic may work.
  - Cystotomy, removal of sand, and flush
- Urolithiasis
  - Surgery to remove stones (White 2001)
  - Antibiosis as it is often accompanied by cystitis
- *E. cuniculi*
  - Co-trimoxazole at 30 mg/kg PO b.i.d. for at least 3 weeks
  - Albendazole at 10 mg/kg PO s.i.d. for 6 weeks
  - Fenbendazole at 10 to 20 mg/kg PO s.i.d. for 1 month

Reproductive disorders

Viral

- Myxomatosis (see *Skin Disorders*)

Bacterial

- *Pasteurella*
- *Staphylococcus*
- *Streptococcus*
- Mycoplasmosis (especially *Mycoplasma pulmonis*)
- Enteric bacteria
- *Leptospira interrogans* (Boucher et al 2001)
- Rabbit syphilis *(Treponema cuniculi)*

Nutritional

- Hypovitaminosis A (see *Nutritional Disorders*)
- Hypovitaminosis E (see *Nutritional Disorders*)

Neoplasia

- Uterine adenocarcinoma (common in entire does over age 3 to 4 years) (Fig. 2-15)
- Testicular neoplasia (Bucks age 5+ years)
- Ovarian tumors
- Mammary adenocarcinomas
- Hypertestosteronism (see *Endocrine Disorders*)

Other noninfectious problems

- Ovarian cysts
- Endometrial hyperplasia

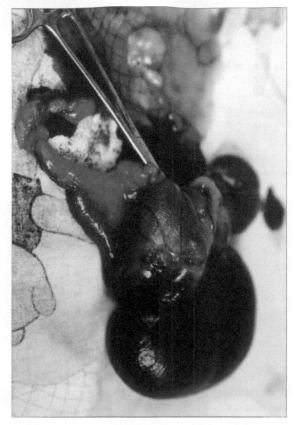

Fig 2-15. Uterine adenocarcinoma.

- Uterine polyps
- Vaginal prolapse
- Uterine torsion
- Hydrometra
- Pseudopregnancy
- Dystocia
- Cystic mastitis (may progress to mammary adenocarcinomas)

Findings on clinical examination

- Septic mastitis: swollen, painful mammary glands; abnormal milk
- Cystic mastitis: glands swollen, firm, not painful; may have a clear or serosanguineous discharge
- High temperature
- Anorexia
- Vaginal discharge
- Apparent hematuria (uterine adenocarcinoma, endometrial venous aneurysms, porphyrinuria)

- Pyometra
- Enlarged palpable viscus (pyometra, uterine adenocarcinoma)
- Epididymitis
- Orchitis
- Vesicles, ulcers, and crusty lesions on the external genitalia; may also be present at the mouth and nares *(T. cuniculi)*
- Poor reproductive performance
- Increased aggression and sexual behavior in castrated male rabbits (hypertestosteronism)

Investigations

1. Radiography
   a. Include thoracic radiographs for metastases from uterine or mammary adenocarcinomas
2. Routine hematology and biochemistry
3. Serology for *T. cuniculi, Mycoplasma pulmonis*
4. Culture and sensitivity
5. Cytology
6. Endoscopy
7. Laparoscopy
8. Ultrasonography
9. Exploratory laparotomy
10. Biopsy

Treatment/specific therapy

- Rabbit syphilis (see *Skin Disorders*)
- Mastitis
  - Septic mastitis (typically *Staphylococcus, Pasteurella,* and *Streptococcus* spp.)
    - Appropriate antibiosis
    - Supportive care including parenteral fluids, analgesia, fostering or hand rearing of young
    - Surgical mastectomy
  - Cystic mastitis
    - Ovariohysterectomy
    - Surgical mastectomy as may progress to adenocarcinomas)
    - Can be associated with uterine hyperplasia and adenocarcinoma
- Metritis and pyometra (typically *Pasteurella,* mycoplasmosis; occasionally *T. cuniculi* and enteric bacteria)
  - Appropriate antibiosis
  - Supportive care
  - Ovariohysterectomy
- Endometrial venous aneurysms
  - Ovariohysterectomy
- Orchitis, epididymitis
  - Appropriate antibiosis
  - Castration

- Uterine adenocarcinoma
  - Ovariohysterectomy
  - Very poor prognosis if metastatic spread
  - Can be seen in neutered females if significant uterine stump remains
  - Recommend routine ovariohysterectomy at 4 months of age
  - Deslorelin implants may prove to be preventative.
- Ovarian tumors or cysts
  - Ovariohysterectomy
- Testicular neoplasia
  - Castration
- Vaginal prolapse
  - Fluid therapy
  - Surgical replacement or resection of prolapse
  - Consider ovariohysterectomy
- Pseudopregnancy
  - Will usually resolve spontaneously within 2 to 3 weeks
  - Hormonal treatment (e.g., proligestone at 10 to 30 mg/kg SC once only)
  - Cabergoline at 5 µg/kg PO s.i.d. for 4 to 6 days
- Dystocia
  - If no obvious obstruction, oxytocin at 1 to 2 IU IM or SC
  - Uterine inertia: 5 to 10 mL 10% calcium gluconate PO 30 min prior to oxytocin
  - Cesarean section

3

Guinea pigs, chinchillas, and degus

Many of the pet rodents presented to the veterinarian belong to the group known as *hystricomorphs*. The following species are the most common as household pets:
- Guinea pig *(Cavia porcellus)*
- Chinchilla *(Chinchilla lanigera)*—the most common chinchilla species kept as pets
- Short-tailed chinchilla *(C. brevicaudata)*
- Degu *(Octodon degus)*

Table 3-1 Guinea pigs, chinchillas, and degus: Key facts

	Guinea pig	Chinchilla	Degu
Average life span (years)	3-8	8-20	5-9
Weight (g)			
Female	600-900	400-600	180-250g (both sexes)
Male	700-1200	400-500	
Body temperature (° C)	37.2-39.5	35.4-38	38
Respiratory rate (per min)	42-150	45-65	75
Heart rate (beats/min)	230-380	100	100-150
Gestation (days)	59-72	111 *(C. lanigera)* 124-128 *(C. brevicaudata)*	90-93
Age at weaning	14-21 days	6-8 weeks	4-6 weeks
Sexual maturity	2-3 months (female) 3-4 months (male)	4-12 months	6 months

Consultation and handling

Hystricomorph rodents are prey animals, so some may respond poorly to handling. All of these rodents are likely to struggle vigorously, and care should be taken to gently restrain them. Always weigh the rodent at every consultation. The earliest sign of dental disease may be weight loss. Guinea pigs and chinchillas rarely bite, although there are always individual exceptions to this; degus are inclined to bite. "Fur slip" in chinchillas is an antipredator response whereby stressed individuals will shed clumps of hair while being handled.

Although both rabbits and guinea pigs are social animals, generally the keeping of guinea pigs with rabbits is not recommended because:
1. Rabbits are often aggressive to guinea pigs and may bite and harass them. Much of this activity occurs at night and may not be noticed by the owner.
2. Guinea pigs require dietary vitamin C (see *Nutritional Disorders*) and may suffer hypovitaminosis if fed on commercial rabbit food only.
3. Rabbits harbor *Bordetella* in their respiratory tract, which can be a significant respiratory pathogen in guinea pigs.

Sexing of chinchillas can be problematic as the female has a pronounced genital papilla that can be easily mistaken as a penis. The vulva lies immediately caudal to this papilla (Fig. 3-1).

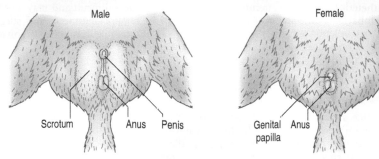

Fig 3-1. Sexing of chinchillas.

Nursing care

For general concepts, see *Nursing Care* in Chapter 2.

Fluid therapy

Small rodents by virtue of their size and the high risk of predation are forced to obtain most of their water from preformed (food) and metabolic sources. Dehydration can be critical for hystricomorph rodents, especially at higher environmental temperatures. For an adult chinchilla, 55.5% of its daily water loss is as urine, 16.7% evaporates from its skin, 22.2% evaporates from its lungs, and 5.6% is lost in the feces. Therefore, 38.9% of its water loss is insensible.

Table 3-2 Guinea pigs, chinchillas, and degus: Fluid therapy

	Guinea pig	Chinchilla	Degu
Daily fluid maintenance requirements (mL/kg per day)	80-100	36	
Subcutaneous (mL/kg) (in divided sites)	10-20	20	10
Intraperitoneal (mL/kg)	20	20	10-15
Shock (mL/kg)	70	70	

Fluids can be given SC, IP, or IO—indeed, if there is marked dehydration, then IP or IO is preferable to SC. Fluids can be given IV either by bolus or by infusion, and all fluids should be warmed to 38° C. For sites for fluid administration, see Table 3-3.

Table 3-3 Guinea pigs, chinchillas, and degus: Sites for fluid administration

Intravenous (guinea pig)	Lateral or medial saphenous and cephalic vein
Intravenous (chinchilla)	Femoral, lateral saphenous, and cephalic vein. Ear veins can be used for IV in some cases, and the use of EMLA cream greatly aids this but is inappropriate if the chinchilla is considered hypothermic.
Intraperitoneal (all three species)	Hold the patient vertically downward and inject into the lower left quadrant.
Intraosseous (all three species)	Under general anaesthesia insert either an intraosseous catheter or a hypodermic needle into the marrow of either the femur (via the greater trochanter) or tibia (through the tibial crest). Fluids, colloids, and even blood can be given IO if necessary.

EMLA, *eutectic mixture of local anesthetics, combination of lidocaine + prilocaine;*
   GA, *general anesthesia.*

Jugular catheterization can be attempted in all species, but it is difficult and may result in respiratory embarrassment. Many of these sites may also require anesthesia and surgical cutdown. In hypovolemic patients, vascular access may be impossible. It is better to consider either IP or IO administration.

Thermoregulation and hypothermia

Use a heat source, such as an electric heat mat plus insulation such as silver foil (reduces heat lost by conduction) and bubble wrap (reduces heat lost by convection). Pay particular attention to the pinnae of chinchillas as these are significant organs of heat loss. Alternatively, maintain in warm air (e.g., incubator) or use a commercial medical warm air generator. If body temperature falls too low, consider the risk of enterotoxemia following massive gut bacterial die-off.

Nutritional status

Many small mammals are presented as emergencies after a prolonged period of ill health that will have affected their food intake (e.g., chinchillas and guinea pigs suffering from undiagnosed chronic dental disease). These rodents are often hypoglycemic—test with a commercial glucometer on a small sample of blood—and IV or IP glucose can be given to these cases once identified.

Analgesia

Table 3-4 Guinea pigs, chinchillas, and degus: Analgesic doses

Analgesic	Dose		
	Guinea pig	**Chinchilla**	**Degu**
Buprenorphine	0.01-0.05 mg/kg SC every 6-12 hours	0.01-0.05 mg/kg SC every 6-12 hours	0.05 mg/kg SC every 8-12 hours
Butorphanol	0.2-2.0 mg/kg SC, IM, IP every 4 hours	0.2-2.0 mg/kg SC, IM, IP every 4 hours	
Carprofen	1.0-4.0 mg/kg SC or PO every 12-24 hours	1.0-5 mg/kg IM SC s.i.d. every 12-24 hours	4.0 mg/kg SC or PO s.i.d.
Ketoprofen	1.0 mg/kg SC or IM every 12-24 hours	1.0 mg/kg SC, IM every 12-24 hours	
Meloxicam	0.1-0.3 mg/kg SC or PO s.i.d.	0.1-0.3 mg/kg SC or PO s.i.d. Chinchillas particularly like meloxicam oral suspension.	
Morphine	2.0-10.0 mg/kg SC or IM every 4 hours		
Pethidine/ meperidine	10-20 mg/kg SC or IM every 2-3 hours		
Nalbuphine	1.0-2.0 mg/kg IM every 2-4 hours		

Anesthesia

Beware of subclinical respiratory infections. There is no need to starve; prolonged fasting can lead to hypoglycemia.

Keep the animal warm; as they have a large surface area compared with volume this results in significant heat loss during surgery, and hypothermia acts as a general depressant and is also immunosuppressive. Merely applying insulation such as bubble wrap is often insufficient—inactive, anesthetized rodents are not generating heat and you may be insulating it from a higher ambient temperature. Place these animals onto a heat mat, onto which is placed an absorptive towel or other material to both protect the mat from becoming wet and reduce the slight risk of localized burns.

Gaseous anesthesia

1. Masking down or placing in an induction chamber is often the safest way to induce anesthesia in a hystricomorph rodent.
2. Guinea pigs will often hypersalivate in response to isoflurane; atropine at 0.1 to 0.2 mg/kg SC may reduce this.
3. Intubation is extremely difficult due to the narrow caudal pharynx, large tongue, and small glottis. Makeshift endotracheal tubes using intravenous catheters readily block with respiratory secretions. It is often more expedient to maintain on a mask or intubate by a tracheotomy if thought necessary.

Parenteral anesthesia

1. Ketamine/medetomidine/butorphanol given IM simultaneously:
   a. Ketamine at 10 mg/kg
   b. Medetomidine at 0.1 mg/kg
   c. Butorphanol at 1.5 mg/kg
2. At end of procedure, reverse medetomidine with atipamezole at 0.75 mg/kg IM, SC.
3. Administering metoclopramide (0.5 mg/kg SC or PO every 6 to 8 hours) postoperatively will help to prevent a postsurgical ileus, especially following painful or abdominal surgery.
4. Monitor feeding and fecal output for 24 hours following surgery.

Cardiopulmonary resuscitation

Respiratory arrest

1. Administer 100% oxygen.
2. Assist ventilation—compress thorax at around 60×/minute.
3. Doxapram sublingual or at 10 mg/kg IV or IP. *Note:* This will increase the animal's oxygen demand.
4. If appropriate, give atipamezole.

Cardiac arrest

1. As for respiratory arrest.
   But also:
2. Compress thorax at around 90×/min.
3. If asystole—give epinephrine at 0.1 mg/kg IV of 1:10,000; 0.003mg/kg IV (guinea pig).
4. If ventricular fibrillation—lidocaine (lignocaine) at 1 to 2 mg/kg IV.

Skin disorders

Chinchillas have extremely dense fur, an attribute that has probably been enhanced by artificial selection. This may be why external parasites are uncommon in the chinchilla.

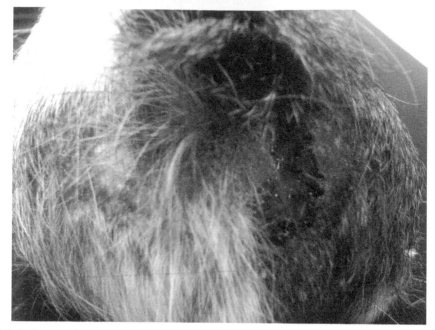

Fig 3-2. Severe self-inflicted trauma in a guinea pig, pruritus secondary to *Trixacarus*.

Pruritus

- Guinea pig
  - *Trixacarus caviae* (sarcoptid mite) (Fig. 3-2): Commonly associated with immunosuppression associated with pregnancy/parturition
  - Other sarcoptids *Sarcoptes muris, Notoedres muris*
  - *Chirodiscoides caviae* and *Myocoptes musculinus* (fur mites)

Alopecia

- Parasitic
  - Mites:
    - *Trixacarus caviae*, the sarcoptid mite (guinea pigs). Commonly associated with immunosuppression associated with pregnancy/parturition
    - Other sarcoptids *Sarcoptes muris, Notoedres muris*
    - *Cheyletiella parasitovorax*
    - *Chirodiscoides caviae* and *Myocoptes musculinus* (fur mites)
    - *Demodex caviae* (significance uncertain)
    - Storage mites: *Acarus farris* (Linek and Bourdeau 2005)
  - Lice:
    - *Gyropus ovalis, Gliricola porcelli* (chewing lice), and *Trimenopon hispidum* (sucking louse). Usually asymptomatic; if heavy infestation, may cause alopecia and a rough coat.

- Bacterial
  - Pyoderma (often secondary infection from scratching)
  - Salmonellosis (Singh et al 2005)
- Fungal
  - Dermatophytosis (*Trichophyton mentagrophytes, Microsporum* spp.); can be asymptomatic
  - *Scopulariopsis brevicaulis,* usually asymptomatic
- Nutritional
  - Hypovitaminosis C (rough hair coat/hair loss in guinea pigs)
  - Fatty acid deficiency (chinchillas—see *Nutritional Disorders*)
  - Pantothenic acid deficiency (chinchillas); may be complicated by zinc deficiency (see *Nutritional Disorders*)
- Other
  - Fur slip: Improper handling/antipredator response seen in chinchillas
  - Cystic ovarian disease (guinea pigs—see *Reproductive Tract Disorders*)
  - Hyperadrenocorticism (Cushing disease—see *Endocrine Disorders*)
  - Barbering/fur chewing (for chinchillas—see also *Endocrine Disorders*); may be linked to lack of dietary fiber
- Very low environmental humidity, such as central heating (chinchillas)
- Linked to intensive breeding of female guinea pigs

Scaling and crusting
- Dermatophytosis (*Trichophyton mentagrophytes, Microsporum* spp.)
- *Scopulariopsis brevicaulis*

Seborrhea
- Dermatophytosis (*Trichophyton mentagrophytes, Microsporum* spp.)

Sebaceous secretions
- Excessive accumulation around the perineal and perianal region in older guinea pig boars

Erosions and ulceration
- Pododermatitis (*Staphylococcus aureus* and *S. epidermidis*)
- *Cryptococcus neoformans*
- Frostbite (chinchillas)

Swellings, nodules, and nonhealing wounds
- Abscess
- Mycobacteriosis
- Aural hematoma (chinchillas)
- Hypovitaminosis E (chinchillas; distinct swellings on abdomen—see *Nutritional Disorders*)
- Cutaneous cysts

Changes in pigmentation
- Yellow ears (chinchillas—see *Nutritional Disorders*)

Neoplasia
- Trichofolliculoma
- Fibrosarcoma
- Sebaceous adenoma

- Lipoma
- Mammary fibroadenoma
- Mammary fibrocarcinoma
- Mammary adenocarcinoma
- Cutaneous papilloma of the foot pad
- Cutaneous hemangioma (Hammer et al 2005)

Other abnormalities

- Bites to pinnae (chinchillas, guinea pigs kept with rabbits)
- Cotton fur syndrome (chinchillas—see *Nutritional Disorders*)
- Degloving of tail in chinchillas and degus (improper handling)

Findings on clinical examination

- Areas of alopecia—may be bilateral (hormonal) or patchy (fatty acid deficiency, pantothenic acid deficiency in chinchillas)
- Swellings, often firm consistency even if abscess. Displacement of normal outline of coat may indicate swelling.
- Texture of hair coat may alter, becoming rougher.
- Cuts and abrasions: these may be self-inflicted in cases of severe pruritus. In guinea pigs, such lesions tend to be over the shoulders and back of the neck where the guinea pig scratches with its hind claws.
- Extreme pruritus
- Seizures may follow episodes of extreme pruritus (guinea pigs with ectoparasites).
- Pododermatitis
  - Ulcerations, erythema, calluses, nail distortions, and abnormalities. Related lymph nodes may be enlarged (especially in guinea pigs).
- Systemic signs
  - Linked to amyloidosis in liver, kidneys, pancreas, spleen, adrenal glands
- Overgrown claws
- Degloved tip of tail (chinchillas and degus)

Investigations

1. Radiography
   a. Pododermatitis—often underlying osteoarthritis
2. Routine hematology and biochemistry
   a. Eosinophilia (ectoparasitism)
3. Bacteriology and mycology: hair pluck or swab lesions for routine culture and sensitivity
4. Fecal swab for salmonellosis
5. Cytology
   a. Fine-needle aspirate followed by staining with rapid Romanowsky stains
   b. Gram stain
6. Microscopy: Examine fur pluck, acetate strips, or skin scrapes to affected area and examine for ectoparasites.
7. Examine teeth. Rodents with dental disease may have difficulty grooming normally.
8. Biopsy obvious lesions.
9. Ultraviolet (Wood's) lamp—positive for *Microsporium canis* only (not all strains fluoresce).

10. Endocrine analysis: thyroxine, estradiol (see *Endocrine Disorders*)
11. If barbering suspected, examine hair under microscope to see if chewed; separate from other animals; supply extra hay.

Treatment/specific therapy

- Treat for any ectoparasites
  - Ivermectin at 200 µg/kg SC or as topical application (Xeno 450, Genitrix Beaphar Anti-Parasite Spot-On for Small Animals, USA); 3 treatments given 2 weeks apart
  - Imidacloprid (Advantage, Bayer) applied as a 40 mg spot-on treatment
  - 40 mg imidacloprid/4.0 mg moxidectin (Advocate, Advantage Multi, Bayer USA) at 0.1 mL per guinea pig (Beck 2007)
  - Permethrin applied as either a dusting powder or shampoo
- *Chirodiscoides caviae*
  - Ivermectin at 0.4 to 0.5 mg/kg SC, repeat after 2 weeks
  - Selamectin at 12 mg/kg topically, 2 treatments, 2 weeks apart
- *Demodex*
  - Ivermectin at 0.4 to 0.5 mg/kg SC or topically every 7 days
  - Amitraz washes at 250 mg/L every 7 days
  - If very pruritic, consider use of NSAIDs.
- Pododermatitis
  - Chronic infections lead to persistent swelling of the feet and gross abnormalities of the feet.
  - *Note*: May also induce amyloidosis in internal organs (see *Hepatic Disorders, Pancreatic Disorders,* and *Endocrine Disorders*)
  - Amelioration of underlying factors (e.g., removal from mesh flooring)
  - Topical and systemic antibiosis
  - Analgesia, such as meloxicam at 0.3 mg/kg PO s.i.d.
  - Amputation of chronic, resistant infections to prevent risk of amyloidosis
- Abscessation
  - Surgical removal (with swab for culture and sensitivity) plus appropriate antibiosis
  - Lancing, debriding, and cleaning of abscesses give poor results compared to surgical resection.
- Salmonellosis
  - Vitamin C supplementation (1 g/kg feed) or 50 to 100 mg/kg PO for guinea pigs
  - Appropriate antibiosis
- Cysts: Surgical resection; may respond to local draining
- Dermatophytosis, *Scopulariopsis,* and *Cryptococcus*
  - Griseofulvin at 15 to 25 mg/kg PO once daily for 4 weeks. Toxic to immature and fetal guinea pigs, so use on adult, nonpregnant guinea pigs only.
  - Miconazole/chlorhexidine (Malaseb) shampoo—bath once daily
  - Itraconazole at 15 mg/kg PO given daily to effect (Van Gestel and Engelen 2004)
  - Lufenuron was found to be ineffective (Van Gestel and Engelen 2004).
  - Often found in young guinea pigs (<6 months old)
- Seborrhea
  - Miconazole/chlorhexidine (Malaseb, Leo) shampoo—bath once daily
- Excessive perianal sebaceous secretion accumulation in older boars
  - Remove manually. Clean regularly with chlorhexidine scrub.

- Neoplasia
  - Surgical resection where possible
- Lacerations/bites to the pinnae
  - If fresh attend to hemostasis.
  - Debride, clean up, and apply topical amorphous hydrogel dressings to encourage secondary healing (e.g., IntraSite Gel, Smith and Nephew Healthcare Ltd).
  - If cartilage is torn, then suturing is unlikely to work.
- Frostbite: Debride, clean, dry thoroughly, and apply antibiotic ointment.
- Hematomas
  - Drain the hematoma.
  - If necessary apply sutures to hold the stretched skin against the pinnal cartilage.
  - Do not use steroids.
- Fur chewing
  - Can be related to poor environmental conditions (e.g., high temperatures, high humidity). In rabbits it is often related to lack of provision of long fiber such as hay.
  - Fur-chewing chinchillas often have hyperthyroidism and hyperactive adrenal glands (see *Endocrine Disorders*).
  - If behavioral, consider fluoxetine at 5 to 10 mg/kg PO s.i.d.
  - Treatment involves elimination of other possible etiologies and correction of environmental conditions.
  - Shaving of the remaining dark-colored short undercoat often encourages regrowth.
- Degloving of tail
  - Apply topical antibacterial preparation if infected. Otherwise encourage granulation using IntraSite Gel or Dermisol cream (Pfizer).
  - Extensive lesions may require amputation.

Respiratory tract disorders

See also *Cardiovascular and Hematologic Disorders*.

Viral

- Adenovirus (guinea pigs)
- Paramyxoviruses, including Sendai virus
- Simian virus 5 (SV5)
- Pneumonia virus of mice (PVM)

Bacterial

- *Bordetella bronchiseptica*
- *Chlamydophila psittaci* (see also *Ophthalmic Disorders*)
- *Mycoplasma caviae* (usually asymptomatic)
- *Mycoplasma pulmonis*
- *Pasteurella*
- *Pneumocystis jiroveci* (usually asymptomatic except with severe immunosuppression)
- *Pseudomonas*
- *Streptobacillus moniliformis*
- *Streptococcus equi zooepidemicus* (pleuritis, hydrothorax, pericarditis)
- *Streptococcus pneumoniae*
- *Streptococcus pyogenes*

Fungal

- *Histoplasma capsulatum* (see *Systemic Disorders*)

Protozoal

- *Toxoplasma gondii* (see *Neurologic Disorders*)

Nutritional

- Hypovitaminosis C (see *Nutritional Disorders*)

Neoplasia

- Bronchogenic and alveologenic papillary adenomas (may be secondary to foreign body inhalation)

Other noninfectious problems

- Trauma (improper handling)
- Pneumothorax
- Diaphragmatic hernia
- Gastric tympany/torsion (see *Gastrointestinal Tract Disorders*)
- Heat stress (see *Systemic Disorders*)
- Dental disease (may resemble upper respiratory tract disease in chinchillas; see *Dental Disorders*)
- Choking (especially chinchillas)
- Cardiovascular disease (see *Cardiovascular and Hematologic Disorders*)
- Inappropriate bedding—wood shavings and sawdust can be a source of irritant essential oils.

Findings on clinical examination

- Dyspnea/tachypnea
- Open-mouth breathing
- Cyanosis
- High temperature
- Increased respiratory sounds
- Anorexia
- Weight loss
- Severe distress (choking)
- Conjunctivitis
  - *Chlamydophila* rarely causes respiratory disease other than conjunctivitis; however, it can occur alongside bacterial pneumonia.
- Nasal discharge
- Vaginal discharge from metritis (guinea pigs with bordetellosis). Pregnant sows may abort.
- Swollen submandibular lymph nodes (*S. moniliformis*)

Investigations

1. Radiography
   a. Lateral and dorsoventral (DV) radiographs
2. Routine hematology and biochemistry
   a. Serology for *Chlamydophila*, *Bordetella*, adenovirus, Sendai virus, SV5, PVM, *Mycoplasma pulmonis*
3. Polymerase chain reaction (PCR) for *Chlamydophila*

4. Culture and sensitivity
5. Cytology
   a. Transtracheal wash
   b. Gram stain
6. Pleural tap and cytology
7. Endoscopy
8. Ultrasonography
9. Biopsy
   a. Intranuclear inclusions (adenovirus)
10. Necropsy

Management

1. Supplement with vitamin C (guinea pigs, degus).
2. Parenteral fluids
3. Gentle soaking and removal of encrusted oculonasal discharges
4. Provide oxygen via mask or chamber.
5. Covering or specific antibiosis. Consider nebulization.
6. Syringe feeding (beware aspiration pneumonia)
7. NSAIDs (e.g., meloxicam 0.3 mg/kg PO s.i.d.) may reduce lung damage.
8. Mucolytics such as bromhexine and *N*-acetylcysteine may be useful.
9. Change bedding to paper-based substrate.

Treatment/specific therapy

- Bordetellosis
  - Appropriate antibiosis
  - *Note:* It is found asymptomatically in the upper respiratory tract of rabbits, which may therefore act as a reservoir of infection for guinea pigs when kept with rabbits.
  - Vaccination with canine *Bordetella* vaccine at 0.2 mL per individual either SC or PO; repeat after 2 to 3 weeks, then give annual or 6-monthly booster according to risk (Huerkamp et al 1996).
- Streptococci
  - Appropriate antibiosis
  - *S. pyogenes* may be spread by biting insects.
  - *S. pneumoniae* is spread by aerosol transmission.
- Sendai virus, SV5, and PVM are usually asymptomatic.
- Adenovirus: Treat symptomatically.
- Mycoplasmosis
  - Appropriate antibiosis
- Choking
  - Often die before treatment initiated
  - Remove or dislodge foreign body (often food item) wedged over glottis.

Dental disorders

Permanent dental formula of the guinea pig and chinchilla

$$I:\frac{1}{1}, \quad C:\frac{0}{0}, \quad PM:\frac{1}{1}, \quad M:\frac{3}{3}$$

For guinea pigs, the maxillar to mandibular ratio is around 1 : 2 (i.e., the mandibular incisors as viewed from the front should be twice the length of the maxillary incisors). Guinea pigs also have an oblique occlusal plane on the cheek teeth of around 40 degrees.

Nutritional

- Lack of long fiber (e.g., hay) in diet
- Hypovitaminosis C (guinea pigs, possibly degus—see *Nutritional Disorders*)
- Inappropriate nutrition

Neoplasia

- Oral neoplasia causing differential wear
- Macrodontia (possibly odontomas—guinea pigs; see Fehr 2014)

Other noninfectious problems

- Fractured incisors (trauma)
- Congenital malocclusion
- Genetic predisposition

Findings on clinical examination

- Chinchilla and degu incisor teeth are naturally highly colored orange or yellow; this often fades with dental disease. Such fading may indicate hypovitaminosis A (see *Nutritional Disorders*).
- Incisor malocclusion
  - Chewing in rodents involves a significant rostrocaudal movement of the mandibles; therefore, the lower incisors in particular are naturally quite long. This should not be mistaken for an abnormality. Compare where possible with another individual.
- Mandibular swellings (unilateral or bilateral) due to bone remodeling to accommodate tooth root overgrowth
- Maxillary swellings rostral to eye; painful on palpation—maxillary root overgrowth (especially chinchillas)
- One or more incisors shortened or fractured
- Excessive salivation/moist fur on chin and ventral neck (slobbers)
- Weight loss
- Anorexia
- Ectoparasitic disease
- Dacryocystitis/conjunctivitis
- Seizures (due to hypoglycemia)

Investigations

1. Otoscopic examination of oral cavity
   a. Normal guinea pig or chinchilla always has a significant amount of food/cecotrophic material in its mouth obscuring the dental arcades; if this is not the case then it is likely to be eating very poorly.
   b. Lingual tilting of mandibular cheek teeth and buccal tilting of maxillary cheek teeth (Fig. 3-3)
   c. The mandibular premolars may form a partial or complete arch over the tongue (guinea pig).
   d. Otoscopic examination does not constitute a complete examination of the oral cavity as structures at the back of the pharynx can be difficult to see due to its depth and the large size of the tongue.

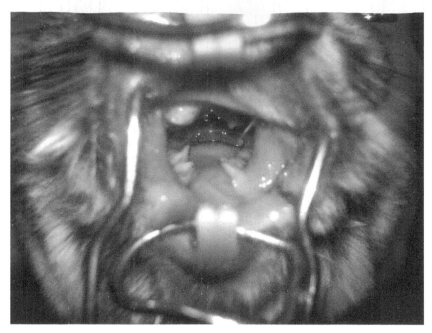

Fig 3-3. Lingual spurs on the lower premolars and molars of a chinchilla.

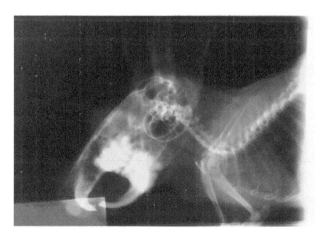

Fig 3-4. Lateral radiograph of a chinchilla with dental disease. Note the divergence of the maxillary tooth roots and the (palpable) bony remodeling of the mandibles associated with cheek tooth root overgrowth.

    e. Spurs on cheek teeth. Often rostral facing on first lower premolars (chinchillas, degus)

    f. Ulceration of tongue

    g. Purulent material in mouth

2. Radiography

    a. Lateral and DV views of skull. *Note:* Skulls often appear osteoporotic (Figs. 3-4 and 3-5).

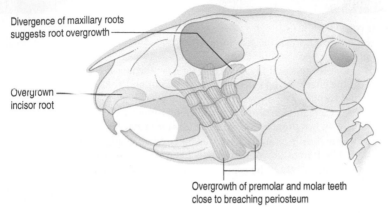

Divergence of maxillary roots
suggests root overgrowth

Overgrown
incisor root

Overgrowth of premolar and molar teeth
close to breaching periosteum

Fig 3-5. Explanatory diagram of skull shown in Figure 3.4.

    b. Left and right lateral oblique views of skull to allow assessment of individual tooth roots. Any divergence of maxillary or mandibular tooth roots away from each other suggests abnormal root elongation.

    c. The mandibles can also be isolated by an open-mouth technique where the animal is placed in sternal recumbency and the mouth opened to its full extent by a bandage placed behind the upper incisors and pulled caudally, with the x-ray beam centered on the molars.

    d. The maxillae are similarly investigated by placing the animal in dorsal recumbency with a roll under the neck, the nose positioned parallel to the plate, and the beam again centered on the molars.

    e. Contrast study on nasolacrimal ducts; difficult in small hystricomorphs

3. Routine hematology and biochemistry
4. Culture and sensitivity
    a. Aerobic and anaerobic culture of abscesses
5. Examination of oral cavity under general anesthesia (GA)
6. Endoscopy

Management

1. Chronic cases often cachexic—may need parenteral fluid support
2. Check blood glucose levels: guinea pig (3.36 to 7.8 mmol/L), chinchilla (3.36 to 6.72 mmol/L).
3. Syringe feeding with commercial feed suspensions (e.g., Oxbow Critical Care or Science Recovery Diet from Supreme Petfoods). May require nasogastric tube or tube feeding
4. Flushing of nasolacrimal ducts where possible
5. Only use antibiotics if indicated. Many cases do not require their use, which can be counterproductive.
6. Gut motility modifiers
7. Metoclopramide at 0.5 mg/kg SC or PO every 6 to 8 hours
8. Cisapride 0.5 mg/kg PO s.i.d. or b.i.d.

Treatment/specific therapy

- Regular coronal reduction
  - Always burr overgrown incisors in preference to clipping due to risk of fracture, pulpal hemorrhage, and infection.
  - For cheek teeth, this will likely necessitate heavy sedation or GA. "Conscious" dental work on the cheek teeth is stressful to the rodent and risks serious trauma to the oral cavity and spine.
  - Often coronal reduction alone is insufficient; often by the time of presentation, dental disease has progressed to a quite advanced stage.
  - Use of a dental drill or equivalent is essential; dental spurs can be clipped but the teeth must be burred down. Clipping is likely to fracture the tooth.
- Incisor extraction—likely to be achieved by extraoral approach
- Cheek teeth extraction—likely to be achieved by extraoral approach and burring of the apical area to attempt complete destruction of the tooth. Regrowth is not uncommon even after apical burring.
- Surgical debridement of tooth root abscesses including removal of infected bone and affected tooth roots, followed by:
  - Packing with antibiotic-impregnated methylmethacrylate (bone cement or similar) *and/or* marsupialization, leaving ostium for recurrent povidone-iodine/antibiotic application during second-intention healing.
  - Antibiosis
    - Usually a broad-spectrum antibiotic such as enrofloxacin at 5 mg/kg PO s.i.d. or co-trimoxazole at 30 mg/kg PO b.i.d. *plus*
    - Anaerobic antibiosis (e.g., metronidazole at 20 mg/kg PO s.i.d.)
  - Drilling out of tooth root apices to initiate tooth root death where extraction is not viable. *Note:* Aggressive dental work in guinea pigs can trigger neuronal degeneration of afferent nerves in the periodontal ligament with subsequent degeneration of the mesencephalic trigeminal nucleus, resulting in dysphagia, postural abnormalities, and death (Azuma et al 1999, Kimoto 1993). See *Neurologic Disorders* and *Cardiovascular and Hematologic Disorders.*
  - Analgesia (e.g., meloxicam at 0.3 mg/kg PO s.i.d.) can be given for many weeks.
- Where possible, wean the animal onto a diet high in long fiber (i.e., grass and hay), as this encourages normal chewing and dental wear on the back teeth. Provision of a pumice stone may encourage gnawing behavior.
  - *Note:* Many chinchillas with dental disease have adrenal hyperplasia (Crossley 2001). See *Endocrine Disorders.*
- Fractured incisors
  - Burr and file back to both the affected tooth and the contralateral to allow normal even wear to occur.

Gastrointestinal tract disorders

It is normal for guinea pigs, chinchillas, and degus to coprophage, especially at night (Kenagy et al 1999).

Disorders of the oral cavity

- Dental disease (see *Dental Disorders*)
- Foreign bodies, especially cheek impactions or under tongue
- Choking (see *Respiratory Disorders*)

- Parotid salivary gland abscessation
- Investigation requires sedation or anesthesia for thorough examination of the oral cavity.
- Foreign bodies and choking require removal of the problem material.
- Parotid salivary gland abscessation requires surgical resection of the abscess; consider bacteriologic culture and sensitivity from the abscess.
- Cheilitis (crusty lesions at corner of mouth in guinea pigs)
  - Hypovitaminosis C (see *Nutritional Disorders*)
  - Secondary bacterial/fungal infection—classically *Staphylococcus* cheilitis
  - Poxvirus
  - Chewing on sharp foods or cage mesh

Differential diagnoses for gastrointestinal disorders

Viral
- Coronavirus (guinea pigs)

Bacterial
- *Clostridium difficile*
- *C. perfringens* Type E (guinea pigs)
- *C. perfringens* Type D and occasionally Type A (chinchillas)
- *C. piliforme* (Tyzzer disease)
- *Escherichia coli*
- *Listeria monocytogenes* (can be asymptomatic in chinchillas, but also has visceral and neurologic presentations—see *Neurologic Disorders*)
- *Campylobacter* spp. (asymptomatic)
- *Citrobacter freundii*
- *Yersinia pseudotuberculosis*
- *Salmonella* spp.
- *Corynebacterium* spp.

Fungal
- *Torulopsis pintolopesii*

Protozoal
- Guinea pig
  - *Eimeria caviae*
  - *Eimeria* spp. (cross-infection with rabbit *Coccidia*)
  - *Cryptosporidium muris* and *C. wrairi*
  - *Entamoeba caviae*
  - *Tritrichomonas caviae*
  - *Giardia caviae*
  - *Balantidium caviae*
- Chinchilla
  - *Giardia*
  - *Trichomonas* (hemorrhagic typhilitis)
  - *Balantidium* (hemorrhagic colitis)
  - *Cryptosporidium*
  - *Eimeria chinchillae*

Parasitic

- Guinea pig
  - *Paraspidodera uncinata* (Heterakidae nematode)
  - Cestodes (from wild rodents)
    - *Fasciola hepatica*
    - *Fasciola gigantica*
- Chinchilla
  - *Physaloptera*
  - *Hymenolepis* spp.
  - *Haemonchus contortus*

Nutritional

- Sudden influx of greens or fruit in diet, probably a carbohydrate overload and fermentation producing gastric dilatation, dysbiosis
- Hypovitaminosis C in guinea pigs (malabsorption, pyogranulomatous enteritis—see *Nutritional Disorders*)
- Constipation (degus and chinchillas on poor diet, possibly too low in short-length fiber)

Neoplasia

Other noninfectious problems

- Iatrogenic dysbiosis (e.g., from antibiotics, especially penicillin, procaine, erythromycin, lincomycin, clindamycin, streptomycin, erythromycin, aureomycin, bacitracin, and spiramycin). Such dysbiosis can result in clostridial overgrowth.
- Intestinal obstruction
  - Neoplasia, foreign body, abscess, impaction
- Colorectal impaction (guinea pigs)
- Cecal impaction
- Cecal dilatation/tympany
- Rectal prolapse
- Gastric ulceration (chinchillas)
- Gastric torsion
- Gastric dilatation
- Aerophagy during anesthetic induction and recovery
- Pregnant, unfasted females especially at risk of dilation/torsion
- Sudden influx of greens in diet (probably carbohydrate overload and fermentation)

Findings on clinical examination

- History of poor diet (e.g., excessive fruit or greens—diarrhea, dysbiosis; coarse or moldy feeds—gastric ulceration)
- Diarrhea
  - Watery diarrhea (*C. piliforme*, hypovitaminosis C)
- Decreased fecal output
  - Constipation
  - Gut stasis
  - Colorectal impaction
  - Obstruction
  - Foreign body
  - Cecal impaction
- Frank blood in feces (severe enteritis)

- Occult blood in feces (hypovitaminosis C)
- Depression
- Hypothermia
- Gut stasis; gastric bloat
- Weight loss
- Impacted rectum; may find inspissated feces, wood shavings, trichobezoars (guinea pigs)
- Flaccid hind-limb paralysis
- Subcutaneous inguinal edema (*C. piliforme* in guinea pigs)
- Dyspnea (compression of thoracic cavity with gastric dilatation, gastric torsion, cecal dilatation)
- Death

Investigations

1. Radiography
   a. Trichobezoars and cecal impactions likely linked to either foreign bodies or poor gut motility
   b. Assess lumbar spine for lesions in cases of colorectal impaction.
2. Routine hematology and biochemistry
3. Serology for *C. piliforme,* coronavirus
4. Culture and sensitivity
5. Fecal examination
   a. Light microscopy (parasites)
   b. Gram stain
   c. Normal gastrointestinal flora is gram positive (i.e., *Bifidobacterium* spp., *Bacteroides* spp., *Eubacterium* spp., and *Lactobacillus* spp.)
   d. Giemsa or acid-fast staining *(Cryptosporidium)*
6. Cytology
7. Electron microscopy
8. Endoscopy
   a. Gastroscopy, colonoscopy
   b. Endoscopic laparoscopy
9. Ultrasonography
10. Biopsy

Management

1. Fluid therapy (see *Nursing Care*)
2. High-fiber diet
3. May need to syringe feed
4. Probiotics. These may be of benefit, but often species specific. One study found no benefit in administering oral *Lactobacillus* spp. as an aid to antibiotic-induced enteritis in guinea pigs (Wasson et al 2000).
5. Transfaunation using caecotrophs from a healthy rodent may help natural gut flora to reestablish.
6. Only use antibiotics if indicated. Many cases do not require their use, which can be counterproductive.
7. Analgesics can be necessary, but avoid those likely to exacerbate gastrointestinal tract ulceration (e.g., flunixin).

Treatment/specific therapy

- Clostridial overgrowth and Tyzzer disease
  - Covering antibiotics, especially cephalosporins, metronidazole (20 mg/kg PO s.i.d.), and vancomycin (20 mg/kg PO s.i.d.) *plus:*
    - Cholestyramine at 100 mg/mL in drinking water
    - Vaccination with clostridial toxoids to reduce mortalities (chinchillas)
- Corona virus:
  - Supportive care only
- *Torulopsis pintolopesii*
  - Nystatin at 100,000 units/kg PO b.i.d.
- *Eimeria* spp.
  - Sulfonamides (e.g., co-trimoxazole at 30 mg/kg PO b.i.d.)
- *Giardia*
  - Metronidazole 20 mg/kg PO s.i.d.
- *Cryptosporidium*
  - Potentiated sulfonamides may be of use
  - Nitazoxanide (Alinia) may prove useful
- Nematodes
  - *Paraspidodera uncinata:* Fenbendazole 20 mg/kg PO s.i.d. for 5 days
- Cestodes and trematodes
  - Praziquantel 5 to 10 mg/kg PO, SC, or IM. Repeat after 10 days.
- Simple constipation
  - Offer liquid paraffin or syrup of figs.
  - Increase fiber in diet.
  - Consider other etiologies.
- Trichobezoars and cecal impactions
  - *Note:* These can be symptomatic of foreign body, gut motility problem, or dehydration.
  - Aggressive fluid therapy
  - Analgesia
  - Gut motility modifiers (e.g., metoclopramide at 0.2 to 1.0 mg/kg SC, PO t.i.d. and cisapride at 0.5 to 1.0 mg/kg PO s.i.d. or b.i.d.)
  - Avoid surgery unless absolutely necessary.
- Colorectal impactions
  - Frequent removal of impacted feces
  - Supplement with B vitamins and vitamin K as caecotrophy will be compromised.
- Rectal prolapse
  - Give fluids and covering antibiosis.
  - Moisten, lubricate, and replace.
  - Keep in place with purse-string suture.
  - May require resection of devitalized area and anastomosis of cut ends
  - Withhold high-fiber foods for a few days.
- Gastric dilatation
  - Tympany: Consider gut motility enhancers such as metoclopramide at 0.5 mg/kg SC or PO every 6 to 8 hours, offering or syringe feeding a high-fiber diet (e.g., Science Recovery Diet or Oxbow Critical Care). Decompress by stomach tube or by paracentesis if severe.
  - Torsion: Can twist >540 degrees; immediate decompression by stomach tube or paracentesis but transabdominal decompression highly likely to initiate a peritonitis.

Early surgical correction to decompress; retorsion and gastric fixation are likely to give best results.

- Fluid therapy
- Feed high-fiber, low-carbohydrate foods.
- Cimetidine at 5 to 10 mg/kg PO, SC, or IM every 6 to 12 hours
- Probiotics (see *Management*)
- Gut stasis, gastric dilation accompanied by hind-limb paralysis in lactating chinchillas often the result of hypocalcemia; usually seen in lactating chinchillas at 2 to 3 weeks postpartum. Calcium gluconate IV or IP at 94 to 140 mg/kg (see *Systemic Disorders*)

- Gastric ulceration
  - Cimetidine at 5 to 10 mg/kg PO, SC, or IM every 6 to 12 hours
- Intestinal obstruction
  - Fluid therapy
  - Covering antibiosis
  - Enemas using warm soapy water
  - Surgical correction/removal of foreign body.

Nutritional disorders

- Hypovitaminosis A (chinchillas—see *Ophthalmic Disorders*)
- Hypovitaminosis C (scurvy—guinea pigs, not proven but often suggested for degus)
- Hypervitaminosis C (may cause heterotrophic bony metaplasia and calcification (metastatic calcification in guinea pigs)
- Hypovitaminosis E (nutritional muscular dystrophy—see *Musculoskeletal Disorders*)
- Hypovitaminosis E or choline or methionine deficiency linked with yellow discoloration of pinna and raised, pigmented lesions in the perineal area and ventral abdomen in chinchillas
- Thiamine deficiency (chinchillas)
- Fatty acid deficiency (chinchillas)
- Pantothenic acid deficiency
- "Cotton fur" (chinchillas)
- Nutritional metabolic bone disease (chinchillas)
- Hepatic lipidosis (see *Hepatic Disorders*)

Findings on clinical examination

- Vague ill health, including weight loss and dehydration
- Dental disease (hypovitaminosis C in guinea pigs)
- Motor abnormalities, including trembling, paralysis, and convulsions
- Pain
- Spontaneous fractures (hypovitaminosis C in guinea pigs)
- Ocular and nasal discharges
- Abortions and stillbirths
- Soft stools/diarrhea (hypovitaminosis C in guinea pigs)
- Spontaneous hemorrhage (hypovitaminosis C in guinea pigs)
- History of guinea pig fed on rabbit food (hypovitaminosis C in guinea pigs)
- Coat abnormalities (cotton-like appearance of fur—cotton fur—and hypovitaminosis A in chinchillas)

- Alopecia (chinchillas—fatty acid deficiency, pantothenic acid deficiency)
- Polydipsia (hepatic lipidosis)
- Edema (hypovitaminosis C, hepatopathy, cardiovascular disease)

Investigations

1. Radiography
   a. Enlarged joints and costochondral junctions, epiphyseal and long bone malformations, pathological fractures (hypovitaminosis C)
   b. Dental abnormalities (hypovitaminosis C—see also *Dental Disorders*)
2. Routine hematology and biochemistry
   a. Anemia
   b. Clotting disorders
3. Culture and sensitivity
4. Cytology
5. Endoscopy
6. Ultrasonography
7. Biopsy

Treatment/specific therapy

- Hypovitaminosis C
  - Supplement with vitamin C (ascorbic acid) at 50 to 100 mg/kg PO daily.
  - Feed with commercial guinea pig food supplemented with vitamin C. Maintenance requirements are 10 mg/kg for adults and 30 mg/kg during pregnancy (Huerkamp et al 1996).
  - Rabbit food fed to rabbit/guinea pig combinations is likely to induce hypovitaminosis in the guinea pig.
  - Guinea pig food that is out of date or has been poorly stored is likely to contain insufficient levels of vitamin C.
  - Degus should be fed either a dedicated degu diet or a vitamin C–supplemented guinea pig food.
- Cotton fur: Excessive protein intake. Alter rations to lower protein (15%) diet.
- Fatty acid deficiency
  - Supplement with unsaturated fatty acids, especially linoleic and arachidonic acid.
  - Recommend feeding 5 to 10 mg/kg evening primrose oil (Richardson 2003).
  - Monitor food storage facilities to prevent rancidity.
- Pantothenic acid deficiency (may be complicated by zinc deficiency)
  - Supplement with dietary pantothenic acid and zinc.
- Nutritional metabolic bone disease
  - Calcium gluconate IM at 94 to 140 mg/kg IV or IP
  - Investigate and correct calcium/phosphorus imbalance in diet.

Hepatic disorders

Bacterial

- Hepatitis
- Yersiniosis (see *Systemic Disorders*)

Fungal

- Ingestion of aflatoxins and mycotoxins in food
- Histoplasmosis (see *Systemic Disorders*)

Protozoal

- *Cryptosporidium* (chinchillas—see *Gastrointestinal Tract Disorders*)

Parasitic

Nutritional

- Hepatic lipidosis (especially degus)

Neoplasia

- Lymphosarcoma
- Other hepatic and biliary tumors

Other noninfectious problems

- Amyloidosis (secondary to chronic infection, especially pododermatitis in guinea pigs)

Findings on clinical examination

- Diarrhea
- Weight loss
- Jaundice
- Polydipsia/polyuria
- Poor blood clotting (hepatic lipidosis)
- Hepatomegaly

Investigations

1. Radiography
    a. Routine hematology and biochemistry
    b. Liver parameters raised
    c. Hyperlipidemia (hepatic lipidosis)
    d. Anemia
    e. Ketones in blood
2. Urinalysis
    a. Ketonuria (hepatic lipidosis)
3. Culture and sensitivity
4. Cytology
5. Endoscopy
6. Ultrasonography
    a. Hepatomegaly (hepatic lipidosis)
7. Biopsy

Management

1. Fluid therapy
2. Milk thistle *(Silybum marianum)* is hepatoprotectant; dose at 4 to 15 mg/kg PO b.i.d. or t.i.d.
3. Lactulose at 0.5 mL/kg PO b.i.d.

Treatment/specific therapy

- Hepatic lipidosis
  - Aggressive fluid therapy
  - Parenteral nutrition with glucose and vitamins
  - Assisted feeding by syringe. Calcium gluconate PO or propylene glycol PO may be of use.
  - Dexamethasone at 0.1 to 0.6 mg/kg IM
- Mycotoxicosis
  - General management of liver disease
  - Prevent exposure to sources of contamination, usually old foods with fungal contamination
- Neoplasia
  - Lymphosarcoma (see *Cardiovascular and Hematologic Disorders*)
  - Hepatic neoplasia
  - Poor prognosis. In some cases surgery may be possible, but euthanasia is more practicable.

Pancreatic disorders

Nutritional
- Congenital manganese deficiency (diabetes mellitus)

Neoplasia
- Islet tumors (benign)

Other noninfectious problems
- Amyloidosis (secondary to chronic infection, especially pododermatitis in guinea pigs)
- Diabetes mellitus (especially degus)

Findings on clinical examination

- Weight loss
- Polydipsia/polyuria
- Bilateral cataracts
- Infertility and other reproductive abnormalities
- Cystitis

Investigations

1. Radiography
2. Routine hematology and biochemistry
   a. Hyperlipidemia
   b. Hyperglycemia (Table 3-5)
   c. Fructosamine (guinea pigs: 134 to 271 µmol/L)
3. Glucose tolerance test

Table 3-5 Guinea pigs, chinchillas, and degus: Hyperglycemia

Species	Normal range for blood glucose (mmol/L)	Diabetic blood glucose (mmol/L)
Guinea pig	3.36-7.8	>20
Chinchilla	3.36-6.72	22
Degu	4.44-5.55	—

Glucose tolerance test for guinea pigs

1. Keep on an 18-hour fast.
2. Take baseline blood glucose sample.
3. Give oral glucose 1.75 g/kg.
4. Repeat blood glucose after 4 hours.
5. Normal blood glucose <1.5 baseline glucose; diabetic = 2 × baseline glucose.

---

4. Urinalysis (see *Urinary Disorders*)
   a. Note that ascorbic acid can interfere with urinary glucose testing.
   b. Glycosuria, ketoacidosis (rare)
5. Cytology
6. Endoscopy
7. Ultrasonography
8. Biopsy

Treatment/specific therapy

- Diabetes mellitus
  - Place on a high-fiber (e.g., hay), low-carbohydrate diet.
  - Insulin usually not required in guinea pigs.
- Spontaneous remissions are common in guinea pigs.
- *Note:* An undiagnosed infectious agent has been linked to induction of diabetes mellitus in Abyssinian guinea pigs (cited in Huerkamp et al 1996).
- For chinchillas, if unable to stabilize by dietary management alone, insulin is initiated at 1 IU/kg b.i.d. and adjusted at 0.1 IU/kg as required, dependent on twice-daily urine analysis (Keeble 2001).
- For degus, place on a low-sugar (low-carbohydrate) diet and substitute vegetables for fruit. Avoid obesity; recommended to keep breeding female degus at around 250 g body weight (Najecki and Tate 1999).

Cardiovascular and hematologic disorders
• •

See also *Respiratory Disorders*.

Viral

- Type C retrovirus

Bacterial

- Endocarditis
- *S. equi zooepidemicus* (pleuritis, hydrothorax, pericarditis)
- *S. pneumoniae* (hemopericardium, pericarditis, pleuritis)
- *S. pyogenes* (hemopericardium, pericarditis, pleuritis)
- *Haemobartonella caviae* (rickettsial)

Nutritional

- Hypovitaminosis C (see *Nutritional Disorders*)
- Copper deficiency
- Heterotrophic bony metaplasia and calcification (see *Systemic Disorders*)

Neoplasia

- Lymphosarcoma/leukemia (usually B cell)
- Mesenchymomas of right atrium
- Cardiac fibrosarcomas
- Splenic hematoma
- Splenic hemangioma

Other noninfectious problems

- Cardiomyopathies (especially chinchillas)
- Poor blood clotting (hepatic lipidosis—see *Hepatic Disorders*)
- 90% of guinea pigs with postural abnormalities following extreme dental extractions showed T-wave inversion on ECG (Azuma et al 1999).

Findings on clinical examination

- Dyspnea
- Abnormal respiratory sounds
- Weight loss
- Dysphagia; cardiomegaly can produce difficulty swallowing.
- Cardiac arrhythmias
- Tachycardia or bradycardia
- Abnormal heart sounds (not always present)
- Spontaneous hemorrhage; bleeding disorders (hypovitaminosis C, copper deficiency, hypokalemia)
- CNS signs (leukemia)

Investigations

1. Radiography
2. Routine hematology and biochemistry
   a. Intraerythrocytic inclusions, anemia, hypoproteinemia, reticulocytosis, increased clotting time *(Haemobartonella caviae)*
   b. Marked lymphocytosis ≥25 × 10^9/L) (leukemia/lymphosarcoma)
3. Culture and sensitivity, including blood culture
4. Cytology
   a. Intraerythrocytic inclusions *(H. caviae)*
   b. Bone marrow aspirate
5. Endoscopy

Table 3-6 Echocardiographic measurements from healthy chinchillas

Variable	Anaesthetized		Awake	
	Range	**Mean ± SD**	**Range**	**Mean ± SD**
Interventricular septum in diastole (cm)	0.15-0.25	0.18 ± 0.03	0.16-0.25	0.20 ± 0.03
Left ventricular free wall in diastole (cm)	0.23-0.32	0.26 ± 0.03	0.18-0.31	0.24 ± 0.04
Left ventricular diastolic dimension (cm)	0.47-0.69	0.64 ± 0.05	0.43-0.75	0.59 ± 0.08
Left ventricular systolic dimension (cm)	0.23-0.45	0.38 ± 0.05	0.18-0.40	0.29 ± 0.06
Fractional shortening (%)	32-51	40 ± 5	35-64	50 ± 8
E-point septal separation (cm)	0.00-0.06	0.03 ± 0.02	0.00-0.09	0.04 ± 0.03
Left atrial diameter (cm)	0.37-0.60	0.49 ± 0.06	0.45-0.67	0.53 ± 0.06
Aortic diameter (cm)	0.27-0.48	0.36 ± 0.05	0.36-0.49	0.41 ± 0.04
Left atrium diameter: Aortic diameter ratio	1.03-1.66	1.38 ± 0.20	1.02-1.52	1.28 ± 0.13
Heart rate (beats/min)	130-220	170 ± 22	130-235	169 ± 32
Aorta peak flow velocity (m/s)	0.33-0.75	0.46 ± 0.10	0.40-1.33	0.81 ± 0.26
Aorta ejection time (ms)	150-225	175 ± 20	110-160	131 ± 13
Pulmonary artery peak flow velocity (m/s)	0.37-1.00	0.61 ± 0.16	0.53-1.47	0.97 ± 0.32
Pulmonary artery ejection time (ms)	125-225	192 ± 34	105-150	129 ± 12
Mitral valve inflow summated (m/s)	—	—	0.50-0.90	0.74 ± 0.10
Mitral valve, E-wave peak flow velocity (m/s)	0.35-0.60	0.48 ± 0.08	—	—
Mitral valve, A-wave peak flow velocity (m/s)	0.17-0.40	0.29 ± 0.07	—	—

6. ECG
7. Ultrasonography
   a. Measure cardiac parameters
   b. Echocardiography (Linde et al 2004, see Table 3-6)
   c. Hepatosplenomegaly (lymphosarcoma)
8. Biopsy
   a. Liver/lymph node (lymphosarcoma)
   b. Bone marrow biopsy

Treatment/specific therapy

- Bacterial diseases
  - Appropriate antibiosis. For *S. pneumoniae* and *S. pyogenes* consider chloramphenicol at 30 to 50 mg/kg PO b.i.d.
- Lymphosarcoma
  - Females > males; usually 2+ years old
  - Cyclophosphamide, as described in Chapter 2 (Table 2.9), may induce remission.
  - Vincristine, methotrexate, and prednisolone have been reported as ineffective.
- Cardiomyopathies and other heart abnormalities
  - Manage as for other species.
  - Examples of suitable medications include taurine at 100 mg/kg PO s.i.d. for 8 weeks.

- Arrhythmias
  - Digoxin at 0.003 to 0.03 mg/kg PO every 12 to 48 hours
  - Lidocaine 1 to 2 mg/kg IV or 2 to 4 mg/kg i.t.
- Congestive heart failure
  - Furosemide 0.3 to 4 mg/kg PO, SC, IM, or IV s.i.d. or b.i.d.
  - Enalapril 0.1-1.0 mg/kg PO every 24-48 hours
  - Nitroglycerin ointment (2%) at 3 mm applied topically to the inner pinna every 6 to 12 hours
- Other medications
  - Atenolol 0.5 to 2 mg/kg PO s.i.d.
  - Verapamil 0.2 mg/kg PO, SC, or IV t.i.d.
  - Diltiazem 0.5 to 1 mg/kg PO b.i.d. or s.i.d.
  - Atropine 0.05 to 0.5 mg/kg SC or IM b.i.d.
  - Glycopyrrolate 0.01 to 0.1 mg/kg SC, IM, or IV
  - Pimobendan at 0.2 mg/kg PO b.i.d.
  - Benazepril at <0.1 mg/kg PO s.i.d.

Systemic disorders

Viral

- Lymphocytic choriomeningitis (LCM)

Bacterial

- *Pseudomonas aeruginosa*
- *Corynebacterium kutscheri*
- *Corynebacterium pyogenes*
- *L. monocytogenes* (chinchilla—see *Neurologic Disorders*)
- *Salmonella*
- *Streptobacillus moniliformis*
- *S. equi zooepidemicus*
- *Streptococcus equi equisimilis*
- *Y. pseudotuberculosis*

Fungal

- *Histoplasma capsulatum*

Protozoal

- *T. gondii* (chinchillas—see also *Neurologic Disorders*)

Nutritional

- Hypovitaminosis C (see *Nutritional Disorders*)
- Heterotrophic bony metaplasia and calcification (metastatic calcification in guinea pigs). Often secondary to high-phosphorus, low-magnesium, and low-potassium diets (may be linked to hypervitaminosis C in guinea pigs)
- Hypervitaminosis C; possible cause of heterotrophic bony metaplasia and calcification (see *Nutritional Disorders*)
- Hypocalcemia (lactating chinchillas—see also *Gastrointestinal Tract Disorders, Neurologic Disorders*, and *Reproductive Tract Disorders*)

Neoplasia

- Lymphoma/leukemia (see *Cardiovascular and Hematologic Disorders*)

Other noninfectious problems

- Hypoglycemia (especially following chronic dental disease)
- Aggressive treatment of dental disease (see *Dental Disorders*)
- Ketosis
- Heat stress (temperatures >27° C).

Findings on clinical examination

- Anorexia/poor physical condition/weight loss
- Fever
- Lethargy
- Conjunctivitis (*Salmonella*, histoplasmosis—see *Ophthalmic Disorders*)
- Marked dental disease/recent history of dental work (guinea pigs)
- Ataxia/weakness
- Central nervous signs (toxoplasmosis, listeriosis)
- Diarrhea (occasionally with salmonellosis)
- Tachypnea, hypersalivation (heat stress, ketosis)
- Hyperthermia (rectal temperature above 41° C)
- Hepatosplenomegaly and enlarged mesenteric lymph nodes palpable (salmonellosis, streptococci, yersiniosis)
- Swollen submandibular lymph nodes (*S. moniliformis*, streptococci, *Yersinia*)
- Sudden death (septicemia, ketosis, heterotrophic bony metaplasia and calcification)
- Multiple signs, including respiratory, mastitis, metritis CNS signs, ocular disease (streptococci)
- Hemorrhagic discharge from nares, mouth, and vagina *(S. equi equisimilis)*
- Disseminated granulomatous disease on postmortem *(Yersinia, Histoplasma)*
- Periparturient female guinea pig (ketosis)
- Prolonged anorexia, especially in obese guinea pigs (ketosis)
- Seizures
- Abortion
- Organ-specific diseases (heterotrophic bony metaplasia and calcification, metastatic calcification)

Investigations

1. Radiography
   a. Signs of heterotrophic bony metaplasia and calcification may be visible.
2. Routine hematology and biochemistry
   a. Hypoglycemia (normal range—guinea pig 3.36 to 7.8 mmol/L; chinchilla 3.36 to 6.72 mmol/L)
   b. Hyperkalemia (normal range—guinea pig 4.0 to 5.0 mmol/L; chinchilla 5 to 6.5 mmol/L)
   c. Hyponatremia (normal range—guinea pig 120 to 152 mmol/L; chinchilla 130 to 155 mmol/L)
   d. Hypochloremia (normal range—guinea pig 90 to 115 mmol/L; chinchilla 105 to 115 mmol/L)
   e. Hyperlipidemia
   f. Hypokalemia (guinea pigs; linked with heterotrophic bony metaplasia and calcification)

     g. Hypocalcemia (guinea pig 2.0 to 3.0 mmol/L; chinchilla 2.5 to 3.75 mmol/L; lactating chinchillas)

     h. Lymphocytosis $\geq 25 \times 10^9$/L) (leukemia/lymphosarcoma)

3. Serology for LCM, toxoplasmosis
4. Culture and sensitivity

     a. May need repeated or bulk fecal samples to isolate intermittent *Salmonella* excreters.

5. Cytology

     a. Gram stain smears from swollen submandibular glands (streptococci: gram-positive; *Yersinia:* gram-negative)

6. Endoscopy

     a. Gastric ulceration (ketosis)

7. Ultrasonography
8. Biopsy

Management

- Supportive treatment, including fluid therapy

Treatment/specific therapy

- Bacterial disease
  - Appropriate antibiosis
  - Carrier animals may exist with salmonellosis.
  - Swollen submandibular lymph nodes may require surgical intervention.
  - Yersiniosis: Transmitted from fecal contamination from wild birds and rodents
  - Pseudomoniasis: Reduce water contamination by acidifying water to pH 2.5 to 2.8 or chlorination at 12 mg/L (cited in Strake et al 1996).
- Histoplasmosis
  - May be linked to soil contaminated with bird droppings
  - Amphotericin B at 0.1 to 1.0 mg/kg IV by infusion s.i.d. 5 days per week for 3 weeks
  - Ketoconazole at 10.0 mg/kg PO every other day <1 year
- Hypoglycemia
  - IV glucose by bolus and infusion
  - Assisted feeding
  - Investigate underlying causes (e.g., dental disease).
- Ketosis
  - Fluid therapy
  - Calcium gluconate 94 to 140 mg/kg IV or IP
  - Dexamethasone 0.1 to 0.6 mg/kg IM
  - Pregnant female guinea pig: Consider cesarean/ovariohysterectomy.
  - Gradual weight reduction using low-calorie, high-fiber diet (e.g., hay)
- Heat stress
  - Monitor core body temperature: Guinea pig 37.2 to 39.5° C (99 to 103.1° F); chinchilla 37 to 38° C (98.6 to 100.4° F); degu 38° C (100° F)
  - Cool (not cold) body (e.g., damp towels, water bath). The pinnae in chinchillas are designed for radiative heat loss, so these can be targeted especially.
  - Dexamethasone at 0.1 to 0.6 mg/kg given IV once only.
  - Supportive treatment such as cool IV fluids; heatstroke may have unforeseen sequelae (e.g., gut stasis).

- Heterotrophic bony metaplasia and calcification
  - No treatment
  - Prevention is by providing an appropriate diet. Dietary recommendations (Huerkamp et al 1996) are:
    - 0.9% to 1.1% calcium; 0.6% to 0.7% phosphorus; Ca:P ratio of 1.5:1.0
    - 0.3% to 0.4% magnesium, 0.4% to 1.4% potassium
  - Associated hypokalemia: Daily supplement with 0.5 to 1.0 mg/kg potassium PO
  - Heterotrophic bony metaplasia and calcification may be linked to hypervitaminosis C.
- Hypocalcemia
  - Usually seen in lactating chinchillas at 2 to 3 weeks postpartum. May be accompanied by gut stasis.
  - Calcium gluconate 94 to 140 mg/kg IV or IP
- Lymphocytic choriomeningitis
  - Potential zoonosis. No treatment. Consider euthanasia.

Musculoskeletal disorders

Bacterial
- Septic arthritis (streptococci, mycoplasmosis)

Fungal
- *Histoplasma capsulatum* (see *Systemic Disorders*)

Nutritional
- Hypovitaminosis C (see *Nutritional Disorders*)
- Hypovitaminosis E (nutritional muscular dystrophy)
- Nutritional metabolic bone disease (see *Nutritional Disorders*)

Neoplasia
- Osteosarcoma

Other noninfectious problems
- Osteoarthritis
- Fractures

Findings on clinical examination

- Pain (osteosarcoma, hypovitaminosis C)
- Swellings associated with limbs and joints
- Abnormal gait
- Lameness
- Infertility problems (hypovitaminosis E)
- Severe muscle spasms of the hind limbs, forelimbs, and face (nutritional metabolic bone disease)

Investigations

1. Radiography
   a. Fractures (trauma, hypovitaminosis C, osteosarcoma)
   b. Long bone and epiphyseal abnormalities (hypovitaminosis C)
   c. Lytic lesions in bone (osteosarcoma)

2. Routine hematology and biochemistry
   a. High creatine kinase levels (hypovitaminosis E)
3. Serology for mycoplasmosis
4. Culture and sensitivity
5. Cytology
6. Endoscopy
7. Ultrasonography
8. Biopsy
   a. Muscle biopsy and liver biopsy and vitamin E analysis (hypovitaminosis E)

Treatment/specific therapy

- Septic arthritis
  - Appropriate antibiosis
  - Joint lavage may be appropriate.
- Hypovitaminosis E
  - Supplement with vitamin E at 5 to 10 mg/kg PO, SC.
  - Normal dietary levels should be 50 mg/kg.
- Osteoarthritis: meloxicam 0.3 mg/kg PO s.i.d.
- Nutritional metabolic bone disease (see *Nutritional Disorders*)
- Fractures
  - Traumatic fractures can be managed:
    - Conservatively by strict rest in confinement, possibly with supportive dressings—although these rodents will tend to gnaw through dressings
    - Surgical repair

Neurologic disorders

Viral

- LCM (arenavirus)

Bacterial

- Otitis media/interna (*S. equi, S. pneumoniae, Bordetella bronchiseptica, Klebsiella, Pseudomonas*, other coliforms); *Pasteurella/Actinobacillus* spp. may be encountered
- *L. monocytogenes*

Fungal

- Ingestion of aflatoxins and mycotoxins (liver damage)

Protozoal

- *Encephalitozoon cuniculi*
- *T. gondii*
- *Frenkelia* spp. (Meingassner and Burtscher 1977)

Parasitic

- *Trixacaris caviae:* Intense pruritus may trigger seizure-like spasms in guinea pigs
- *Baylisascaris procyonis* (cerebral nematodiasis)

Nutritional

- Eclampsia in periparturient guinea pigs (see *Reproductive Tract Disorders*)
- Thiamine deficiency (chinchillas—see *Nutritional Disorders*)

Neoplasia

Other noninfectious problems

- Heavy metal poisoning
- Neuronal degeneration in the mesencephalic trigeminal nerve nucleus following dental work in guinea pigs (Kimoto 1993)
- Lymphosarcoma (meningeal infiltration—see *Cardiovascular and Hematologic Disorders*)
- Renal disease
- Hypocalcemia in lactating chinchillas (see *Systemic Disorders* and *Gastrointestinal Tract Disorders*)
- Epilepsy-like conditions

Findings on clinical examination

- CNS signs
- Progressive flaccid paralysis
- Closure of the ear canal with debris and inflammatory tissue (otitis media)
- Otitis interna evidenced by torticollis, rolling, and nystagmus
- Drooping ears (chinchillas)
- Seizures
- Pneumonia
- Progressive deterioration following dental work, accompanied by ataxia, postural abnormalities, dysphagia/inability to chew (guinea pigs; trigeminal motor neuron degeneration—Azuma et al 1999)
- Self-inflicted lesions, especially over the shoulders *(Trixacaris caviae)*

Investigations

1. Otoscopic examination of the ear canals
2. Radiography
   a. Skull radiography to assess tympanic bullae for otitis interna
3. Routine hematology and biochemistry
   a. Blood levels for heavy metals (e.g., zinc and lead)
4. Serology for LCM, *E. cuniculi,* and *Toxoplasma*
5. Culture and sensitivity
6. Cytology
7. Endoscopy
   a. Examination of the ear canal
8. Ultrasonography
9. Biopsy
   a. Heavy metal levels in liver tissue
10. Postmortem

Management

- Supportive treatment, including fluid therapy, assisted feeding, and covering antibiosis

Treatment/specific therapy

- Otitis media/interna
  - Very guarded prognosis—treatment often unsuccessful
  - Appropriate antibiosis
  - Bulla osteotomy
- *L. monocytogenes*
  - Usually poor response to therapy
  - Prophylactic treatment of in-contact chinchillas with autogenous vaccine or antibiotics
  - Trigeminal mesencephalic neuron degeneration following dental work in guinea pigs
  - Supportive treatment only; usually requires euthanasia
- *E. cuniculi*
  - Co-trimoxazole at 30 mg/kg PO b.i.d. for at least 3 weeks
  - Albendazole at 10 mg/kg PO s.i.d for 6 weeks
  - Fenbendazole at 10 mg/kg PO s.i.d for 1 month
- *Toxoplasma* and *Frenkelia* spp.
  - Co-trimoxazole at 30 mg/kg PO b.i.d. for at least 3 weeks
- *Trixacaris caviae* (see *Skin Disorders*)
- *Baylisascaris procyonis* (cerebral nematodiasis)
  - Treatment difficult; consider ivermectin as anthelmintic plus NSAID (e.g., meloxicam at 0.1 mg/kg PO, SC s.i.d.).
  - Adult roundworms found in raccoon
- Hypocalcemia
  - Gut stasis and gastric dilation and hind-limb paralysis in lactating chinchillas often the result of hypocalcemia; usually seen in lactating chinchillas at 2 to 3 weeks postpartum. Calcium gluconate at 94 to 140 mg/kg IV or IP (see *Systemic Disorders*)
- LCM
  - No treatment. Consider euthanasia.
- Thiamine deficiency
  - Supplement with thiamine at 1 mg/kg food.
- Heavy metal poisoning
  - Calcium disodium edetate at 30 mg/kg b.i.d. for 5 days (Richardson 2003)
- Epilepsy-like conditions
  - Epilepsy is a diagnosis of exclusion. Attempt to control with pediatric phenobarbital preparations at 1 to 3 mg/kg b.i.d. PO (Richardson 2003).

Ophthalmic disorders

Bacterial

- *Chlamydophila psittaci*
- *S. equi zooepidemicus*
- *Salmonella*

Fungal

- *Histoplasma capsulatum* (see *Systemic Disorders*)

Protozoal

- *Encephalitozoon cuniculi* (uveitis)

Nutritional

- Protein deficiency (cataracts—guinea pigs)
- Fed on cow's milk (cataracts—guinea pigs)
- Hypovitaminosis A (chinchillas)
- Hypervitaminosis C (heterotrophic bony metaplasia and calcification)

Neoplasia

Other noninfectious problems

- Diabetes mellitus (cataracts—see *Pancreatic Disorders*)
- Aging changes (cataracts and asteroid hyalosis in chinchillas)

Findings on clinical examination

- Conjunctivitis (*Chlamydophila, Salmonella,* hypovitaminosis A in chinchillas)
- Panophthalmitis/uveitis
- Exophthalmos (retrobulbar abscess/retroorbital lymphadenopathy; *S. equis zooepidemicus*)
- Cataracts (chinchillas—hypovitaminosis A)
- Systemic signs (salmonellosis, hypovitaminosis A in chinchillas)
- Bony spicules surrounded by fibrous tissue present in the ciliary body (hypervitaminosis C)

Investigations

1. Full ophthalmic examination
   a. Bilateral cataracts (degu—diabetes mellitus)
2. Radiography
3. Routine hematology and biochemistry
4. Serology for *E. cuniculi*
5. PCR for *Chlamydophila*
6. Culture and sensitivity
7. Cytology
   a. Gram stain
8. Endoscopy
9. Ultrasonography
10. Biopsy

Treatment/specific therapy

- *Chlamydophila*
  - Enrofloxacin at 5 mg/kg s.i.d. or b.i.d.
  - Ofloxacin ophthalmic drops topically q.i.d.
  - Chlortetracycline ointment topically t.i.d.
- Other bacterial causes
  - Appropriate topical and systemic antibiosis
- *E. cuniculi*
  - Co-trimoxazole at 30 mg/kg PO b.i.d. for at least 3 weeks
  - Albendazole at 10 mg/kg PO s.i.d. for 6 weeks
  - Fenbendazole at 10 mg/kg PO s.i.d. for 1 month

- Hypovitaminosis A
  - Supplement with vitamin A at 2000 IU/chinchilla/day SC, PO for 7 days and then every 7 to 14 days.
- Heterotrophic bony metaplasia and calcification of the ciliary body: No treatment. Assess vitamin C status.
- Other nutritional causes: Identify and correct.

Endocrine disorders

- Amyloidosis of the adrenal glands and pancreatic islets (secondary to chronic infection, especially pododermatitis in guinea pigs)
- Diabetes mellitus (see *Pancreatic Disorders*)
- Cystic ovarian disease (see *Reproductive Tract Disorders*)
- Hyperadrenocorticism (see also *Skin Disorders*)
- Adrenal hyperplasia often accompanies dental disease and fur chewing in chinchillas (Crossley 2001).
- Thyroid hyperplasia can be associated with fur chewing in chinchillas.

Findings on clinical examination

- Alopecia (see *Skin Disorders*)
  - Bilateral symmetrical often nonpruritic (guinea pigs—cystic ovarian disease, hyperadrenocorticism)
- Fur chewing (chinchillas; possibly associated with thyroid hyperplasia or adrenal hyperplasia)

Investigations

1. Blood cortisol levels (guinea pig)
   a. These are biphasic in guinea pigs. Peak at 1600 and 0400 hours; low points at 0800 and 2400 hours (Fujieda et al 1982)
   b. Normal free plasma cortisol = 0.6 to 5.8 µg/dL. This represents 6.1% to 14.5% of total cortisol levels (Fujieda et al 1982).
   c. Mean salivary cortisol = 6.6 ± 3.4 ng/mL. After ACTH stimulation: 157 ± 53 ng/mL (Zeugswetter et al 2007)

ACTH response test in guinea pigs

1. Collect blood or saliva for basal cortisol.
2. Inject 20 IU ACTH IM.
3. Repeat blood or saliva collection at 4 hours post ACTH.

---

2. Thyroid hormone levels (guinea pig)
   a. Total serum T_4 = 2.5 ± 0.3 to 3.2 ± 0.8 µg/dL (Castro et al 1986)
   b. Free T_4 = 1.26 to 2.03 ng/dL (% free T_4 = 0.046% to 0.068%)
   c. Total T_3 = 39 to 44 ng/dL
   d. Free T_3 = 0.221 to 0.260 ng/dL (% free T_3 = 0.521% to 0.638%)
3. Radiography
4. Routine hematology and biochemistry
   a. Low potassium levels (guinea pig normal levels: 4.5 to 8.8 mmol/L)

5. Culture and sensitivity
6. Endoscopy
7. Biopsy
8. Ultrasonography
   a. Guinea pig: Normal size adrenal glands around 14×4 mm (left); 13×6 mm (right) (Zeugswetter et al 2007). Enlarged adrenal glands were 15×7 mm (left) and 16×9 mm (right).

Treatment/specific therapy

- Hyperadrenocorticism
  - Trilostane at 2 to 4 mg/kg PO s.i.d.
  - Attempt management and treatment as in other species.

Urinary disorders

Bacterial

- Cystitis
- *S. pyogenes,* staphylococci, fecal coliforms
- Pyelonephritis may follow metritis or abortion.

Protozoal

- *Klossiella cobayae (caviae)*

Neoplasia

Other noninfectious problems

- Amyloidosis (often linked to chronic inflammatory conditions, such as pododermatitis)
- Urethral obstruction with coagulated seminal vesicle secretions or other proteinaceous concretions in males (guinea pigs)
- Urinary calculi (triple phosphate, $CaCO_3$, $CaPO_4$, calcium oxalate—guinea pigs)
- Hydronephrosis
- Idiopathic glomerulonephropathy
- Hypertensive nephrosclerosis (linked to Ca:P imbalance—see "Heterotrophic Bony Metaplasia and Calcification" in *Systemic Disorders*)
- Chronic renal failure
- Balanoposthitis (see *Reproductive Tract Disorders*)
- Diabetes mellitus (see *Pancreatic Disorders*)

Findings on clinical examination

- Polydipsia/polyuria
- Perineal dermatitis (urine scalding)
- Urinary tenesmus
- Obvious pain and discomfort; vocalization (guinea pigs)
- Hematuria
- Glycosuria, ketonuria (diabetes mellitus)
- Hemorrhagic discharge from vagina
- Anorexia, listlessness
- Weight loss

- Gross swelling of the abdomen (urine retention/obstruction)
- Cystitis may be asymptomatic.

Investigations

1. Urinalysis (Table 3-7)
2. Culture and sensitivity
3. Sediment examination/cytology
4. Radiography
   a. Lateral and ventrodorsal views
   b. Contrast studies
   c. Intravenous pyelography
5. Routine hematology and biochemistry
   a. Raised renal parameters
6. Endoscopy
7. Laparoscopic endoscopy
8. Ultrasonography
9. Biopsy
   a. Renal biopsy

Table 3-7 Normal urine parameters for guinea pigs and chinchillas

Value	Guinea pig	Chinchilla
Volume (mL/adult per day)	20-25	
pH (average)	9.0	8.5
Urine gravity	>1.045	
Protein	Negligible	
Crystals	Triple phosphate, $CaCO_3$	
Glucose	Negative (mild glycosuria may be masked by ascorbic acid excretion)	
Ketones	Negative	
Other	The cysts of *Klossiella cobayae* may occasionally be observed.	

Management

- Fluid therapy
- Covering broad-spectrum antibiosis if appropriate (e.g., enrofloxacin at 5 mg/kg PO or SC s.i.d.

Treatment/specific therapy

- Urinary calculi
- Surgical removal via cystotomy
- Predisposed by reduced fluid intake, nutritional imbalance, bacterial cystitis, and anatomic abnormalities
- Ureteral calculi advanced gently into bladder for removal via cystotomy

- Triple phosphate calculi may be prevented by high supplementation with ascorbic acid to acidify the urine.
- Oxalates: Avoid high-oxalate foods such as rhubarb.
- Select a lower calcium diet. Calcium requirement = 4 mg/kg per day.
- Supplementing with magnesium hydroxide at 4 mg/kg may protect against calcium uroliths (cited in Huerkamp et al 1996).
- Cystitis
  - Appropriate antibiosis
  - Supplement with vitamin C.
  - Exacerbated by diabetes mellitus

Reproductive tract disorders

Bacterial

- Wide variety of bacteria causing metritis, pyometra, and mastitis
- In guinea pigs consider *Bordetella* (see *Respiratory Disorders*), erysipelas, and *S. equi equisimilis* (mastitis/metritis), as well as other infections (*E. coli*, *Klebsiella*, *Proteus*, staphylococci, and other streptococci).
- Preputial gland abscess (chinchillas)

Neoplasia

- Ovarian teratoma
- Ovarian cystadenoma
- Leiomyoma (often concurrent with cystic ovarian disease)
- Mammary tumors (fibroadenomas, fibrocarcinomas)

Other noninfectious problems

- Balanoposthitis—often secondary to foreign body (e.g., hair ring, bedding particles)
- Mastitis secondary to bites or abrasions from bedding/cage furniture
- Cystic ovarian disease (Nielsen et al 2003)
- Cystic endometrial hyperplasia, endometritis, mucometra (often concurrent with cystic ovarian disease)
- Pregnancy toxemia (see "Ketosis" in *Systemic Disorders*)

Findings on clinical examination

- Vaginal discharge from metritis, pyosalpinx, abortion, stillbirths (guinea pigs with bordetellosis, erysipelas, *S. equi equisimilis*)
- Abdominal enlargement (cystic ovarian disease)
- Hyperemic or even blackened vulva with discharge (metritis—chinchillas)
- Paraphimosis
- Mastitis
  - Slight increase in size and firm texture (localized disease)
  - Marked swelling, pain, discoloration, fever, anorexia, depression, weight loss, litter abandonment, high mortality rate (systemic disease)
- Other clinical signs, such as pneumonia (systemic disease)
- High temperature
- Nonpruritic alopecia (cystic ovarian disease)
- Large, palpable masses in the abdomen (cystic ovarian disease, neoplasia)

Investigations

1. Radiography
2. Routine hematology and biochemistry
   a. Leukopenia suggests endotoxin production (with mastitis).
3. Culture and sensitivity
4. Cytology
5. Endoscopy
   a. Endoscopic laparotomy
6. Ultrasonography
   a. Cystic structures visible, often bilateral but asymmetrical. Can be several centimeters in diameter (cystic ovaries especially in guinea pigs)
7. Biopsy

Management

- Supportive treatment, such as fluid therapy and assisted feeding

Treatment/specific therapy

- Metritis
  - Vaginal/uterine irrigation with warm saline and antibiotic solution
  - Oxytocin at 1 IU/guinea pig SC or IM
  - Antibiosis
  - Ovariohysterectomy
- Preputial gland abscess
  - Lance and flush. Use appropriate antibiosis.
- Balanoposthitis
  - Remove any foreign bodies, hair, etc.
  - Clean daily with dilute chlorhexidine solution.
  - Antibiosis
- Paraphimosis
  - As for balanoposthitis
  - Attend to other underlying conditions, such as urethral calculi or fur ring (chinchillas).
  - If fur ring, gently extrude penis and remove accumulated fur; wash down with dilute chlorhexidine solution.
- Mastitis
  - Broad-spectrum antibiosis (e.g., co-trimoxazole at 30 mg/kg PO b.i.d. or enrofloxacin at 5 mg/kg PO or SC s.i.d.)
  - Fluid therapy
  - Wean or foster any young as soon as possible.
- Cystic ovarian disease
  - Ovariohysterectomy (treatment of choice)
  - hCG 1000 IU weekly for 1 to 3 weeks
  - Draw fluid off by paracentesis.
- Neoplasia
  - Surgery

Reproductive failure

Viral
- Caviid herpesvirus type 1 (cytomegalovirus—guinea pigs)
- Caviid herpesvirus type 2 (Epstein-Barr–like virus—guinea pigs)
- Caviid herpesvirus type 3 (guinea pigs)

Bacterial
- A variety of bacterial infections, including mycoplasmosis, can lead to reproductive failures, abortions, and stillbirths.
- Puerperal septicemia

Protozoal
- *T. gondii*

Parasitic
- *Trixacarus caviae* infestation (abortion in extreme cases—see *Skin Disorders*)

Nutritional
- Hypovitaminosis C (see *Nutritional Disorders*)
- Hypocalcemia (eclampsia)

Neoplasia
Other noninfectious problems
- Diabetes mellitus (see *Pancreatic Disorders*)
- Ketosis
- Retained fetus
- Fetal mummification
- Dystocia
  - Fetal malpresentation
  - Fetal oversize
  - Uterine inertia
- Agalactia

Findings on clinical examination

- Abortion (caviid herpesviruses, toxoplasmosis)
- Vulvar hemorrhage (vaginitis, pyometra, toxoplasmosis)
- Anorexia
- Depression
- Muscle spasms, seizures in pregnant or lactating female guinea pigs (eclampsia)
- Young may be palpable in abdominal cavity.
- Failure to breed

Investigations

1. Radiography
2. Routine hematology and biochemistry
   a. Blood calcium (guinea pig: 2.0 to 3.03 mmol/L; chinchilla: 2.5 to 3.75 mmol/L)
   b. Anemia, hypoglycemia, hyperkalemia, hyponatremia, hypochloremia, and hyperlipidemia (ketosis)

3. Serology for toxoplasmosis
4. Culture and sensitivity
5. Cytology
6. Endoscopy
7. Ultrasonography
8. Biopsy
9. Postmortem
   a. Hepatic lipidosis, enlarged adrenal glands, empty stomach/gut (ketosis)
   b. Hepatic lipidosis

Management

- Fluid therapy
- Keep warm.

Treatment/specific therapy

- Caviid herpesviruses: Infection is transplacental, sexually transmitted, and possibly via urine and saliva. Caviid herpesvirus 2 can be transmitted via fomites.
- Toxoplasmosis
  - Co-trimoxazole at 30 mg/kg PO b.i.d. for at least 3 weeks or, alternatively, try a combination therapy consisting of:
    – Co-trimoxazole at 30 mg/kg PO b.i.d.
    – Pyrimethamine at 0.5 mg/kg PO b.i.d.
    – Folic acid at 3.0 to 5.0 mg/kg PO s.i.d.
- Eclampsia
  - Usually periparturient or postparturient females affected
  - Calcium gluconate at 94 to 140 mg/kg IV or IP to response/as needed
  - Supplement pregnant female guinea pigs with calcium.
  - Early weaning of young
  - Gut stasis and gastric dilation and hind-limb paralysis in lactating chinchillas are often the result of hypocalcemia; usually seen in lactating chinchillas at 2 to 3 weeks postpartum. Give calcium gluconate at 94 to 140 mg/kg IV or IP to response/as needed (see *Systemic Disorders*).
- Retained fetus; mummified fetus and dystocia
  - If birth takes longer than 4 hours (chinchilla), may require intervention
  - Radiography
  - If radiographs appear normal, attempt calcium at 0.5 mL of 20% calcium solution followed by oxytocin 1 IU/guinea pig. IM, can be repeated after 30 minutes.
  - If no improvement, consider cesarean section.
- Puerperal septicemia
  - Antibiotics
  - Fluid therapy
  - Uterine irrigation
- Agalactia
  - Usually due to an underlying problem, so investigate for this.
  - Oxytocin at 1 IU/guinea pig to encourage milk letdown
  - Foster or hand-rear kits.
- Dystocia
  - Radiography
  - If uterine inertia, try oxytocin 1 IU/guinea pig; IM, can repeat after 30 minutes; otherwise consider cesarean section.

Small rodents

Small rodents are popular not only as children's (and adult's) pets but also as show animals. Rats in particular have a very enthusiastic following. Those species that are likely to be encountered in the veterinary surgery are:

- Mice *(Mus musculus)*
- Rats *(Rattus norvegicus)*
- Mongolian gerbils *(Meriones unguiculatus)*
- Hamsters
  - Syrian (golden) hamster *(Mesocricetus auratus)*
  - Russian hamster *(Phodopus sungorus)*
  - Roborovski hamster *(Phodopus roborovskii)*
  - Chinese hamster *(Cricetulus griseus)*
  - Hamster species differ in their standard husbandry. Syrian hamsters are solitary and will fight if kept together. *Phodopus* spp. are highly sociable and fare best in small groups and, indeed, live longer if kept that way. The Chinese hamster falls between the two and is best kept in pairs.

Table 4-1 Small rodents: Key facts

	Mouse	Rat	Gerbil	Syrian hamster	Russian hamster	Chinese hamster
Average life span (years)	2-3	3-4	2-3	2-3	9-15 (months)	2
Weight (g)						
Male	20-40	250-1000+	117	85-130	30-35	30-35
Female				100	95-150	
Body temperature (°C)	37.5	38	38	36-37.4		
Respiratory rate (breaths/min)	100-250	70-150	90-140	75		
Heart rate (beats/min)	500-600	300-450	200-360	300-600		
Gestation (days)	19-21	21-23	24-26	15-16	18-20	20-21
Age at weaning (days)	21-28	21-28	21-24	21-28	21-28	21
Sexual maturity (weeks)	5-8	6-8	10-12	6-8	6-8	7-14

Consultation and handling

Small rodents are prey animals and may become stressed by the presence of potential predators such as cats, dogs, and unfamiliar people; this includes auditory and olfactory signals, so where possible they should be housed separately from such animals, and hands should be well cleaned to remove other species' odors before handling.

Many small rodents move quickly and unpredictably, and care should be taken to prevent unwanted escapes or potentially disastrous leaps to the floor. Gently wrapping in a towel will often help with the handling and control of an excitable rodent. A sure way to annoy a pet rat (and alienate its owner) is to attempt to grasp it by the scruff of the neck. Most are used to being gently handled and are unlikely to bite. If in doubt, use a towel. Do not attempt to pick up a hamster straight from its bed; they are territorial of this and are likely to bite. Instead, gently tease or tip it out. Recalcitrant hamsters are more easily scruffed and, although this will help with an examination of the teeth, it may upset the rodent.

Hamsters are permissive hibernators and may attempt hibernation if temperatures fall consistently below 4.5° C. Poor food availability, altered photoperiod, and other factors may also induce hibernation, although this varies among individuals. Hibernation is not continuous but is interrupted every 2 or 3 days by bouts of normal activity, including foraging. During hibernation, hamsters remain sensitive to tactile stimulation and can be gently aroused. Exposure to normal room temperatures (18 to 22°C) and lighting (12 to 14 hours) are unlikely to trigger hibernation. Many owners misinterpret clinical signs of illness (lack of movement and lethargy, anorexia) with hibernation, often delaying presentation to the veterinary surgeon.

Nursing care

See *Nursing Care* in Chapter 2 for general principles.

Small rodents by virtue of their size and the high risk of predation are forced to obtain most of their water from preformed (food) and metabolic sources. Dehydration can be a real issue, especially at higher environmental temperatures (Table 4-2).

Fluids can be given SC, IP, or IO. For small rodents, the intravenous route (Fig. 4-1) for fluid administration is largely impractical, but Table 4-3 gives suggested sites.

Jugular catheterization can be attempted in all species, but it is difficult and may result in respiratory embarrassment. Many of these sites may also require anesthesia and surgical cutdown, which may not be appropriate for the welfare of the patient. In hypovolemic patients vascular access may be impossible. It is better to consider either IP or IO administration.

Table 4-2 Small rodents: Nursing care

Species	Weight (g)	Maintenance daily water intake (mL/kg per day)	Approximate volumes for fluid replacement therapy (mL/kg body weight)		
			Subcutaneous	Intraperitoneal	Shock
Syrian hamster	85-130 (M)	100	30	30	65-80
	95-150 (F)				
Gerbil	45-130 (M)	Allow 3-4 mL/day	20-40	40-60	60-85
	50-85 (F)				
Rat	267-520 (M)	0.8-1.1	25	25	50-70
	250-325 (F)				
Mouse	20-40 (M)	1.5	30-60	60	70-80
	25-63 (F)				

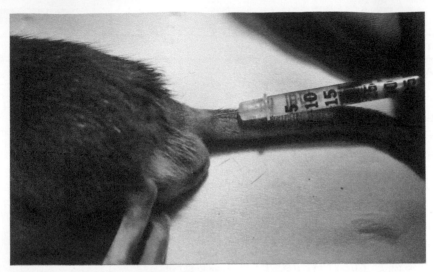

Fig 4-1. Intravenous fluids given through the lateral tail vein.

Table 4-3 Small rodents: Sites for fluid administration	
Intravenous (rat and mouse)	Lateral tail vein (helps if warm!) (Fig. 4-1)
Intravenous (hamster)	Very difficult: lateral tarsal vein, anterior cephalic vein, and lingual vein
Intravenous (gerbil)	Lateral tail vein or saphenous vein
Intraperitoneal (all three species)	Hold the patient vertically downward and inject into the lower left quadrant
Intraosseous (all three species)	Under GA to insert either an intraosseous catheter or a hypodermic needle into the marrow of either the femur (via the greater trochanter) or tibia (through the tibial crest). Fluids, colloids, and even blood can be IO if necessary.

Hypothermia

Much endogenous body heat is generated by gut and muscle activity; sick, inactive, or anesthetized rodents are prone to hypothermia (Jepson 2004). Use a heat source, such as an electric heat mat, plus insulation such as silver foil over the feet, pinnae, and tail (reduces heat lost by conduction) and bubble wrap (reduces heat lost by convection). Maintain in warm air (e.g., incubator) or use a commercial medical warm air generator.

Nutritional status

Many small rodents are presented as emergencies after a prolonged period of ill health that has affected their food intake. These animals are often hypoglycemic—test with a commercial glucometer on a small sample of blood—and IV or IP glucose can be given to these cases once identified.

131

Analgesia

Table 4-4 Small rodents: Analgesic doses

Analgesic	Dose			
	Rat	**Mouse**	**Hamster**	**Gerbil**
Buprenorphine	0.05-0.1 mg/kg SC or IP every 6-12 hours	0.05-0.1 mg/kg SC or IP b.i.d.	0.1 mg/kg SC every 6-12 hours	0.1 mg/kg SC every 6-12 hours
Butorphanol	0.2-2.0 mg/kg SC every 2-4 hours	1.0-2.0 mg/kg SC every 2-4 hours		
Carprofen	1.0-5.0 mg/kg SC or PO s.i.d. or b.i.d.	1.0-5.0 mg/kg SC or PO s.i.d. or b.i.d.		
Ketoprofen	2.0-5.0 mg/kg SC or IM every 12-24 hours	2.0-5.0 mg/kg SC or IM every 12-24 hours		
Meloxicam	0.5-2.0 mg/kg SC or PO s.i.d.	1.0-2.0 mg/kg SC or PO s.i.d.		
Morphine	2.0-5.0 mg/kg SC or IM every 4 hours	2.0-5.0 mg/kg SC or IM every 4 hours		
Meperidine/ pethidine	10-20 mg/kg IM, SC, or IP q.i.d.	10-20 mg/kg IM, SC, or IP q.i.d.	10-20 mg/kg IM, SC, or IP q.i.d.	10-20 mg/kg IM, SC, or IP q.i.d.
Nalbuphine	4.0-8.0 mg/kg SC every 2-4 hours	4.0-8.0 mg/kg SC every 2-4 hours		

Anesthesia

Small rodents may have subclinical respiratory infections.

It is important to keep small rodents warm as they have a large surface area compared with volume, which results in significant heat loss during surgery. This also applies during anesthesia—hypothermia acts as a general depressant and is also immunosuppressive. Merely applying insulation such as bubble wrap is often insufficient—inactive, anesthetized rodents are not generating heat and you may be insulating it from a higher ambient temperature. Place these animals onto a heat mat, onto which is placed an absorptive towel or other material to both protect the mat from becoming wet and reduce the slight risk of localized burns.

Use reflective foil over hairless areas where heat loss can occur, e.g., tails, feet, pinnae on mice and rats.

There is no need to starve—prolonged fasting can lead to hypoglycemia.

Premedication

1. Premedication is rarely used, but it does permit easier, smoother anesthetic induction; this should be balanced against increased recovery times where short operations are performed.
2. Suitable premedications include:
   a. Acepromazine: 0.5 to 5.0 mg/kg IM or IP
   b. Diazepam: 2.5 to 5.0 mg/kg IM or IP
   c. Midazolam: 2.5 to 5.0 mg/kg IM or IP
3. Premedicate 45 to 60 minutes before gaseous anesthesia.
4. Mask down or use induction chamber with isoflurane. Induction is usually quick due to high respiratory rates.

Parenteral anesthesia

1. Always weigh accurately.
2. Always supply oxygen by face mask.
3. Many rodents fail to lose withdrawal reflex and may respond to surgical stimuli; therefore, you may need to use low concentration of inhalation anesthetic or infiltrate with local anesthetic.
4. There is a range of published anesthetic regimens. The author has found the following of use:
   a. Ketamine: 50 to 100 mg/kg plus xylazine 2.0 to 10 mg/kg IP
   b. Ketamine: 50 to 100 mg/kg plus medetomidine 0.25 to 1.0 mg/kg IP

Cardiopulmonary resuscitation

For respiratory arrest

1. Administer 100% oxygen.
2. Assist ventilation—compress thorax at around 60×/min.
3. Doxapram sublingual or at 10 mg/kg IV or IP. *Note:* This will increase the animal's oxygen demand.
4. If appropriate, give atipamezole.

For cardiac arrest

1. As for respiratory arrest. *But also:*
2. Compress thorax at around 90×/min.
3. If asystole—give epinephrine at 0.1 mg/kg IV, IO, repeat if necessary every 3-5 minutes of 1:10,000.
4. If ventricular fibrillation—lidocaine (lignocaine) at 1 to 2 mg/kg IV, IO, Intratracheal; repeat after 3-5 minutes if needed.

Skin disorders

Syrian hamsters have large, bilaterally symmetrical hip glands; these are scent glands used for marking burrow walls; in males they can be particularly pronounced in both size and the amount of sebaceous secretion they produce. These are frequently mistaken as skin lesions. Dwarf hamsters and gerbils possess ventral scent glands visible on the abdomen.

Pruritus

- Ectoparasites (Fig. 4-2)
- Otitis externa (ear mites)
- Pyoderma (see also "Abscessation" below)
- Diet-associated dermatitis (mouse, see *Nutritional Disorders*)
- Allergic dermatitis
  - Swollen feet, palpebral swelling, ocular discharge, and sneezing (hamsters)
- Contact allergy to nickel (mouse)—typically see inflammation on nose, feet, and tail
- Nasal dermatitis (gerbil)

Alopecia

- Ectoparasites (see below)
- Dermatophytosis (rat, mouse—often asymptomatic)
- *Trichophyton* spp. and *Microsporum* spp.
- Barbering (usually done by dominant individual in group)
- Muzzle alopecia—secondary to repetitive rubbing of muzzle against bars during cage-bar chewing
- *Staphylococcus aureus* dermatitis (gerbil)—localized alopecia and erythema around the external nares

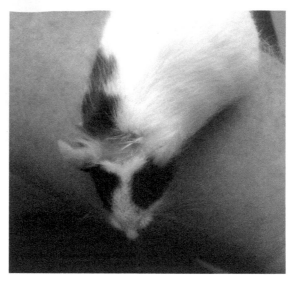

Fig 4-2. Trauma from *Myobia musculi* infestation in a mouse.

- Nasal dermatitis (gerbil): Alopecia and pruritic reddened scabs appear first around the external nares, mainly on the upper lip. May spread over the head and to the forepaws.
- Wood shaving and sawdust bedding made from treated wood
- Low-protein diet (<16%; hamster)
- Hormonal alopecia, especially hyperadrenocorticism in hamsters (see *Endocrine Disorders*)
- Cystic ovaries (see *Reproductive Disorders*)
- Satinization in hamsters: Individuals homozygous for the satin gene may have only a thin coating of hair.

Scaling and crusting

- Ectoparasites (*Radfordia*—rats; *Demodex, Notoedres*—hamsters)
- Dermatophytosis (rat, mouse; often asymptomatic)
- Build-up of wax and debris in the ear canals (ear mites, otitis externa)

Erosions and ulceration

- *Notoedres* (hamsters)
- On the dorsum of mice (ectoparasitic: *Myobia musculi* and *Mycoptes musculinus*). Resultant self-inflicted trauma can be severe. Black-coated strains of mice may be more prone to hypersensitivity reactions to these mites
- Bite wounds
- Sores and ulcers on the medial aspect of the legs of hamsters—abrasions secondary to wire wheel

Nodules and nonhealing wounds

- Ectromelia virus (mousepox); *Orthopoxvirus*
- Rat poxvirus *(Orthopoxvirus)*
- Hamster polyomavirus (HaPV, papovavirus)

- Self-inflicted trauma
- Abscessation, often resulting from bites; can be from pyoderma or bacteremic spread. *Staphylococcus aureus* is a common isolate, but others include *Streptococcus* spp., *Pasteurella* spp., and, in the mouse, *Actinobacillus* spp. and *Corynebacterium* spp. as well
- Rats with *Corynebacterium kutscheri* may have slightly enlarged cervical lymph nodes in addition to mild to severe respiratory disease.
- *Streptobacillus moniliformis* is a rare oral commensal in rats that can cause abscessation in rats following rats bites and rat-bite (Haverhill) fever in man.

Changes in pigmentation

- Rash (ectromelia virus in the mouse); nickel contact allergy (mouse)
- Seborrhea (especially older adult male rats)

Ectoparasites

- Rat
  - Mites: *Radfordia ensifera* (fur mite), *Myobia musculi* (fur mite), *Sarcoptes scabiei*, *Demodex nanus*, *Ornithonyssus bacoti* (tropical rat mite)
  - Ear mites: *Notoedres muris*—may infest the pinnae, face, tail, and extremities
  - Lice: *Polyplax spinulosa* (sucking louse)
  - Fleas: *Ctenocephalides felis*, *Xenopsylla* spp., *Leptosylla* spp., *Nosopsyllus* spp.
- Mouse
  - Mites: *Myobia musculi* (fur mite), *Mycoptes musculinus* (fur mite), *Radfordia affinis* (fur mite); *Sarcoptes scabiei* (rare), *Psorergates simplex* spp. (follicular mite—rare)
  - Ear mites: *Notoedres muris*
  - Lice: *Polyplax serrata* (sucking lice), *P. spinulosa*
  - Fleas: *Ctenocephalides felis*
- Hamster
  - *Demodex criceti* and *D. aurati*. Infestation more common than disease
  - *Sarcoptes scabiei*
  - *Ctenocephalides felis*
  - Ear mites: *Notoedres notoedres* and *N. cati* (but can have a more generalized distribution, including the face, genitalia, limbs, and tail)
  - *Ornithonyssus bacoti* (tropical rat mite; Fox et al 2004)
- Gerbil
  - Mites: *Demodex meroni*, *Liponyssoides sanguineus* (especially Egyptian gerbils, *Meriones libycus*); rarely *Sarcoptes scabiei* and *Notoedres muris*
  - Storage mites *(Acarus farris)* on cereal-based foods may occasionally cause irritation.

Neoplasia

- Squamous cell carcinoma
- Mammary adenocarcinomas (mouse—see *Reproductive Disorders*)
- Melanoma
- Hemangiosarcomas
- Trichoepitheliomas (in hamsters, may be related to HaPV infection)
- Dermal lymphoma (Kubiak and Denk 2014)

Necrosis of extremities

- Shortening of extremities secondary to necrosis (mouse—ectromelia virus)
- Ringtail (annular constrictions of the tail—rats)

Other

- Anemia, debilitation (*Ornithonyssus bacoti*, the tropical rat mite; heavy infestations of lice)
- *Note:* Lice (*Polyplax* spp.) can be vectors for *Encephalitozoon cuniculi, Eperythrozoon coccoides,* and *Haemobartonella muris.*
- Fleas (*Xenopsylla* spp. and *Nosopsyllus* spp.) can be vectors for *Yersinia pestis* (plague) and *Rickettsia typhus* and can act as intermediate hosts for *Hymenolepis* spp. (see *Gastrointestinal Tract Disorders*).

Findings on clinical examination

- Areas of alopecia
- Swellings, often firm consistency even if abscess. Displacement of normal outline of coat may indicate swelling.
- Cuts and abrasions
- Extreme pruritus
- Systemic signs
- Overgrown claws
- Pododermatitis—swelling and abscessation of the soles of the feet, especially the hind feet
- Areas of inflammation and excoriation around the nares in gerbils (nasal dermatitis, staphylococcal dermatitis)
- Hair loss and sores on legs of hamsters (repetitive trauma from wire wheel)
- Hair loss on one side of mouth (persistent bar gnawing)
- Seborrhea
- Multiple small lumps around neck in hamsters (with subsequent ulceration), weight loss; mortalities (can be up to 15% to 20%) (HaPV)

Investigations

1. Microscopy: examine fur pluck, acetate strips, or skin scrapes to affected area, and examine for ectoparasites.
2. Examine teeth. Rodents with dental disease may have difficulty grooming normally.
3. Radiography
   a. Pododermatitis—often underlying osteoarthritis
4. Routine hematology and biochemistry
   a. Eosinophilia (ectoparasitism)
5. Serology for ectromelia virus
6. Bacteriology and mycology: hair pluck or swab lesions for routine culture and sensitivity
7. Cytology
8. Gram stain
   a. Fine-needle aspirate followed by staining with rapid Romanowsky stains
9. Biopsy obvious lesions.
10. Ultraviolet (Wood's) lamp—positive for *Microsporium canis* only (not all strains fluoresce). Also porphyrins fluoresce (nasal dermatitis in gerbils).
11. Endocrine analysis: Thyroxine (see *Endocrine Disorders*), estradiol
12. If barbering suspected, examine hair under microscope to see if chewed; separate from other animals; supply extra hay.

Management

1. Pododermatitis
   a. Soft bedding
   b. Covering antibiosis
   c. Regular cleansing
   d. Application of topical amorphous hydrogel dressings, such as IntraSite Gel (Smith and Nephew Healthcare Ltd), encourages secondary healing.
   e. Attend to any underlying osteoarthritis with NSAIDs (e.g., meloxicam).

Treatment/specific therapy

- Poxviruses (including ectromelia virus)
  - No treatment; supportive only. Consider euthanasia. Rat poxvirus is a potential zoonosis.
- HaPV (papovavirus)
  - No treatment
  - Transmitted via the urine
  - Cull affected and in-contact animals.
- *Corynebacterium kutscheri* (pseudotuberculosis)
  - Appropriate antibiosis. Prevalence is variable.
- Dermatophytosis
  - Griseofulvin at 25 mg/kg PO once daily for 30 to 60 days
  - Miconazole/chlorhexidine (Malaseb, Leo) shampoo—bath once daily.
  - Itraconazole 5 mg/kg PO s.i.d. for 30 days
  - Improve ventilation.
- Ectoparasites
  - Ivermectin at 0.2 mg/kg SC or as topical (450 μg/tube) spot-on (Beaphar Anti-Parasite Spot-On for Small Animals, USA, Genitrix Xeno 450, UK) weekly for 3 to 4 weeks
  - Dust with pyrethrin powder.
  - For cases of severe self-inflicted trauma, NSAIDs plus prophylactic toe clipping may be necessary to reduce excoriation, plus antibiotics to control secondary infections.
- *Notoedres* in Syrian hamsters (Beco et al 2001)
  - Ivermectin at 400 μg/kg SC every 7 days for a minimum of 8 weeks
  - Moxidectin at 400 μg/kg PO every 7 days for a minimum of 8 weeks
- *Demodex* mites
  - Amitraz as wash at 100 mg/L applied topically every 7 days until resolution
  - Ivermectin as for *Notoedres*
  - Some mice may fail to respond to treatment; it is thought that some of these individuals may have inherent, genetic immune deficits while others may develop a hypersensitivity to mite antigen that is difficult to control.
- Storage mites
  - Topical fipronil spray applied with a cotton bud
  - Dispose of affected foods and clean storage containers.
- *Ornithonyssus bacoti* is a potential zoonosis (Beck and Pfister 2004).
- Ringtail
  - Surgical removal of affected part. Linked to low humidity (relative humidity <40%), so increase to 50% to 70%.

- Allergic dermatitis
  - Separate from all potential allergens, and where appropriate seek alternatives, including beddings, certain foods (see below), metallic objects (including caging), environmental triggers such as cigarette smoke.
  - For suspected dietary allergies an elimination protocol can be developed—remove all high-risk triggers (e.g., sunflower seeds, peanuts, colored dog biscuits) and replace with cooked rice, maize flakes, and fruits, including dried fruits (Richardson 2003).
- Diet-associated dermatitis
  - Change food to more appropriate ingredients (see *Nutritional Disorders*).
- NSAIDs to control pruritus
- Abscessation
  - Systemic antibiosis
  - Bathe wounds and apply topical antibiosis.
  - May require surgical removal
- Neoplasia
  - Surgical removal
  - Where surgery is considered nonviable, accessible cutaneous tumors can be treated by injecting cisplatin directly into the tissue mass on a weekly basis as a debulking exercise.
- Dermal lymphoma
  - Excision followed by chlorambucil 6 mg/kg PO every 3 days and prednisolone 3.0 mg/kg PO s.i.d. (Kubiak and Denk 2014) appeared to have an effect. Weekly hematology was carried out.
- Staphylococcal dermatitis
  - Topical and systemic antibiosis
  - Environmental modification: High humidity, fighting, and trauma are thought to predispose.
- Nasal dermatitis
  - May be linked to focal hyperplasia of the harderian glands and increased lachrymal secretion
  - Environmental modification; may be associated with trauma from burrowing into certain beddings; provision of sand may improve the condition.
  - Topical ophthalmic treatment may be beneficial.
- Sores on legs from wire wheel
  - Treat with topical preparations and switch to a solid backed and rimmed wheel.
- Seborrhea
  - Treat symptomatically with appropriate shampoos.

Respiratory tract disorders

Respiratory disease is a common presentation of pet rats. Typically it is multifactorial with concurrent bacterial and viral infections and so is often referred to as rat pneumonia complex.

Viral

- Paramyxovirus
- Sendai virus (rats and mice; forms part of rat pneumonia complex)
- Sialodacryoadenitis virus (SDAV; coronavirus—rats; see also *Gastrointestinal Tract Disorders* and *Ophthalmic Disorders*)
- Mouse hepatitis virus (MHV—mouse; see also *Gastrointestinal Tract Disorders*)

Bacterial

- *Pasteurella pneumotropica*
- Mycoplasmosis, esp. *M. pulmonis* (rats and mice; forms part of rat pneumonia complex)
- Cilia-associated respiratory bacillus (CAR; part of rat pneumonia complex)
- *Streptococcus pneumoniae* (rats—see also *Cardiovascular and Hematologic Disorders*)
- *Corynebacterium kutscheri* (pseudotuberculosis); often subclinical (rats and mice)
- Listeriosis (bushy-tailed jirds, *Sekeetamys calurus*); acute pneumonitis (see also *Gastrointestinal Tract Disorders*)

Fungal

Neoplasia

- Alveologenic carcinoma
- Pulmonary metastases from other neoplasias, especially uterine adenocarcinomas

Other noninfectious problems

- Allergic disorders (e.g., to fine sawdust)
- Heart disease (see *Cardiovascular and Hematologic Disorders*)
- High environmental ammonia levels

Findings on clinical examination

- Upper respiratory signs, such as sneezing, porphyrin staining around the eyes (Fig. 4-3)
- Swollen neck and eyes; ophthalmic lesions (SDAV in rats)

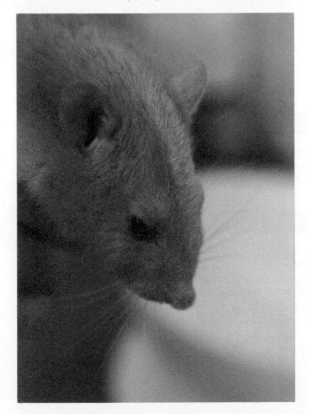

Fig 4-3. Porphyrin-stained tears in a rat.

- Respiratory distress—can be severe
- Cyanosis of mucous membranes, feet, nares, and tails (rats and mice)
- Tachypnea: Estimates for the normal respiratory rates of small mammals can be achieved with the following formula:

$$\text{Respiratory rate} = 53.5 \times wt^{-0.26}, \text{ where } wt = \text{body weight in kg}$$

- Dyspnea
- Marked lung sounds
- Rhinitis and nasal discharge
- Torticollis, circling, and other neurologic disorders (see *Neurologic Disorders*)
- Weight loss, anorexia
- Pyrexia

Investigations

1. Differentiate porphyrin staining from blood by either using blood "dipstick" tests or UV light (porphyrins fluoresce).
2. Radiography
   a. Pneumonia
3. Routine hematology and biochemistry
4. Polymerase chain reaction (PCR) for *M. pulmonis,* Sendai virus, CAR, SDAV, MHV
5. Culture and sensitivity (including from tracheal wash)
6. Cytology from tracheal wash
7. Pleural tap and cytology
8. Culture and sensitivity
9. *Mycoplasma* culture
10. Cytology
    a. Gram staining of discharges or effusions
11. Endoscopy
12. Ultrasonography

Management

- A clean, well-ventilated, but not drafty, air space is necessary.
- Some of the smaller module-based rodent housing has poor ventilation, which can produce areas of high humidity and high ammonia levels. Both of these can predispose to respiratory disease.

Treatment/specific therapy

- Viral infections
  - Control of secondary infections
  - For SDAV, MHV, and Sendai virus, attempt removal from breeding colonies by euthanizing all unweaned and weanling young and preventing breeding for 8 weeks. This allows immunocompetent adults to seroconvert and eradicate these viruses.
- Bacterial disease, including mycoplasmosis
  - Appropriate antibiosis
  - *M. pulmonis* infections may be exacerbated by concurrent SDAV.
- Rat pneumonia complex
  - Broad-spectrum antibiotics
  - NSAIDs (e.g., meloxicam)

- Mucolytics such as bromhexine and *N*-acetylcysteine may be useful.
- Improved environmental conditions (i.e., sanitation and ventilation)
- Often cure is impractical; control of the condition is often the case.
- Allergic disease
  - Often only one in a group affected.
  - Consider NSAIDs or antihistamines as a control.
  - Avoid suspected antigens.

Gastrointestinal tract disorders

Disorders of the oral cavity

In small rodents, the cheek teeth either grow very slowly or not at all, so dental disease involving these is rare. Gnawing in rodents involves a significant rostrocaudal movement of the lower jaw relative to the upper; therefore, the lower incisors are naturally long. True indicators of incisor malocclusion include uneven wear, sloping of the cutting edges, fractured teeth, altered pigmentation, and obvious pathological overgrowth.

The hemimandibular junction is flexible, and it is normal for the lower incisors to be able to deviate from each other during manipulation.

Permanent dental formula of a rodent

$$I:\frac{1}{1}, \quad C:\frac{0}{0}, \quad PM:\frac{0}{0}, \quad M:\frac{3}{3}$$

Dental disorders

- Incisor malocclusion—secondary to fractures, developmental problems, hereditary predisposition
- In some cage bar–chewing rodents the cutting edges of the incisors may show a slope to one side associated with uneven wear due to repetitive gnawing on vertical bars.
- Some rodents with grossly overgrown incisors may present with weight loss secondary to extreme incisor malocclusion that results in an inability to physically close the mouth for mastication.
- Dental caries can be common in rodents fed treats high in sugar and other carbohydrates or acidic foods.
- Burr back overgrown incisors. Avoid rotation of tooth during this process to reduce risk of trauma.
- Provide something to gnaw on (e.g., safe wood or dog biscuit).
- Incisor extraction: Significant risk of mandibular fracture
- Tooth root abscessation
  - Surgical debridement and covering antibiosis.

Cheek pouches

Very well developed in hamsters and some other rodents (e.g., chipmunks)
- Cheek pouch impaction
  - Food accumulation; may begin to autolyze and secondary infection ensues. Empty under general anesthesia (GA).
- Cheek pouch eversion/prolapse/neoplasia (Fig. 4-4)
  - Some cases may respond to gentle replacement.
  - Requires surgical resection

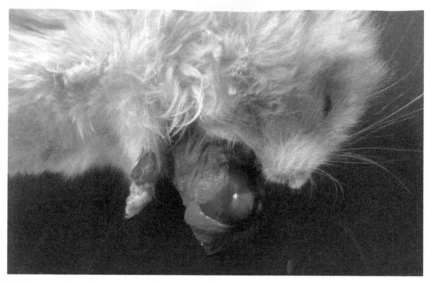

Fig 4-4. Prolapsed cheek pouch secondary to neoplasia.

Foreign bodies

- The rodent may display an apparent malocclusion, hypersalivation, and discomfort around the mouth. Require removal, possibly under GA

Differential diagnoses for gastrointestinal disorders

Coprophagy is commonly practiced by many small rodents. Hamsters have a stomach divided into two compartments: an aglandular forestomach (which allows some pregastric fermentation to occur, especially of ingested feces) and the true glandular stomach.

Viral

- SDAV (coronavirus—rats; see also *Respiratory Tract Disorders* and *Ophthalmic Disorders*)
- MHV (coronavirus—mouse; see also *Respiratory Tract Disorders*)
- Rotavirus (mouse)
- Reovirus (mouse)

Bacterial

- *Citrobacter freundii* (mouse)
- *Clostridium piliforme* (Tyzzer disease—all rodents, especially gerbils)
- Salmonellosis, especially *Salmonella enteriditis* and *S. typhimurium*
- Listeriosis (bushy-tailed jirds, *Sekeetamys calurus*); disease characterized by acute deaths without clinical signs
- Proliferative ileitis or wet-tail in hamsters
- *Lawsonia intracellularis*
- *Campylobacter* spp.
- *Escherichia coli*
- *Yersinia pseudotuberculosis*
- *Pasteurella* (enteritis in hamsters)

Protozoal

- Rat
  - *Cryptosporidium parvum*
  - *Eimeria* spp. (rare)
  - *Giardia muris*
  - *Spironucleus muris*
- Mouse
  - *Cryptosporidium muris, C. parvum*
  - *Eimeria* spp., common in wild mice *(E. falciformis, E. musculi, E. schueffneri, E. krijgsmanni, E. keilini, E. hindlei)*
  - *G. muris*
  - *Trichomonas muris*
  - *Spironucleus muris*
  - *Entamoeba muris*
- Hamster
  - *Cryptosporidium* spp. (see "Proliferative Ileitis" in *Treatment/Specific Therapy* below)
  - *Giardia* spp.
  - *Balantidium coli* and *B. caviae*
  - *Spironucleus muris*
  - *Tritrichomonas muris*
  - *Entamoeba muris*

Parasitic

- Rat
  - Nematodes: *Aspiculuris tetraptera, Syphacia muris* (pinworms), *Trichosomoides crassicauda*
  - Cestodes: *Hymenolepis nana* and *H. diminuta*
- Mouse
  - Nematodes: *A. tetraptera, Syphacia obveolata, Trichuris muris*
  - Cestodes: *H. nana, H. diminuta,* and *H. microstoma*
- Gerbil
  - Nematodes: *S. muris* and *S. obveolata* (pinworms), *Dentostomella translucida* (oxyurid)
  - Cestodes: *Hymenolepis nana*
- Hamster
  - Nematodes: *S. obveolata* (pinworms) and *A. tetraptera*
  - Cestodes: *H. nana*

Nutritional

- Sudden change in dietary composition (e.g., influx of vegetable material)

Neoplasia

- Intestinal polyps
- Forestomach papillomas
- Intestinal adenocarcinoma

Other noninfectious problems

- Antibiotic-induced enterotoxicosis (often secondary to *Clostridium difficile*)
- Intussusception
- Rectal prolapse
- Gut stasis/impaction

Findings on clinical examination

- Diarrhea, soiling around the perineum
- Nonspecific signs of ill health (e.g., hunched posture, ruffled coat)
- Weight loss
- Rectal prolapse (*C. freundii* in mice)
- Death
- Cervical thickening (swollen salivary glands, lymph nodes), ocular swelling (swollen lachrimal glands), and ocular discharge (SDAV in rats)
- CNS signs (e.g., head tilt, ataxia indicate neurologic involvement such as with *Clostridium piliforme*)
- Testicular enlargement suggestive of salmonellosis in gerbils (Laber-Laird 1996)
- Proliferative ileitis (wet-tail) in hamsters
  - Acute: Acute enteritis with profuse and often hemorrhagic diarrhea
  - Subacute: Stunting, dehydration and diarrhea, palpable abdominal viscus, mortalities
  - Chronic: Few overt, clinical signs; palpable ileal lesions, sudden death. This may explain some outbreaks without contact with other hamsters.

Investigations

1. Fecal examination
   a. Microscopy of wet prep; flotation
2. *Aspiculuris* ova are symmetrical; *Syphacia* are asymmetrical (slightly banana shaped). *Syphacia* deposits eggs around anus while *Aspiculuris* does not, so use acetate strip test for *Syphacia*.
3. *H. diminuta* and *H. microstoma* ova have polar filaments. *H. nana* and *H. diminutia* eggs have three pairs of hooks.
4. *Spironucleus muris*—look for cysts in feces (shaped like Easter eggs); trophozoites in small intestine (wet mounts, histology). Usually subclinical
5. Radiography
   a. Intestinal obstruction (parasites, neoplasia, foreign bodies)
   b. Ileus (obstruction, compromise of gut motility, dietary-induced gut disorder)
6. Routine hematology and biochemistry
7. PCR for *C. piliforme*, SDAV, MHV
8. Culture and sensitivity
9. Ultrasonography
10. Endoscopy
11. Biopsy
    a. Wet-tail without ileal hyperplasia may be caused by *E. coli*.
12. Postmortem
    a. Gross thickening of colon and rectum (*C. freundii* in mice)
    b. Yellowish foci in the liver and myocardium *(C. piliformis)*
    c. Multiple microabscessation, especially liver and spleen *(Yersinia)*

Management

- Fluid therapy
- In cases of severe disruption of the gut environment and its commensal flora, consider supplementation with vitamin B compounds.
- Probiotics may be of benefit.

Treatment/specific therapy

- Bacterial diseases, including *C. freundii*
  - Appropriate antibiosis
  - Address any stress factors (e.g., environmental temperatures and overcrowding).
- *C. piliformis* (Tyzzer disease)
  - Appropriate antibiosis and supportive care
- *Yersinia*
  - Appropriate antibiosis
  - Strict sanitation
  - Prevent access of wild rodents and birds to pet rodent food/living areas.
- Proliferative ileitis (wet-tail) in hamsters
  - Fluid therapy plus good nursing care (see *Nursing Care*)
  - Appropriate antibiosis
    - Enrofloxacin at 5 mg/kg PO or SC or as 10 mg/100 mL fresh drinking water daily
    - Erythromycin at 100 mg/L fresh (distilled or de-ionized) drinking water
    - Oxytetracycline at 400 mg/L fresh drinking water
  - *Cryptosporidium:* No effective treatment. Consider potentiated sulfonamides or nitazoxanide (100mg/kg PO b.i.d. for 3 days).
  - Strict sanitation
- Protozoa
  - Sulfamethazine at 0.2% in drinking water for 7 to 10 days
  - Metronidazole at 2.5 mg/mL in drinking water
- Nematodes
  - Ivermectin at 0.2 mg/kg SC or as topical (450 µg/tube) spot-on (Beaphar Anti-Parasite Spot-On for Small Animals, USA, Genitrix Xeno 450, UK) weekly for 3 to 4 weeks
  - Topical emodepside plus praziquantel preparations (Profender, Bayer) at 0.004 mL/30 g body weight (Mehlhorn et al 2005a)
  - Topical imidacloprid and moxidectin compound (Advocate Cat, Bayer) reduced *T. muris* burdens by up to 95% at a concentration of 128 mg imidacloprid and 32 mg moxidectin/kg body weight (Mehlhorn et al 2005b).
- Cestodes, including *Hymenolepis* spp.
  - Praziquantel at 5 to 10 mg/kg PO or SC. Repeat after 10 days.
  - *Note:* All species have intermediate arthropod hosts, but *H. nana* can have a direct life cycle. Zoonotic hazard, especially with *H. nana*, as no intermediate host required.
- Sudden dietary changes
  - Switch to dried food only.
  - If pronounced diarrhea, consider fluid therapy (see *Nursing Care*)
  - Do not use antibiotics unless specifically indicated, as these may retard the reestablishment of the normal gut flora.
- Antibiotic-induced enterotoxicosis
  - As for "Sudden dietary changes" above
  - Cease antibiotic administration.
  - Supplementation with probiotics *may* be useful.
  - Vitamin B supplementation
- Intussusception
  - Especially seen in hamsters
  - Euthanasia or surgical correction

- Rectal prolapse
  - May be secondary to diarrhea or intussusception
  - Surgical correction
  - Supportive nursing
- Gut stasis/impaction
  - May be linked to systemic disease, dry foods, and foreign bodies (e.g., bedding fibers)
  - Laxatives and gut motility enhancers (e.g., metoclopramide at 0.2 to 1.0 mg/kg PO, SC) may be of benefit.
  - Surgical removal of foreign bodies

Nutritional disorders

- Diet-associated dermatitis (mouse), possibly linked to high sunflower and nut diet (Richardson 2003)
- Hypovitaminosis E in hamsters (see *Musculoskeletal Disorders* and *Reproductive Disorders*)

Findings on clinical examination

- Pruritus in mice (diet-associated dermatitis)

Treatment/specific therapy

- Diet-associated dermatitis
  - NSAIDs (e.g., meloxicam)
  - Place on simpler diet or proprietary pelleted mouse food.

Hepatic disorders

A gallbladder is present in the mouse, gerbil, and hamster but absent in the rat.

Bacterial
- Listeriosis (gerbils)
- Salmonellosis

Neoplasia
- Hepatic carcinoma

Other noninfectious disorders
- Amyloidosis (see *Systemic Disorders*)

Findings on clinical examination

- Vague signs of ill health
- Diarrhea
- Weight loss
- Jaundice
- Polydipsia/polyuria
- Poor blood clotting (hepatic lipidosis)
- Hepatomegaly

Investigations

1. Radiography
2. Routine hematology and biochemistry
3. Culture and sensitivity
4. Endoscopy
5. Biopsy
6. Ultrasonography

Management

- Fluid therapy
- Milk thistle *(Silybum marianum)* is hepatoprotectant; dose at 4 to 15 mg/kg PO b.i.d. or t.i.d.
- Lactulose at 0.5 mL/kg PO b.i.d.

Treatment/specific therapy

1. Bacterial infections
   a. Guarded prognosis
   b. Antibiosis

Pancreatic disorders

Diabetes mellitus (see *Endocrine Disorders*)

Cardiovascular and hematologic disorders

Cardiac disease is considered very common in Syrian hamsters, such that heart failure may represent a common aging-related cause of mortality (Schmidt and Reavill 2007). Rodent heart rates are fast. As a guide the normal heart rate of a rodent can be reasonably estimated with the following formula:

$$\text{Heart rate} = 241 \times wt^{-0.25} \text{ where } wt = \text{body weight in kg}$$

Viral

- Encephalomyocarditis virus (hamsters)
- Hamster leukemia virus

Bacterial

- *Streptococcus pneumoniae* (rats—see also *Respiratory Tract Disorders*)
- *Bacillus piliformis* (Tyzzer disease)
- *Erysipelothrix rhusiopathiae* (see *Systemic Disorders*)
- Septicemia (phlebothrombosis) with, for example, *Salmonella* spp.
- Myocarditis (suppurative)

Fungal

Protozoal

- *Haemobartonella muris* (rat)
- *Eperythrozoon coccoides* (mouse)

Parasitic

Dietary

Neoplasia

- Lymphocytic leukemia

Other noninfectious problems

- Cardiomyopathy (Syrian hamsters)
  - Autosomal recessive in the Bio 14.6 strain
  - Inherited dilated cardiomyopathy in Bio TO-2 strain
- Congenital cardiac and aortic anomalies (Syrian hamsters)
- Atrial thromboses (Syrian hamsters)
- Calcifying vasculopathy (Syrian hamsters)
- Myocardial fibrosis (acute and chronic)
- Polyarteritis nodosus (rat)—can cause aneurysms, thrombus formation, and stenosis of blood vessels, leading to multiple organ disruption or failure
- Anemia secondary to other causes (e.g., hemorrhage, hemolytic anemias, anemia of chronic disease, neoplasia, chronic renal disease)

Findings on clinical examination

- Anemia
- Exercise intolerance
- Heart abnormalities (e.g., arrhythmias, abnormal heart sounds)
- Exaggerated breathing postures (air hunger) and other respiratory signs
- Pulmonary edema
- Cyanosed extremities
- Splenomegaly, hepatomegaly
- Lymphadenopathy
- Sudden death (may be due to rupture of aneurysms formed in polyarteritis nodosus)

Investigations

1. Radiography
   a. Pericardial effusions *(S. pneumoniae)*
2. Routine hematology and biochemistry
3. Culture and sensitivity
   a. Gram stain effusions *(S. pneumoniae)*
4. Endoscopy
5. Ultrasonography
6. ECG

Management

- Supportive treatment, including vitamin B_{12} for anemia

Treatment/specific therapy

- Cardiomyopathies
  - Benazepril at <0.1 mg/kg PO s.i.d.
  - Furosemide 0.3 to 4 mg/kg PO, SC, IM, or IV s.i.d. or b.i.d.

- Intraerythrocytic protozoa
  - *H. muris* and *E. coccoides* transmitted by *Polyplax* lice (see *Skin Disorders*), so control by treatment for these.
- Hamster leukemia virus
  - No effective treatment

Systemic disorders
• •

See also *Endocrine Disorders*.

Viral
- Ectromelia virus (mouse pox; *Orthopoxvirus*)
- LCM virus (arenavirus)
- HaPV (papovavirus—see also *Skin Disorders*)

Bacterial
- Salmonellosis, especially *Salmonella enteritidis*
- *Streptobacillus moniliformis*
- *Erysipelothrix rhusiopathiae* (rare—see also *Cardiovascular and Hematologic Disorders*)

Neoplasia
- Lymphoma (in hamsters can be related to HaPV)

Other noninfectious problems
- Dental disease (see *Gastrointestinal Tract Disorders*)
- Amyloidosis
- Dystrophic calcification
- Polyarteritis nodosa (rat)—can cause aneurysms, thrombus formation and stenosis of blood vessels, leading to multiple organ disruption or failure
- Pregnancy toxemia in hamsters
- Polycystic disease in hamsters
- Hypothermia

Findings on clinical examination

- Extreme weight loss
- Hunched posture, staring, ruffled fur
- Loss of interest in surroundings
- Overgrowth of incisors, causing masticatory difficulties
- Arthritis, limb abnormalities, distal limb necrosis (mice—streptobacillosis, ectromelia virus; see *Skin Disorders*)
- Stunting of mice, renal disease (LCM virus)
- Sudden death
- Multiple small lumps around the neck area in hamsters (HaPV—see *Skin Disorders*)
- Polyarthritis, myocarditis, and endocarditis (erysipelas)
- Subnormal body temperature (using rectal thermometer and/or remote thermal sensing)

Investigations

1. Radiography
2. Routine hematology and biochemistry
3. Serology for LCM virus
4. Culture and sensitivity
5. Endoscopy
6. Biopsy
7. Ultrasonography
8. Postmortem
   a. Multifocal necrosis of liver, lymphoid tissue, intestine, spleen, integument, and other organs (mouse—ectromelia virus)
   b. One to many cysts in one or more organs. Cysts contain an amber fluid (hamster—polycystic kidney disease).
   c. Polyarthritis, myocarditis, endocarditis (erysipelas)

Management

- Supportive care, including fluid therapy, covering antibiosis where applicable

Treatment/specific therapy

- LCM virus: Potentially fatal zoonosis, so consider euthanasia.
- Salmonellosis: Can consider treatment with appropriate antibiosis but is potential zoonosis.
- Streptobacillosis: Appropriate antibiosis. Asymptomatically carried by rats in the oral cavity; is potentially zoonotic as rat-bite fever
- Erysipelas
  - Appropriate antibiosis
- Pregnancy toxemia
  - Similar to ketosis seen in guinea pigs (see "Ketosis" in Chapter 3)
- Polycystic disease
  - Hereditary disorder, rare in hamsters below age 1 year
  - No treatment
- Hypothermia
  - See *Nursing Care.*

Musculoskeletal disorders

Viral
- LCM virus

Nutritional
- Hypovitaminosis E (see also *Reproductive Disorders*)

Neoplasia
Other noninfectious problems
- Limb bone fractures
- Spinal trauma

- Myopathies in hamsters
- Progressive hind-limb paralysis in hamsters
- Kinked tail in mice (inherited)
- See also *Neurologic Disorders*.

Findings on clinical examination

- Muscle weakness and paralysis
- Reproductive problems in hamsters (hypovitaminosis E)

Investigations

1. Radiography
2. Routine hematology and biochemistry
3. Culture and sensitivity
4. Endoscopy
5. Biopsy
6. Ultrasonography

Treatment/specific therapy

- LCM virus: Potentially fatal zoonosis, so consider euthanasia.
- Hypovitaminosis E
  - Supplement with dietary vitamin E.
- Fractures
  - Closed fractures can be treated conservatively with cage rest and analgesia.
  - Internal fixation may be possible in some cases using a hypodermic needle as an intramedullary pin; external fixation and supportive dressings are likely to be chewed and damaged.
  - Open fractures may require amputation.
- Myopathies in hamsters
  - Often strain specific
  - Affected hamsters have shortened life spans.
  - Not all muscle groups are affected equally; the limb adductor muscles are the first and most severely affected.
- Progressive hind-limb paralysis in Syrian hamsters
  - Sex-linked, occurs in males; Bio 12.14 strain; a degenerative peripheral neuropathy

Neurologic disorders

Viral

- Murine encephalitis virus, or MEV; (rare—mouse, rat)
- Rabies (very rare—wild rodents)

Bacterial

- *Mycoplasma pulmonis* (rat, mouse—see *Respiratory Tract Disorders*)
- *Streptococcus pneumoniae* (rat, mouse—see *Respiratory Tract Disorders*)
- *Clostridium piliforme* (see *Gastrointestinal Tract Disorders*), especially gerbil

Protozoal

- *Encephalitozoon cuniculi* (rats)

Neoplasia

- Pituitary hyperplasia/adenomas in rats (see *Endocrine Disorders*)

Other noninfectious problems

- Trauma
- Radiculoneuropathy (spinal nerve root degeneration)
- Seizures—inherited predisposition in gerbils, possibly linked to a deficiency of glutamine synthetase
- Streptomycin administration in gerbils (causes neuromuscular blockade, paralysis, and death)
- See also *Musculoskeletal Disorders*.

Findings on clinical examination

- Torticollis (including otitis media/interna)
- Circling (including otitis media/interna)
- Weakness
- Flaccid paralysis of hind legs
- Seizures; in gerbils can last for up to 5 minutes.

Investigations

1. Radiography
2. Routine hematology and biochemistry
3. Serology for MEV, *E. cuniculi*, rabies (very rare)
4. Culture and sensitivity
5. Endoscopy
6. Biopsy
7. Ultrasonography

Management

- Supportive care, including hand feeding and attending to sores and abrasions

Treatment/specific therapy

- Viral disorders
  - Rare; if diagnosed, consider euthanasia.
- Rabies: Euthanasia
- Otitis media
  - Treat with appropriate antibiotics, both topical and systemic. Ensure eardrum is intact before treatment.
- Otitis interna
  - Appropriate systemic antibiosis depending on etiology
  - If bulla osteotomy is required, swab for culture and sensitivity.

- *E. cuniculi*
  - Co-trimoxazole at 30 mg/kg PO b.i.d. for at least 3 weeks
  - Albendazole at 10 mg/kg PO s.i.d. for 6 weeks
  - Fenbendazole at 10 mg/kg s.i.d. PO for 1 month
- Radiculoneuropathy
  - Consider euthanasia. Small "carts" have been used to support the back-end of rats with similar disorders, thereby allowing some voluntary movement. The ethics of this should be considered carefully.
- Seizures
  - Phenobarbital at 10 to 20 mg/kg PO b.i.d.
  - Phenytoin at 25 to 50 mg/kg PO b.i.d.

Ophthalmic disorders

In rats, mice, and gerbils the harderian gland can produce tears rich in porphyrins when the rodent has a concurrent illness. These porphyrins can stain the fur around the eyes and external nares a reddish-brown color—this can be mistaken by owners for hemorrhage; differentiate either by exposing to UV light (porphyrins fluoresce) or by testing on a urine dipstick (Fig. 4-3).

Viral

- SDAV (coronavirus—rats)

Bacterial

- Uveitis

Parasitic

- *Rhabditis orbitalis* (rare)

Neoplasia
Other noninfectious problems

- Allergies
- Prolapse (especially Syrian hamsters)
- Glaucoma (possibly inherited in Campbell's Russian hamsters)
- Keratitis sicca
- Microphthalmia/anophthalmia (recessive disorder in black-eyed white, white-bellied, and dominant-spot Syrian hamsters—see Richardson 2003)
- Diabetes mellitus (Russian and Chinese hamsters)

Findings on clinical examination

- Porphyrin secretion around the eyes (SDAV in rats)
- Suborbital swelling (SDAV in rats)
- Keratitis
- Uveitis
- Cataracts (see *Endocrine Disorders*)
- Corneal ulceration
- Deaths in weanling rats (SDAV in rats)
- Upper respiratory tract signs and swollen neck/salivary glands (SDAV in rats—see *Gastrointestinal Tract Disorders* and *Respiratory Tract Disorders*)

- Swollen globe (glaucoma); may prolapse and/or ulcerate
- Nematodes present on the cornea *(Rhabditis orbitalis)*

Investigations

1. Routine ophthalmic examination
2. Radiography
3. Routine hematology and biochemistry
4. Culture and sensitivity
5. Endoscopy
6. Biopsy
7. Ultrasonography
8. Tonometry
    a. Rat: 13.9 ± 4.2 mm Hg (Lewis rats)
    b. Mice: 13.7 ± 0.8 mm Hg (C3H strain); 12.3 ± 0.5 mm Hg (B6 strain); 9.4 ± 0.5 mm Hg (A/J strain); 7.7 ± 0.5 mm Hg (BALB/c strain)

Treatment/specific therapy

- Uveitis
    - Topical ophthalmic steroid or NSAID preparations
    - Topical ophthalmic antibiotic preparations plus systemic antibiosis if appropriate
    - Enucleation if severe
- Prolapse/ulceration
    - Tarsorrhaphy
- Glaucoma
    - Enucleation (hereditary form)
    - Otherwise treat as for uveitis.
- Keratitis sicca
    - Topical cyclosporine A ointment
    - Covering antibiosis
- *Rhabditis orbitalis*
    - Ivermectin at 400 µg/kg SC, topically; repeat weekly as necessary.

Endocrine disorders

Neoplasia

- Thyroid neoplasia
    - C-cell tumors (rats)
    - Follicular cell adenomas (mice)
- Hyperadrenocorticism (Cushing disease)
    - Adrenocortical adenoma/carcinoma
    - Pituitary adenoma
- Insulinomas

Other noninfectious problems

- Hypothyroidism
- Diabetes mellitus (inherited in Russian and Chinese hamsters)
- Iatrogenic hyperadrenocorticism (glucocorticoid therapy)

Findings on clinical examination

- Bilateral symmetrical alopecia of flanks
- Weight loss
- Ataxia, head tilt, and other CNS signs (pituitary hyperplasia/adenomas)
- Thin skin (hyperadrenocorticism)
- Alopecia, hyperpigmentation, cold intolerance, thick skin, and lethargy (hypothyroidism in hamsters)
- Hyperpigmentation
- Polydipsia, polyuria, polyphagia (hyperadrenocorticism, diabetes mellitus)
- Cataracts, weight loss (diabetes mellitus)
- Secondary infections and parasitic infestations (diabetes mellitus)
- Intermittent weakness, collapse, seizures (insulinoma)
- Pseudopregnancy, mammary gland hyperplasia/neoplasia (pituitary hyperplasia/adenomas in rats—see also *Reproductive Disorders*)

Investigations

1. Radiography
2. Routine hematology and biochemistry
   a. Diabetes mellitus (Table 4-5)
   b. Hyperadrenocorticism (Table 4-6). *Note:* Hamsters may secrete both cortisol and corticosterone, so diagnosis on cortisol levels alone may be inaccurate.
   c. Hypothyroidism (Table 4-7)

Table 4-5 Small rodents: Diabetes mellitus

Species	Blood glucose: normal range (mmol/L)	Blood glucose: diabetic (mmol/L)
Syrian hamster	3.6-7.0	>16
Gerbil	2.8-7.5	
Rat	4.7-7.3	
Mouse	3.3-12.7	

Table 4-6 Small rodents: Hyperadrenocorticism

Species	Blood cortisol		ALP (IU/L)	
	Normal range (nmol/L)	Hyperadrenocorticism (mmol/L)	Normal range	Hyperadrenocorticism
Syrian hamster	13.8-27.6	<110.4	8-18	>40
Rat			39-216	
Mouse			28-94	

Table 4-7 Small rodents: Serum thyroxine levels

Species	$T_{4(total)}$ nM/L	$T_{3(total)}$ nM/L	$T_{4(free)}$ pM/L	$T_{3(free)}$ pM/L
Syrian hamster	46.3	0.7		
Mouse	39.7-61.0	1.3-1.7		
Rat	43.8-80.0	0.8-1.2	15.0-36.0	1.7-16.0
After Hulbert (2000).				

3. Culture and sensitivity
4. Urinalysis
   a. Ketonuria occasionally seen in diabetic hamsters
5. Endoscopy
6. Biopsy
7. Ultrasonography
   a. Enlarged adrenal gland(s)

Treatment/specific therapy

- Diabetes mellitus
  - Provide a high-fiber, low-fat diet.
  - Oral hypoglycemic agents such as glyburide may prove useful in hamsters.
  - The author has used the oral hypoglycemic metformin hydrochloride oral solution 500 mg/5ml at 0.1 mL b.i.d. in a rat with diabetes mellitus.
  - In rats, Keeble (2001) reports that twice-daily treatment with a medium duration insulin product at 1.0 IU/kg SC can give stabilization, combined with twice daily urinary glucose monitoring.
  - In hamsters, neutral protamine Hagedorn (NPH) insulin may be useful, but titration and subsequent dosage may prove difficult long term at home.
  - In gerbils diabetes mellitus is associated with obesity and high sunflower intake.
- Insulinoma
  - Surgical resection
  - Glucocorticoid therapy may give palliative results for a period of time.
- Hyperadrenocorticism
  - Pituitary hyperplasia/adenomas in rats
    - Toremifene at 12 mg/kg PO s.i.d.
    - Early ovariohysterectomy may prevent adenoma formation.
  - Surgical adrenalectomy
  - Hamsters (Keeble 2001): Metyrapone 8 mg PO s.i.d. for 4 weeks
    - Mitotane 5 mg PO s.i.d. for 4 weeks
    - Trilostane 2-4 mg/kg PO every 24 hours
  - Palliative and supportive treatment
- Hypothyroidism
  - Supplement with thyroxine (e.g., levothyroxine) at 10 µg/kg daily in divided doses.
- Thyroid neoplasia in rats
  - Usually involves C-cells and, therefore, does not produce typical thyroid disease–associated signs.

Urinary disorders

Viral
- LCM virus (arenavirus—mouse, hamster)

Bacterial
- Cystitis
- Leptospirosis (wild rodents); usually asymptomatic but is significant zoonosis

Parasitic
- *Trichosomoides crassicauda* (bladder threadworm)
- *Encephalitozoon cuniculi* (rats)

Neoplasia
- Can be related to *T. crassicauda* infestations in the rat

Other noninfectious problems
- Glomerulosclerosis, with an interstitial fibrosis (rats)
- Glomerulonephritis
- Amyloidosis
- Urolithiasis (especially hamsters)

Findings on clinical examination

- Nonspecific signs of ill health (e.g., hunched posture, ruffled coat, reduced appetite)
- Weight loss
- Polydipsia, polyuria
- Ascites
- Fibrous osteodystrophy
- Dysuria
- Hematuria
- Preputial hemorrhage
- Uroliths may be palpable in the penile urethra of males (especially hamsters)
- Hairlike nematode visible in rat urine *(T. crassicauda)*

Investigations

1. Urinalysis (Table 4-8)
2. Radiography
3. Calculi (may accompany *T. crassicauda* infestations in the rat)
4. Routine hematology and biochemistry
   a. Rats with glomerulosclerosis, biochemistry findings may show elevated urea (normal, 2.2 to 8.3 mmol/L) and creatinine (normal, 17.7 to 70.7 μmol/L).
   b. Eosinophilia *(T. crassicauda)*
5. Serology for LCM virus
6. Culture and sensitivity
7. Endoscopy
8. Ultrasonography
9. Biopsy

Table 4-8 Small rodents: Typical urinalysis values

Value	Rat	Syrian hamster
Urine volume	5.5 mL/100 g per day	Around 7.0 mL/day total
Crystals		Triple phosphate and calcium carbonate crystals (in some cricetids allantoin is excreted)
Protein	<0.5 g/L. *Note:* By 12-14 months old, up to 50% of rats will have a proteinuria >2.0 g/L.	0-3 g/L; >30 g/L reported for renal disease
Urine gravity		1.014-1.060
pH		≈ 8.5
WBCs	Few	
Parasites	*Trichosomoides crassicauda* (bladder threadworm). Bioperculated, light brown, larvated ova in urine. May be accompanied by urinary WBCs	

Management

- Supportive care, especially fluid therapy
- Feed more natural diet; rats fed more refined foods tend to develop chronic renal disease earlier (Fallon 1996).

Treatment/specific therapy

- LCM virus: Potentially fatal zoonosis so consider euthanasia
- *T. crassicauda*
  - Combination therapy (Bowman et al 2004):
    - Ivermectin at 0.2 mg/kg SC weekly for 3 weeks
    - Fenbendazole at 20 mg/kg PO s.i.d. for 5 days
  - Thorough and repeated cage sanitation
- Urolithiasis
  - Cystotomy and/or urethrotomy
  - Hamsters especially prone as they naturally produce triple phosphate and calcium carbonate crystals in their urine.

Reproductive disorders

The mammary tissue in small rodents, especially rats and mice, can be quite extensive and may extend laterally up the neck, flanks, and perineum.

Viral

- Mouse mammary tumor viruses (MMTV; retroviruses)
- LCM virus (hamster, mouse—see *Systemic Disorders*)

Bacterial

- *Mycoplasma pulmonis* (endometritis, pyometra; rats—see *Respiratory Tract Disorders*)
- *Staphylococcus aureus* (preputial gland abscess—mouse, rat)

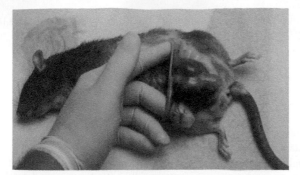

Fig 4-5. Postmortem showing uterine neoplasm in a rat.

- *Streptococcus* spp.; streptococcal mastitis in hamsters
- *Pasteurella pneumotropica* (preputial gland abscess, pyometra—mouse, rat, hamster)
- Salmonellosis (cause of testicular hyperplasia in gerbils—see *Gastrointestinal Tract Disorders*)
- Mastitis

Nutritional
- Hypovitaminosis E in hamsters

Neoplasia
- Uterine neoplasia (Fig. 4-5)
- Preputial gland neoplasia
- Mammary gland adenocarcinomas and carcinomas (especially mice); may be triggered by MMTV
- Mammary gland fibroadenomas (especially rats); can grow extremely large and suffer significant abrasions
- Ovarian neoplasia
- Interstitial cell tumors and other testicular neoplasia
- Pituitary hyperplasia/adenoma (rat—see *Endocrine Disorders*)

Other noninfectious problems
- Uterine prolapse (mouse—rare)
- Ovarian follicular cysts (cystic ovaries)
- Pseudopregnancy
- Physiologic postestrus vaginal discharge (hamster). This is clear and should not be mistaken for a vaginitis.
- Pregnancy toxemia (see *Systemic Disorders*)

Findings on clinical examination

- Swollen viscus palpable in females (uterine neoplasia, pyometra, pregnancy)
- Swollen abdomen (pregnancy, phantom pregnancy, abdominal mass, ascites)
- Symmetrical alopecia (cystic ovaries)
- Bilateral swelling around penis (preputial gland abscess—mouse, rat)
- Unilateral swelling next to penis (preputial gland neoplasia)

- Single or multiple swellings of mammary tissue. *Note:* In rats and mice the distribution of mammary tissue can be extensive, spreading some way up the flank, neck, and perineal area.
- Mastitis
- Pseudopregnancy, mammary gland hyperplasia/neoplasia, CNS signs, hyperadrenocorticism (pituitary hyperplasia/adenomas in rats—see also *Endocrine Disorders*)
- Male sterility, abnormal gestation, muscular weakness, and paralysis in hamsters (hypovitaminosis E)
- Testicular enlargement
  - If unilateral consider neoplasia. This appearance may be exacerbated as the other testicle may also reduce in size. Occasionally a hard mass may be palpable in an otherwise normal testicle.
  - Bilateral in gerbils—salmonellosis

Investigations

1. Radiography
   a. Enlarged uterus (pyometra, neoplasia)
2. Ovarian cysts
3. Routine hematology and biochemistry
4. Serology for LCM virus (hamster)
5. Culture and sensitivity
6. Endoscopy
7. Biopsy
8. Ultrasonography
   a. Ovarian cysts

Treatment/specific therapy

- Bacterial diseases
  - Appropriate antibiosis
  - Bacterial infections (e.g., pyometra) may follow an outbreak of respiratory disease
- LCM virus may induce pyometra
- Preputial gland abscess
  - Lance, flush, and drain. Administer appropriate antibiosis.
- Preputial gland neoplasm
  - Surgical removal
- Mammary gland neoplasia
  - Surgical resection
  - Implantation with the GnRH-agonist deslorelin (Suprelorin) at the time of surgery may prevent or delay the recurrence of further mammary neoplasia in rats.
  - Early implantation with deslorelin may prevent the formation of mammary neoplasia in rats.
  - Early ovariohysterectomy may reduce incidence of mammary neoplasia in rats.
- Other neoplasia
  - Surgical removal where practical
- Uterine prolapse
  - Replace uterus and apply suture to retain; poor prognosis; may require ovariohysterectomy

- Mastitis
  - Systemic antibiosis
  - May require debriding and application of antibiotics or medications to enhance healing (e.g., topical amorphous hydrogel dressings to encourage secondary healing such as IntraSite Gel from Smith and Nephew Healthcare Ltd)
- Pseudopregnancy
  - In hamsters, lasts 7 to 13 days; usually resolves spontaneously
- Ovarian cysts
  - Ovariohysterectomy (treatment of choice)
  - Draw fluid off by paracentesis
  - Attempt hCG at 1000 IU/kg SC weekly for 1 to 3 weeks
- Hypovitaminosis E in hamsters
  - Supplement with vitamin E.

5

Common or cotton-eared marmosets

The common marmoset is probably the most commonly kept primate. Its small size and ready availability mean that it has branched out from zoo and laboratory collections into the pet trade. Its tiny, humanlike face and features attract attention, but unfortunately many owners equate these with human characteristics too, and appear to base their expectations of marmoset behavior and care more on children's and comedy movies than the realities of keeping a nonhuman primate. Marmosets cannot be toilet-trained, have multiple scent glands that are used liberally, and if kept individually as a household pet are highly likely to develop behavioral abnormalities. There is also a significant zoonosis and reverse zoonosis risk. Kept in appropriate family groups in aviary-type accommodation, they can make fascinating pets, however.

Table 5-1 Common or cotton-eared marmosets: Key facts

Average life span (years)	8-12
Weight (g)	350-450 (adult)
	60-150 (weaning)
	25-35 (newborn)
Body temperature (°C)	38.4-39.1
Respiratory rate (per min)	36-44
Heart rate (beats per min)	230 ± 26 (unrestrained)
	348 ± 51 (restrained)
Gestation (days)	141-145
Age at weaning (days)	40-120
Sexual maturity (months)	8-12 (puberty)
	18-24 (sexual and social)

Consultation and handling

Common marmosets vary in their acceptance of handling, and one should also be mindful of the risk of bites and zoonosis. They can be restrained using a towel or with two or more handlers. Sedation with ketamine at 10 to 20 mg IM/adult marmoset, or masking with isoflurane, should be undertaken to enable further examination and sample taking.

Blood sampling

Femoral vein: No more than 1% body weight every 2 to 3 weeks. Apply pressure to prevent a hematoma forming. Smaller volumes can be taken from the saphenous vein.

Nursing care

Thermoregulation

Individual marmosets, with their small body size, can be prone to hypothermia. For general principles, see "Thermoregulation" under *Nursing Care* in Chapter 2.

Fluid therapy

Either intravenously via the saphenous (will need restraint) or subcutaneously. Volumes up to 3% to 4% body weight can be given subcutaneously in 4 to 5 divided amounts. Select fluids as for other small mammals.

Nutritional support

Marmosets in recovery can be given commercial omnivore supportive foods; it is thought that marmosets require 150 to 160 kcal/kg body mass per day (Morin 1980). The National Research Council (1978) recommends 3.5 to 4.5 g/kg body mass per day of high-quality protein for small primate species. This is particularly so for marmosets with marmoset wasting syndrome (see *Marmoset Wasting Syndrome*). These should be fed a high-protein, gluten-free diet; such marmosets also appear to need extra calcium (possibly to compensate for reduced uptake).

Analgesia

Table 5-2 Common or cotton-eared marmosets: Analgesic doses

Analgesic	Dosage
Paracetamol (acetaminophen)	5-10 mg/kg PO q.i.d. Pediatric suspensions are palatable and usually readily accepted.
Asprin (acetylsalicylic acid)	5-10 mg/kg PO every 4-6 hr
Ibuprofen	20 mg/kg PO daily
Carprofen	2-4 mg/kg PO daily to b.i.d.
Meloxicam	0.2 mg/kg PO daily
Buprenorphine	0.005-0.03 mg/kg IM or IV b.i.d. to q.i.d.
Butorphanol	0.01-0.02 mg/kg IM, SC, or IV b.i.d. to q.i.d. Can cause profound respiratory depression.
Morphine	1-2 mg/kg SC or IM q.i.d.
Naloxone	0.01-0.05 mg/kg IM or IV for opioid reversal

Anesthesia

Several anesthetic protocols have been described. The author finds the following combination useful, given IM combined in the same syringe:
- Ketamine 5.0 mg/kg *plus*
- Medetomidine 0.01 mg/kg
- Reverse medetomidine with atipamezole (same volume) IM

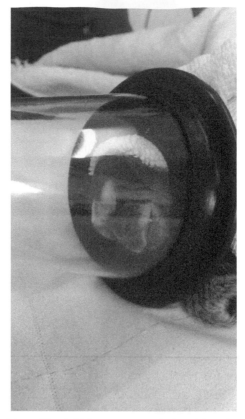

Fig 5-1. An induction mask is used to administer gaseous anesthetic and for maintenance with a marmoset.

As an alternative for longer procedures:

Parenteral anesthesia

1. Analgesia/premedication: buprenorphine
2. Ketamine 15.0 to 20.0 mg/kg IM
3. Propofol induction 2.0 to 5.0 mg/kg IV
4. Intubate and maintain on isoflurane.

For cesareans

1. Atropine at 0.02-0.05 mg/kg SC
2. Induce with isoflurane with mask (Fig. 5-1) or in induction chamber.

Mean arterial blood pressure = 95 ± 9 mm Hg

- Intraoperative care
  - Keep warm (see "Thermoregulation").
  - Fluids (see "Fluid Therapy")
- Postoperative aftercare
  - Reverse medetomidine (if used) with atipamezole at same volume as medetomidine IM.
  - Analgesia—as for other small mammals (see "Analgesia")

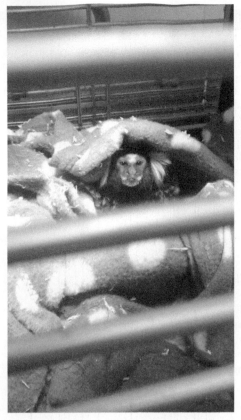

Fig 5-2. Postoperative aftercare for marmosets should include providing a warm, dark, quiet area, such as blankets to hide in that bear the marmoset's scent, to minimize stress for these intelligent animals.

- Animal must be offered food as soon as it recovers. Hypoglycemia is common in marmosets postoperatively.
- Keep warm and place in darkened, quiet area. Provide a hide or blankets for the marmoset to hide in (Fig. 5-2) as well as some furniture or material from its home cage that bears its scent.

Cardiopulmonary resuscitation

1. Intubate and ventilate at 20 to 30 breaths/min.
2. Reverse medetomidine (if used) with atipamezole at 0.4 to 1.0 mg/kg IM.
3. If cardiac arrest, external cardiac massage at around 100 compressions/min.
4. Epinephrine at
   a. 0.2 to 0.4 mg/kg diluted in sterile saline intratracheal
   b. 0.2 mg/kg intracardiac, IV, or IO
5. Fluid therapy (see "Fluid Therapy")
6. If bradycardic, atropine at 0.05 mg/kg IV or 0.05 to 0.1 mg/kg intratracheal

---

Skin disorders

Olfaction is a very important sense for marmosets, and common marmosets possess three areas high in scent glands—the sternal, suprapubic, and circumgenital areas—with the circumgenital fields being especially large and the sternal glands remaining small. The scent marks left are functionally the calling card for each individual, giving information on identity, social rank, and reproductive status (including the ovarian suppression of other females by the dominant female). They are also used for territorial definition and intergroup spacing. Wild common marmosets scent mark 0.19 to 0.45 scent marks/hour (Lazaro-Perea et al 1999), although this is much lower in captive marmosets. Scent marks should be left to accumulate in the enclosure, and when moving the marmoset, it should be accompanied by something bearing its scent.

Pruritus

- Ectoparasites
- Dermatitis

Alopecia

- Tail alopecia (see *Marmoset Wasting Syndrome*)
- Dermatophytosis
- Poor nutrition
- *Trichospirura* (see *Pancreatic Disorders*)
- Zinc deficiency

Scaling and crusting

- Dermatophytosis
- Zinc deficiency

Erosions and ulceration

- Monkeypox (poxvirus—see also "Disorders of the Oral Cavity" in *Gastrointestinal Tract Disorders*)
- Marmoset poxvirus
- Bite wounds

Nodules and nonhealing wounds

- Calcinosis circumscripta (see *Systemic Disorders*)
- Blastomycosis (see *Respiratory Disorders*)
- *Anatrichosoma cutaneum* (nematode)

Changes in pigmentation

- Measles virus (see *Systemic Disorders*)
- Vitiligo

Ectoparasites

- *Sarcoptes*/sarcoptiform mites
- *Demodex*
- Fleas

Neoplasia

Findings on clinical examination

- Discolored lesions in the skin and nasal cavity *(Anatrichosoma cutaneum)*

Investigations

1. Microscopy: Examine fur pluck, acetate strips, or skin scrapes to affected area and examine for ectoparasites, *Anatrichosoma* eggs.
2. Bacteriology and mycology: Hair pluck or swab lesions for routine culture and sensitivity.
3. Fine-needle aspirate followed by staining with rapid Romanowsky stains
4. Biopsy obvious lesions.
5. Ultraviolet (Wood's) lamp—positive for *Microsporium canis* only (not all strains fluoresce)
6. Radiography
7. Routine hematology and biochemistry
8. Culture and sensitivity
9. Endoscopy
10. Biopsy
11. Ultrasonography

Treatment/specific therapy

- Monkeypox
  - Treat symptomatically.
  - Smallpox vaccine will protect against monkeypox.
  - Potential zoonosis
- Marmoset poxvirus
  - In new imports
  - As for monkeypox
  - Not known if zoonosis
- *Anatrichosoma cutaneum*
  - Ivermectin 0.2 mg/kg SC or topically; repeat after 4 weeks.
- Bite wounds
  - Covering antibiosis
  - May require surgery for primary closure to reduce risk of self-mutilation; use subcuticular pattern.
- Dermatophytosis
  - Griseofulvin 20 mg/kg PO daily for 30 to 60 days
  - Itraconazole 5 to 10 mg/kg PO b.i.d.
- Vitiligo
  - Unknown etiology
- *Sarcoptes/Demodex*
  - Ivermectin 0.2 mg/kg SC or topically; repeat after 4 weeks.
- Fleas
  - Commercial flea treatments at cat dose rates
  - Rare
- Zinc deficiency
  - Add zinc to drinking water.

Respiratory tract disorders

Viral
- Paramyxovirus type 1, 2 (simian virus 5 (SV5) and SV41), and 3 (simian agent 10)
- Myxovirus (influenza type A and A2)
- Measles virus (see *Systemic Infections*)

Bacterial
- *Bordetella bronchiseptica*
- *Klebsiella pneumoniae*
- Tuberculosis *(Mycobacterium tuberculosis)*
- *Mycobacterium avium*
- *Streptococcus (Diplococcus) pneumoniae*
- *Ureaplasma* (see *Urinary Disorders*)

Fungal
- *Blastomyces dermatitidis* (blastomycosis)
- *Coccidioides immitis* (coccidiomycosis)
- *Cryptococcus neoformans* (see *Neurologic Disorders*)

Protozoal
- *Toxoplasma gondii* (see *Systemic Disorders*)
- *Pneumocystis* spp.

Parasitic
- *Strongyloides stercoralis* (pulmonary migration)

Neoplasia

Other noninfectious problems

Findings on clinical examination

- Sneezing
- Coughing
- Dyspnea
- Mucopurulent nasal discharge (bordetellosis, toxoplasmosis)
- Pneumonia
- Pyrexia
- Ocular and nasal discharges
- Anorexia
- Sudden death (bordetellosis, toxoplasmosis)
- Diarrhea (*Klebsiella*, myxovirus)
- Peritonitis, septicemia *(Klebsiella)*
- Neurologic signs *(S. pneumoniae)*

Investigations

1. Tracheal wash/bronchoalveolar lavage
2. Culture and sensitivity

3. Cytology
4. Pleural tap and cytology
5. Radiography
6. Serology for paramyxoviruses
7. Intradermal skin test (tuberculosis)
   a. The site for this test is the eyelid, but the small size of the palpebrum means that only a minute volume (0.05 mL) of tuberculin can be injected intradermally. *M. avium* can cause a false positive so the other eyelid can be used to test for *M. avium* reaction.
   b. The injection site is examined at 24, 48, and 72 hours and is graded.

Table 5-3 Common or cotton eared marmoset: tuberculin intradermal skin test grading

Grade	Description	Remarks
1	Slight bruising of the eyelid	Negative
2	Erythema of the palpebrum without swelling	Negative
3	Variable degree of erythema with minimal swelling	Indeterminate
4	Obvious swelling, with drooping of the eyelid and erythema	Positive
5	Marked swelling and/or necrosis of the eyelid	Positive

Ludlage et al, 2003

8. Endoscopy
9. Biopsy
10. Ultrasonography

Management

1. Supportive treatment (e.g., fluids, covering antibiosis)
2. Mucolytics (e.g., 0.5 mg/kg PO bromhexine) may prove beneficial.
3. Reduce stress levels. Hospitalize away from dogs and noisy cats; keep in darkened position.
4. Oxygen therapy if appropriate

Treatment/specific therapy

- Paramyxoviruses
  - Clinical signs vary from mild upper respiratory tract signs to severe rhinotracheobronchitis and interstitial pneumonia.
  - Supportive treatment
  - Humans are commonly the source.
  - May be more severe in animals younger than age 1 year
- Myxoviruses (influenza)
  - Treat symptomatically.
  - Mortalities can occur from secondary infections.
  - Avoid contact with humans with colds—face masks should be worn to reduce risk of transmission.

- *Bordetella bronchisepticum*
  - Transmitted by aerosol droplets
  - Appropriate antibiosis and as described in "Management" above
  - Treatment may resolve signs but become subclinical.
- Tuberculosis
  - Marmosets with grade 3 result on tuberculin test can be retested every fortnight for 6 weeks until 3 consecutive negative results are obtained. If this fails, euthanize.
  - Significant zoonosis. Euthanize.
- *Mycobacterium avium*
  - As for tuberculosis
- Coccidiomycosis, *Blastomyces,* and mucormycosis
  - Miconazole/chlorhexidine (Malaseb, Leo) shampoo—bathe once daily.
  - Griseofulvin at 25 mg/kg PO daily for 21 to 30 days
  - Itraconazole at 5.0 to 10 mg/kg PO daily for 30 days
  - Ketoconazole at 10 to 30 mg/kg PO daily for 60 days
- *Pneumocystis* spp.
  - Potentiated sulfonamides at 30 mg/kg PO b.i.d.

Gastrointestinal tract disorders

Permanent dental formula

Callithrix jacchus

$$I : \frac{2}{2} \quad C : \frac{1}{1} \quad PM : \frac{3}{3} \quad M : \frac{2}{2}$$

Dental disease is common in marmosets and is usually associated with inappropriate diet, particularly high levels of fruit with concomitant high levels of sugars (see *Nutritional Disorders*). The high incidence of metabolic bone disease can mean that the periodontal bone is substandard (Johnson-Delaney 2008). Also, although occasionally requested to reduce the risk of injury to the owner, canine removal is not appropriate and represents an unnecessary mutilation. An annual dental checkup is recommended, with preventative work being undertaken.

Disorders of the oral cavity

Dental disease is common and is managed as one would with other small animals.
- Dental disease
  - Buildup of tartar and calculus
  - Gingivitis
  - Dental fractures
  - Caries
  - Periodontal disease
  - Osteomyelitis
- Tooth root abscess
  - Typically swelling beneath eye
  - Purulent material on aspiration
  - Radiography to assess for underlying pathology
  - Dental extraction
  - Antibiosis—*Note:* Anaerobes often involved too.

- Hypovitaminosis C—gingival inflammation with hemorrhage and loosening of the teeth (see *Nutritional Disorders*)
- Papules and ulcers on oral mucosa, accompanied by skin lesions (monkeypox—see *Skin Disorders*)
- *Anatrichosoma cutaneum* (see *Skin Disorders*)
- *Gongylonema pulchrum*
  - Nematode—severe inflammation and edema of the lips; severe pruritis leads to aggravation of the condition. May be in mouth and esophagus.
  - Transmitted by cockroaches, so encourage good pest control.

Differential diagnoses for gastrointestinal disorders

Viral

- Measles virus (see *Systemic Disorders*)

Bacterial

- *Escherichia coli*
- *Campylobacter* spp.
- *Yersinia enterocolitica*
- *Shigella sonnei*
- *Clostridium perfringens*
- *Helicobacter*
- Leptospirosis

Fungal

- *Candida*

Protozoal

- *Cryptosporidium parvum*
- *Entamoeba histolytica*
- *Balantidium coli*

Parasitic

- *Strongyloides stercoralis*
- *Acanthocephala* spp.
  - *Prostenorchis elegans*
  - *Moniliformis clarki*
- *Pentastoma* spp.
- *Pterygodermatites nycticebi* (spirurid)

Nutritional

Neoplasia

- GI tract lymphoma
- Small intestine carcinoma

Other noninfectious problems

- Inflammatory bowel disease (IBD—see *Marmoset Wasting Syndrome*)
- Inflammatory fibroid polyp (Yokouchi et al 2013)
- Gastric bloat

Findings on clinical examination

- Acute hemorrhagic diarrhea (*E. coli,* worms)
- Chronic, progressive diarrhea (*E. coli,* worms)
- Watery diarrhea, colitis *(Campylobacter, Cryptosporidium)*
- Swollen lymph nodes *(Yersinia enterocolitica)*
- Rectal prolapse
- Dehydration
- Abdominal distension, peritonitis *(Prostenorchis elegans)*
- Abdominal mass (small intestinal carcinoma, other abdominal lesions)

Investigations

1. Fecal examination
   a. Gram stain
   b. MZN staining for *Cryptosporidium*
   c. Motile flagellated protozoa *(Giardia)*
   d. Motile ciliated protozoa *(Balantidium)*
   e. Worm eggs
      i. Spirurid nematode eggs *(Trichospirura leptostoma,* but could be *Pterygodermatites*— see *Pancreatic Disorders;* capillaria eggs—see *Hepatic Disorders)*
2. Radiography
   a. Foreign body
3. Routine hematology and biochemistry
4. Culture and sensitivity
5. ELISA *(Giardia, Cryptosporidium)*
6. Endoscopy
7. Biopsy
   a. Lymphoma
   b. GI tract carcinoma
8. Ultrasonography

Management

1. Fluid therapy (see *Nursing Care*)
2. If vomiting:
   a. Do not feed for 6 to 12 hours and use antiemetics (e.g., metoclopramide at 0.2-0.5 mg/kg SC t.i.d.).
   b. Monitor blood glucose—consider dextrose/saline fluids.

Treatment/specific therapy

- *E. coli*
  - As in "Management" above
  - Antibiotics
  - Asymptomatic carriers common
  - Potential serious zoonosis

- *Campylobacter* spp.
  - Supportive symptomatic treatment
  - May resolve spontaneously
  - Zoonotic
- *Yersinia enterocolitica*
  - As in "Management"
  - Appropriate antibiosis
  - In temperate climates tends to be seasonal, with peaks in late winter and early spring
- *Helicobacter*
  - Appropriate antibiosis
  - Gastroprotectants (e.g., sufalcrate)
  - Cimetidine 5.0 to 10.0 mg/kg PO
- Leptospirosis
  - A cause of severe gastroenteritis
  - Appropriate antibiosis
  - Potential zoonosis
  - Prevent rodent egress.
- *Candida*
  - Occasionally follows prolonged antibiotic treatment
  - Nystatin at 100,000 IU/kg PO daily for 10 days
- *Giardia*
  - Common, typically asymptomatic
  - Potential zoonosis, so treat with metronidazole 30 to 50 mg/kg daily for 5 to 10 days.
  - Tinidazole 2 doses given 4 days apart; first dose at 150 mg/kg PO with second dose at 77 mg/kg (Kramer et al 2009)
- *Entamoeba histolytica*
  - As for *Giardia*
- *Balantidium coli*
  - As for *Giardia*
- *Cryptosporidium*
  - More common in marmosets <1 year old
  - Difficult to treat
  - Paromomycin 15 mg/kg PO b.i.d. for 28 days reported successful on 2 marmosets (Hahn and Capuano 2010)
  - Consider nitazoxanide at 5.0 mg/kg PO per day
  - Insect vectors (e.g., cockroaches and flies) may be important for the spread of this disease and should be controlled as part of the management of this problem.
  - Potential zoonosis
- *Entamoeba histolytica*
  - Metronidazole at 10 to 20 mg/kg PO b.i.d.
- *Pterygodermatites nycticebi*
  - Cockroach is intermediate host, so must control insects
  - Mebendazole at 22 mg/kg PO daily for 3 days, repeat after 3 weeks
- *Enterobius vermicularis*
  - Reverse zoonosis
  - Often asymptomatic; can cause enteritis or even fatalities in high infestations

- *Strongyloides stercoralis*
  - Fenbendazole 50 mg/kg PO daily for 5 days
  - Autoinfective life cycle
  - Rarely a problem, but in early stages they may show bristling fur, respiratory signs, and a reduced appetite.
  - Potential zoonosis
- *Acanthocephala* spp.
  - Common; can cause colitis and peritonitis
  - Albendazole at either 50 mg/kg PO b.i.d. for 16 days or 100 mg/kg b.i.d. for 3 days, then repeated twice weekly for 4 treatments (Weber and Junge 2000)
  - *Prostenorchis elegans* may require surgical removal, as it is often resistant to anthelmintics.
  - Indirect life cycle using cockroaches or beetles, so insect control important
- *Pentastoma* spp.
  - Common
  - Can cause enterocolitis
  - Ivermectin 0.2 mg/kg SC, topically; repeat after 4 weeks.
- GI tract lymphoma
  - Typically secondary to oncogenic viral infections such as Callitrichine herpesvirus 3 (CalHV-3) and herpes simplex virus (HSV—see *Systemic Disorders*)
  - Concentrate on identifying source of underlying viral etiology.
- Small intestinal carcinoma
  - Consider surgical resection.
- Gastric bloat
  - Unknown etiology but may accompany episodes of diarrhea
  - Requires decompression by passing a gastric tube
  - May need surgical correction

Nutritional disorders

Marmoset nutrition

1. Common marmosets are gumnivores/omnivores. Tree gums often contain high levels of calcium and little phosphorus.
2. Calcium to phosphorus ratio: 1.5 to 2:1 with a daily intake of 250 mg/kg dietary calcium
3. Recommended vitamin D_3 intake: 100 IU/kg
4. Feed a commercially available marmoset food plus vegetables with minimal fruit. Modern fruit varieties are selected for their human palatability and contain excessive sugar levels, whereas vegetables contain sugar levels more like those of wild fruits.

Hypoglycemia

- From starvation or postoperative (see *Pancreatic Disorders* for management)

Zinc deficiency

- See *Skin Disorders.*

Metabolic bone disease

- Typically a lack of dietary calcium, an incorrect calcium to phosphorus ratio, or inadequate vitamin D_3 linked to failure to provide UVB or full-spectrum lighting; often a combination of these. There may be a link with marmoset wasting syndrome (Jarcho et al 2013—see *Marmoset Wasting Syndrome*).

- In youngsters it presents as rickets with bending of long bones and swollen metaphyses. Adults will develop osteomalacia with skeletal deformities; pathological fractures, including those of the lumbar vertebrae causing acute-onset hind-limb paralysis; and tetany. Other nonspecific signs include lethargy, reduced appetite, and anemia.
- Diagnosis is on radiography and biochemistry—typically a decreased ionized calcium level or inverse calcium to phosphorus ratio. Normal values: calcium 2.05 to 2.6 mmol/L; ionized calcium 1.08 to 1.28 mmol/L; phosphorus 0.87 to 2.75 mmol/L; 25-hydroxyvitamin D >124.8 nmol/L.
- Treat with oral and injectable calcium supplements such as calcium glubionate at 1.0 mL/kg PO b.i.d.
- Vitamin D_3 at 2000 IU/kg added to the diet
- Salmon calcitonin at 10 IU/kg every 48 hours for 3 weeks. *Note:* The marmoset must be normocalcemic.
- Reassess environment and diet.
- Supplement during periods of high calcium stress such as pregnancy and lactation. There is some evidence to suggest that reproductively active females increase their calcium intake (Power et al 1999) and that vitamin D_3 marginal individuals show a degree of preference for calcium solutions over plain water.

Obesity

- Very common in captive marmosets
- Linked to poor diet, sedentary existence, and single pet
- Defined (Tardif et al 2009) as:
  - Total body fat or relative body fat >14% (58.2 g) in males and >17% (73.4 g) in females
  - Average HDL: <1.08 mmol/L
  - Average fasting glucose: 12.15 mmol/L or average HbA_{1c} 0.055% total hemoglobin
  - Triglyceride concentration: >0.055 mmol/L
- Reassess diet; reduce carbohydrate intake.
- See also "Hepatic Lipidosis" in *Hepatic Disorders* and "Diabetes Mellitus" in *Pancreatic Disorders*.

Hypovitaminosis C

- A lack of vitamin C causes scurvy.
- Seen in marmosets not supplemented properly or fed out-of-date commercial diets
- Signs include swelling of the epiphyses of long bones, gum hemorrhages, loosening teeth, periosteal hemorrhages, and cephalohematoma.
- Radiography is useful in diagnosis.
- Treat with vitamin C supplements up to 25 mg/kg PO body weight b.i.d. PO for 5 days in severe cases.
- Maintenance levels regarded as are 1.0 to 4.0 mg/kg PO body weight daily.

Hypovitaminosis E

- Linked to anemia, myopathies, and pansteatitis (Juan-Sallés et al 2003)
- Signs include weight loss, fecal retention, diarrhea, difficulty in moving, anemia, hypoproteinemia, or hypoalbuminemia.
- Biochemistry: raised creatine kinase, lactate dehydrogenase, and alanine transaminase and renal failure with hypercholesterolemia
- Supplement with vitamin E.

Coprophagy

- Usually secondary to inadequate nutrition, especially low-protein diets
- Correct any dietary deficiencies.
- Install a grate into the bottom of the cage to reduce access to feces.

Hepatic disorders

Viral

- Lymphocytic choriomeningitis (LCM, arenavirus)
- Yellow fever (Flavivirus)
- Hepatitis G virus (GB virus C)—see *Systemic Disorders*)

Bacterial

- *Yersinia pseudotuberculosis* (see *Systemic Disorders*)

Parasitic

- *Capillaria hepatica*

Nutritional

Neoplasia

Noninfectious disorders

- Amyloidosis (see *Systemic Disorders*)
- Cholelithiasis (Smith et al 2006)
- Fatty liver disease/steatohepatitis (Kramer et al 2015)/hepatic lipidosis

Findings on clinical examination

- Reduced appetite or loss of appetite
- Vague signs of ill health
- Abnormal feces, diarrhea
- Emesis
- Hepatomegaly
- Weight loss, lethargy, hepatomegaly (amyloidosis)
- Jaundice
- Ascites
- Dyspnea
- Bile-tinged (green) diarrhea
- Abnormal gait
- Seizures
- Hemorrhages

Investigations

1. Fecal examination
   a. *Capillaria hepatica* eggs (typical bipolar)
2. Radiography

3. Routine hematology and biochemistry
   a. Raised liver enzymes
   b. Leukocytosis
   c. Anemia
4. Culture and sensitivity
5. Virus isolation (yellow fever)
6. Endoscopy
7. Biopsy
8. Ultrasonography

Management

1. Fluid therapy (see *Nursing Care*)
2. Lactulose at 0.25-1.1 ml/kg PO b.i.d or t.i.d.
3. Milk thistle *(Silybum marianum)* is hepatoprotectant. Dose at 4 to 15 mg/kg PO b.i.d. or t.i.d.

Treatment/specific therapy

- LCM
  - Transmitted by ingestion of rodents, either wild rodents or pinkies given as part of diet
  - Attempt treatment with general supportive care (see "Management" above).
  - Zoonosis, so consider euthanasia.
  - Prevent access to rodents, and assess sources of dietary rodents.
- *Capillaria hepatica*
  - Fenbendazole 50 mg/kg PO every 2 weeks until clear
  - Avoid rodents (primary host).
- Hemosiderosis
  - Unexpected mortalities
  - Linked to diet (Miller et al 1997); may be due to excessive scavenging of dietary iron in a species that feeds naturally on an iron-deficient diet; the lack of naturally occurring tannins may also be important.
  - May also be related to feeding of homemade diets, possibly with high fruit/vitamin C. Alternatively can be triggered by chronic inflammatory disease. Hypervitamosis C and chronic inflammation can increase transferrin levels.
  - Minimize fruit in diet (see *Nutritional Disorders*); if using human milk substitutes for hand-rearing, choose a low-iron formula.
- Yellow fever
  - Marmosets are relatively resistant but may still show signs.
  - Outbreaks typically follow importation/arrival; if die-offs occur within 10 days with appropriate signs, then consider yellow fever.
  - Protect from mosquito vectors.
  - Potential zoonosis; vaccinate staff.
- Cholelithiasis
  - Surgical removal
  - Covering antibiosis and as for *Management*
  - Dietary reappraisal; in Smith et al (2006) the stones were found to be largely pigment stones, although two were cysteine.

- Fatty liver disease/steatohepatitis/hepatic lipidosis
  - Can be linked to obesity combined with anorexia
  - Aggressive fluid therapy
  - Parenteral nutrition with glucose and vitamins
  - Calcium gluconate PO or propylene glycol PO may be of use.
  - Dexamethasone at 0.2 mg/kg IV, SC, or PO. Can be repeated after 24 hours if necessary.
  - See also "Obesity" in *Nutritional Disorders*.

Splenic disorders

- Splenomegaly
  - Hemangiosarcoma and hemangioma
  - Cardiac disease (see *Cardiovascular and Hematologic Disorders*)
  - Lymphoma/lymphosarcoma (see *Systemic Disorders*)
  - Idiopathic splenomegaly

Treatment

- Address underlying cause.
- Splenectomy
  - Hypersplenism
  - Splenic rupture
  - Splenic torsion
  - Neoplasia
  - Splenitis

Pancreatic disorders

Parasitic

- *Trichospirura leptostoma* (spururid nematode)

Neoplasia
Other noninfectious problems

- Diabetes mellitus type II (Juan-Sallés et al 2002)
- Insulin resistance (Juan-Sallés et al 2002)

Findings on clinical examination

- Ataxia and hind-limb paresis
- Lethargy
- Hypersalivation
- Vomiting
- Abdominal distension
- Pain
- Weight loss and emaciation despite normal appetite, alopecia, muscle weakness, ataxia, hind-limb paralysis *(T. leptostoma)*
- Poor weight gain in juveniles and increased mortality of newborns *(T. leptostoma)*
- Obesity

Investigations

1. Radiography
2. Fecal examination: spirurid nematode eggs *(T. leptostoma)*
3. Routine hematology and biochemistry
   a. *T. leptostoma* can trigger a subclinical pancreatitis with secondary pancreatic insufficiency.

Table 5-4 Common or cotton-eared marmoset: blood glucose and insulin levels.

	Normal range	Obesity
Blood glucose normal resting (mmol/L)	6.9-14.3	>12.15
Blood glucose normal fasting (mmol/L)	5.3-5.8	
Normal insulin (pmol/L)	35-70	
Mean fasting insulin (pmol/L)	35	

1. Tardif et al, 2011
2. Ziegler et al, 2013

   b. Hyperglycemia/glycosuria (diabetes mellitus/insulin resistance)
4. Glucose tolerance curve (from Fox 2002)

Table 5-5 Common or cotton-eared marmoset: normal glucose curve.

Animal	Fasting blood glucose (mmol/L) (urine glucose on dipstick)	30 minutes	60 minutes	120 minutes
1	5.3 (negative)	9.2 (negative)	6.2 (negative)	5.6 (negative)
2	5.8 (negative)	12.9 (positive)	7.3 (trace)	4.4 (negative)

5. Culture and sensitivity
6. Urinalysis
   a. Glycosuria/ketonuria
7. Endoscopy
8. Exploratory surgery and biopsy
9. Ultrasonography

Management

1. Treatment of hypoglycemia (see box)

Hypoglycemia

1. Rub honey or sugared water onto the gingiva, taking care not to get bitten.
2. 0.5- to 2.0-mL total volume bolus IV of 50% dextrose solution given slowly
3. Fluid therapy (see *Nursing Care*) with 5% dextrose infusion
4. If marmoset fails to respond, can give shock dose of dexamethasone at 4 to 8 mg/kg IV or IM onceonly.
5. Diazepam at 1 to 2 mg IV as needed to control if seizures persistent

Treatment/specific therapy

- Diabetes mellitus
  - May be controlled by limiting carbohydrate in diet. Feeding snacks high in unsaturated fats and protein (cashew nuts and waxworms) appeared to improve glucoregulation (Ziegler et al 2013b).
  - Oral antidiabetic drugs: metformin at 5.0 to 10.0 mg/kg PO b.i.d.
  - If necessary start on neutral protamine Hagedorn (NPH) insulin at a starting dose of 0.1 IU/marmoset SC b.i.d. until stablized. Monitor blood glucose levels.
  - Maintain on daily ultralente insulin.
  - Linked to obesity, sedentary lifestyle, lack of socialization, and early weaning. Obese marmosets can develop type II diabetes mellitus from age 5 years on.
- *T. leptostoma*
  - Fenbendazole 50 mg/kg PO s.i.d. for 14 days.
  - Cockroaches *Blatella germanica* and *Supella longipalpa* are intermediate hosts, so they need to be eliminated.

Cardiovascular and hematologic disorders

Bacterial

- Bacteremia/septicemia
- Endocarditis (especially staphylococci—Chamanza et al 2006)
- Pericarditis

Protozoal

- *Toxoplasma gondii* (myocarditis—see *Systemic Disorders*)
- *Trypanosoma cruzi*
- *Dipetalonema*

Nutritional

- Atherosclerosis

Neoplasia

- Lymphoma (see *Systemic Disorders*)
- Myelofibrosis

Other noninfectious problems

- Myocardial fibrosis
- Cardiomyopathy
  - Dilative
- Chronic/focal myocarditis
- Femoral artery hematoma
- Perivasculitis/vasculitis
- Mineralization
- Ectopic thyroid
- Valvular heart disease
- Congenital disorders
- Anticoagulant drug poisoning (rodenticides)

Findings on clinical examination

- Cyanosis or pallor of the mucous membranes
- Slow capillary refill time
- Dyspnea
- Precordial thrill
- Abnormalities of femoral arterial pulse, including weakness, irregularities, pulse deficits
- Arrhythmia
- Lack of thoracic percussion with auscultation
- Abnormal lung sounds
- Abnormal heart sounds
- Exercise intolerance
- Ascites
- Hepatomegaly, splenomegaly *(Trypanosoma cruzii)*
- Weight loss
- Sudden death
- Swelling of medial aspect of quadriceps muscle; obvious hematoma following phlebotomy (femoral artery hematoma)

Investigations

1. Auscultation
2. Blood pressure
3. ECG

Table 5-6   Normal lead II ECGs

Parameter	*Callithrix jacchus* (Davies 1969)	*Callithrix penicillata* (Giannico et al 2013)
Heart rate (beats/min)	224 (206-245)	264 ± 74
Frontal plane mean electrical axis (degrees)	+41 (+18 to +91)	—
P duration (sec)	0.025 (0.021-0.029)	0.034 ± 0.006
P amplitude (mV)	—	0.132 ± 0.051
PR interval (sec)	0.057 (0.052-0.062)	0.056 ± 0.011
QT interval (sec)	0.117 (0.088-0.156)	0.130 ± 0.026
QS interval (sec)	0.024 (0.020-0.029)	0.035 ± 0.007
QRS complex duration (sec)		35 ± 7
T wave (sec)	0.101 (0.091-0.112)	—
T amplitude (mV)	—	0.19 ± 0.083
R amplitude (mV)	1.07 (0.83-1.37)	0.273 ± 0.269
QT interval (sec)	0.117 (0.088-0.156)	0.130 ± 0.026

4. Routine hematology and biochemistry
   a. Pancytopenia, leukoerythroblastosis, anisocytosis, poikilocytosis, giant platelets (myelofibrosis)
   b. Smear *(T. cruzii, Dipetalonema)*

5. Serology for *Toxoplasma, T. cruzi*
6. PCR *T. cruzi*
7. Culture and sensitivity
8. Endoscopy
9. Biopsy
    a. Marrow: fibrosis, atypical megakaryocytes (myelofibrosis)

Management

- Reduce stress (e.g., keep in a cool, shaded, or darkened area away from potential stressors such as dogs).
- Provide a high-oxygen environment.
- For pleural effusion, consider tube thoracostomy.

Treatment/specific therapy

Specific treatments for cardiac disease not described, so consult human literature as well as established veterinary protocols.

- Cardiomyopathy
    - Dilated (congestive) cardiomyopathy
        - Furosemide at 1 to 4 mg/kg PO, SC b.i.d.
        - Enalapril at 0.5 mg/kg PO every 48 hours
        - Benazepril 0.25 to 0.5 mg/kg PO daily; less nephrotoxic than enalapril
        - Digoxin at 0.01 mg/kg PO daily
        - Nitroglycerin at 3 mm of 2% ointment applied to skin daily or b.i.d.
        - Pimobendan at 0.2 mg/kg PO daily
- Valvular heart disease
    - Treat as for dilated cardiomyopathy
- Myelofibrosis
    - Very guarded prognosis
    - If diagnosed antemortem, consider blood transfusions, erythropoetic growth factors, and prednisolone (1 mg/kg PO daily). Consult present recommendations for human medicine.
- *T. cruzi*
    - Transmitted by trauma, direct exchange of bodily fluids, and transplacental
    - Can be transmitted by insects, so good insect control needed
    - Benzimidazole 5.0 to 7.5 mg/kg PO b.i.d. for 60 days
    - Nifurtimox 15 to 20 mg/kg PO t.i.d. for 90 days
    - Potential zoonosis
- *Dipetalonema* spp.
    - Microfilariae found in peripheral blood smears
    - Adults found in pleural cavity and peritoneum.
    - Ivermectin at 0.2 mg/kg SC or PO; repeat after 4 weeks.
    - Transmitted by blood-sucking fleas and ticks, so ectoparasite control is essential.
- Femoral artery hematoma
    - If noticed immediately, then apply a pressure bandage.
    - If long-standing, may require surgical resection; may need blood transfusion prior to surgery.

- Anticoagulant drug poisoning
  - Treat with vitamin K IV and PO.
  - Consider transfusion if necessary.
  - General supportive care.

Systemic disorders

Viral

- Herpes simplex virus 1 (HSV-1)
- Herpesvirus tamarinus
- Herpesvirus saimiri (HVS)
- Herpesvirus ateles
- Epstein-Barr virus (EBV)
- Callitrichine herpesvirus 3 (CalHV-3)
- GB virus A (flavivirus)
- LCM (see *Hepatic Disorders*)
- Measles virus (morbillivirus)
- Eastern equine encephalitis virus (EEEV)

Bacterial

- *Franciscella tularensis*
- *Streptococcus zooepidemicus*
- *Yersinia pseudotuberculosis*
- *Clostridium botulinum* (botulism)

Protozoal

- *Toxoplasma gondii*

Parasitic

- *Trichospirura leptostoma* (see *Pancreatic Disorders*)
- *Dipetalonema* spp. (see *Cardiovascular and Hematologic Disorders*)

Nutritional

- Hypovitaminosis E (see *Nutritional Disorders*)

Neoplasia

- Lymphoma
  - Malignant T-cell lymphoma (Yamaguchi et al 2013)

Other noninfectious problems

- Amyloidosis
- Calcinosis circumscripta (Wachtman et al 2006)

Findings on clinical examination

- Fever, lethargy, and anorexia followed by conjunctivitis and salivation due to oral vesicles; commonly progresses to ataxia, paresis, blindness, seizures, and death (HSV-1, herpesvirus tamarinus)

- Lethargy, anorexia, abdominomegaly, lymphadenopathy, exophthalmos (malignant lymphoma, HVS, herpesvirus ateles, EBV)
- Anorexia, weight loss, diarrhea, and abdominal masses (CalHV-3)
- Swollen lymph nodes, lethargy, anorexia *(Franciscella tularensis)*
- Wasting and muscle atrophy *(Trichospirura leptostoma)*
- Weight loss, lethargy, hepatomegaly (amyloidosis)
- Polylymphadenopathy (lymphoma, *Streptococcus*)
- Firm subcutaneous mass (calcinosis circumscripta)
- Splenitis, enteritis *(Streptococcus)*
- Diarrhea, lethargy, depression, abortions, stillbirths, and septicemia

Investigations

1. Radiography
   a. Radiodense mass; bone density (calcinosis circumscripta)
2. Routine hematology and biochemistry
3. Normochromic, normocytic anemia, hypoalbuminemia, raised alkaline phosphatase
4. Abdominal centesis and cytology
5. Serology for toxoplasmosis, herpesviruses, EBV
6. Culture and sensitivity
7. Virus isolation from infected tissue
8. Endoscopy
9. Biopsy/necropsy
   a. Liver biopsy (amyloidosis—beware hemorrhage)
10. Ultrasonography
    a. Hypoechoic areas (amyloidosis)
    b. Splenic enlargement; organ enlargement (lymphoma)

Management

- See *Nursing Care.*

Treatment/specific therapy

- HSV-1, herpesvirus tamarinus
  - Very guarded prognosis: 76% to 100% mortaility with herpesvirus tamarinus
  - Attempt treatment with acyclovir, famciclovir, or lysine.
  - Marmosets should be kept separate from squirrel monkeys and Cebus monkeys (natural hosts) to prevent transmission of herpesvirus tamarinus to marmosets.
  - Avoid contact with humans with active herpes lesions (cold sores).
- Herpesvirus ateles, HVS, EBV, CalHV-3
  - Malignant lymphoma
  - 40% to 60% captive common marmosets seropositive for CalHV-3 but clinically asymptomatic.
  - Viral etiology is likely to make chemotherapy ineffective.
  - Consider euthanasia.
- GB virus A
  - Typically asymptomatic but can cause acute liver failure
  - May reduce immunity of host

- Measles virus
  - Hemorrhagic diarrhea with consequential hypothermia, dehydration, and death
  - Edema of periorbital area
  - Skin erythema and respiratory signs may be absent in marmosets.
  - Highly likely to be fatal
  - Human attenuated vaccines are suitable.
- Eastern equine encephalitis virus
  - Experimentally infected marmosets may be asymptomatic or develop a progressive anorexia, eventually becoming inactive, somnolent, either not blinking or repeatedly blinking their eyes, and exhibiting a depressed posture (Adams et al 2008).
  - Avoid exposure to mosquitoes.
  - Consider euthanasia.
- *Streptococcus zooepidemicus*
  - Linked to exposure to raw meat
  - Appropriate antibiosis
- *Franciscella tularensis*
  - Appropriate antibiosis
- *Yersinia pseudotuberculosis*
  - Appropriate antibiosis
  - Vaccination (autogenous)
  - Control rodent and bird vectors.
- Botulism
  - Paralysis of laryngeal and respiratory muscles
- Toxoplasmosis
  - Primary host is cat, so prevent access to cat feces.
  - Can be transmitted by rodents (ingestion of wild rodents) or on insects (e.g., cockroaches), so control of these essential
  - Clindamycin at 12.5 mg/kg PO b.i.d. for at least 2 weeks
  - Combination therapy consisting of:
    - Co-trimoxazole at 30 mg/kg PO b.i.d.
    - Pyrimethamine at 0.5 mg/kg PO b.i.d.
    - Folic acid at 3.0 to 5.0 mg/kg PO daily
      or
    - Co-trimoxazole at 30 mg/kg PO daily
    - Toltrazuril at 7.0 mg/kg PO daily for 2 consecutive days
    - Treat for 3 weeks.
- Amyloidosis
  - Often follows chronic inflammatory conditions
  - Control by attending to underlying problem.
- Lymphoma
  - Very guarded prognosis
  - Steroids (e.g., prednisone 1 mg/kg PO s.i.d.) may give temporary improvement.
  - Modification of existing chemotherapeutic protocols as described for other animals or humans may be considered.
- Calcinosis circumscripta
  - Surgical resection
  - Investigate possible underlying etiologies: inflammation/biochemical imbalance.

Marmoset wasting syndrome (MWS)

MWS is an extremely common condition characterized by weight loss, diarrhea, and alopecia, with some cases also developing neurologic signs such as hind-limb paresis. This becomes more common after age 10 years. The several suggested etiologies and the inconsistent clinical signs may indicate a varied spectrum of the same disorder or may be due to misidentification of the condition with something that gives a similar clinical outcome. It may be that the reduction in digestive deficiency seen in MWS also contributes to the development of metabolic bone disease by reducing the absorption of dietary vitamin D_3 and calcium (Jarcho et al 2013); see *Nutritional Disorders*.

Parasitic

- *Trichospirura leptostoma* (see *Pancreatic Disorders*)

Nutritional

- Hypovitaminosis E (see *Nutritional Disorders*)
- Gliadin/gluten allergy
- Dietary protein deficiency (see Nutritional Support)

Neoplasia

- GI tract lymphoma
- Small intestinal carcinoma

Other noninfectious problems

- Amyloidosis (see *Systemic Disorders*)
- Renal disease (see *Urinary Disorders*)
- Tubulointerstitial nephritis (Brack and Rothe 1981)
- Inflammatory bowel disease (IBD)
  - Chronic lymphocytic enteritis (LCE; lymphoplasmacytic inflammation)
    - Protein deficiency
    - Food allergy (e.g., gliadin/gluten)

Findings on clinical examination

- Chronic, progressive weight loss
- Occasional diarrhea
- Reduced activity
- Muscle wastage
- Weakness
- Tail alopecia
- Necrosis of the extremities is not uncommon with MWS.

Investigations

1. Body weight
   a. Adult weight <325 g (LCE)
2. Routine hematology and biochemistry
   a. A serum albumin below 35 g/L
   b. Macrocytic normochromic anemia (LCE)
3. Culture and sensitivity

4. Cytology
5. Radiography
6. Serology
   a. Raised antigliadin IgA antibodies
7. Endoscopy
8. Biopsy (enteric)
9. Ultrasonography

Management

- Supportive treatment (e.g., fluids, covering antibiosis)
- Supportive nutrition—see "Nutritional Support" in *Nursing Care*.
- Reduce stress levels. Hospitalize away from dogs and noisy cats; keep in darkened position.

Treatment/specific therapy

- Routine worming if marmoset has access to cockroaches *(Trichospura)*
- Remove sources of gliadin/gluten from diet. Kuehnel et al (2013) found an improvement of gastrointestinal signs on withdrawal of gluten.
- Sources of gliadin/gluten are likely to include pelleted foods; other possible sources of gliadin include maize/corn, millet, and rice (Gore et al 2001).
- Otovic et al (2015) suggest the following for marmosets meeting the criteria for LCE (weight <325 g and/or serum albumin <35 g/L):
  - Prednisolone 1 mg/kg PO s.i.d. subsequently adjusted to response to therapy.
  - Budesonide at 0.5 mg per animal PO daily for 8 weeks. If no response to therapy the dose is increased to 0.75 mg for a further 8 weeks.

Musculoskeletal disorders

Viral
- Herpes simplex virus 1 (see *Systemic Disorders*)
- Herpesvirus tamarinus (see *Systemic Disorders*)

Bacterial
- *Clostridium tetani* (tetanus) (see *Neurologic Disorders*)

Protozoal
- *Sarcocystis*

Neoplasia
- Rhabdomyosarcoma (Tochitani et al 2013)

Other noninfectious problems
- Traumatic fractures
- Any causes of weakness
  - See *Neurologic Disorders*.
  - See *Cardiac and Hematologic Disorders*.
  - See *Systemic Disorders*.

Findings on clinical examination

- Pain
- Lameness
- Swelling
- Hind-leg paresis/paralysis
- Small rounded mass at tip of tail (chordoma)

Investigations

1. Radiography
2. Osteolysis, pathological fractures (multiple myeloma)
3. Traumatic fractures
4. Routine hematology and biochemistry
5. Culture and sensitivity
6. Endoscopy
7. Biopsy
8. Ultrasonography

Treatment/specific therapy

- Multiple myeloma
  - No treatment recorded
- Traumatic fractures
  - Repair using standard small animal techniques.

Neurologic disorders

Viral

- Herpes simplex virus 1 (see *Systemic Disorders*)
- Herpesvirus tamarinus (see *Systemic Disorders*)
- EEEV (see *Systemic Disorders*)
- Rabies
  - Common marmosets have their own rabies variant (Favoretto et al 2001).

Bacterial

- Bacterial meningitis or other CNS infection
- Otitis media/interna
- *Clostridium tetani* (tetanus)
- *Listeria monocytogenes* (see *Reproductive Disorders*)
- *Streptococcus (Diplococcus) pneumoniae* (see *Respiratory Disorders*)

Fungal

- *Cryptococcus neoformans*

Protozoal

- *Toxoplasma gondii* (see *Systemic Disorders*)
- *Encephalitozoon cuniculi*

Parasitic

- *Balisascaris*

Other noninfectious problems

- Trauma
- Hypoglycemia (see *Pancreatic Disorders*)

Findings on clinical examination

- Apparent weakness
- Neurologic signs, fever (meningitis—*Cryptococcus*)
- Posterior paralysis/paresis
- Stiff gait, extensor rigidity, opisthotonos (tetanus)
- Anxiety, lethargy, constipation, bladder atony, posterior paresis, aggression (rabies)
- Epileptiform seizures

Investigations

1. Full neurologic examination
2. Radiography
3. Routine hematology and biochemistry
4. Serology for toxoplasmosis
5. Culture and sensitivity
6. Endoscopy
7. Biopsy
8. Ultrasonography

Management

- Important to differentiate from other causes of weakness (insulinoma, lymphoma, etc.)

Treatment/specific therapy

- *Encephalitozoon cuniculi*
  - Co-trimoxazole at 30 mg/kg PO b.i.d. for at least 3 weeks
  - Albendazole at 10 mg/kg PO for 6 weeks
  - Fenbendazole 10 to 20 mg/kg PO s.i.d. for 1 month
  - Combination therapy consisting of:
    - Co-trimoxazole at 30 mg/kg PO b.i.d.
    - Pyrimethamine at 0.5 mg/kg PO b.i.d.
    - Folic acid at 3.0 to 5.0 mg/kg PO daily
- *Baylisascaris*
  - Racoon is the natural host.
  - Direct life cycle
  - Larva migrans can cause neurologic signs.
  - Fenbendazole at 50 mg/kg PO daily for 5 days
  - Antiinflammatories
  - Consider euthanasia.
- Tetanus
  - Treat symptomatically.
  - Tetanus antitoxin may help.
  - Reduce risk of accidental soil contamination.

- *Cryptococcus*
  - Amphotericin B, at 150 µg/kg i.v. 3 times weekly for 2-4 months
- Rabies
  - Risk of exposure from bites by infected bats, dogs, or other reservoir species in endemic areas or while they are held before export
  - Killed vaccines have unknown efficacy but can be used.
  - Control risk of infection by barrier methods of protection, safe handling procedures, and prompt and appropriate follow-ups.
  - Important zoonosis. Euthanize suspected individuals.

Ophthalmic disorders

Viral

- HVS
- Measles virus (see *Systemic Disorders*)

Bacterial

Fungal

- *Cryptococcus* (see *Neurologic Disorders*)

Protozoal

- Toxoplasmosis (see *Systemic Disorders*)

Other noninfectious problems

- Hereditary cataracts
- Idiopathic cataracts
- Retinal degeneration (may be hereditary)
- Periorbital edema (measles virus)
- Trauma

Findings on clinical examination

- Corneal ulceration
- Conjunctivitis
- Nasal discharge
- Uveitis
- Corneal edema, hypopyon, and synechiae
- Cataracts
- Exophthalmos (retrobulbar lymphoma—HVS)
- Megaglobus/glaucoma
- Night blindness (hypovitaminosis A, retinal degeneration)
- Cataracts (hereditary, idiopathic)

Investigations

1. Ophthalmic examination
   a. Schirmer tear test: Mean = -0.46 ± 3.41 mm/min (*Callithrix penicillata*—Lange et al 2012)
2. Topical fluorescein to assess extent of ulceration

3. Tonometry
   a. Intraocular pressure 14.5 ± 3.27 mm Hg
4. Skull radiography
5. Routine hematology and biochemistry
6. Serology for toxoplasmosis
7. Culture and sensitivity
8. Biopsy
9. Ultrasonography

Treatment/specific therapy

- Corneal ulceration
  - Topical and systemic antibiosis
  - Once infection is cleared, treat as for other small animals (e.g., scarification to encourage healing, conjunctival grafts, etc.).
- Uveitis
  - Topical ophthalmic steroid or NSAID preparations
  - Topical ophthalmic antibiotic preparations plus systemic antibiosis if appropriate
  - Enucleation if severe
- Cataracts
  - Treat for any uveitis as above.
  - Cataract removal either surgically or by phacoemulsification
- Neoplasia
  - Enucleation
- Toxoplasmosis—see *Neurologic Disorders*

Endocrine disorders

All primates are highly susceptible to stress; in the common marmoset the most reliable indicators of stress are fecal cortisol and lymphocyte count (Kuehnel et al 2012).

Table 5-7 Cotton or cotton-eared marmoset: lymphocyte count and fecal cortisol levels.

Parameter	Base values	Stress values	Recovery values (4 weeks post stressor)
Lymphocyte count × 10⁹/L	1.87 (1.17-2.70)	1.70 (0.82-1.85)	2.30 (1.61-3.30)
Fecal cortisol (ng/g)	57.20 (19.62-122.32)	130.28 (66.66-223.45)	52.01 (33.75-182.64)

Kuehnel et al, 2012

Hyperthyroidism or hypothyroidism has not been described clinically. Normal values (Mano et al 1985) are as follows:
- Thyroxine (total T_4): 140.1 nmol/L
- Thyroid-stimulating hormone: 38.1 mIU/L

Urinary disorders

Bacterial

- Cystitis
- Pyelonephritis
- Ureaplasmas (Furr et al 1979)

Nutritional

- Oxalate nephropathy (Vanselow et al 2011)

Neoplasia

- Lymphoma (see *Systemic Disorders*)
- Malignant nephroblastoma (Zöller et al 2008)

Other noninfectious problems

- Tubulointerstitial nephritis (see *Marmoset Wasting Syndrome*)
- Chronic interstitial nephritis (often part of MWS—see *Marmoset Wasting Syndrome*)
- Glomerulonephropathy (Yamada et al 2013)

Findings on clinical examination

- Depression
- Anorexia
- Weight loss
- Polydipsia/polyuria
- Oral ulceration
- Hematuria (urolithiasis, cystitis, neoplasia)
- Hind-leg weakness
- Melena
- Dysuria/polyuria
- Urine dribbling, wet perineum, constant licking at genitalia (urolithiasis)
- Death

Investigations

1. Urinalysis (normal urine parameters extracted from Yamada et al 2013)

Table 5-8	Common or cotton-eared marmoset: Normal urine parameters
pH	5.0-8.5
Protein	++
Blood	Negative /trace
WBCs	Negative
Glucose	Negative
Crystals	Negative
Epithelial cells	Negative
Casts	Negative
Yamada et al, 2013	

Management

- Fluid therapy (see *Nursing Care*)
- Appropriate antibiosis
- For protein-losing nephropathies, consider telmisartan at 1.0 mg/kg body weight PO.

Treatment/specific therapy

- Ureaplasmas
  - Unknown significance
  - Standard anti-*Mycoplasma* antibiotics should be effective.
  - Flurofamide, a potent bacterial urease inhibitor, also eliminated ureaplasmas from marmosets. Dose used: 25 mg/animal PO every 12 hours for 3 doses
- Cystitis
  - As for other small animals
  - Appropriate antibiosis and analgesia
- Pyelonephritis
  - Fluid therapy
  - Appropriate antibiosis

Reproductive disorders

Reproduction in common marmosets can be controlled by surgical means such as castration, vasectomy, fallopian tube ligation, or ovarohysterectomy or chemically. Castration or ovariohysterectomy does not reduce aggression in marmosets.

Chemical methods of reproductive control

- Deslorelin implant (Suprelorin) available as a 4.7-mg or 9.4-mg implant, which should give at least 6 months' and 12 months' contraception, respectively: A GnRH analog, it can cause initial stimulation of the HPG axis before downregulation occurs, so sexes are best not mixed for 3 weeks, or an alternative control must be used. This is probably the safest.
- Progesterone-containing implants: Act by altering uterine environment to prevent embryo implantation
- MGA (melengestrol acetate) implant (only available in the United States)
- Etonogestrel 68 mg implant.
- Porcine zona pellucida (PZP) vaccine: Not effective until at least 2 injections have been given, 2 to 4 weeks apart; then another 2 weeks before mixing sexes

Bacterial

- *Listeria monocytogenes*
- Prostatitis
- Metritis/pyometra
- Mastitis

Neoplasia

- Prostatic hyperplasia
- Mammary carcinoma
- Uterine carcinoma
- Testicular neoplasia

Other noninfectious problems

- Endometrial hyperplasia
- Endometritis
- Pyometra
- Abortion
  - Stress
  - Toxoplasmosis (see *Systemic Disorders*)
  - Listeriosis
  - Leptospirosis (see *Gastrointestinal Tract Disorders*)
- Placenta previa
- Dystocia
  - Physical abnormalities
  - Large young (single baby)
  - Deformed/anasarca young
  - Maternal pelvic abnormalities (e.g., history of metabolic bone disease)
  - Placenta previa

Findings on clinical examination

- Abortion, sick neonates; meningoencephalitis in young (see also *Neurologic Disorders* and *Neonatal Disorders*)
- Obvious dystocia (Fig. 5-3)

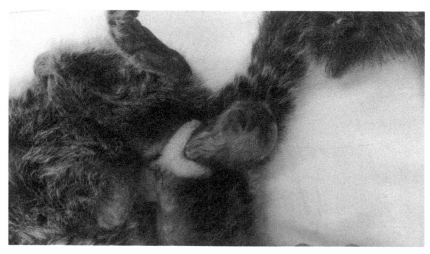

Fig 5-3. An obvious case of dystocia in a common marmoset. This singleton was too big for this primiparous female to give birth to.

Investigations

1. Radiography
   a. Dystocia
2. Routine hematology and biochemistry
   a. Calcium levels—metabolic bone disease

3. Urinalysis
4. Culture and sensitivity
5. Endoscopy
6. Biopsy
7. Ultrasonography
   a. Prostatic hyperplasia/cysts
   b. Metritis/pyometra
   c. Dystocia

Management

1. Supportive care as outlined in *Nursing Care*
2. Prophylactic antibiotics

Treatment/specific therapy

- Prostatic hyperplasia
  - Common in aging males. Usually asymptomatic.
- Testicular neoplasia
  - Castration
- Endometrial hyperplasia, endometritis, and pyometra may be linked to hormonal implants.
- Endometritis
  - Induce uterine contractions with 0.5 mg prostaglandin $F_{2\alpha}$ SC.
  - Antibiosis
- Pyometra
  - Ovariohysterectomy
  - Antibiosis
- Neoplasia
  - Mammary carcinoma: Mastectomy
  - Uterine carcinoma: Ovariohysterectomy
- Mastitis
  - Antibiosis and fluids
  - NSAIDs may have antiendotoxin effects (see "Analgesia" in *Nursing Care*).
  - Debride or surgically resect affected mammary tissue.
  - Fostering young may spread pathogens to other females.
- Abortion
  - Investigate causes.
  - Supportive care of the dam
- Placenta previa
  - Placenta covers entrance to cervix.
  - Will initiate a cesarean
- Dystocia
  - Birth is usually quick and occurs at night. Typically twins; occasionally triplets and quadruplets are produced.
  - If young obviously still in pelvic canal are discovered in the morning, the babies are likely to be dead.
  - Stabilize with fluids, calcium, and covering antibiosis.

- Consider immediate cesarean if young likely to be alive. However, if considered dead (ultrasonography, excessive time before presentation) and radiography reveals no obstruction or pelvic abnormality (e.g., from historical metabolic bone disease), then can try oxytocin at 1.0 to 2.0 IU IM, repeated every 20 minutes for 4 injections.
- Place somewhere warm, dark, and quiet.
- If this fails or there are other complications, consider cesarean.
- Use subcuticular sutures; an abdominal bandage may need to be applied to prevent interference with the sutures postoperatively.
- Provide analgesics.
- The female may need to be kept separate from her normal group during recovery, as other group members may interfere with the sutures while grooming. However, one should not allow social bonds to break down, so housing her in sight, scent, and ear shot of the rest will help, although make sure they cannot access her through cage mesh.

Neonatal disorders

Marmosets typically produce twins, but occasionally triplets may be born. The weakest one will usually die within 1 week of birth unless either hand-reared or given supplemental feeds. In such situations human milk substitutes are generally adequate but require the addition of extra protein, carbohydrate, and total lipids, plus a small amount of fish oil to improve the fatty acid composition.

Table 5-9 Common or cotton-eared marmoset: Composition of milk

Parameter	Composition/100 mL
Protein (g)	3.6
Lactose (g)	7.5
Total lipids (g)	7.7
Sodium (mg)	21.4
Potassium (mg)	54.3
Calcium (mg)	92.2
Phosphorus (mg)	22.8
Magnesium (mg)	5.0
Chloride (mg)	52.2
Osmotic pressure (mOsm/kg water)	354

Turton et al, 1978

Bacterial

- *Listeria monocytogenes*

Other noninfectious problems

- Hypothermia (especially in first few weeks as young are unable to thermoregulate). If hand-rearing, maintain temperatures at 35° to 42° C.
- Lack of maternal milk
- Mastitis (see *Reproductive Disorders*)
- Maternal metritis (see *Reproductive Disorders*)
- Maternal systemic illness

Findings on clinical examination

- Lethargy
- Failure to feed
- History of lack of maternal care
- Failure to grow
- Diarrhea (may not be apparent as female continually licks clean)
- Neurologic signs in neonates (listeriosis)

Investigations

1. Weigh young daily
2. Radiography
3. Routine hematology and biochemistry
4. Culture and sensitivity
5. Endoscopy
6. Biopsy
7. Ultrasonography

Management

- Nursing care, especially provision of warmth and fluids, is extremely important with neonates.

Treatment/specific therapy

- Lack of maternal milk production
  - Supplement with commercial milk substitute, altered as outlined above.
  - Foster only if appropriate to do so (may transfer pathogens between females).
  - Investigate underlying problem in the dam.
- *Listeria monocytogenes*
  - Appropriate antibiosis and supportive treatment
  - Prevent contamination of feed.

CHAPTER 6

Hedgehogs

African pygmy hedgehogs, or four-toed hedgehog *Atelerix albiventris* (APH), have become popular pets over the past decade or so and are more frequently presented to the clinician. There are four *Atelerix* spp. native to Africa, and *A. albiventris* originates from central and eastern Africa; in the United States and Europe this is the pet hedgehog, although in Europe the European hedgehog *Erinaceus europaeus* (EH) will be occasionally encountered as a wildlife casualty. Their susceptibility to important diseases such as foot and mouth disease mean that wild importations from Africa are severely restricted or prohibited, which may have consequences regarding a reduced genetic pool and possible increased risk of genetic disorders becoming prevalent.

Table 6-1 Hedgehogs: Key facts

Parameter	African pygmy hedgehog (*Atelerix albiventris*)	European hedgehog (*Erinaceus europaeus*)
Average life span (yr)	3-8 (occasionally >10)	3-6 (occasionally >10)
Weight (g)	500-600 (male) 250-400 (female)	600-1200 (the high weights are typically immediately prior to hibernation)
Body temperature (° C)	36.1-37.2	35.0 31.5-34 for unweaned hoglets
Respiratory rate (per min)	25-30	25-30
Heart rate (beats per min)	180-280	200-280
Gestation (days)	32	31-39
Age at weaning (weeks)	4-6	5-6
Sexual maturity (months)	2-6 (male) 6-8 (female)	6-12

Consultation and handling

Most hedgehogs can be handled reasonably easily, although this can vary between individuals. African pygmy hedgehogs are commonly well handled and will tolerate a basic clinical examination. European hedgehogs are often much more variable in their acceptance.

Anting, or anointing, is a behavior seen when the hedgehog tastes or mouths a novel food or substance. Excessive salivation is triggered that, when it has been mouthed into a thick substance, is then spread along the hedgehog's sides and back. Many reasons have been suggested for this, including antipredation, but its true function remains unclear.

Hedgehogs can be asymptomatic carriers of ringworm, so caution should always be exercised when handling them. Wearing gloves will help protect from ringworm plus reduce the risk of an urticarial reaction from the pinpoint pressure from particularly prickly hedgehogs can produce on the palms of your hands.

African pygmy hedgehogs should kept at an environmental temperature of 24° to 30° C; at temperatures below 18° C or above 30° C they may enter torpor. For European hedgehogs true hibernation is triggered by temperatures falling consistently below 15° to 17° C, and arousal is triggered by temperatures rising above 12° C.

Blood sampling

Under general anesthesia, use the jugular vein for larger volumes. Small amounts can be taken from the cephalic, lateral saphenous, and femoral veins. The vena cava can be accessed, but the heart lies further rostral in hedgehogs so care should be taken when using this method.

Nursing care

Thermoregulation

For general principles see "Thermoregulation" under *Nursing Care* in Chapter 2. Keep African pygmy hedgehogs at 24° to 30° C; avoid temperatures below 18° C as this may induce torpor even in healthy hedgehogs.

Fluid therapy

Fluids can be given subcutaneously up to 100 mL/kg beneath the loose skin over the dorsum, although absorption may take some time. Vascular access is difficult. The cephalic vein may be accessible for bolus fluids; otherwise consider intraosseus administration into the trochanteric fossa or proximal tibia. Intraperitoneal injections can be given; the optimum site is just to the right of the umbilicus.

Nutritional support

Hedgehogs need to be fed a high-quality diet. Normal diet should be a mixture of high-quality dried cat foods, live invertebrate prey such as mealworms, and some vegetable material. Do not give milk as this can trigger diarrhea. Anorexic hedgehogs can be offered or fed on commercially available supportive powdered carnivore or omnivore diets or on high-calorie wet foods as available for cats.

Analgesia

Table 6-2 Hedgehogs: Analgesic doses

Analgesic	Dose
Buprenorphine	0.01-0.5 mg/kg SC or IM every 6-12 hr
Butorphanol	0.05-0.4 mg/kg IM every 6-12 hr
Carprofen	1.0 mg/kg SC, PO every 12-24 hr
Meloxicam	0.1-0.2 mg/kg SC or PO every 24 hr

Anesthesia

Starve for 4 hours maximum to reduce risk of regurgitation.

Gaseous anesthesia
- Premedicate with atropine at 0.01 to 0.05 mg/kg SC to prevent hypersalivation.
- Induction with gaseous isoflurane in an induction chamber
- Maintain either with a mask or intubate with small-diameter endotracheal tube (<2 mm) or suitable intravenous catheter.

Parenteral anesthesia

- Ketamine at 5.0 to 10.0 mg/kg IM
- Medetomidine at 0.05 to 0.2 mg/kg SC or IM

- Intraoperative care
  - Keep warm (see "Thermoregulation"). It is crucial that body temperature is maintained to ensure a good recovery.
  - Fluids (see "Fluid Therapy")
- Postoperative aftercare
  - Reverse medetomidine (if used) with atipamezole at 0.4 to 1.0 mg/kg IM
  - Analgesia—as above
  - Must be offered food as soon as recovers
  - Keep warm.

Cardiopulmonary resuscitation

1. Intubate and ventilate at 20 to 30 breaths/min.
2. Reverse medetomidine (if used) with atipamezole at 0.3 to 1.0 mg/kg IM.
3. If cardiac arrest, external cardiac massage at around 100 compressions/min
4. Epinephrine at
   a. 0.2 mg/kg IV or diluted in sterile saline intratracheal
   b. 0.003 mg/kg intracardiac, IV, or IO
5. Fluid therapy (see above)
6. If bradycardic, atropine at 0.05 to 0.2 mg/kg IV or 0.05 to 0.1 mg/kg intratracheal

---

Skin disorders

General

The hairs on hedgehogs are modified into quills that cover the dorsal surface. There is a narrow spineless tract that runs from the crown of the head rostrocaudally for around 2 cm or so. The skin of the back has a thin epidermis that overlies a thick dermal fibrous layer, and underneath this there is a loose layer of fat and subcutaneous tissue. Although often used for subscutaneous fluid administration, vascularization here is poor. Sweat glands and sebaceous glands are present in the haired regions and on the soles of the feet. Newborn hedgehogs sport a pelage of white soft spines that harden within a few hours. A second set of harder and darker spines emerges 2 days after birth. In APH quills are replaced at 4, 6, 9, and 12 weeks.

Hedgehogs do not tolerate Elizabethan collars. They are avid groomers.

Differential diagnoses of skin disorders

Pruritus

- Mites
- Bacterial dermatitis (including *Staphylococcus* spp.)
- Epitheliotropic T-cell lymphoma (mycosis fungoides—Chung et al 2014)

Alopecia and quill loss

- Dermatophytosis (ringworm)—*Trichophyton mentagrophytes* var. *erinacei*, *Arthroderma benhamiae* var. *erinacei*, *Microsporum* spp.
- Mites

- Bacterial dermatitis
  - *Staphylococcus simulans* (Han et al 2011)
- Epitheliotropic T-cell lymphoma (mycosis fungoides—Chung et al 2014)
- Ectoparasites

Scaling and crusting

- Ringworm—*Trichophyton mentagrophytes* var. *erinacei*, *Arthroderma benhamiae* var. *erinacei*, *Microsporum* spp.
- Epitheliotropic T-cell lymphoma (mycosis fungoides—Chung et al 2014)
- Ectoparasites

Erosions and ulceration

- Bite wounds
- Burst abscesses
- Foot and mouth disease

Nodules and nonhealing wounds

- Papillomas (suspected viral etiology)
- Pododermatitis
- Abscesses

Changes in pigmentation

- Dermatophytosis
- Mites
- Neoplasia

Ectoparasites

- Mites
  - *Caparinia erinacei*, *C. tripilis* (Moreira et al 2013)
  - *Notoedres oudesmani*
  - *Notoedres cati* (Pantchev and Hofmann 2006)
  - *Chorioptes* spp.
  - *Otodectes cyanotis* (ear mites)
  - *Demodex erinacei*
  - *Sarcoptes* spp.
  - *Neotrombicula* spp. (chiggers)
- Ticks
  - *Rhipicephalus sanguineus* (APH)
  - *Haemaphysalis erinacei* (APH)
  - *Ixodes ricinus* (EH)
  - *Ixodes hexagonus* (EH)
- Fleas
  - *Archeopsylla erinacei*
- Myiasis
  - *Lucilia* spp.
  - *Calliphora* spp.

Neoplasia

- Mast cell tumor
- Mammary tumors

- Squamous cell carcinoma
- Sebaceous carcinoma (Kim et al 2010)
- Neurofibroma
- Extraskeletal osteosarcoma (Phair et al 2011)
- Epithelioid variant of hemangiosarcoma (Finkelstein et al 2008)
- Epitheliotropic T-cell lymphoma (Chung et al 2014; Spugnini et al 2008)

Otitis externa

Pinnal dermatitis

Cutaneous emphysema

Other findings on clinical examination

- Discharge from ear canal; unpleasant smell from ear (otits externa)
- Crusty areas on pinnae, especially around margins (pinnal dermatitis)
- Quill loss, hyperkeratosis (dermatophytosis, bacterial dermatitis—Fig. 6-1)
- Quill loss, chronic pruritic dermatitis leading to self-trauma, scabs, lethargy, dehydration, and weight loss (*Caparinia* mites)
- Vesicles or open lesions on feet, muzzle, perineum, and tongue (foot and mouth disease)

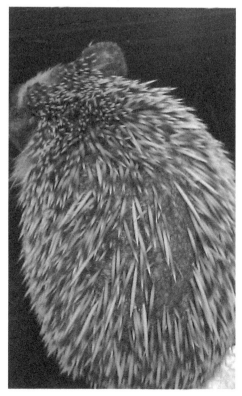

Fig. 6-1. Hedgehog exhibiting quill loss secondary to a bacterial dermatitis.

Investigations

1. Microscopy: Examine fur pluck, acetate strips, or skin scrapes to affected area and examine for ectoparasites and ringworm.
2. Cytology: Stain with lactophenol blue for ringworm.
3. Examine material from ear canals for *Otodectes cynotis*.
4. Bacteriology and mycology: Hair/quill pluck or swab lesions for routine culture and sensitivity.
5. Fine-needle aspirate followed by staining with rapid Romanowsky stains
6. Biopsy obvious lesions.
7. Ultraviolet (Wood's) lamp: Positive for *Microsporium canis* only (not all strains fluoresce)
8. Radiography
9. Routine hematology and biochemistry
10. Endoscopy
11. Biopsy
12. Ultrasonography

Treatment/specific therapy

- Bite wounds
  - Clean and debride; hedgehogs may self-mutilate, so primary closure with subcuticular suture pattern is preferred.
- Abscesses
  - Drain and debride; some may require surgical removal.
  - Be aware of possibility of mycobacteriosis.
- Bacterial dermatitis
  - Appropriate antibiosis
  - Clean lesions with topical antibacterial preparations (e.g., chlorhexidine/F10).
- Papillomas
  - Likely benign; surgical resection if required
- Dermatophytosis (ringworm)
  - Systemic antifungals
    - Itraconazole at 5 to 10 mg/kg PO every 12 to 24 hours
    - Ketoconazole 10 mg/kg PO b.i.d.
    - Griseofulvin 25 to 50 mg/kg PO daily
  - Potential zoonosis
- Mites
  - *Caparinia* infestations are often highly pruritic and may require antiinflammatories to control pruritis and covering antibiosis for secondary skin infections.
  - Ivermectin 0.2 to 0.5 mg/kg SC every 2 weeks for 3 treatments
  - Selamectin topically at 15 mg/kg, 2 doses at 30-day interval (Delk et al 2013)
  - Topical 10% imidacloprid plus 1.0% moxidectin spot-on (Advocate for Cats (UK), Advantage Multi (US), Bayer) at 0.1 mL/kg (Kim et al 2012)
  - Moxidectin 0.3 mg/kg SC; repeat after 10 days (Pantchev and Hofmann 2006)
  - Permethrin 1%, apply once only
  - Amitraz 0.3% dip every 7 to 10 days
- Fleas
  - As for mites; also environmental control as for other small animal species

- Ear mites
  - Topical antiparasitic ear preparations, although the small size of the ear canal may prevent effective treatment.
  - Selamectin spot-on at 6 mg/kg as a topical spot-on preparation
  - Cross-infection with dogs and cats in the same household may occur.
- Ticks
  - Unlikely in captive APH; common in wild hedgehogs of all species
  - Manual removal; may need general anesthetic to allow access to all areas if high tick burden
  - Ivermectin at 0.2 mg/kg SC or topically repeat after 2 weeks
  - *Note:* Ticks in both APH and EH are implicated in harboring rickettsial infections.
- Myiasis
  - Physical removal of maggots
  - Ivermectin 0.2 to 0.5 mg/kg SC once only, but can be repeated after 2 weeks.
  - Fluids
  - Covering antibiosis; analgesics
- Neoplasia
  - Surgical resection
  - Some may respond to chemotherapy. Consult contemporary small animal protocols according to histopathologic classification.
  - Epitheliotropic T-cell lymphoma: May respond to chemotherapy if diagnosed sufficiently early
- Pododermatitis
  - Radiography to assess underlying bone involvement
  - Clean and debride if appropriate.
  - Covering antibiosis
  - Analgesia
  - Soft substrate
- Otitis externa
  - Systemic antibiosis/antifungals according to culture
  - Topical otic preparations if tympanic membrane known to be intact
- Pinnal dermatitis
  - No one etiology identified; associated variously with dermatophytosis (see above), acariasis (see "Mites" above), nutritional deficiency, low-humidity conditions, and dry skin
- Cutaneous emphysema
  - Etiology often difficult to ascertain; may be linked to mediastinal injury (e.g., rib fracture), allowing air to escape subcutaneously; deep-seated gas-producing infections
  - Air/gas in subcutaneous tissues
  - Release/aspirate gas aseptically; may need to be repeated
  - Covering antibiosis and analgesia
- Foot and mouth disease—see *Gastrointestinal Tract Disorders*

Respiratory tract disorders

Bacterial

- *Pasteurella*
- *Corynebacterium*
- *Bordetella bronchisepticum*

Fungal
- Histoplasmosis (see *Splenic Disorders*)

Parasitic
- *Capillaria aerophilum* (EH)
- *Crenosoma striatum* (EH)

Neoplasia
- Bronchoalveolar carcinoma
- Squamous cell carcinoma
- Pulmonary adenocarcinoma

Other noninfectious problems
- Aspiration pneumonia (Pei-Chi et al 2015)
- Pulmonary hemorrhage (Pei-Chi et al 2015)
- Cardiac disease (see *Cardiovascular Disorders*)

Findings on clinical examination

- Dyspnea
- Respiratory noise
- Nasal discharge
- Lethargy
- Inappetence
- Sudden death

Investigations

1. Tracheal wash/bronchoalveolar lavage
2. Fecal microscopy (lungworm eggs)
3. Culture and sensitivity
4. Cytology
5. Pleural tap and cytology
6. Radiography
7. Endoscopy
8. Biopsy
9. Ultrasonography

Management

1. Supportive treatment (e.g., fluids, covering antibiosis)
2. Reduce stress levels. Hospitalize away from dogs and noisy cats; keep in darkened position.

Treatment/specific therapy

- Bacterial pneumonia
  - Appropriate antibiosis
  - NSAIDs

- High-oxygen environment
- Mucolytics may be useful.
- Lungworms
  - Consider covering antibiosis and NSAIDs, as rapid die-offs of worms following treatment can cause serious lung damage and increase risk of pneumonia.
  - Ivermectin at 0.2 mg/kg PO topically body weight; repeat after 2 weeks.
  - Fenbendazole at 50 mg/kg PO body weight; repeat after 2 weeks.
  - *Crenosoma* spp. carried by snails. Prepatent period of 21 days before eggs are shed. Prevent access to mollusk hosts. *Crenosoma* can cross placental barrier.

Gastrointestinal tract disorders

Permanent dental formula

A. albiventris and *E. europeus*

$$I : \frac{3}{2} \quad C : \frac{1}{1} \quad PM : \frac{3}{2} \quad M : \frac{3}{3}$$

In *A. albiventris* the deciduous teeth begin to erupt at 18 days and are complete by 9 weeks old. The permanent teeth begin to erupt at around age 7 to 9 weeks. The upper incisors slot into a gap between the lower incisors, which are forward-projecting.

Disorders of the oral cavity

An anesthetic will be required for a good oral examination
- Dental disease
  - Periodontal disease
    - Antibiosis
    - Tartar removal under general anesthetic
    - Dental extractions

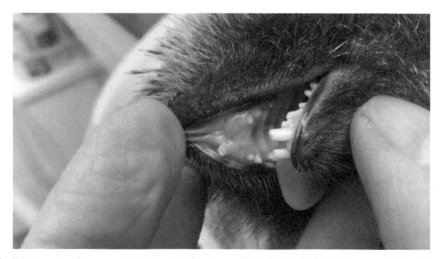

Fig 6-2. A good oral exam on a hedgehog requires an anesthetic. This hedgehog lost an upper incisor; the resultant tooth root abscess caused a unilateral discharge that triggered the initial presentation.

  - Attempt prophylaxis by feeding self-cleaning, abrasive diets such as chitinous insects, adding charcoal or powdered bone to feed, or hard kibble.
- Fractured tooth
  - Extraction
- Tooth root abscess
  - Extraction
  - Antibiosis
- Mandibular osteomyelitis
  - *Actinomyces naeslundii* (Martínez et al 2005)
  - Appropriate antibiosis (e.g., potentiated sulfonamides)
  - High risk of systemic spread
- Bone cysts (mandibular swelling)
- Neoplasia
  - Undifferentiated sarcoma (Fig. 6-3)
- Neoplasia
  - Squamous cell carcinoma
  - Poorly differentiated tumor
  - Fibrosarcoma plasmacytoma
  - Mucoepidermoid carcinoma of the parotid gland (Pei-Chi et al 2015)

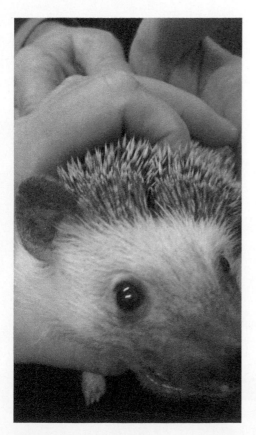

Fig 6-3. Hedgehog exhibiting an undifferentiated sarcoma of the gums of the lower mandible visible as an asymmetric swelling of the mandible.

Differential diagnoses for gastrointestinal disorders

Viral

- Foot and mouth disease
- Parvovirus

Bacterial

- Bacterial enteritis
- *Salmonella*

Fungal

Protozoal

- *Cryptosporidium erinacei* (Kváč et al 2014a)
- *Eimeria rastegaiv*
- *Isospora erinacei*

Parasitic

- Nematodes
  - *Capillaria erinacei*
  - *Capillaria* spp.
  - *Physaloptera* spp. (stomach worms)
  - *Gonglyonema* spp. (esophageal worms)
- Acanthocephalans (thorny-headed worms)
  - *Echinorhynchus erinacei; E. roase* (EU)
  - *Moniliformis cestodiformis, M. moniliform* (APH)
- *Hymenolepis erinacei* (tapeworm)
- *Brachylaemus erinacei* (fluke)

Nutritional

- Milk (lactose intolerance)
- Dietary indiscretion

Neoplasia

- Squamous cell carcinoma (oral)
- Fibrosarcoma plasmacytoma (oral)
- Plasmacytoma (intestinal)
- Acinic cell carcinoma (intestine)
- Adenocarcinoma
- Intestinal lymphosarcoma

Other noninfectious problems

- Foreign body (e.g., carpet fibers)
- Gastric ulceration (Pei-Chi et al 2015)
- Gastroesophageal intussusception (Lee and Park 2012)
- Megaesophagus (Lee and Park 2012)
- Liver disease

Findings on clinical examination

- Diarrhea
  - Green mucoid diarrhea (*Capillaria* spp.)

- Reduced or absent feces (obstruction, constipation, inappetence)
- Vesicular lesions on the tongue, snout, and feet (foot and mouth disease)
- Sudden death *(Cryptosporidium)*
- Anorexia, vomiting, collapse (foreign body)
- Hemorrhagic diarrhea (lymphosarcoma)
- Melena, restlessness (flukes)
- Vesicular and abraided lesions on tongue, around muzzle, feet, and perineum (foot and mouth disease)

Investigations

1. Fecal examination
   a. MZN staining for *Cryptosporidium*
   b. Bipolar eggs (*Capillaria* spp.—but see also lungworm in *Respiratory Tract Disorders*)
   c. Proglottids (tapeworm)
   d. Unipolar eggs (flukes)
   e. Grass seedlike worms; embryonated eggs with hooks visible (acanthocephalans)
2. Radiography
   a. Foreign body
3. Routine hematology and biochemistry
   a. Pronounced leukocytosis with neutrophilia and lymphocytosis (intestinal lymphosarcoma—Helmer 2000)
4. Culture and sensitivity
5. PCR (parvovirus)
6. Endoscopy
7. Biopsy
8. Ultrasonography

Management

1. Fluid therapy (see *Nursing Care*)
2. If vomiting:
   a. Do not feed for around 6 hours and use antiemetics (e.g., metoclopramide at 0.2 to 1.0 mg/kg SC t.i.d.
   b. Monitor blood glucose; consider dextrose/saline fluids.

Treatment/specific therapy

- Foot and mouth disease
  - Notifiable in United Kingdom, and reportable in United States
  - Euthanasia
- Parvovirus
  - Symptomatic treatment
- Bacterial enteritis
  - See "Management" above.
  - Appropriate antibiosis
- *Salmonella*
  - Potentially zoonotic
  - Discuss implications of zoonotic risk with owner.

- *Cryptosporidium*
  - Often subclinical, but described as a cause of sudden death (Graczyk et al 1998). Postmortem revealed a catarrhal gastroenteritis.
  - Prepatent period 4 to 5 days; patent period >20 days (Kváč et al 2014a)
  - No effective treatment recognized
  - Potentiated sulfonamides may be of use, as may nitazoxanide at 5 mg/kg PO s.i.d.
  - Potential zoonosis (Kváč et al 2014b), so consider euthanasia.
- *Eimeria* and *Isospora*
  - Toltrazuril at 10 mg/kg PO daily for 2 days, repeated weekly for 3 weeks
  - Potentiated sulfonamides
- *Capillaria* spp.
  - As for lungworm in *Respiratory Tract Disorders*
- Acanthocephalans
  - Praziquantel at 25 mg/kg PO
  - Covering antibiosis and analgesia for heavy burdens
- Tapeworm
  - Usually asymptomatic
  - Prevent access to beetles (intermediate hosts).
  - Praziquantel at 5 to 10 mg/kg PO or SC; repeat monthly if required.
- Fluke
  - As for tapeworm
- Foreign body
  - Likely to need surgical removal
- Gastric ulceration
  - As for other species: Consider antibiosis, H_2 blockers (e.g., cimetidine, ranitidine), and gastroprotectants (e.g., sucralfate).
- Gastroesophageal intussusception
  - Attempt surgical correction; poor prognosis
  - Treat underlying causes, typically esophagitis.

Nutritional disorders

Hedgehogs are invertebrate predators with omnivore leanings, so the natural diet of hedgehogs consists largely of invertebrates such as insects and terrestrial mollusks, with some fruits and roots taken. Recommended fat and protein levels are 5% and 22%, but with mealworms having 33% fat and 53% protein, offering a diet largely of these commercially available insects is likely to lead to obesity. In addition there is a risk of hypocalcemia unless balanced with suitable calcium supplements. Hence the following recommendations are made:

Hedgehog nutrition

1. Low-calorie dry cat or dog kibble foods are recommended. The dental self-cleaning nature of these foods helps to reduce dental disease (see *Gastrointestinal Tract Disorders*), and the lower calorific value reduces the risk of obesity.
2. Only a small percentage of insect-based foods such as mealworms should be offered.
3. A small proportion of vegetable material is recommended.
4. Adjust portion size to that consumed overnight.

Table 6-3 Hedgehogs: normal serum calcium and phosphorus

Parameter	APH *Atelerix albiventris*	EH *Erinaceus europeus*
Calcium (mmol/L)	2.2 ± 0.4	3.1
Phosphorus (mmol/L)	1.6 ± 0.5	1.5

APH, *African pygmy hedgehog*; EH, *European hedgehog*.

- Obesity
  - Common with captive diets; likely an imbalance between high caloric intake and reduced energy expenditure (reduced exercise, nonbreeding, nonhibernation)
  - Weigh weekly and record the weights so as to avoid obesity.
  - Limit amount offered so that all is consumed overnight with none left over.
- Hypoglycemia from starvation (see *Pancreatic Disorders* for management)
- Hepatic lipidosis
  - Linked to anorexia, especially in obese individuals
  - Aggressive fluid therapy
  - Parenteral nutrition with glucose and vitamins
  - Assisted feeding by syringe (see *Nursing Care*)
  - Calcium gluconate PO or propylene glycol PO may be of use.
  - Dexamethasone at 0.2 mg/kg IV, SC, or PO once only
- Thiamine (vitamin B_1) deficiency
  - Possibly linked to feeding diets deficient in or compromised for vitamin B_1 (e.g., frozen milk) or due to chronic gut environment abnormalities (e.g., diarrhea)
  - Signs include weight loss, ataxia and paresis, lethargy, and muscle weakness.
  - Vitamin B complex at 1 to 2 mg/kg thiamine content as needed IM
  - Supplement with thiamine at 300 mg/hedgehog/day.
- Hypovitaminosis A (see *Ophthalmic Disorders*)
- Hypovitaminosis D_3
  - Stunted growth, shortened deformed limbs, squatting gait
  - Anorexia, ataxia, hyperpnea, weight loss, diarrhea
  - Deformation of vertebrae and ribs; pathological fractures of long bones
  - Biochemistry (Table 6-3)
  - Supplement with dietary vitamin D_3 and calcium.

Hepatic disorders

Viral
- Herpesvirus (EH)

Nutritional
- Hepatic lipidosis
- Ketosis (see *Reproductive Disorders*)

Neoplasia
- Lymphoma/lymphosarcoma (see *Systemic Disorders*)
- Metastases (e.g., insulinoma)

- Hemangiosarcoma
- Adenocarcinoma
- Hepatocellular adenoma
- Hepatocellular carcinoma
- Bile duct cyst adenoma
- Biliary carcinoma

Other noninfectious problems

- Lymphocytic hepatitis
- Cholangiohepatitis
- Chylous ascites (Roh et al 2014)
- Cirrhosis (Roh et al 2014)

Findings on clinical examination

- Reduced appetite or loss of appetite
- Vague signs of ill health
- Abnormal feces
- Hepatomegaly
- Jaundice (rare)
- Ascites
- Bile-tinged (green) diarrhea
- Seizures

Investigations

1. Radiography
2. Routine hematology and biochemistry
3. Culture and sensitivity
4. Abdominal tap
   a. Milky white fluid with triglyceride <1.24 mm/L (chylous ascites)
5. Endoscopy
6. Biopsy
7. Ultrasonography

Management

1. Fluid therapy (see *Nursing Care*)
2. Lactulose at 150 to 750 mg/kg PO b.i.d. or t.i.d.
3. Milk thistle *(Silybum marianum)* is hepatoprotectant. Dose at 4 to 15 mg/kg PO b.i.d. or t.i.d.

Treatment/specific therapy

- Herpesvirus (see *Systemic Disorders*)
- Hepatic lipidosis (see *Nutritional Disorders*)
- Cirrhosis
  - General management as for other species

- Chylous ascites
  - Regular abdominal drainage
  - General liver management
  - Low-fat foods
  - Very poor prognosis

Splenic disorders

Fungal
- *Histoplasma capsulatum* (Snider et al 2008)

Neoplasia
- Hemangiosarcoma and hemangioma
- Lymphoma/lymphosarcoma (Burballa et al 2012—see *Systemic Disorders*)

Noninfectious disorders
- Cardiac disease (see *Cardiovascular and Hematologic Disorders*)

Findings on clinical examination

- Loss of appetite, weakness, lethargy, weight loss (histoplasmosis)

Investigations

- Radiography
  - Splenomegaly
- Routine hematology and biochemistry
  - Anemia, thrombocytopenia, leukopenia, hypoproteinemia, hypoglycemia (histoplasmosis)
- Culture and sensitivity
- Endoscopy
  - Splenomegaly, disseminated granulomatous infiltration (histoplasmosis)
- Exploratory surgery and biopsy
  - As for endoscopy
- Ultrasonography

Treatment

- *Histoplasma capsulatum*
  - Itraconazole 5 to 10 mg/kg PO daily
- Neoplasia
  - Hemangiosarcoma/hemangioma: Surgical resection
  - Chemotherapy for lymphoma/lymphosarcoma if generalized

Pancreatic disorders

Neoplasia
- Adenoma
- Islet cell tumor

Findings on clinical examination

- Abdominal distension
- Pain
- Abdominal mass palpable
- Lethargy
- Weight loss

Investigations

1. Radiography
2. Routine hematology and biochemistry
   a. Normal glucose: APH 3.1 to 6.9 mmol/L; EH 1.3 to 5.9 mmol/L
3. Culture and sensitivity
4. Urinalysis
5. Endoscopy
6. Exploratory surgery and biopsy
7. Ultrasonography

Management

1. Treatment of hypoglycemia (see box)

Hypoglycemia

1. Rub honey or sugared water onto the gingiva, taking care not to get bitten.
2. 0.5 to 2.0 mL IV bolus of 50% dextrose solution given slowly
3. Fluid therapy (see *Nursing Care*) with 5% dextrose infusion
4. If hedgehog fails to respond, can give shock dose of dexamethasone at 4 to 8 mg/kg IV or IM once only.
5. Diazepam at 1 to 2 mg/kg IV as needed to control if seizures persistent

---

Treatment/specific therapy

- Pancreatic neoplasia
  - Symptomatic treatment of clinical signs (e.g., hypoglycemia)
  - Surgical resection possible if discrete and away from pancreatic duct area

Cardiovascular and hematologic disorders

Cardiovascular disease is common in APH and can reach an incidence of 40%.

Bacterial

- Bacteremia/septicemia
- Endocarditis
- Pericarditis

Parasitic

- *Trypanosoma* spp.

Neoplasia

- Lymphoma (see *Systemic Disorders*)
- Hemangioma

Other noninfectious problems

- Cardiomyopathy
- Congenital disorders
- Endocardiosis (Hedley et al 2013)
- Erythropoietic porphyria (Wolff et al 2005)

Findings on clinical examination

- Cyanosis or pallor of the mucous membranes
- Anaemia
- Slow capillary refill time
- Dyspnea
- Precordial thrill
- Abormalities of femoral arterial pulse, including weakness, irregularities, and pulse deficits
- Arrhythmia
- Lack of thoracic percussion with auscultation
- Abnormal lung sounds
- Abnormal heart sounds
- Exercise intolerance
- Ascites
- Hepatomegaly, splenomegaly
- Weight loss
- Sudden death
- Hematuria, proteinuria (*Trypanosoma* spp.)
- Renal disease
- Pink-stained urine; urine, teeth, quills fluoresce under ultraviolet light (erythropoietic porphyria)
- Icterus

Investigations

1. Auscultation
2. Radiography (Table 6-4)
   a. Cardiomegaly
   b. Pulmonary edema
   c. Hydrothorax
   d. Hepatomegaly
3. Ultrasonography/echocardiography (Table 6-5)
4. Culture and sensitivity, including blood cultures
5. Endoscopy
6. Biopsy
7. Spectroscopic analysis of urine and fecal pigments (erythropoietic porphyria)

Table 6-4 Radiographic cardiac values for healthy anesthetized African hedgehogs (*Atelerix albiventris*)

Variable	Mean ± SD	Median	CV%	First quartile	Third quartile	Range
AB/CD	1.38 ± 0.11	1.41	8.23	1.29	1.46	1.24-1.59
AB/H	0.88 ± 0.07	0.88	8.43	0.84	0.90	0.74-1.01
AB/R5-7	1.89 ± 0.29	1.85	16.14	1.75	1.92	1.55-2.73
CD/H	0.63 ± 0.04	0.63	8.23	0.60	0.67	0.58-0.70
VHS	8.16 ± 0.48	8.25	5.86	8.00	8.50	7.25-8.75
L/W	1.40 ± 0.11	1.41	7.68	1.38	1.48	1.16-1.55
L/C	1.64 ± 0.25	1.56	15.08	1.46	1.77	1.38-2.13
W/T	0.60 ± 0.03	0.59	5.23	0.58	0.62	0.55-0.66
W/C	1.17 ± 0.17	1.09	14.14	1.05	1.26	1.00-1.45

Values taken from lateral radiograph:

AB, *Apicobasilar length of the heart (as measured from the long axis of the heart); CD, the maximum width of the heart perpendicular to AB; R5-7, distance from the cranial edge of the fifth rib to the caudal edge of the seventh rib; H, the vertical depth of the thorax from the ventral border of the spine to the dorsal border of sternum at the level of the tracheal bifurcation; VHS, vertebral heart score. AB and CD are each lined up with the vertebrae starting with T4 and the distances measured to the nearest 0.25 of a vertebra. These two values are then added to produce the VHS.*

On the ventrodorsal view, the following values were taken:

L, *The heart length as measured along the long axis of the heart; W, the maximum heart width perpendicular to L; T, the thoracic width at the level of the articulation of the sixth rib with the vertebral column; C, length of the clavicle.*

(After Black et al 2011.)

Management

- Reduce stress (e.g., keep in a cool, shaded or darkened area away from potential stressors such as dogs).
- Provide a high-oxygen environment.
- For pleural effusion, consider tube thoracostomy.
- *Note:* Renal disease is common with cardiomyopathies (Raymond and Garner 2000).

Treatment/specific therapy

- Cardiomyopathies
  - Dilated (congestive) cardiomyopathy
    - Furosemide at 1 to 5 mg/kg PO, SC t.i.d. or q.i.d. (see Delk et al 2013)
    - Enalapril at 1.0 mg/kg PO every 24 hours (Delk et al 2013)
    - Benazepril 0.25 to 0.5 mg/kg PO daily should be considered; less nephrotoxic than enalapril
    - Pimobendan at 0.3 mg/kg PO b.i.d.
    - L-carnitine at 50 mg/kg PO b.i.d. (Delk et al 2013)

Table 6-5 Echocardiographic values for healthy anesthetized African hedgehogs (*Atelerix albiventris*)

Variables	Mean ± SD	Median	CV%	First quartile	Third quartile	Range
IVSd (cm)	0.15 ± 0.01	0.15	7.40	0.14	0.16	0.13-0.17
IVSs (cm)	0.22 ± 0.02	0.22	6.97	0.21	0.23	0.19-0.24
LVIDd (cm)	0.74 ± 0.05	0.74	6.65	0.71	0.77	0.67-0.84
LVIDs (cm)	0.58 ± 0.03	0.58	5.98	0.57	0.59	0.54-0.65
LVFWd (cm)	0.16 ± 0.01	0.16	7.84	0.15	0.16	0.14-0.18
LVFWs (cm)	0.23 ± 0.02	0.23	11.04	0.21	0.24	0.19-0.27
FS (%)	21.45 ± 2.50	22.10	11.65	19.90	22.55	17.40-26.80
EPSS (cm)	0.11 ± 0.02	0.10	15.49	0.10	0.12	0.09-0.14
AO (cm)	0.36 ± 0.02	0.36	6.90	0.35	0.38	0.31-0.40
LA (cm)	0.56 ± 0.04	0.56	7.05	0.52	0.60	0.51-0.62
LA/AO	1.55 ± 0.16	1.49	10.48	1.47	1.56	1.37-1.92
LVOT (cm/s)	48.86 ± 10.76	46.20	22.02	42.80	55.95	29.60-66.20
RVOT (cm/s)	33.50 ± 9.43	28.90	28.16	26.80	40.95	23.60-51.20

AO, *Aortic diameters during diastole;* EPSS, *E-point-to-septal separation length;* FS, *fractional shortening;* IVSd, *interventricular septal thickness in diastole;* IVSs, *interventricular septal thickness in systole;* LA, *left atrium internal dimension;* LVFWd, *left ventricular free wall thickness in diastole;* LVFWs, *left ventricular free wall thickness in systole;* LVIDd, *left ventricular internal dimension in diastole;* LVIDs, *left ventricular internal dimension in systole;* LVOT, *maximum velocity of the left ventricular outflow;* RVOT, *maximum velocity of the right ventricular outflow.*
(After Black et al 2011.)

- Hypertrophic cardiomyopathy
  - Atenolol at 0.5 to 2.0 mg/kg PO daily
  - Diltiazem at 0.5 to 1.0 mg/kg PO b.i.d.
- Valvular heart disease
  - Treat as for dilated cardiomyopathy
- Erythropoietic porphyria
  - Treat symptomatically.
  - Wolff et al (2005) report affected hedgehog showed few signs of ill health. Lack of expected photodermatitis possibly due to nocturnal nature of APH.
  - Presumed autosomal recessive as in other species
- Bacterial infections
  - Appropriate antibiosis

Systemic disorders

Viral

- Retrovirus (possible cause of lymphoma)
- Pneumonia virus of mice (PVM—Madarame et al 2014)
- Herpesvirus

Bacterial

- Bacteremia/septicemia
- Mycobacteriosis
  - *M. bovis*

Fungal

- *Histoplasma capsulatum* (see *Splenic Disorders*)

Nutritional

Neoplasia

- Lymphosarcoma (multicentric, gastrointestinal)
- Myeloproliferative disease/myelogenous leukemia

Other noninfectious problems

- Torpor (see *Neurologic Disorders*)
- Levamisole toxicity

Findings on clinical examination

- Weight loss
- Hind-leg weakness (wobbly hedgehog syndrome, intervertebral disease—see *Neurologic Disorders*)
- Chronic upper respiratory infections, dyspnea, general lethargy, wasting, and lymphadenopathy (lymphoma)
- Palpable abdominal masses (splenomegaly, mesenteric and/or gastric lymph nodes—lymphoma)
- Seizures
- Ataxia
- Circling
- Hyperesthesia, twitching, dyspnea, hypersalivation, and possibly cyanosis (levamisole toxicity, metaldehyde poisoning)
- Bluish colored feces or vomit (metaldehyde poisoning)
- Sudden death; signs of pain and discomfort and rapid death (herpesvirus)

Investigations

1. Radiography
   a. Mediastinal masses, pleural effusions, abdominal masses (lymphoma)
2. Routine hematology and biochemistry
3. Bone marrow aspirate/lymph node cytology (lymphoma)
4. Abdominal centesis and cytology
5. Culture and sensitivity
6. Endoscopy
7. Biopsy/necropsy
   a. Lymphoma (especially mesenteric lymph node, peripheral lymph nodes, spleen, liver, and any abnormal organs)
8. Ultrasonography

Management

- See *Nursing Care.*

Treatment/specific therapy

- Rabies
  - Significant zoonosis. Euthanize.
- Bacteremia/septicemia
  - Appropriate antibiosis
  - Supportive therapy as necessary (see *Nursing Care*)
- Mycobacteriosis
  - Zoonosis; notifiable in UK
  - Euthanasia
- Lymphoma/lymphosarcoma
  - Chemotherapy protocols for small animals are regularly altered and updated, so if in doubt, consult a veterinary oncologist.
  - Palliative treatment for lymphoma:
    - Prednisolone at 0.5 mg/kg PO b.i.d., increasing to control signs. *Note:* Prednisolone treatment alone is likely to make the lymphoma refractory to chemotherapy.
    - Regular annual CBC to screen for lymphoma
- PMV
  - Recorded as strongly suspected cause of encephalitis by Madarame et al 2014
- Levamisole toxicity
  - Treat symptomatically.
- Metaldehyde poisoning
  - Typically seen in EH following direct ingestion of slug bait; indirect ingestion (i.e., consumption of poisoned slugs) appears to have minimal effects.
  - Control hyperesthesia/convulsions (e.g., diazepam at 2 to 3 mg/kg SC, PO, per rectum body weight).
  - Consider apomorphine as an emetic.
  - Supportive therapy (e.g., fluids, gastric lavage)
- Herpesvirus
  - If diagnosed antemortem, consider acyclovir or famciclovir.
  - Poor prognosis

Musculoskeletal disorders

A unique property of hedgehogs is their ability to roll into an almost closed ball and position their spines into an erect position. This is achieved by a combination of the frontodorsalis and caudodorsalis muscles, which respectively move the spines down over the rump and forehead. The panniculus carnosus muscle rolls the hedgehog up, while the orbicularis muscle pulls the mantle of spines together like a drawstring.

Bacterial

- Myositis

Parasitic

- Pentastomids
  - *Lingulata* spp.
  - *Armillifer armillatus*

Neoplasia

- Osteosarcoma (Benoit-Biancamano et al 2006; Rhody and Schiller 2006)

Other noninfectious problems

- Bone cysts (see *Gastrointestinal Disorders*)
- Traumatic fractures
- Orbicularis muscle prolapse
- Osteoarthritis
- Foreign body/annular fiber around digit/extremity
- Any causes of weakness
  - See *Neurologic Disorders*
  - See *Cardiac and Hematologic Disorders*
  - See *Systemic Disorders*
  - See *Pancreatic Disorders*

Findings on clinical examination

- Pain
- Lameness
- Swelling
- Hind-leg paresis/paralysis
- Mandibular swelling (bone cysts)
- Self-mutilation of hind feet (spinal osteosarcoma—Rhody and Schiller 2006)
- Apparent paralysis; the hind legs and pelvis protrude backward and sideways from below spiny coat, with the tail and anus pulled up over the back. The orbicularis muscle is found to lie above (dorsal to) the pelvis (orbicularis muscle prolapse).

Investigations

1. Radiography
   a. Osteolysis, pathological fractures (multiple myeloma)
   b. Spinal cord compression (osteosarcoma)
2. Traumatic fractures
3. Routine hematology and biochemistry
4. Culture and sensitivity
5. Endoscopy
6. Biopsy
7. Ultrasonography

Treatment/specific therapy

- Traumatic fractures
  - Repair using standard small animal techniques.
  - May respond well to strict rest (close confinement), especially if bone density suspect (See "Hypovitaminosis D_3" in *Nutritional Disorders*)
- Neoplasia
  - Surgical resection, amputation, chemotherapy, or radiation therapy as for other small animals

- Annular fiber
  - Remove under general anesthesia; may require digital amputation if extremity not considered viable
- Pentastomids
  - Incidental finding in peritoneum
  - Surgical removal
- Osteoarthritis
  - Analgesics/antiinflammatories (see "Analgesia" in *Nursing Care*)
- Myositis
  - If bacterial, use appropriate antibiosis; otherwise analgesia
- Orbicularis muscle prolapse
  - Under anesthesia, pull the muscle back into position. It will usually stay in place.

Neurologic disorders

Viral
- Herpes simplex virus 1
- Rabies

Bacterial
- Bacterial meningitis or other CNS infection
- Otitis media/interna

Nutritional
- Hypoglycemia
- Thiamine deficiency (see *Nutritional Disorders*)
- Malnutrition (see "Hedgehog Nutrition" in *Nutritional Disorders*)

Neoplasia
- Cortical carcinoma (of the nerve sheath)
- Schwannoma
- Lymphoma (Burballa et al 2012)

Other noninfectious problems
- Toxins
- Trauma
- Torpor
- Intervertebral disc disease (Raymond et al 2009)
- Other spinal lesions (e.g., fractures)
- Wobbly hedgehog syndrome

Findings on clinical examination

- Apparent weakness
- Posterior paralysis/paresis
- Seizures
- Otitis externa (see also "Ear Mites" in *Skin Disorders*)
- Exposure to possible source of herpes simplex (e.g., owner with cold sores)

Investigations

1. Full neurologic examination
2. Radiography
   a. Intervertebral disc collapse, spondylosis (intervertebral disc disease)
3. Routine hematology and biochemistry
4. Serology for toxoplasmosis
5. Culture and sensitivity
6. Endoscopy
7. Biopsy
8. Ultrasonography

Management

- Important to differentiate from other causes of weakness (insulinoma, lymphoma, etc.)

Treatment/specific therapy

- Herpes simplex virus 1
  - Unlikely to be diagnosed premortem
  - If diagnosed, attempt treatment with oral lysine at 250-500 mg/kg PO or acyclovir at 40 to 100 mg/kg PO daily.
- Rabies
  - Significant zoonosis; euthanasia
- Bacterial CNS infection
  - Appropriate antibiosis
  - Supportive care
- Fungal infections see Dermatophytosis in Skin disorders
- Hypoglycemia
  - For management of hypoglycemic episodes, see *Pancreatic Disorders.*
- Orthopedic conditions
  - Treat as for other small animals.
- Torpor
  - Check environmental temperatures. For APH it should be above 18° C.
  - Hedgehogs will initially use external heat sources to begin reversal of torpor before initiating physiologic heat generation.
  - During torpor, hedgehogs do not thermoregulate but allow their body temperature to fluctuate with the ambient temperature.
  - In the related A. *frontalis*, torpor is believed to be an energy-saving strategy rather than directly linked to low temperatures (Hallam and Mzilikazi 2011); lighter individuals had shorter bouts of torpor than heavier ones, possibly due to reduced levels of fat reserves.
- Wobbly hedgehog syndrome
  - Progressive hind-limb ataxia and muscle wastage
  - Eventually tetraparesis
  - Death within 18 to 25 months following onset of signs
  - Ameliorative treatment—consider NSAIDs, B vitamin supplementation.
  - Unknown etiology. Some lines appear more susceptible than others, suggesting a genetic predisposition.

- Intervertebral disc disease
  - NSAIDs
  - Surgical decompression

Ophthalmic disorders

Hedgehogs have shallow orbits and large eyelid fissures, which can predispose them to proptosis, especially combined with excessive amounts of retrobulbar fat due to obesity.

Bacterial

- *Salmonella* spp.
- *Mycobacterium* spp.
- Osteomyelitis of the nares/socket

Protozoal

Nutritional

- Obesity
- Hypovitaminosis A

Neoplasia

- Carcinoma of the ocular globe
- Acinic cell carcinoma (Fukuzawa et al 2004)

Other noninfectious problems

- Idiopathic cataracts
- Retinal degeneration
- Foreign body
- Trauma

Findings on clinical examination

- Corneal ulceration
- Conjunctivitis
- Nasal discharge
- Uveitis
- Corneal edema, hypopyon, and synechiae
- Cataracts
- Exophthalmos proptosis (obesity, retrobulbar lesion, acinic cell carcinoma, panophthalmitis)
- Megaglobus/glaucoma
- Cataracts
- Keratoconjunctivitis sicca, conical deformation of eyeball, and discoloration (hypovitaminosis A)

Investigations

1. Ophthalmic examination
2. Schirmer tear test (STT)
   a. In long-eared hedgehogs *(Hemiechinus auritus)*, the mean STT = 1.7 ± 1.2 mm/1 min with a range of 0 to 4 mm/1 min. For males the STT was 2.2 ± 1.2 mm/1 min; for females, 1.3 ± 1.1 mm/1 min (Ghaffari et al 2012).

3. Topical fluorescein to assess extent of ulceration
4. Tonometry
5. In long-eared hedgehogs (*Hemiechinus auritus*), the intraocular pressure (IOP) = 20.1 ± 4.0 mm Hg (range, 11.5 to 26.5 mm Hg). For males the IOP was 18.2 ± 4.0 mm Hg; females, 22.0 ± 3.2 mm Hg (Ghaffari et al 2012).
6. Skull radiography
7. Routine hematology and biochemistry
8. Culture and sensitivity
9. Biopsy
10. Ultrasonography

Treatment/specific therapy

- Proptosis
  - Typically involves orbital cellulitis, corneal perforation, and panophthalmitis (Wheler et al 2001). The lens may be absent, extruded through a corneal lesion.
  - Enucleation
  - Covering antibiosis
  - Consider protective tarsorraphy of the remaining eye, as bilateral proptosis is possible.
- Corneal ulceration
  - Topical and systemic antibiosis
  - Once infection cleared, treat as for other small animals (e.g., scarification to encourage healing, conjunctival grafts etc.).
- Uveitis
  - Topical ophthalmic steroid or NSAID preparations
  - Topical ophthalmic antibiotic preparations plus systemic antibiosis if appropriate
  - Enucleation if severe
- Cataracts
  - Treat for any uveitis as above.
  - Cataract removal either surgically or by phacoemulsification
- Neoplasia
  - Enucleation
- Hypovitaminosis A
  - Supplement with vitamin A.
  - Topical lubricants and antibiosis if keratoconjunctivitis sicca present

Endocrine disorders

Neoplasia
- C-cell carcinoma (thyroid gland)
- Follicular adenoma (pituitary gland)
- Adenocarcinoma (parathyroid gland)
- Adrenal adenoma
- Adrenocortical carcinoma (Juan-Sallés et al 2006)
- Pheochromocytoma

Findings on clinical examination

- Palapable mass on ventral neck (thyroid carcinoma)
- Dysphagia, weight loss, tetraplegia (thyroid carcinoma—Miller et al 2002)

Investigations

1. Radiography
2. Routine hematology and biochemistry
   a. Thyroxine (T_4) in EH varies with season from 2.4 nmol/L (winter) to 16.0 nmol/L (summer)—Augee et al 1979
3. Low-dose dexamethasone suppression test (hyperadrenocortism)
4. Culture and sensitivity
5. Endoscopy
6. Biopsy
7. Ultrasonography

Treatment/specific therapy

- Hyperadrenocorticism
  - Trilostane at 2.0 mg/kg PO daily initially, can increase to 6.0 mg/kg daily

Urinary disorders

Bacterial
- Cystitis
- Leptospirosis

Neoplasia
- Lymphoma (see *Systemic Disorders*)

Other noninfectious problems
- Urolithiasis
- Cystitis
- Nephrosis
- Intrarenal calcinosis
- Renal calculi
- Nephritis
- Nephrocalcinosis
- Tubular necrosis
- Glomerulosclerosis
- Renal infarcts
- Glomerulonephropathy

Findings on clinical examination

- Depression
- Anorexia

- Weight loss
- Polydipsia/polyuria
- Oral ulceration
- Hematuria (urolithiasis, cystitis, uterine neoplasia, endometrial polyps—see *Reproductive Disorders*)
- Hind-leg weakness
- Melena
- Dysuria/polyuria
- Pinkish urine (erythropoietic porphyria—see *Cardiovascular and Hematologic Disorders*)
- Urine dribbling, wet perineum, constant licking at genitalia (urolithiasis)
- Painful urination, stranguria (urolithiasis, cystitis)
- Green urine (leptospirosis)
- Death
- Palpable abnormalities
  - Distended bladder (urethral obstruction)

Investigations

1. Urinalysis (normal urine parameters, see Table 6-6)
   a. Ketonuria (ketosis—see *Reproductive Disorders*)
   b. Leptospires may be seen in urine.
2. Radiography
   a. Useful to differentiate uncomplicated cystitis from urolithiasis
   b. Contrast studies (pyelography, double contrast bladder studies, pneumocystography)
3. Routine hematology and biochemistry (Table 6-7)
   a. Serology for leptospirosis
4. Cytology
5. Culture and sensitivity

Table 6-6 Hedgehogs: Urinalysis

pH	Acidic
Protein	Negative
Ketones	Negative
Glucose	Negative
Crystals	Negative

Table 6-7 Hedgehogs: renal blood parameters

Parameter	APH	EH
Creatinine (μmol/L)	35.4 ± 17.7	26.5 ± 8.8
Urea (mmol/L)	9.3 ± 3.2	7.5 ± 2.1
Uric acid (μmol/l)	35.7 ± 5.9	—

APH, *African pygmy hedgehog*; EH, *European hedgehog*.

6. Endoscopy
7. Biopsy
8. Ultrasonography

Management

1. Fluid therapy (see *Nursing Care*)
2. Reduction of proteinuria with angiotensin retention blocker (e.g., telmisartan at 1 mg/kg PO once daily)
3. Anabolic steroids may be useful.
4. Appropriate antibiosis

Treatment/specific therapy

- Leptospirosis
  - Often subclinical
  - Experimental infection of EH with *L. pomona* (Webster 1957) causes intermittent fever, jaundice, and abortion.
  - Appropriate antibiosis
- Urolithiasis
  - May be linked to dried cat food–based diet
  - If urethral obstruction:
    - Attempt catheterization (can be difficult in males due to J-shaped os penis).
    - Cystocentesis
    - Surgical cystotomy
    - If unable to clear urethra, create a perineal urethrostomy.
- Cystic calculi
  - Cystotomy
  - Submit any stones/sand for analysis.
  - Antibiosis (usually has accompanying cystitis) and other supportive care
  - May be linked to dried cat food-based diet
  - Change diet based on results of stone analysis.
- Neoplasia
  - Neoplasia of the bladder: Surgery difficult because it is often diffuse. Chemotherapy may prove useful.

Reproductive disorders

Females have two pairs of nipples on the chest and one on the abdomen; some females may have extra. Ovulation is induced.

Bacterial
- Mastitis

Nutritional
- Ketosis/pregnancy toxemia

Neoplasia
- Mammary tumors
- Granulosa cell tumor

- Adenoma/adenosarcoma
- Leiomyosarcoma
- Adenocarcinoma
- Adenoleiomyosarcoma
- Spindle cell tumor
- Neurofibrosarcoma
- Endometrial stromal sarcomas
- Endometrial polyps

Other noninfectious problems

- Dystocia
  - Physical abnormalities
  - Large hoglets
  - Maternal pelvic abnormalities

Findings on clinical examination

- Hemorrhagic vaginal discharge (endometrial polyps, uterine/vaginal neoplasia)
- Swollen, painful, discolored mammary glands (acute mastitis, neoplasia)
- Swollen but otherwise normal mammary glands (chronic mastitis)
- Lethargy and dehydration in pregnant female. Melena may be present (pregnancy toxemia).

Investigations

1. Radiography
2. Routine hematology and biochemistry
3. Urinalysis
   a. Ketonuria (ketosis)
4. Culture and sensitivity
5. Endoscopy
6. Biopsy
7. Ultrasonography

Management

1. Fluid therapy (see *Nursing Care*)
2. Prophylactic antibiotics

Treatment/specific therapy

- Mastitis
  - Acute mastitis
    - Antibiosis and fluids
    - NSAIDs may have antiendotoxin effects (see "Analgesia" in *Nursing Care*).
    - Debride or surgically resect affected mammary tissue.
    - Fostering of young may spread pathogens to other females.
  - Chronic mastitis
    - Often nonresponsive to therapy.

- Ketosis
  - Usually linked to period of anorexia/starvation during pregnancy
  - In some cases linked to large litters
  - Supportive treatment, including fluids, warmth, and IV glucose/force feeding (see *Nursing Care*)
  - Perform cesarean as soon as possible.
  - Foster or euthanize young as they are hard to hand-rear and recovering female is unlikely to lactate.
- Dystocia
  - Large or deformed hoglets, pelvic abnormalities, and other anomalies
  - If pelvis normal, consider 0.2 to 3.0 units oxytocin SC, IM. If no result, either repeat treatment or undertake cesarean.
  - Cesarean

Neonatal disorders

- Some normal parameters of hedgehog neonates are shown in Table 6-8.

Other noninfectious problems

- Hypothermia (especially up to 100 g body weight, after which the hoglets become more active and are better thermoregulators)
- Lack of maternal milk
- Mastitis (see *Reproductive Disorders*)
- Maternal systemic illness
- Maternal aggression/cannibalism

Findings on clinical examination

- Lethargy
- Failure to feed
- History of lack of maternal care
- Failure to grow
- Diarrhea (may not be apparent as female continually licks clean)

Investigations

1. Weigh young.
2. Radiography
3. Routine hematology and biochemistry

Table 6-8 Hedgehogs: Normal parameters of neonates

	E. europeus	*A. albiventris*
Approximate weight at birth (g)	8-25	10
Approximate weight at 40 days (g)	120-350	—
Age of eyes opening (days)	14	14
Age of weaning (days)	38-44	35-48

4. Culture and sensitivity
5. Endoscopy
6. Biopsy
7. Ultrasonography

Management

- Nursing care, especially provision of warmth and fluids, is extremely important with neonates.

Treatment/specific therapy

- Lack of maternal milk production
  - Hedgehogs have been raised on a variety of milk replacers, including artificial bitch and cat milk and goat milk.
- Hypothermia
  - Place in warm environment initially, with temperatures up to 35° C.

Sugar gliders

7

Sugar gliders *(Petaurus breviceps)* are a relatively new addition to the pet-keeping hobby. Native to Australia, Papua New Guinea, and parts of Indonesia, with seven subspecies recognized, it is likely to represent a species complex rather than a single wide-ranging species. It is a gliding possum that is highly nocturnal. Sugar gliders are highly social animals and can suffer depression if kept individually, not stimulated, or kept incorrectly (see Jones et al 1995).

At the time of writing only limited baseline information on this species is available, so the clinician may have to make inferences when dealing with sugar gliders. This is expected to change over the next few years as their popularity grows and they are presented to the veterinarian more frequently.

In the United States state permits may be required for the possession, breeding, trade, or display of sugar gliders. The same is true for Canada and Australia.

Table 7-1 Sugar gliders: Key facts

Average life span (yrs)	9-15
Weight (g)	Males: 115-160
	Females: 90-130
Body temperature (°C) (see "Thermoregulation")	36.2 ± 0.4
Respiratory rate (per min)	16-40
Heart rate (beats per min)	200-300
Gestation (days)	16
Average litter size	2
Time in pouch (weeks)	10
Age at weaning	110-120 days (35-60 days out of pouch)
Sexual maturity (months)	Males: 12-14
	Females: 8-12

Consultation and handling

Sugar gliders vary markedly in their tolerance of routine handling and examination. Some are used to handling; others will bite and make efforts to escape. They are fast and can grip extremely well and can readily elude the veterinarian's grasp. A loose sugar glider can be covered with a towel and restrained gently but firmly through the towel, simultaneously minimizing the risk of a bite. A sugar glider is small enough to be restrained in one hand, facing out from the palm with a thumb under the jaw and index finger on top of the head and the body cupped in the palm of the hand. A thorough clinical examination may require sedation or anesthesia.

Some individuals may develop a mild urticarial reaction triggered by the sharp points of sugar glider claws.

Blood sampling

Up to 1% body weight (g) can be safely taken. The preferred site is the cranial vena cava at the thoracic inlet. Alternatively the medial tibial artery just distal to the stifle.

Nursing care

Thermoregulation and torpor

Sugar gliders should be kept at an ambient temperature of 24° to 27°C, with nighttime temperatures not dropping below 21°C. They maintain their body temperature by a combination of social thermoregulation (huddling), good insulation, and low-cost locomotion. Core body temperature fluctuates naturally between 32° and 34°C at rest, increasing up to 38°C when active (Körtner and Geiser 2000).

Cool sugar gliders may exhibit torpor; this appears to be a physiologic adaptation to minimize energy consumption at times of poor energy availability—in wild sugar gliders, torpor is triggered on cold and wet days, typically when environmental temperatures fall below 10°C, although heavy rain can trigger torpor at temperatures of 15°C or below (Körtner and Geiser 2000).

Torpor should be distinguished from lethargy or shock; a good clinical history especially with regard to ambient environmental conditions, as well as response to gentle warming, should help to differentiate torpor from clinical conditions. Periods of torpor usually last between 2 and 23 hours.

For general principles see "Thermoregulation" under *Nursing Care* in Chapter 2.

Fluid therapy

Fluid requirements are 60 to 100 mL/kg per day. Subcutaneous fluids can be given at 2% of body weight 2 to 4 times daily; note that fluids may pool in the patagium. Hyaluronidase (150 IU/mL) 0.5 to 1.0 mL/L of fluids may improve fluid absorption. Intraosseous fluids can be given into the femur; alternatively, small bolus volumes may be given into the cephalic or lateral saphenous vein.

Nutritional support

Use commercial powdered recovery diets that reconstitute into a paste. Some sugar gliders may accept fruit juice, yogurt, or baby foods (0- to 3-month-old fruit purees—avoid milk-containing products) fortified with vitamins and/or calcium.

$$\text{Basal energy requirements (BER)} = 49\,(\text{BW in kg}^{0.75})$$

(Note the different constant for marsupials.)

$$\text{Actual energy requirement (MER)} = 1.25\,(\text{BER})$$

because the glider's actual energy requirements will vary from 1 to 2 times the BER depending on the condition.

Analgesia

Analgesics are especially important to prevent postoperative self-mutilation.

Table 7-2 Sugar gliders: Analgesic doses

Drug	Dose
Buprenorphine	0.01-0.03 mg/kg PO, SC b.i.d.
Meloxicam	0.20 mg/kg PO SC s.i.d.
Flunixin	1 mg/kg SC or IM every 12-24 hr, up to 3 days
Butorphanol	1.7 mg/kg PO or SC
Acepromazine	• 1.7 mg/kg SC combined with butorphanol 1.7 mg/kg immediately postoperative to control self-mutilation • 1 mg/kg with ketamine 10 mg/kg SC for postoperative analgesia to control self-mutilation

Anesthesia

Ideally starve for 4 hours prior to surgery. Induction and maintenance with isoflurane are safe and effective. Initiate anesthesia in an induction chamber and maintain with a small mask. Atropine at 0.02 to 0.04 mg/kg can be given to control salivation during induction.

Parenteral anesthesia with tiletamine–zolazepam at doses ranging from 8.4 to 12.8 mg/kg IM is cited as being safe (Carboni and Tully 2009), although the same combination at 10 mg/kg has been linked with neurologic signs and death in the related squirrel gliders *(Petaurus norfolcensis)* (Fig. 7-1).

- Intraoperative care
  - Keep warm (see "Thermoregulation").
  - Fluids (see "Fluid Therapy")
- Postoperative aftercare
  - Analgesia (see "Analgesia" above)
  - Must be offered food as soon as recovers
  - Keep warm.

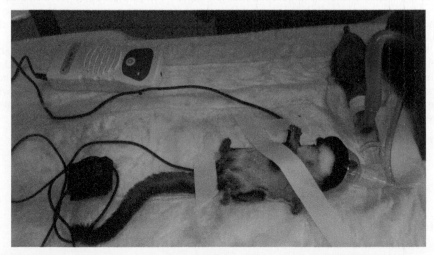

Fig 7-1. Anesthetic monitoring of small mammals like sugar gliders can be challenging. Note the cloacal thermometer and Doppler ultrasound probe taped to the chest to monitor heart rate. *(Courtesy of Sophie Jenkins, MRCVS.)*

Cardiopulmonary resuscitation

1. Intubate and ventilate at 20 to 30 breaths/min.
2. If cardiac arrest, external cardiac massage at around 100 compressions/min.
   a. Epinephrine at 0.2 mg/kg intracardiac, IV, or IO
3. Fluid therapy (see above)
4. If bradycardic, atropine at 0.05 mg/kg IV.

Behavioral disorders

Sugar gliders are communal animals that need the company of conspecifics where possible, and if kept individually they need a great deal of attention. Social deprivation can lead to loss of appetite, irritability, and self-mutilation and has been used experimentally to induce a serotonin-deficient model for the study of depression (Jones et al 1995). Where possible keep at least two sugar gliders; if not possible or as a temporary arrangement (e.g., after the loss of a companion), give plenty of time and attention, plus multiple toys to distract and provide environmental enrichment. Self-mutilation may also be triggered by stress, as well as postoperative irritation (see "Analgesia"). Fluoxetine 1 mg/kg PO every 12 hours may prove useful, but treatment is likely to take 4 to 8 weeks. Collars may need to be fashioned to temporarily prevent self-mutilation, although this is not a remedy in itself, and underlying issues need to be addressed.

Other stressors include unsuitable diet, sexual frustration, overcrowding, and unsanitary conditions.

Skin disorders

Sugar gliders have a thick fur covering. They possess a patagium on each side—a skin flap well supplied with muscles that connects the lateral edge of the foreleg with the tarsi to provide a gliding plane when outstretched (Fig. 7-2). Sugar gliders possess a well-developed tibiocarpalis muscle along the most lateral area of the patagium. This patagium largely consists of the humerodorsalis and tibioabdominalis muscle complex. The tibiocarpalis bundle and the humerodorsalis and tibioabdominalis muscle complex probably serve as a membrane controller while gliding. There is a thin membranous structure between the cutaneous and deeper muscles of the patagium (Endo et al 1998). The tail is used as a rudder during gliding flight.

Male sugar gliders have a scent gland at the base of the neck ventrally (gular scent gland) (Fig. 7-3) and over the frontal bone between the eyes (frontal scent gland); these, especially the frontal gland, should not be confused with an area of alopecia. These glands are under sex hormonal influence; the size varies with reproductive status and is reduced following castration (Stoddart and Bradley 1991). Both sexes possess an anal gland. Females have a scent gland in their pouch (marsupium), which also contains four teats.

Pruritus

- Ectoparasites
- Self-mutilation (see *Behavioral Disorders*)
- Aberrant visceral larval migrans (see *Gastrointestinal Disorders*)
- *Parastrongyloides* (see *Gastrointestinal Disorders*)

Alopecia

- Self-inflicted trauma
- Dermatophytosis (*Trichophyton* spp.)
- Hair loss at base of tail/head

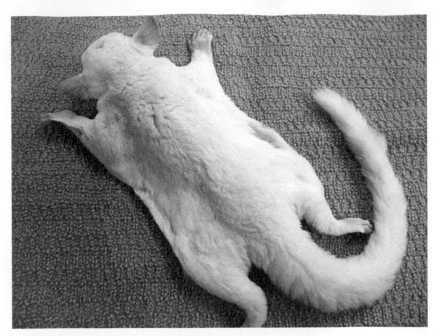

Fig 7-2. The patagium, or gliding membrane, of sugar gliders stretches between the front and hind legs. *(From Ness RD, Johnson-Delaney CA. 2012. Sugar gliders. In: Quesenberry KE, Carpenter JW (eds.). Ferrets, rabbits, and rodents: Clinical medicine and surgery, 3rd ed. Saunders, St. Louis.)*

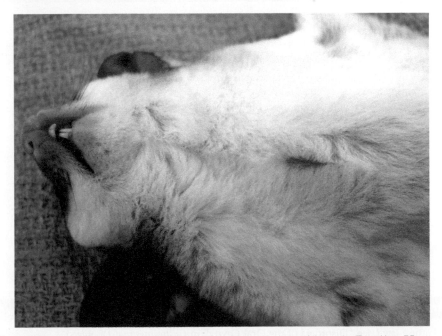

Fig 7-3. The male glider also has a gular scent gland, located at the base of the neck. *(From Ness RD, Johnson-Delaney CA. 2012. Sugar gliders. In: Quesenberry KE, Carpenter JW (eds). Ferrets, rabbits, and rodents: Clinical medicine and surgery, 3rd ed. Saunders, St. Louis.)*

Scaling and crusting

- Dermatophytosis (*Trichophyton* spp.)

Erosions and ulceration

- Bite wounds

Nodules and nonhealing wounds

- Lumpy jaw (*Actinomyces*—see *Gastrointestinal Disorders*)
- Abscessation
- *Pasteurella multocida* abscess

Ectoparasites

- Rare in captive sugar gliders
  - *Choristopsylla tristis* (flea)
  - *Acanthosylla pavida* (flea)
  - *Guntheria kowanyam* (trombiculid mite)
  - *Petauralges rackae* (astigmatid mite)
  - Atopomelid mites
  - *Ixodes tasmani* (tick)

Neoplasia

- Cutaneous lymphosarcoma (Hough et al 1992); see also *Systemic Disorders*
- Dermal hemangiosarcoma (Rivas et al 2014)

Other findings on clinical examination

- Damage to the partagium (laceration, bite wounds)

Investigations

1. Microscopy: Examine fur pluck, acetate strips, or skin scrapes to affected area and examine for ectoparasites and ringworm.
2. Cytology: Stain with lactophenol blue for ringworm.
3. Bacteriology and mycology: Hair/quill pluck or swab lesions for routine culture and sensitivity.
4. Fine-needle aspirate followed by staining with rapid Romanowsky stains
5. Biopsy obvious lesions.
6. Ultraviolet (Wood's) lamp: Positive for *Microsporium canis* only (not all strains fluoresce).
7. Radiography
8. Routine hematology and biochemistry
9. Endoscopy
10. Biopsy
11. Ultrasonography

Treatment/specific therapy

- Lumpy jaw (see "Disorders of the Oral Cavity" in *Gastrointestinal Disorders*)
- Patagial damage
  - Repair; covering antibiosis if bite wound/infected

- Abscessation
  - Remove intact if possible; lance, debride, and flush if not.
  - Appropriate antibiosis
  - May be secondary to skin-penetrating injury
- Dermatophytosis
  - Griseofulvin 20 mg/kg PO s.i.d. for 30 to 60 days
  - Itraconazole 5 to 10 mg/kg PO b.i.d.
- Hair loss at tail base/head
  - Linked with increased sexual activity
- Ectoparasites
  - Ivermectin 0.2 mg/kg PO or SC once; repeat after 2 weeks.
  - Selamectin 6 to 18 mg/kg applied topically; repeat in 30 days.
  - Carbaryl powder in nest
- Ticks
  - Physical removal of individual ticks
  - Ivermectin 0.2 mg/kg PO or SC once; repeat after 2 weeks.
- Neoplasia
  - Surgical resection
  - Chemotherapy

Respiratory tract disorders

Bacterial
- Pneumonia
  - *Pasteurella multocida*
  - *Streptococcus pneumoniae*
  - *Klebsiella* spp.
- Mycobacteriosis (see *Systemic Disorders*)

Fungal
- Cryptococcosis (see *Systemic Disorders*)

Protozoal
- Toxoplasmosis (see *Neurologic Disorders*)

Parasitic
- *Marsupostrongylus* spp. (lungworm)
- *Rileyella petauri* (pentastomes)

Neoplasia
Other noninfectious problems
- Trauma
- Aspiration pneumonia
- Cardiovascular disease (see *Cardiovascular and Hematologic Disorders*)
- Iron storage disease (see *Nutritional Disorders*)

Findings on clinical examination

- Dyspnea
- Cyanosis

- Abnormal lung sounds
- Abnormal heart sounds (see *Cardiovascular and Hematologic Disorders*)
- Ocular and nasal discharge

Investigations

1. Tracheal wash/bronchoalveolar lavage
2. Culture and sensitivity
3. Cytology
4. Pleural tap and cytology
5. Radiography
6. Serology
7. Endoscopy
8. Biopsy
9. Ultrasonography

Management

1. Supportive treatment (e.g., fluids, covering antibiosis)
2. Nebulization either with antibiotics or general antimicrobial (e.g., F10, Health and Hygiene Ltd.)
3. Oxygen therapy if needed
4. Reduce stress levels. Hospitalize away from dogs and noisy cats; keep in darkened position.

Treatment/specific therapy

- Bacterial pneumonia
  - As for other small animal species including antibiosis, anti-inflammatories
  - Nebulization
  - *Pasteurella* often associated with stress
- Pentastomes *(Rileyella)*
  - Believed to have direct life cycle (Spratt 2003)
  - Ivermectin at 0.2 mg/kg SC, topically repeated every 2 weeks for three injections
  - Anti-inflammatories may reduce risk of inflammation following parasite die-off.
- *Marsupostrongylus*
  - Fenbendazole at 20 to 50 mg/kg PO in a single daily dose for 3 days; repeat after 2 weeks.
  - Ivermectin 0.2 mg/kg PO or SC once; repeat after 2 weeks.
  - Selamectin 6 to 18 mg/kg applied topically; repeat in 30 days.
  - Consider covering antibiotics and anti-inflammatories as large worm mortalities can trigger a serious pneumonia.
- *Parastrongyloides trichosuri*
  - Parasite of the brush-tailed possum *Trichosurus vulpecula*; experimentally readily infects sugar gliders
  - Parasitic adults found in small intestine.
  - Eggs passed out in feces; develop into free-living adults; in conditions of starvation and crowding infective L3 larvae develop that penetrate skin and seek out the small intestine, where they become parasitic adults.

Gastrointestinal tract disorders

Sugar gliders are diprotodont and are considered primarily as insectivore/gumnivores and have a fairly simple gastrointestinal tract, although the cecum is enlarged for gum fermentation.

Permanent dental formula

$$I:\frac{3}{2} \quad C:\frac{1}{0} \quad PM:\frac{3}{3} \quad M:\frac{4}{4}$$

Sugar gliders have teeth designed for stripping bark off branches. The teeth do not grow continuously; they have distinct anatomical roots. The mandibular incisors are longer than the maxillary. The molars are larger and wider than the premolars.

Disorders of the oral cavity

- Dental disease
  - Periodontal disease: Can be plaque-induced. Radiography to assess root resorption/ bone disease. Clean and polish; extract problem teeth. Incisor extraction frequently results in mandibular fracture.
- Oral abscesses
  - Typically in young sugar gliders
  - Usually enteric bacteria isolated
  - Lance, debride, and administer appropriate antibiosis.
  - Thought to be initiated from fecal bacteria on claws introduced during scratching of head and mouth
- Lumpy jaw (*Actinomyces* spp.)
  - Radiography to assess extent of underlying pathology
  - Associated tooth extraction
  - Surgical resection
  - Debride as much as possible if unable to resect completely.
  - Appropriate antibiosis; clindamycin-impregnated methylmethacrylate beads may be useful (Brust 2013).

Differential diagnoses for gastrointestinal disorders

Bacterial

- *Actinomyces* (lumpy jaw)
- *Fusobacterium necrophorum* (lumpy jaw)
- Bacterial overgrowth
- *Clostridium* spp.
- *Yersinia pseudotuberculosis*
- *Salmonella* spp.
- Paracloacal and cloacal abscessation

Protozoal

- *Cryptosporidium*
- *Giardia*
- *Trichomonas*
- Coccidiosis

Parasitic

- Worms (see also "Pruritus" in *Skin Disorders* and *Neurologic Disorders*)
  - *Parastrongyloides* spp. (Nolan et al 2007)
  - *Paraustrostrongylus* spp.
  - *Paraustroxyuris* spp.
  - *Capillaria* spp.

Nutritional

- Excess sugar content in diet

Neoplasia

- Transitional cell carcinoma (Marrow et al 2010)
- Cloacal and paracloacal gland enlargement

Other noninfectious problems

- Constipation
- Obstruction
- Rectal prolapse
- Megacolon

Findings on clinical examination

- Vomiting
- Diarrhea
- Lack of feces (reduced food consumption, constipation, obstruction)
- Dehydration
- Lethargy
- Swelling of mandible/maxilla (lumpy jaw)
- Rectal mucosa prominent (rectal prolapse)
- Swollen abdomen, lethargy, dehydration, (intussusception, megacolon/gastric dilatation–volvulus (GDV)/impaction/constipation)
- Palpable mass, straining to defecate, reduced appetite, self-mutilation of the perineal skin (neoplasia)
- Swellings around cloaca, pain, dyschezia (cloacal/paracloacal gland enlargement/abscessation)

Investigations

- Fecal examination
  - Gram stain
  - Modified Ziehl-Neelsen staining for *Cryptosporidium*
  - Motile flagellated protozoa *(Trichomonas, Giardia)*
  - Worm eggs
- Radiography
  - Foreign body
  - Osteomyelitis/osteolysis of maxilla/mandible (lumpy jaw)
  - Cloacal narrowing, intestinal and colonic distension (pericloacal neoplasia)
  - Intussusception/megacolon/GDV
- Routine hematology and biochemistry

- Culture and sensitivity
- Endoscopy
- Biopsy
- Ultrasonography

Management

1. Fluid therapy (see *Nursing Care*)
2. Gut motility enhancers (e.g., cisapride 0.25 mg/kg PO daily to q.i.d.)
3. Gastroprotectants (e.g., sucralfate)
4. If vomiting:
   a. Use antiemetics (e.g., metoclopramide at 0.05-0.1 mg/kg SC t.i.d.).
   b. Monitor blood glucose; consider dextrose/saline fluids.

Treatment/specific therapy

- Lumpy jaw (see *Disorders of the Oral Cavity*)
- Bacterial overgrowth
  - Appropriate antibiosis
  - Correct any dietary predisposing factors.
- Cloacal and paracloacal abscessation
  - Appropriate antibiosis
  - Lance and debride if appropriate.
- Excess dietary sugar
  - Diarrhea may be due to bacterial overgrowth.
  - Possible osmotic diarrhea
  - Correct diet and consequential disease.
- "Stress diarrhea" of joeys—see *Neonatal Disorders*
- Coccidiosis
  - Potentiated sulfonamides at 15 mg/kg PO b.i.d.
  - Toltrazuril 7.0 mg/kg PO for 2 days; repeat weekly for 3 weeks.
- *Cryptosporidium*
  - No effective treatment recognized
  - Potentiated sulfonamides may be of use, as may nitazoxanide at 5 mg/kg PO s.i.d.
  - Potential zoonosis, so consider euthanasia.
- *Trichomonas*
  - Metronidazole at 10 to 20 mg/kg PO daily.
- Giardia
  - Metronidazole 25 mg/kg PO b.i.d.
- Intestinal worms
  - Fenbendazole at 20 to 50 mg/kg PO in a single dose for 3 days; repeat after 2 weeks.
  - Ivermectin 0.2 mg/kg PO or SC once; repeat after 2 weeks.
- Rectal prolapse
  - Replace under general anesthesia.
  - May need vertical sutures to temporarily retain; ensure that the urinogenital slit remains unobstructed.
  - Analgesia: meloxicam 0.2 mg/kg PO daily. An E-collar may be needed.
  - Feed low-bulk foods during recovery.

- Megacolon
  - No etiology elucidated.
  - Stool softeners and cisapride 0.25 mg/kg PO daily to q.i.d. may prove useful.
- Intussusception
  - Secondary to chronic diarrhea; more common in younger gliders
  - Surgical correction
- GDV
  - Surgical correction
- Constipation
  - Laxatives (e.g., soft paraffin-based gut lubricants, lactulose)
  - Gut motility enhancers (see "Management")
  - Surgery
  - Possible causes include insufficient dietary liquids or fiber, generally overall diet, stress, lack of exercise, or gut disease/problems.
- Pericloacal neoplasia
  - If caught sufficiently early, may respond to surgery/chemotherapy
  - Likely to require euthanasia

Nutritional disorders

Note that sugar gliders will seasonally gain weight, peaking in the late autumn and winter, with weight increases as much as 20 to 30 g (Holloway and Geiser 2001).

Sugar glider nutrition

In total, aim to offer approximately 15% to 20% of the sugar glider's body weight.

Diet 1

1. 75% sugar glider kibble/pellet. Should be available at all times.
2. 25% fresh fruit and vegetables, placed in the enclosure at night and removed each morning. Items should not be diced or chopped to maintain moisture content.
3. A calcium-based multivitamin should be sprinkled over fresh fruits or vegetables 3 to 4 times per week.

Diet 2

1. 50% Leadbeater's Mixture
2. 50% insectivore/carnivore diet/pellet

Leadbeater's Mixture:
- 150 mL warm water
- 150 mL honey
- 1 shelled hard-boiled egg
- 25 g high-protein baby cereal
- 1 tsp vitamin/mineral supplement

Mix warm water and honey. In a separate container, blend the egg until homogenized, then gradually add honey/water mixture followed by the vitamin powder, then baby cereal. Blend after each addition until smooth. Refrigerate.

- Aflatoxicosis (see *Hepatic Disorders*)
- Iron storage disease (Clauss and Paglia 2012)
  - Sudden-onset dyspnea and death
  - May be due to excessive scavenging of dietary iron in a species that feeds naturally on an iron-deficient diet; the lack of naturally occurring tannins may also contribute.

- May also be related to feeding of homemade diets, possibly with high dietary vitamin C. Linked with obesity also; alternatively can be triggered by chronic inflammatory disease. Hypervitaminosis C and chronic inflammation can increase transferrin levels.
- Recommended dietary iron levels of 50 μg/g of dry diet and 100 mg/kg vitamin C.
- Dierenfeld et al (2006) report postfeeding trial iron levels of 1.5 ± 0.7 μmol/L, which they consider to be elevated.
- Iron was also detected in the feces of sugar gliders.
- Metabolic bone disease (nutritional osteodystrophy)
  - Muscle weakening of hind legs, progressing to paralysis; lameness (pathological fractures); seizures
  - Pneumonia, heart disease
  - Radiography: Pathological fractures; poor bone density
  - Biochemistry: Normal blood calcium 2.1 to 2.2 mmol/L;
       phosphorus 1.4 to 2.0 mmol/L;
       normal range of 25-hydroxyvitamin D unknown, but Dierenfeld et al (2006) report a range of 44.9 to 132.3 nmol/L.
  - Strict rest for fractures
  - Emergency treatment
    - Calcium gluconate 100 mg/kg SC b.i.d. for 3 to 5 days followed by calcium glubionate 23 mg/kg PO daily
    - If normocalcemic then calcitonin at 50 IU/kg weekly for 3 weeks (see Corriveau 2015)
  - Dietary calcium and vitamin D_3 supplementation
- Obesity
  - Common with captive diets; likely an imbalance between high caloric intake and reduced energy expenditure (reduced exercise, nonbreeding)
  - Weigh weekly and record the weights so as to avoid obesity.
  - Limit amount offered so that all is consumed overnight with none left over.
- Polioencephalomalacia (see *Neurologic Disorders*)
- Hepatic lipidosis
  - Likely associated with obesity and anorexia
  - Aggressive fluid therapy
  - Parenteral nutrition with glucose and vitamins
  - Assisted feeding by syringe (see *Nursing Care*)
  - Calcium gluconate PO or propylene glycol PO may be of use.
  - Dexamethasone at 0.2 mg/kg IV, SC, or PO

Hepatic disorders

Bacterial
- Hepatitis
- Listeriosis (see *Neurologic Disorders*)

Parasitic
- *Athesmia* spp. (trematode—liver fluke)

Nutritional
- Aflatoxicosis
- Hepatic lipidosis
- Iron storage disease (see *Nutritional Disorders*)
- Ketosis (see *Reproductive Disorders*)

Neoplasia

- Lymphoma/lymphosarcoma (see *Systemic Disorders*)
- Hepatic adenocarcinoma

Other noninfectious problems

- Lymphocytic hepatitis
- Cholangiohepatitis

Findings on clinical examination

- Reduced or loss of appetite
- Vague signs of ill health
- Abnormal feces
- Hepatomegaly
- Jaundice (rare)
- Ascites
- Seizures
- Anorexia, anemia, jaundice, lethargy, and diarrhea

Investigations

1. Radiography
2. Fecal examination
   a. Trematode eggs (*Athesmia* spp.)
3. Routine hematology and biochemistry
4. Culture and sensitivity
5. Endoscopy
6. Biopsy
7. Ultrasonography

Management

1. Fluid therapy (see *Nursing Care*)
2. Lactulose at 150 to 750 mg/kg PO b.i.d. or t.i.d.
3. Milk thistle *(Silybum marianum)* is hepatoprotectant. Dose at 4 to 15 mg/kg PO b.i.d. or t.i.d.

Treatment/specific therapy

- Hepatitis
  - General supportive management (see *Management*)
  - Appropriate antibiosis
- *Athesmia* spp.
  - Praziquantel at 5 to 10 mg/kg PO or SC single dose
- Aflatoxicosis
  - Treat as above in *Management*.
  - Typical sources include contaminated foodstuffs (e.g., peanuts; also crickets fed on contaminated sources), so investigate possible sources. Change all suspect food items for fresh.
- Hepatic lipidosis (see *Nutritional Disorders*)

Splenic disorders

Splenomegaly
- Hemangiosarcoma and hemangioma
- Cardiac disease (see *Cardiovascular and Hematologic Disorders*)
- Lymphoma/lymphosarcoma (see *Systemic Disorders*)
- Splenic erythroid hyperplasia
- Idiopathic splenomegaly

Treatment
- Address underlying cause.
- Splenectomy
  - Splenic rupture
  - Splenic torsion
  - Neoplasia
  - Splenitis

Pancreatic disorders

Neoplasia
- Pancreatic exocrine adenocarcinoma

Investigations

1. Radiography
2. Routine hematology and biochemistry
3. Culture and sensitivity
4. Urinalysis
5. Endoscopy
6. Exploratory surgery and biopsy
7. Ultrasonography

Treatment/specific therapy

- Pancreatic exocrine adenocarcinoma
  - Readily metastasize; surgery is a possible option but metastasis highly likely before diagnosis is confirmed.

Cardiovascular and hematologic disorders

Bacterial
- Bacteremia/septicemia
- Endocarditis

Protozoal
- *Toxoplasma gondii* (myocarditis—see *Neurologic Disorders*)
- *Hepatozoon* spp.

Parasites

- *Ophidascaris robertsi* (larva migrans) (Gallego Agúndez et al 2014)

Neoplasia

- Lymphoma (see *Systemic Disorders*)

Other noninfectious problems

- Cardiomyopathy
- Valvular heart disease
- Congenital disorders

Findings on clinical examination

- Cyanosis or pallor of the mucous membranes
- Anemia
- Slow capillary refill time
- Dyspnea
- Precordial thrill
- Arrhythmia
- Lack of thoracic percussion with auscultation
- Abnormal lung sounds
- Abnormal heart sounds
- Exercise intolerance
- Ascites
- Hepatomegaly, splenomegaly
- Weight loss
- Sudden death
- Nematodes in heart chambers (ultrasound/postmortem—*Ophidascaris* spp.)

Investigations

1. Auscultation
2. Blood pressure
3. ECG
4. Radiography
5. Ultrasonography/echocardiography
6. Routine hematology and biochemistry
7. Serology for *Toxoplasma*
8. Culture and sensitivity
9. Endoscopy
10. Biopsy

Management

- Reduce stress (e.g., keep in a cool, shaded, or darkened area away from potential stressors such as dogs).
- Provide a high oxygen environment.
- For pleural effusion, consider tube thoracostomy.

Treatment/specific therapy

- Cardiomyopathies
  - Dilated (congestive) cardiomyopathy
    - Furosemide at 1 to 4 mg/kg PO, SC b.i.d.
    - Enalapril at 0.2-0.5 mg/kg PO s.i.d.
    - Digoxin at 0.01 mg/kg PO daily
    - Pimobendan at 0.2 mg/kg PO daily
- Valvular heart disease
  - Treat as for dilated cardiomyopathy.
- *Ophidascaris robertsi*
  - History of potential indirect contact with usual snake host
  - Ivermectin at 0.2 mg/kg SC, topically repeated every 2 weeks for three injections
  - Treatment may trigger thromboembolism.
  - Ivermectin given monthly may be preventative.

Systemic disorders

Bacterial
- Bacteremia/septicemia
- *Pasteurella multocida*
- Mycobacteriosis

Fungal
- Cryptococcosis

Parasitic
- *Ophidascaris robersti* (larva migrans—see *Cardiovascular and Hematologic Disorders*)

Neoplasia
- Lymphoma/lymphosarcoma

Other noninfectious problems
Findings on clinical examination:
- Multiple abscesses, sudden death (pasteurellosis)
- Chronic weight loss, also possibly dyspnea, lameness, abscesses, neurologic signs, and blindness (mycobacteriosis)
- On postmortem: multiple organ abscessation (pasteurellosis, mycobacteriosis, cryptococcosis)
- Polylymphadenopathy (lymphoma/lymphosarcoma)

Investigations

1. Radiography
2. Routine hematology and biochemistry
3. Abdominocentesis and cytology
4. Endoscopy

5. Biopsy/necropsy
6. Ultrasonography

Management

- See *Nursing Care.*

Treatment/specific therapy

- Bacteremia/septicemia
  - Appropriate antibiosis
  - Supportive therapy as necessary (see *Nursing Care*)
- Mycobacteriosis
  - Potential zoonosis, so consider euthanasia.
- Cryptococcosis
  - Itraconazole at 5 to 10 mg/kg SC PO b.i.d.
- Lymphoma/lymphosarcoma
  - Typically affects liver and lymph nodes
  - Treat as for other small animals. Steroids may give temporary remission, but gliders are very susceptible to the effects of glucocorticoids (Bradley and Stoddart 1990).
  - For potential chemotherapy, consult modern chemotherapeutic protocols.

Musculoskeletal disorders

Nutritional

- Metabolic bone disease (see *Nutritional Disorders*)
- Polioencephalomalacia (vitamin B_1 deficiency—see *Neurologic Disorders*)

Neoplasia
Other noninfectious problems

- Traumatic fractures
- Toe injuries
- Any causes of weakness
- See *Neurologic Disorders.*
- See *Cardiac and Hematologic Disorders.*
- See *Systemic Disorders.*

Findings on clinical examination

- Pain
- Lameness
- Swelling
- Hind-leg paresis/paralysis

Investigations

1. Radiography
   Traumatic fractures

2. Routine hematology and biochemistry
3. Culture and sensitivity
4. Endoscopy
5. Biopsy
6. Ultrasonography

Treatment/specific therapy

- Traumatic fractures
  - Repair using standard small animal techniques.
- Toe injuries
  - Usually require digit amputation; dressings poorly tolerated
- Neoplasia
  - Surgical resection, amputation, chemotherapy, or radiation therapy as for other small animals

Neurologic disorders

Bacterial
- Bacterial meningitis or other CNS infection
- *Clostridium piliforme*
- *Pasteurella multocida*
- *Listeria monocytogenes*
- Otitis media/interna

Protozoal
- Toxoplasmosis

Parasitic
- Self-mutilation (aberrant visceral larva migrans—see *Gastrointestinal Disorders*)

Nutritional
- Hypoglycemia
- Polioencephalomalacia (possibly vitamin B_1 deficiency)
- Hind-limb paralysis syndrome (see "Metabolic Bone Disease" in *Nutritional Disorders*)
- Head tilt, ataxia, depression *(Pasteurella)*

Neoplasia
Other noninfectious problems
- Toxins
- Spinal lesions—e.g., intervertebral disc prolapse, fractures
- Polioencephalomalacia

Findings on clinical examination

- Apparent weakness
- Posterior paralysis/paresis

- Inappetence, weight loss, lethargy, weakness, ataxia, disorientation, tremors, and gradual paralysis (polioencephalomalacia)
- Otitis externa (see also "Ectoparasites" in *Skin Disorders*)
- Ataxia, tremors, head tilt, diarrhea, inappetence and weight loss, loss of energy, hypothermia, dyspnea, and sudden death (toxoplasmosis)
- CNS signs, vomiting, self-mutilation, pinpoint necrosis of liver (listeriosis)

Investigations

1. Full neurologic examination
2. Radiography
3. Routine hematology and biochemistry
4. Serology for *Toxoplasma*
5. Culture and sensitivity
6. Endoscopy
7. Biopsy
8. Ultrasonography

Management

- Seizures: Diazepam at 2.0 mg/kg PO, IV, or IM to effect

Treatment/specific therapy

- Bacterial CNS infection (including *Pasteurella, Clostridium piliforme,* and listeriosis)
  - Appropriate antibiosis
  - Supportive care
  - *Note:* Listeriosis is a zoonosis.
- Toxoplasmosis
  - Clindamycin at 12.5 mg/kg PO b.i.d. for at least 2 weeks.
  - Combination therapy consisting of:
    - Co-trimoxazole at 30 mg/kg PO b.i.d.
    - Pyrimethamine at 0.5 mg/kg PO b.i.d.
    - Folic acid at 3.0 to 5.0 mg/kg s.i.d. daily
    Or
    - Co-trimoxazole at 30 mg/kg PO daily
    - Toltrazuril at 7.0 mg/kg PO daily for 2 consecutive days
    - Treat for 3 weeks.
- Polioencephalomalacia
  - May respond to vitamin B_1 supplementation
- Aberrant visceral larva migrans
  - Larvae in CNS
  - Treat with fenbendazole (see *Gastrointestinal Disorders*)
  - Treat neurologic signs symptomatically.
- Hypoglycemia
  - For management of hypoglycemic episodes, see *Pancreatic Disorders*.
- Orthopedic conditions
  - Treat as for other small animals.

Ophthalmic disorders

As a nocturnal marsupial, sugar gliders have relatively large and pronounced eyes, which can lead to an increased risk of trauma.

Bacterial

- Uveitis

Protozoal

- Toxoplasmosis (see *Neurologic Disorders*)

Nutritional

- Poor nutrition (blindness, cataracts)
- Corneal fat deposits

Neoplasia

Other noninfectious problems

- Corneal trauma/damage
- Idiopathic cataracts
- Idiopathic uveitis
- Senescent cataracts

Findings on clinical examination

- Corneal ulceration
- Corneal trauma
- Corneal fat deposits in young
- Cataracts (poor nutrition, idiopathic)

Investigations

1. Ophthalmic examination
2. Topical fluorescein to assess extent of ulceration
3. Tonometry
4. Skull radiography
5. Routine hematology and biochemistry
6. Serology for *Toxoplasma*
7. Culture and sensitivity
8. Biopsy
9. Ultrasonography

Treatment/specific therapy

- Corneal ulceration
  - Topical and systemic antibiosis
  - Once infection is cleared, treat as for other small animals (e.g., scarification to encourage healing, conjunctival grafts, etc.).
- Corneal trauma
  - As for corneal ulceration
  - May require tarsorrhaphy

- Uveitis
  - Topical ophthalmic steroid or NSAID preparations
  - Topical ophthalmic antibiotic preparations plus systemic antibiosis if appropriate
  - Enucleation if severe
- Cataracts
  - May be seen in hand-reared young and in joeys from obese mothers. Hypovitaminosis A may be involved.
  - Supplement with vitamin A.
- Neoplasia
  - Enucleation
- Toxoplasmosis—see *Neurologic Disorders*

Endocrine disorders

None described as yet, but the clinician should remain aware of the possibility, especially thyroid and adrenal disease.

Urinary disorders

Bacterial

- Nephritis
- Cystitis

Protozoal

- *Klossiella*

Nutritional

- Urolithiasis

Neoplasia

Other noninfectious problems

- Bladder rupture secondary to urinary obstruction

Findings on clinical examination

- Depression
- Anorexia
- Weight loss
- Polydipsia/polyuria
- Oral ulceration
- Hematuria (urolithiasis, cystitis, neoplasia)
- Hind-leg weakness
- Melena
- Dysuria/polyuria
- Urine dribbling, wet perineum, constant licking at genitalia (urolithiasis)
- Painful urination, stranguria (urolithiasis, cystitis)
- Death

Investigations

1. Radiography
   a. Useful to differentiate uncomplicated cystitis from urolithiasis
2. Routine hematology and biochemistry
   a. Creatinine 41.6 to 52.2 µmol/L; urea 5.4 to 6.5 mmol/L
3. Cytology
   a. Renal casts, neoplastic cells
4. Culture and sensitivity
5. Endoscopy
6. Biopsy
7. Ultrasonography

Management

1. Fluid therapy (see *Nursing Care*)
2. Appropriate antibiosis

Treatment/specific therapy

- *Klossiella* spp.
  - Asymptomatic
  - Attempt treatment with toltrazuril at 7.0 mg/kg PO once daily for 2 days; repeat weekly over 3 weeks.
- Nephritis
  - As for "Management"
  - Treat as for other small animals.
- Urolithiasis
  - If urethral obstruction:
    - Attempt catheterization (can be difficult in males due to J-shaped os penis)
    - Cystocentesis
    - Surgical cystotomy
    - If unable to clear urethra, create a perineal urethrostomy.
- Cystic calculi
  - Cystotomy
  - Submit any stones/sand for analysis.
  - Antibiosis (usually has accompanying cystitis) and other supportive care
  - Address dietary change depending on urolith analysis/assess water management.
- Neoplasia
  - Guarded prognosis
  - As for other small animal species

Reproductive disorders

Male sugar gliders have a pendulous scrotum that hangs cranial to the penis (Fig. 7-4). The penis is bifurcated. Castration will prevent breeding but also reduces odor and urine marking behavior and reduces the development (and the associated hair loss) of the scent glands on the head and chest.

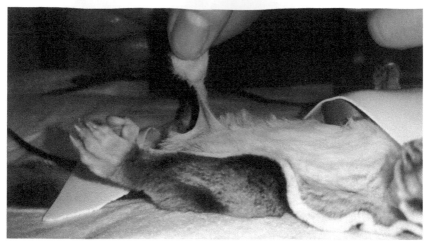

Fig 7-4. Sugar gliders have a pendulous scrotum located cranial to the penis. *(Courtesy of Sophie Jenkins, MRCVS.)*

Female sugar gliders have an usual reproductive tract anatomy—a single urogenital sinus branches into a single median and two lateral vaginas. Of surgical significance is that the left and right lateral vaginas encircle the ureter on that side before rejoining the median vagina proximally at the cervices. Therefore ovariohysterectomy necessitates careful avoidance of the ureters. Approach via a midline abdominal incision, although this is complicated by the ventrally located pouch. Females possess a marsupium. Pregnancies may be palpable as abdominal masses. One to two joeys are born at a time (Fig. 7-5).

Bacterial
- Pouch infections

Fungal
- Candidiasis (pouch infection)

Neoplasia
- Mammary carcinoma (Keller et al 2014)

Other noninfectious problems
- Dry/necrotic penis (septicemia/trauma)

Findings on clinical examination

- Irritation and/or unpleasant smell from pouch (pouch infection)
- Firm mammary swelling (mammary carcinoma)

Investigations

1. Radiography
2. Routine hematology and biochemistry
3. Urinalysis
4. Culture and sensitivity
5. Endoscopy

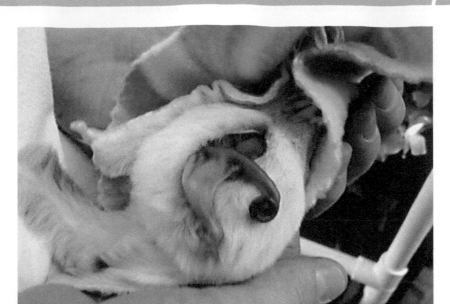

Fig 7-5. The female sugar glider raises one or two joeys in its pouch. *(From Ness RD, Johnson-Delaney CA. 2012. Sugar gliders. In: Quesenberry KE, Carpenter JW (eds.). Ferrets, rabbits, and rodents: Clinical medicine and surgery, 3rd ed. Saunders, St. Louis.)*

6. Biopsy
7. Ultrasonography
    a. Prostatic hyperplasia/cysts

Management

1. Fluid therapy (see *Nursing Care*)
2. Prophylactic antibiotics

Treatment/specific therapy

- Necrotic penis
    - Amputate (does not impede urination).
    - Covering antibiotics and analgesia
- Pouch infections
    - Appropriate antibiosis
    - Itraconazole 5 to 10 mg/kg PO b.i.d.
    - Topical antibiotics/antifungals
- Testicular neoplasia
    - Castration
- Metritis
    - Induce uterine contractions with 0.5 mg prostaglandin $F_{2\alpha}$ SC.
    - Antibiosis

255

- Pyometra
  - Ovariohysterectomy
  - Antibiosis
- Mastitis
  - Acute mastitis
    - Antibiosis and fluids
    - NSAIDs may have anti-endotoxin effects (see "Analgesia" in *Nursing Care*)
    - Debride or surgically resect affected mammary tissue.
    - Fostering joeys may spread pathogens to other females, so may need to hand-rear (see *Neonatal Disorders*)
  - Chronic mastitis
    - Often nonresponsive to therapy
  - Joeys may need supplemental feeding (see *Neonatal Disorders*).

Neonatal disorders

- Some normal developmental parameters of joeys (after Brust 2009) are shown in Table 7-3.

Table 7-3	Sugar gliders: Normal developmental stages
Days 0-7	8-18 g body weight; no fur, eyes closed
Days 8-14	12-22 g body weight; very fine fur, eyes closed
<Day 28	18-35 g body weight; fur becoming more prominent; tail starting to fluff out; animal is weaning
<Day 56	23-75 g body weight; self-sufficient; very active at night

Young gliders below the age of 100 days rely largely on heat from the adults to maintain a relatively high body temperature but are able to cope temporarily with temperatures down to 10° C as a survival strategy that allows the female to forage, leaving young in the nest (Holloway and Geiser 2000). By age 100 days the young can no longer access the pouch and must be able to thermoregulate individually.

Other noninfectious problems

- Stress diarrhea (Brust 2013)
- Hypothermia (especially in first 2 weeks as joeys unable to thermoregulate)
- Lack of maternal milk
- Mastitis (see *Reproductive Disorders*)
- Maternal systemic illness
- Maternal aggression/cannibalism
- Poor maternal nutrition

Findings on clinical examination

- Lethargy
- Failure to feed
- History of lack of maternal care
- Failure to grow

- Diarrhea (may not be apparent as female continually licks clean)
- Apparent visual problems

Investigations

1. Weigh joeys.
2. Radiography
3. Routine hematology and biochemistry
4. Culture and sensitivity
5. Endoscopy
6. Biopsy
7. Ultrasonography

Management

- Nursing care, especially provision of warmth and fluids, is extremely important with neonates.

Treatment/specific therapy

- Lack of maternal milk production
  - Hand-rear joeys. Use a commercial milk replacer for small mammals that does not contain lactose (Table 7-4).

Table 7-4 Sugar gliders: hand-rearing guide

Stage	Diet
Furless	Milk formula. Need feeding every 3 hours.
Just furring	Milk formula but start to offer soft fruits. Feed every 4-6 hours.
Short thick fur	Milk formula plus offer usual adult foods (see *Nutritional Disorders*). Feed every 6-8 hours. Give water as is now lapping.
Thick fur	Feed every 8-12 hours. Offer usual adult foods. Provide water.
Thick fur and active at night only	Need only 1 milk formula feed per day. Offer other normal adult foods and provide access to water.
Weaning	Offer usual adult foods once daily at night, and provide water.

Parks and Wildlife Commission of the Northern Territory 2015.

  - Investigate underlying problem in the dam.
- Stress diarrhea
  - Typically follows either a major change in surroundings/environment or a change in diet
  - Give supportive fluids (see "Fluid Therapy" in *Nursing Care*) and gut motility enhancers (see *Gastrointestinal Disorders*).
  - Always transition diets slowly over several days.
- Poor maternal nutrition
  - Females fed a low-protein diet (8%) had young that developed visual discrimination defects compared with those from females fed an adequate diet (32% protein)—Punzo et al 2003

Parrots and related species

Members of the parrot family are the most common avian pet and, therefore, the most likely to be presented to the veterinarian. Table 8-1 shows the most commonly encountered species.

Consultation and handling

Psychologically, most pet birds are little different from their wild ancestors—the veterinary surgeon constitutes a potential predator, so the bird is likely to exhibit a flight or fight response when handled. Exceptions to this are hand-reared parrots (or imprinted raptors and owls). However, in extremis, birds vary in their susceptibility to stress, and while some, such as the larger psittacines, can be handled relatively safely, others, such as canaries, carry a greater risk.

A great many captive-bred, hand-reared birds can be superficially examined while perched on the owner or on a freestanding perch, thereby minimizing stress. If care and patience are used, then auscultation of the lungs and air sacs, plus some assessment of body condition, can be achieved in this way.

It is important to weigh parrots at every consultation (Fig. 8-1); tame birds can be accurately weighed using a small perch designed to fit onto standard weighing scales.

Aggressive birds, or birds unused to handling, may need to be "toweled" in order to examine them. Use a large towel that will cover most of the bird. Drop or place it over the bird such that the head is covered and the bird cannot see your hands. With one hand, grab the bird's head or neck from behind so that there is control of the beak, and use the other hand to gather up the rest of the bird into the towel. Do not in any way compress the sternum, as this will seriously compromise the bird's breathing.

Birds will attempt to mask signs of illness and so may not exhibit clinical signs until a disease course is quite advanced. It is important to observe the bird from a distance for several minutes prior to handling, as a relaxed bird is more likely to show signs of ill health.

Important nonspecific clinical signs in parrots

- Heavy lidded/dark periorbital coloring
- Fluffed up/feather plucking
- Abnormal or absent feeding/drinking behavior
- Polydipsia/polyuria
- Lethargy
- Abnormal activity
- Change from normal perching activity or on floor of cage
- Abnormal profile
- Abnormal breathing action
- Abnormal vocalization
- Tail-bobbing. A sign of dyspnea. Respiratory rates of psittacines are high, but a recovery time exceeding 3 min would be considered abnormal.
- Regurgitation

From Malley (1996).

Table 8-1 Parrots and related species: Key facts

	African grey parrot	Blue-fronted Amazon parrot	Blue and gold macaw	Moluccan cockatoo	Peach-faced lovebird	Cockatiel	Budgerigar
Average life span (years)	50-70	40-50+	50-80+	50+	10+	10-20+	4-13
Weight (g)	300-400	320-460	950-1175	640-1025	50-61	80-90	45-50 (60+ for large show budgerigars)
Sexing	DNA or surgical sexing	DNA or surgical sexing	DNA or surgical sexing	DNA or surgical sexing. Also males have black irides, females have reddish brown.	DNA sexing	The small, ventral (true) tail feathers (not the overlying longer remiges) are barred in females (hard to assess in Lutinos). The red-orange color of the cheek patches is more pronounced in males.	Cere is blue and smooth in males; brown and rough in females. Young blue mutation females may have a pastel-blue cere.
Estimating age	Young <5 months have dark gray irides; adults have yellow irides.	In very young birds the irides are black or dark brown; adults have yellowish irides.	Young birds have dark brown irides.	Younger birds are a duller color with less yellow and blue on the head.	Young birds have dark/black saddle marks on the mandible and maxilla.	Resemble females but the tail is shorter and the cere is pinkish rather than gray	Young birds (<6 weeks) have barred feathering on the forehead
Normal clutch size	3-4	3-4	2-3	2	3-8	4-7	3-8
Incubation (days)	28	30	28	30 days	21-24	17-23	17-20 (begins with the second egg)

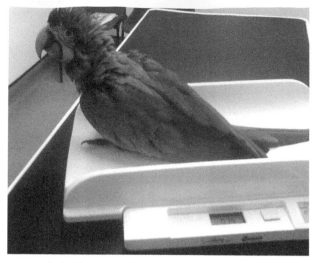

Fig. 8-1. Weighing a young harlequin macaw (hybrid blue and gold × green-wing).

Avian emergencies

1. It is best to attempt an initial assessment *before* handling a stressed or extremely ill bird, as this may allow you to take some diagnostic shortcuts, thereby reducing handling time.

2. Remove the bird to as quiet and darkened an area as possible so as to reduce stress, preferably into a heated chamber such as an incubator, and supply oxygen as close to the bird's head as possible.

3. Allow the bird a few minutes to relax in this warm, high-oxygen environment before continuing with the examination.

4. If it is imperative to handle the bird, *warn the owner first* that although you must do this, there is a chance of losing the bird. If necessary ask the owner to sign a consent form.

5. Handle the bird either with your hands or with a towel. Never use gloves or gauntlets. With larger psittacines, if necessary, have an assistant grip the head firmly from behind if you are concerned about being bitten. Do not grip around or otherwise compress the sternum as this will compromise respiration.

6. Consider either sedation or inducing anesthesia by masking the bird down with isoflurane or sevoflurane for a more detailed examination. For those birds with respiratory or cardiovascular compromise, the relative risks and benefits of anesthesia need to be considered.

Nursing care

Thermoregulation

Avian core body temperature often exceeds 40.5° C, and birds have a large surface area relative to body mass, which means that they must expend a great deal of energy in thermal homeostasis. Feathers act as an insulative layer but do not grow back as readily as mammalian fur, so as few as possible should be removed, should surgery be indicated.

Heat loss and, therefore, energy conservation can be reduced by placing the bird close to a heat source—vivarium heat mats are ideal for this. Place a towel or similar over the mat to prevent burns and protect the mat from fluids. Young chicks are unable to thermoregulate, so they must be maintained in an incubator.

Fluid therapy

Birds are primarily uricotelic which, as in reptiles, predisposes them to gout-related problems. Blood volume is between 4.4 and 8.3 mL/100 g body weight in chickens. In some species, it can be as high as 14 mL/100 g.

Dehydration

1. Most critically ill birds should be assumed to be 5% to 10% dehydrated.
2. Increased skin turgor over the foot or upper eyelid, collapse or poor filling of the ulnar vein, sunken or glazed eyes, dry and tacky mucous membranes, tachycardia, depression, and red or wrinkled skin in psittacine neonates all indicate dehydration.
3. The daily maintenance water requirement for psittacine birds is around 50 mL/kg per day, with that of passerines and young birds being much higher.
4. A 500-g (0.5-kg) bird with 10% (0.1) dehydration, therefore, requires (0.5 × 0.1) liters = 0.05 L = 50 mL fluid. As in other species, which fluids are given depends on the reason for giving fluids. Half of the fluid deficit should be replaced within the first 12 to 24 hours. The remaining 50% is divided over the following 48 hours, to be given alongside the daily maintenance.

Fluid administration

- *Per cloaca*. Water can be absorbed from the cloaca (and naturally from material refluxed into the colon), so this can be used as route for rehydrating with small volumes when there is a risk of aspiration pneumonia (Table 8-2).
- *Oral fluids* are usually given by crop tube. Not suitable for birds that are regurgitating, recumbent, or fitting.
- *Intravenous*. Birds can tolerate fluid replacement rates of up to 10 mL/kg given in a bolus, if given slowly over 5 to 7 minutes. Sites include the right jugular vein, brachial vein (Fig. 8-2), and the medial metatarsal vein. Intravenous catheters are difficult to maintain in birds, so bolus administration is preferred. Isotonic solutions should be administered slowly at a rate of 10 to 15 mL/kg. A "shock" dose of 90 mL/kg can be used if large volumes are needed rapidly. Suggested individual bolus volumes are listed in Table 8-3.

Table 8-2 Parrots and related species: Cloacal fluid administration

Species	Suggested volumes for cloacal administration (mL)
Budgerigar	0.5
Cockatiel	1
Amazon	4
Macaw	6-7

Table 8-3 Parrots and related species: Suggested individual bolus volumes

Species	Bolus volume (mL)
Budgerigar	1-2
Cockatiel	2-3
Conure	4-6
Amazon	8-10
Macaw	15-25

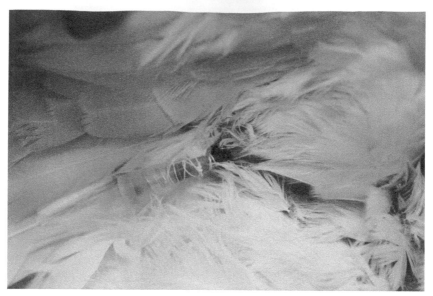

Fig. 8-2. Placement of an intravenous catheter into the brachial vein of a cockatoo. Use a collar if it is to be kept in place for several days.

- *Subcutaneous fluids* can be given into the interscapular area (not caudal neck to avoid the cervicocephalic air sac) or the inguinal region. Small volumes (5 to 10 mL/kg) should be given at each site, and absorption may be poor.
- *Intraosseous.* Distal ulna and proximal tibiotarsus. Strict asepsis and anesthesia. All types of fluids, including blood transfusions. Do not administer very acidic, alkaline, or hypertonic solutions IO without diluting them first.

Choice of parenteral fluids

- Crystalloids. Only 25% of a crystalloid solution remains in the peripheral vasculature 30 minutes after administration. Hartmann's solution contains lactate that is converted to bicarbonate by the liver and so may help correct acidosis but is contraindicated with hypernatremia.
- Hypertonic saline solution at 3% to 7.5% will help to correct circulatory collapse by triggering fluid shifts from the interstitial space into the circulation, followed quickly by isotonic solutions to prevent tissue dehydration. Do not use hypertonic solutions if cranial hemorrhages are suspected.
- Colloids. Bolus administration of hetastarch at 10 to 15 mL/kg IV t.i.d. for up to 4 treatments may be safe and effective for hypoproteinemia.
- Oxyglobin can be given at a dose rate of up to 15 mL/kg IV or IO.
- Whole blood. Birds are tolerant of anemia, but a transfusion should be considered if the PCV falls below 15.0 L/L. Use blood from the same or similar species; blood groups have been only poorly investigated.

Nutritional supplementation

If the bird is eating normally, then supply its usual diet. For short-term management, recovery diets commercially available for dogs and cats (nonmilk-based) may be crop-tubed for carnivorous, insectivorous, or omnivorous birds. Dextrose can be given orally, by subcutaneous injection up to 2.5%, or IV. It is a metabolic acidifying agent and may be contraindicated in cases of metabolic acidosis. Note that most birds are diurnal and will not feed in the dark. For parrots, hand-rearing formula can be used.

Wing clipping of pet parrots

A badly clipped bird is not only at increased risk of damage to itself, but such clipping may also predispose to feather-picking and self-mutilation. Wing clipping can be controversial, but the major justification for wing clipping is that it facilitates the necessary interaction between a pet parrot and the other family members, allowing the bird to become involved with, and behave as, part of the family (or "flock") rather than being confined to its cage. However, the ideal would be that the bird is left fully flighted and controlled verbally, using commands such as "step up," "step down," "leave," and "no."

Wing clipping

1. Both wings should be clipped, allowing the bird to maintain its balance.
2. It is the primary flight feathers that allow lift, and it is these that should be trimmed such that the cut end is tucked beneath the coverts.
3. Developing "pin" feathers should not be cut as these will hemorrhage; instead leave alone and leave a feather alongside it or on either side for support to prevent accidental damage.

Microchipping

1. Microchips are placed into the left pectoral musculature.
2. Occasionally hemorrhage may occur, but usually digital pressure is sufficient for hemostasis.
3. Microchips inserted SC, although potentially less traumatic, are readily palpable and are subject to removal and fraud.

Analgesia

Table 8-4 Parrots and related species: Analgesic doses

Analgesic	Dose
Butorphanol	0.5-4.0 mg/kg IM every 2-4 hr
Carprofen	1.0-4.0 mg/kg SC or PO b.i.d.
Ketoprofen	1.0-5.0 mg/kg IM b.i.d. or t.i.d.
Meloxicam	0.1-0.5 mg/kg SC or PO s.i.d.
Morphine	0.1-3.0 mg/kg IV

Sedation

- Midazolam 0.5 to 3.0 mg/kg IM or intranasal
- Diazepam 0.2 to 2.0 mg/kg intranasal. IM administration likely to be irritant with delayed absorption (Mans 2014)
- Butorphanol 1.0 to 3.0 mg/kg IM or intranasal
- Midazolam 1 to 2 mg/kg plus butorphanol 1 to 2 mg/kg IM if heavier sedation is required. Macaws usually require this combination to gain adequate sedation for clinical procedures (Mans 2014).
- Benzodiazepines can be reversed by flumazenil at 0.01 to 0.1 mg/kg PO.

From a practical point of view, induction and maintenance with gaseous anesthesia are of choice. Atropine can be given as premedication at 0.05 to 0.1 mg/kg SC. This reduces mucus and counters bradycardia from vagal stimulation during surgery.

Gaseous anesthetic protocol

1. Hold the bird's head into a mask or place into an induction chamber. Isoflurane offers a rapid induction and recovery (as does sevoflurane).
2. Intubate (uncuffed endotracheal tube) whenever possible.
3. During anesthesia, regularly give positive-pressure ventilation to reduce risk of CO_2 buildup in the abdominal air sacs.
4. Main sources of heat loss are the extremities (especially the feet) and the air sacs. Wrap the feet with silver foil and maintain the bird on an external heat source.
5. If using halothane, start at low concentrations (0.5% to 1.0%) and gradually increase to 3.0% to 4.0%. Induction at high concentrations can lead to dangerously high levels of halothane present in posterior air sacs. Attempts to resuscitate bird by flushing through with oxygen or manual ventilation will only force this reservoir of halothane through the lungs, further increasing blood concentrations.

Parenteral anesthesia

1. Always weigh the bird accurately before using parenteral anesthesia, and always intubate and maintain on oxygen whenever possible.
2. A range of anesthetic protocols are available from the literature. The ones the author has used include:
   a. Ketamine at 5 to 30 mg/kg IV or IM. No analgesic effect. Avoid birds with potential liver/kidney complications.
   b. Ketamine 5 mg/kg plus xylazine 0.25 to 1.0 mg/kg IV or IM
   c. Ketamine 5 to 20 mg/kg plus midazolam 0.25 mg/kg IV or IM. This gives good sedation, muscle relaxation, and recovery.
   d. Ketamine 3 to 6 mg/kg plus medetomidine 25-100 µg/kg IV or IM
   e. Both medetomidine and xylazine can be reversed with atipamezole at 5 × medetomidine dose.

Air sac perfusion anesthesia

Avian respiratory anatomy means that the trachea can be "bypassed" by insertion of a suitable cannula into one of the caudal air sacs (abdominal or caudal thoracic) for delivery of oxygen and anesthetic gases. This technique is suitable for oral or tracheal obstructions or if surgery is required at or around the oral cavity. Glottal or tracheal foreign bodies or other obstructions will usually give their presence away by producing a whistling sound during the respiratory cycle. These birds are extremely liable to sudden death. The main priority is to establish a patent airway as quickly as possible, therefore the need to anesthetize and insert an air sac tube.

Air sac perfusion anesthesia technique

1. Use soft tube with holes in walls.
2. Use a 4-mm-diameter tube for a 350-g bird, increasing pro rata.
3. A left lateral approach is used with the left leg extended cranially and a small incision made behind the last rib and ventral to the flexor cruis medialis muscle (Fig. 8-3).
4. A small pair of hemostats can then be used to enter the coelom in a craniomedial direction, which will provide access to the caudal thoracic air sac.
5. A tube is then secured in place with a suture and attached to the anesthetic machine. *Note:* A higher airflow rate (>50% above normal) will be required to maintain anesthesia this way.
6. The tube can be left in situ for 1 to 3 weeks.

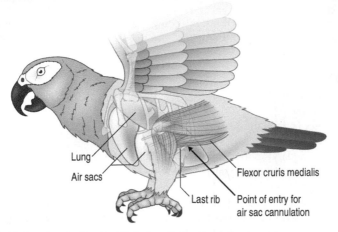

Fig. 8-3. Anatomical markers for the placement of an air sac tube.

Recovery
- Keep quiet.
- Wrap wings gently in towel/paper toweling to reduce injury from flapping.
- Keep warm, preferably mid-20s° C.
- Recovery must be fast from anesthetic—birds under 100 g should be eating within 30 minutes.

Cardiopulmonary resuscitation
1. Can use doxapram at 5 to 7 mg/kg IM or sublingually.
2. Intubate if not already done.
3. Intermittent positive-pressure ventilation once every 5 seconds.
4. If in cardiac arrest, begin rapid chest compressions.
5. Give epinephrine at 0.5 to 1.0 mL/kg of 1:1000 intrathecal, intracardiac, IO, or intraperitoneal.

Skin disorders

Avian skin is very thin, with the epidermis only up to 10 cells thick in feathered areas. There are few cutaneous glands:

1. Uropygial gland. Not present in all species (e.g., Amazon parrots and *Pionus* parrots). When present, it lies dorsally near the tip of the tail. There can be up to 18 orifices depending on the species. Usually bare except for a tuft of down feathers known as *uropygial wick*. Secretes a lipoid sebaceous secretion—sebum—that is water repellent. It also helps to keep plumage supple and smooth, contains vitamin D_3 precursors, has antibacterial and antifungal properties, and enhances feather coloration. However, most sebum is produced from epidermal cells that contain keratin-bound phospholipids that coat the skin and feathers.
2. Small wax-secreting glands are present in the external wall of the auditory meatus.
3. There are mucus-secreting vent glands.
4. There are no sweat glands.

Commensal bacterial numbers on the skin of birds are considered to be lower than those found on mammals. Yeasts are infrequent commensals. *Malassezia* is not isolated from normal or self-mutilating birds (Preziosi et al 2006); in the same study, *Candida albicans* was isolated but significance was unclear.

Feathers serve a number of functions, including insulation, protection from trauma, accessories to flight, species recognition patterns, and display. There are several types and subgroups of feathers.

Feather types

1. Contour feathers are divided into:
   a. Flight feathers
      i. Remiges (carried on the wing)
         (1) Primary—borne on the manus
         (2) Secondary—borne on the antibrachium
      ii. Retrices (carried on the tail)
   b. Body feathers
   c. Coverts—cover the bases of the retrices or remiges
   d. Ear coverts—screen the external opening of the ear and improve hearing
2. Other feathers include down feathers, filoplumes, bristles, and semi-plumes. Various intermediate forms of feathers will be encountered. Powder feathers usually structured like down feathers, occasionally semi-plumes, and contours shed a fine white powder of keratin onto contour feathers to provide waterproofing. Particularly obvious in African grey parrots and cockatoos.

Signs of skin disease

Pruritus

- Flies
  - Hippoboscids (flat flies/louse flies) occasionally encountered, especially with aviary birds. Can transmit hemoparasites such as *Haemoproteus* and *Leukocytozoon*, as well as transferring mites and lice among individuals.
- Lice: Can reach significant numbers on debilitated birds
- Ticks: Occasionally on new imports. Sudden death associated with tick attachment to head. Suggested etiologies include hypersensitivity reactions, toxin injection, or a tickborne infection. Can also transmit other diseases such as haemoprotozoan parasites, *Borrelia* spp., and louping ill
- Red mite *(Dermanyssus avium)* and other species
- Northern fowl mite *(Ornithonyssus* spp.)
- Feather mites: Found between the barbs on the ventral surfaces of feathers. Often niche specific so in the budgerigar, *Protolichus lunula* is found on the wing and tail feathers, whereas *Dubininia melopsittaci* occurs on the smaller body feathers.
- Quill mites: Live inside quills
- Sarcoptid mites present on the feather shafts may be encountered occasionally. Treat as above.
- Quill wall mites
- Skin mites
- Epidermoptid mites
- Knemidocoptid mites. Common is *Knemidocoptes pilae* (scaly face/scaly leg)
- Harpirhynchid mites: Attach to feather bases. May induce hyperkeratotic epidermal cysts
- Cheyletiellid mites: Rare
- Polyfolliculitis: Common in lovebirds. Multiple feathers arise from single feather follicle.

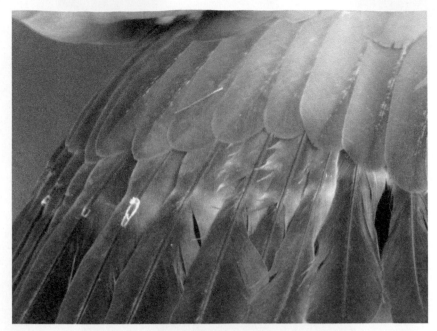

Fig. 8-4. Stress lines in the primary and secondary flight feathers in an African grey parrot. Note also the abnormal red pigmentation.

Ulceration/folliculitis

- Erysipelas
- *Staphylococcus*
- *Aspergillus*

Feather damage, pathology, and loss

- "Stress" lines (see "Findings on Clinical Examination" below and Fig. 8-4)
- Dystrophic feathers sometimes occur secondary to folliculitis.
- Polyomavirus (papovavirus): Usually presents in chicks but is carried asymptomatically by adults. Signs include a distended abdomen, lack of or malformed down feathers, multifocal follicular and feather pulp hemorrhages, and retarded growth of tail and contour feathers (infected budgie chicks may be referred to as "walkers"). There may be a urate-soaked vent because the virus also infects the liver and the kidneys. Also slow weight gain, slow emptying crop, and vomiting. This virus is responsible for budgerigar fledgling disease, which usually is rapidly fatal.
- Psittacine beak and feather disease (PBFD, circovirus; Fig. 8-5). Usually affects birds younger than age 3 years. Signs include loss of feathers, decrease in down feathers on flanks, retained pin feathers, short clubbed feathers, and deformed feathers. Beak may change in color, grow abnormally, and become necrotic, beginning with a palatine crust in the maxillary beak. Secondary bacterial infections make the condition worse. Older, chronically infected African grey parrots may produce red feathers in abnormal position such as the covert feathers (Fig. 8-6).

Diet

- In macaws especially, thinning of the feathers and retention of keratin sheaths of pin feathers, in particular the flight and tail feathers, is linked to poor diet.

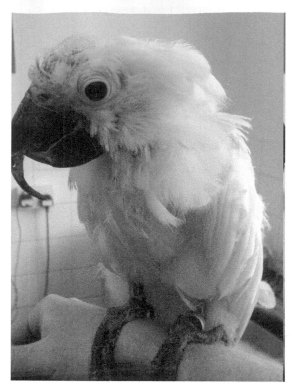

Fig. 8-5. Psittacine beak and feather disease in a sulfur-crested cockatoo.

- Unsupplemented seed diets are deficient in minerals, sulfurous amino acids, and vitamins; birds on unsupplemented diets show increased feather replacement intervals (Wolf et al 2003) and may exhibit old, tattered feathers.

Self-trauma
- Secondary to ectoparasites
- Hand-reared parrots may never learn the normal species-specific methods of preening.
- Grossly abnormal feathers in budgerigars—called *feather dusters* or *chrysanthemum disease*—are a genetically recessive condition.
- Chewing at extremities; can be secondary to topical irritations

Scaling and crusting
- Papillomavirus: Reported in Timneh African grey parrots. Proliferative cutaneous lesions seen on head, especially eyelids, beak commissure, and skin contiguous with lower beak
- Herpesvirus: Described in cockatoos and macaws as dry proliferative lesions on the toes that are limited to extremities; not life-threatening
- Hyperkeratosis of the plantar surfaces of the feet—hypovitaminosis A (see *Nutritional Disorders*)

Erosions and ulceration
- Neoplasia (squamous cell carcinoma; Klaphake et al 2006)

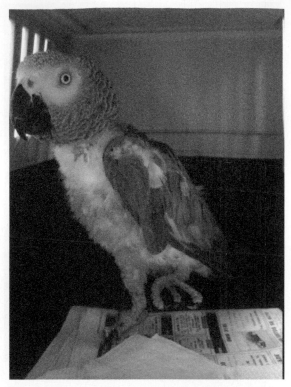

Fig. 8-6. Abnormal red pigmentation in an African grey parrot with psittacine beak and feather disease.

Nodules and nonhealing wounds

- Avian pox virus (skin pox)
  - Wartlike lesions of the skin. Yellowish nodules form on the beak, eyelids, and other areas of the skin that disintegrate and discharge a serosanguineous fluid. The areas then scab over. When present on the feet, lesions may occlude distal vasculature, resulting in tissue necrosis of the lower extremities. *Note:* Can occur in a diphtheritic form or a septicemic form.
- *Staphylococcus* may occasionally be encountered as a cause of dermatitis. More often it is isolated as a secondary invader in bumblefoot.
- Candidiasis has been seen as focal raised lesions as well as more generalized ulcerations. Head lesions have been reported in eclectus parrots, Amazon parrots, and cockatiels. *Aspergillus* lesions, *Trichosporon asahii*, and dermatophytosis are occasionally encountered.
- Feather cysts: Secondary to follicle damage; the developing feather is unable to emerge and forms a large, cystlike structure.
- Cryptococcosis (Berrocal 2004)
- Mycobacteria (Ferrer et al 1997)
- Bumblefoot: Typically chronic infection and abscessation of the feet, especially the plantar surfaces. Often due to staphylococci or streptococci.

Changes in pigmentation

- *Erysipelothrix* infections may cause an erythema of the skin in an acute infection with sudden death.

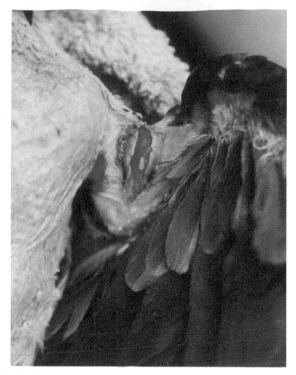

Fig. 8-7. Prepatagial chronic ulcerative dermatitis in an African grey parrot.

Chronic ulcerative dermatitis (CUD)

- Usually associated with chronic conditions such as mycobacteriosis, tumors, abscesses, or xanthomas. Poor nutrition may also contribute. Four main presentations are:
  - Prepatagial CUD: Wing web area. Possibly linked to *Giardia* or hypovitaminosis E. Usually very pruritic and painful. Patagium may also be affected. Commonly seen in chronic self-mutilating African greys (Fig. 8-7)
  - Proventer CUD: Keel area; common in African greys and large Amazons. Secondary to trauma following hard landings. Bruises or splits forming ulcers.
  - Postventer CUD: Between cloaca and tail. Possibly similar etiology to proventer CUD. Poor nutrition also implicated
  - Squamous cell carcinoma (Klaphake et al 2006)
- Ectoparasites (see "Pruritus" above)

Alopecia

- Pruritic (self-mutilation) versus nonpruritic. PBFD is provisionally differentiated from self-inflicted trauma in single birds as feathers on head also affected; normally bird cannot reach these to self-damage.

Neoplasia

- Lipomas (Fig. 8-8), fibrosarcomas, liposarcomas, and squamous cell carcinomas are some of the more common skin neoplasms reported in birds. Xanthomas are common, especially in budgerigars. These are nonneoplastic yellowish nodules or plaques caused

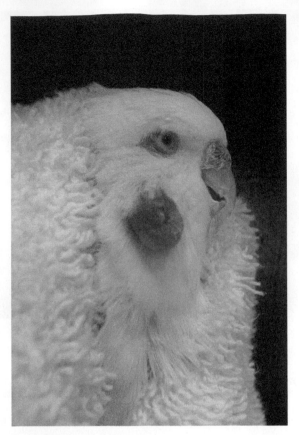

Fig. 8-8. Lipoma in a budgerigar.

by an accumulation of cholesterol and fats. Can be ulcerative. Often found over an area of pathology such as a lipoma.

Allergies

- There is a strong suggestion that allergies may be the cause of skin disease in some cases, especially in Old World psittacines.

Findings on clinical examination

- Observe bird in cage or at rest on owner. Assess if it show signs of a typical sick bird—ruffled, fluffed up feathers, sleepiness, and tail "pumping." Is it pruritic?
- Assess the surroundings. Are feces normal? Stress or sudden influx of fruit may trigger very loose feces.
- Handle the bird:
  - Examine nares, beak, eyes, and buccal cavity, including choana. Look particularly for signs of vitamin A deficiency (see *Nutritional Disorders*).
  - Examine skin; note signs of inflammation, hyperkeratosis, ulceration, and trauma.
- Assess feather quality:
  - Stress lines—lines visible on the vanes of the feather that denote areas of poor quality of the barbs. Thought to be linked to release of endogenous corticosteroid.

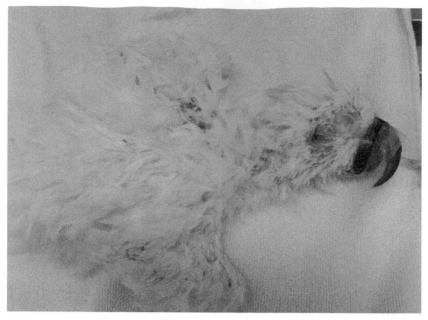

Fig. 8-9. Anesthesia of a cockatoo for further skin investigation.

- Frayed, dirty, or matted feathers: Inappropriate size caging may cause repeated damaged to the retrices of those birds with long tails such as parakeets and macaws.
  - Abnormal feather coloration may result from nutritional deficiencies, hepatopathies, or PBFD.
- Examine for parasites:
  - Pluck one or two feathers for examination under a light microscope for ectoparasites and feather pulp examination.
- Examine uropygial (preen) gland, cloaca, and feet.
- Auscultate heart, lungs, and air sacs.
- Palpate abdomen.
- Anesthesia may be required with birds difficult to handle safely (Fig. 8-9).

Investigations

1. Routine hematology and biochemistry
   a. Zinc and lead levels may be appropriate to investigate low-grade heavy metal poisoning. Collect samples for zinc in either heparin or plain tube (without gel as this may contain zinc). Although blood levels can be indicative of zinc toxicity, there is no absolute correlation between blood zinc levels and clinical signs. As a general rule, if zinc levels are >32 to 50 µmol/L and there are consistent clinical signs (see *Neurologic Disorders* and *Gastrointestinal Tract Disorders*), then zinc toxicity should be suspected. Significant zinc levels are often accompanied by an absolute or relative monocytosis.
2. Aseptic collection of samples for bacteriology/mycology
3. Cytology

4. Radiography: A standing view using horizontal beam is useful for detecting metallic foreign bodies in the conscious bird; otherwise lateral and ventrodorsal views, under general anesthesia (GA), are required for meaningful radiography.
5. Endoscopy
6. Serology for PBFD, polyomavirus, *Aspergillus* antigen, and *Chlamydophila* antigen should be taken if thought necessary.
7. Fresh fecal samples for parasitic examination; look for *Giardia*, nematode eggs, etc. Smears can be dried and stained.
8. Bulk fecal samples (collected over 3 to 5 days) can be submitted for *Chlamydophila* polymerase chain reaction (PCR).
9. Diagnostic imaging, including radiography and endoscopy
10. Biopsy
    a. *Note:* Eosinophilic dermatitis linked to *Trichosporon asahii* infection.

Management

- Optimize diet: Consider converting to pelleted foods, using multivitamin supplements, reducing seed intake, and increasing fruit consumption where appropriate.
- Where there is significant feather loss, consider supplementary heating to counter loss of insulation.
- Covering broad-spectrum antibiotics may be useful if there are obvious skin lesions.
- If pruritic, consider analgesia—meloxicam (Metacam) oral suspension at 0.1 mg/kg body weight b.i.d. Do not use steroids.
- Collars
  - Collars are inherently very stressful to parrots; they interfere with normal feeding (many parrots transfer their food to their mouth with a foot), flight, climbing, and crop function. They are heavy relative to the weight of the bird and generally alienate the bird from its immediate surroundings. They also do not address any underlying cause or pathology, and if these are not addressed then feather plucking/self-mutilation may resume when the collar is removed.
  - Therefore, collars should be used judiciously and on a case-by-case basis.
  - If possible, hospitalize the parrot for 24 to 48 hours to enable the bird to get used to the collar, as well as allowing any minor adjustments and reassessments to be made.
  - A collar should be removed only after the bird has been clinically well for a reasonable period of time, as it is likely that, as in other species, abnormal or triggering sensations will persist for some time following the clinical resolution of lesions. Early removal often results in repeat damage.

Treatment/specific therapy

- Ectoparasites
  - Ticks: Treat with ivermectin or fipronil. Remove ticks manually where possible.
  - Red mite and other species
    - Ivermectin at 0.2 mg/kg PO, SC, or IM. Repeat monthly as required
    - Light dusting with pyrethrin powder
    - Treat environment in case of red mite; painting woodwork may "seal in" mites.
  - Feather mites
    - Cis-permethrin powder
    - Fipronil spray applied to cotton wool; beware hypothermia in small birds due to evaporation of carrier.
    - Treat quill mites, sarcoptid mites, and quill wall mites as for feather mites.

- Knemidocoptid mites (e.g., *Knemidocoptes pilae*):
  - Ivermectin at 0.2 mg/kg PO, SC, or IM. A small drop may be applied topically over the jugular vein or onto the back of the neck and seems to work well. Injection is not recommended in birds weighing <500 g due to problems with toxicity. Treat harpirhynchid, epidermoptid, and cheyletellid mites as for knemidocoptid mites.
- Giardiasis
  - Metronidazole at 25 mg/kg PO b.i.d. for 5 to 10 days
- Bacterial infections: Appropriate antibiosis
- Mycobacterial infections
  - Potential zoonosis, so consider euthanasia.
  - For treatment, see *Respiratory Tract Disorders.*
- Candidiasis
  - Nystatin at 300,000 IU/kg PO b.i.d. for 10 days
  - Amphotericin B at 1 mg/kg PO b.i.d.
- *Aspergillus* and *Trichosporon asahii* infection
  - Ketoconazole at 30 mg/kg PO b.i.d. for 7 to 14 days
- Avian pox: Supportive treatment only
- PBFD
  - Supportive treatment
  - In early viremic form avian interferon has been used successfully, but no data exist for its use in more cases showing dermatologic signs. PBFD-positive birds that show no feather abnormalities may be transiently viremic and so should be retested. If negative after 90 days then they are clear of the infection.
- Herpesvirus and papillomavirus
  - Supportive treatment, including covering antibiosis to prevent secondary infections
- CUD
  - Covering antibiosis and meloxicam at 0.2 mg/kg PO, IM body weight once daily. Do not use steroids. Investigate and address underlying factors.
- Suspected allergies
  - Consider meloxicam at 0.2 mg/kg PO, IM body weight once daily as an initial treatment.
  - Chlorpheniramine 0.75 to 3.0 mg/kg PO daily
  - Systemic and topical steroids should be used with extreme caution.
- Neoplasia
  - Surgical resection or debulking
  - Cisplatin given intralesional at 17.5 mg/m^2 (Klaphake et al 2006). Cisplatin is potentially nephrotoxic and ototoxic and has been linked with anorexia, diarrhea, seizures, peripheral neuropathies, and hematologic disturbances. A dose rate of 30 mg/m^2 has been linked with fatal toxicity (Manucy et al 1998)
- Lipomas in budgerigars can respond to L-carnitine supplementation at 1000 mg/kg of feed (De Voe et al 2004)
- Xanthomas typically occur over other lesions, such as neoplasms, or sites of previous hemorrhage and trauma such as at wing tips. Often require surgical excision.
- Polyfolliculitis: Antibiotics, NSAIDs, surgical removal of affected follicles
- Feather cysts require surgical removal.
- Polyomavirus: In some countries such as the United States, vaccination may be available. The virus may persist in the environment for some time, so testing with PCR should be undertaken.
- Bumblefoot: Usually requires surgical intervention; bird may need supportive dressing on affected foot to prevent reinfection of surgical site. If the condition is unilateral, be

aware of pressure sores and other sequelae affecting the good leg due to bird shifting weight onto it.

The self-mutilating parrot

Self-mutilation, like stereotypies, is a form of abnormal repetitive behavior exhibited in captive parrots. Often psychological in origin, the alternative of an underlying causal disease should not be ruled out, either as differential diagnoses or as contributing factors. Epidemiologic evidence (Garner et al 2005) points toward there being an inherited susceptibility, an increased incidence in females, and a link to certain stressful environmental conditions. There are no "quick fixes," and investigation is often prolonged and expensive. A methodical and holistic approach is required. This should take into account the background of the bird, its environment, its disease status, and its psychological well-being.

Background

- Species
  - Most common in African grey parrots and cockatoos (*Cacatua* spp.—Jayson et al 2014).
  - Macaws and cockatiels often begin with the wings and legs.
  - Amazon parrots and Moluccan cockatoos tend to mutilate skin rather than feathers.
  - African greys will denude all areas of skin from neck down.
- Captive-bred/hand-reared (CBHR) or wild-caught? Wild-caught individuals may be more prone to parasitic or psychological causes, while nutritional causes may be more common in CBHR birds. Hand-reared parrots may never learn the normal, species-specific methods of preening.
- Single or with others? If with others, are any of them showing similar signs?
- House bird or aviary? Again parasites are more common in aviary than living rooms. If aviary, are others affected? Positioning the cage next to a wall is associated with increased risk of feather plucking (Jayson et al 2014).
- Is the parrot a recent introduction/acquisition of unknown clinical history, or a long-standing pet of known clinical history that has not been exposed to any new birds? *Note:* Even long-standing pets can be at risk of "new bird" problems if introduced or exposed to other birds it has not previously been with (e.g., if the owner buys another bird or the parrot is boarded at the local pet shop). Length of ownership also increases the risk of feather plucking (Jayson et al 2014).
- How long has the bird been self-mutilating?
- Is it constant or recurrent, and if recurrent, is it associated with anything (time of year, owner holidays, perceived periods of sexual activity)? Does it occur at a particular time of day?
- Was there an apparent initial trigger? Building work? New dog/child/partner? Birds not used to change may not tolerate it well.
- Does the bird self-mutilate when owner is present? Or when absent? Self-mutilation is associated with owners who have one or more holidays per year (Jayson et al 2014). If seen, how does bird behave while self-mutilating? Does it appear pruritic, vocalize or scream, or even interrupt a favored activity to self-mutilate?
- Try to find out what the bird's normal demeanor is. Is the bird normally relaxed, fearful, aggressive?
- How has the self-mutilation progressed? Where did the bird start plucking and how did it progress?
- How does the owner respond? In some psychological cases the noisy excitable response of the owner can become a reward for this behavior!

Environmental

Lighting

- Photoperiod: Many of the birds kept as pets are equatorial in origin and so are physiologically attuned for a 12-hour day/night cycle. African grey parrots exposed to longer than 12 hours of darkness are more likely to feather pluck (Jayson et al 2014).
- Intensity: The majority of psittacines are open scrub (budgerigars) or high canopy (parrots) species that are exposed to high-intensity sunlight. This would include UV light that may act as a natural antiparasiticide, bactericide, and fungicide.
- Spectrum: UV lighting in particular may be important with vitamin D_3 synthesis from precursors excreted by the uropygial gland. In mammals vitamin D is important for normal skin function, and this may also be the case in birds.

Diet

- Seed-based diets are inappropriate for sole, long-term maintenance of many psittacines. Fat and hence energy levels are too high and protein levels relatively low and of poor quality. They are also low in vitamin levels.
- Attempt to wean onto newer pelleted diets. This can be difficult to do, plus anecdotally there seem to be occasional behavioral reactions to colorings used. Otherwise some basic research may be needed to ascertain suitable foods.

Water

- Amazons, African greys, and many others are from humid, tropical rainforest areas. A daily dowsing with water and consequent necessary preening may encourage normal feather and skin integrity. Daily spraying with lukewarm water or access to a bath is appreciated by many birds.

Environmental toxins

- Zinc, often from galvanized caging or cheap metallic toys: Blood levels can be indicative of zinc toxicity, but as with lead, there is no absolute correlation between blood zinc levels and clinical signs. As a general rule, if zinc levels are >32.0 to 50.0 µmol/L and there are consistent clinical signs (see *Neurologic Disorders* and *Gastrointestinal Tract Disorders*), then zinc toxicity should be suspected. Significant levels often accompanied by an absolute or relative monocytosis. Feather plucking can be associated with chronic low-grade zinc toxicity; gut problems may be seen as toxicity and can cause gut stasis. Acute poisonings can damage liver and kidneys, causing vomiting, polyuria, and hematuria. Consider radiography to look for metallic foreign bodies in the gizzard.
- Other heavy metals such as lead, copper, and iron may cause similar signs.

Treatment for zinc toxicity

- Sodium calcium edetate at 35 mg/kg IM b.i.d. for 5 days, stop for 3 to 4 days, and then repeat. Continue until zinc levels fall.
- Dimercaptosuccinic acid (DMSA) at 30 mg/kg PO b.i.d. for 10 days or 5 days per week for 3 to 5 weeks
- Penicillamine at 55 mg/kg PO b.i.d. for 7 to 14 days

- Tobacco smoke: May predispose to brittle feather production, as may an excessively dry atmosphere
- Toys: Psittacines are gregarious creatures. Most live as a pair within a flock and are constantly interacting with their flock members. All single psittacines should have a toy "friend" that they can feed, huddle up to, beat up, and generally completely dominate.

Other toys should be rotated or changed with great frequency. Particularly useful toys are:

- Wooden objects, as these can be systematically destroyed, exercising the beak and claws, and occupying valuable time
- Toys into which food can be placed and with which the parrot must work to obtain its food

Findings on clinical examination

- Note if the condition is symmetrical. Self-mutilation due to psychological causes is often not symmetrical in early stages.
- Handle the bird:
  - Examine nares, beak, eyes, and buccal cavity, including choana. Look particularly for signs of vitamin A deficiency.
  - Examine skin; note signs of inflammation, hyperkeratosis, ulceration, trauma, and seborrhea.
- Assess feather quality:
  - Stress lines—lines visible on the vanes of the feather that denote areas of poor quality of the barbs—may indicate that a significant stressor has happened to the bird at a crucial point in the development of that feather. This may have been a disease or nutritional deficiency.
  - Frayed, dirty, or matted feathers: Inappropriate size caging may cause repeated damage to the retrices of those birds with long tails such as parakeets and macaws.
  - Abnormal coloration may result from nutritional deficiencies, hepatopathies, or PBFD.
- Examine for parasites:
  - Pluck one or two feathers for examination under a light microscope for ectoparasites and feather pulp examination.
- Feather scoring:
  - This allows a structured approach to defining and monitoring the extent of the self-mutilation. A final score is arrived at and noted, allowing an objective view of improvement or deterioration to be assessed. Feather scoring may prove difficult with a recalcitrant bird and should GA be needed (e.g., for radiography), this would provide an ideal opportunity to assess this (Fig. 8-10).

Investigations

1. A general blood screen is highly recommended. Especially interested in WBC count and differential, liver and kidney biochemistry, and zinc levels.
2. Blood samples for PBFD or polyomavirus PCR
3. *Chlamydophila* serology
4. Fresh fecal samples for parasitic examination; look for *Giardia*, nematode eggs, etc.
5. Bulk fecal samples (collected over 3 to 5 days) can be submitted for *Chlamydophila* PCR.
6. Diagnostic imaging, including radiography and endoscopy
7. Aseptic collection of samples for bacteriology/mycology
8. Biopsy

Pathological causes of self-mutilation

Refer to *Skin Disorders*.
   Otherwise significant conditions include:

- Chlamydophilosis
- *Staphylococcus* has been linked to feather-picking in a budgerigar and feather loss in an unspecified psittacine (Hermans et al 2000).

BODY AND LEGS	Score	Chest and flank	Back	Legs
All or most feathers removed, down removed and skin exposed, evidence of skin or tissue injury	0			
All or most feathers removed, down removed and skin exposed, no evidence of skin or tissue injury	0.25			
All or most feathers removed, some down removed, patches of skin exposed	0.5			
All or most feathers removed, down exposed and intact *or* Feathers removed from more than half the area, some down removed, patches of skin exposed	0.75			
Feathers removed from less than half the area, some down removed and skin exposed	1.0			
Feathers removed from more than half the area, down exposed and intact	1.25			
Feathers removed from less than half the area, down exposed and intact	1.5			
Feathers intact with fraying and breakage	1.75			
Feathers intact with little or no fraying and breakage	2.0			
WINGS				
All or most primaries, secondaries and coverts removed, down removed, skin exposed, evidence of skin or tissue injury			0	
All or most primaries, secondaries and coverts removed, down removed, skin exposed, no evidence of injury			0.5	
More than half of coverts removed, down exposed and intact *or* more than half of primaries and secondaries removed, down exposed and intact			1.0	
Fewer than half of coverts removed, down exposed and intact *or* fewer than half of primaries and secondaries removed, down exposed and intact or primaries and secondaries intact with significant breakage and fraying			1.5	
Feathers intact with little or no fraying or breakage			2.0	
TAIL				
All or most tail feathers removed or broken			0	
Some tail feathers removed or broken *or* Significant fraying of tail feathers			1.0	
Feathers intact with little or no fraying or breakage			2.0	

Fig. 8-10. Feather scoring system. *From Meehan et al 2003a.*

- *Aspergillus*
- Avian bornavirus (proventricular dilatation disease, PDD)
- Other diseases, including hepatopathies and renal disease
- Endocrinologic
  - Hypothyroidism—rare (see *Endocrine Disorders*)
  - Sex hormone disturbances: Self-mutilation can be associated with seasonal changes or sexual activity. May pick at leggings. It is normal in many species to remove a patch of feathers ventrally at nesting time to form the brood patch whereby eggs can be kept warm. Consider measuring serum estrogen or androstenedione levels. Possible sex predisposition toward females.

Psychological causes of self-mutilation

- Frequently overdiagnosed. Should only be considered when other etiologies have been reasonably eliminated.
- True cause not yet elucidated. Adverse environmental stimuli likely to be involved in many cases (see Garner et al 2005); may in some cases be linked to commercial bird-rearing techniques and practices that nestling parrots are exposed to at a time of neurologic development with high psychological sensitivity and receptivity
- Suggested manifestations include:
  - Attention seeking: Abnormal behavior is reinforced by the owner paying attention when bird self-mutilates.
  - Displacement behavior: In the wild stressful situations can be avoided by flying off. In captivity this may not be an option, and so fear/aggression may be channeled into exaggerated "normal" behavior such as preening.
  - Boredom, including the concept of time budgets: In the wild, a parrot will spend a significant amount of time flying to and from roosts and food sources, interacting with flock mates, avoiding predators, and so on. In captivity this time void can be filled by extending other normal behavioral repertoires that it can undertake, such as eating (especially Amazon parrots) or preening.
  - Separation anxiety: The high intelligence of parrots suggests that this could be quite common.
  - Obsessive-compulsive disorders: Akin to stereotypic disorders—bird will stop favored activity just to pluck.

Psychotropic drugs

These should not be considered a first line of action; their use should be considered once a physical or environmental problem has been reasonably ruled out or addressed. Suggested medications include:
1. Amitriptyline at 1.0 to 5.0 mg/kg PO b.i.d.
2. Doxepin at 0.6 mg/kg IM or IV daily 0.5-2 mg/kg PO every 12 hours, or 2 drops of 5.0 mg/kg solution per 30 mL drinking water
3. Fluoxetine at 0.4 mg/kg PO daily
4. Haloperidol at 0.1 to 0.4 mg/kg PO daily
   a. Alternatively, dilute 3.0 mg into 1 L of fresh drinking water, offered fresh daily; increase the dose progressively by double dosing every 2 weeks until a dose of 12.0 mg/L is achieved.
   b. Continue treatment for at least 3 to 4 months before gradually withdrawing over a period of time.
   c. May induce Parkinson-like tremors, which disappear when drug is withdrawn
   d. Haloperidol works reasonably well with self-mutilating birds; behavior of the bird is likely to alter for the better long before feather improvements are seen.

Management

1. Correct diet. Ideally change to pelleted foods. At the very least, begin supplementation with multivitamin and/or calcium (if appropriate).
2. Address any environmental issues such as photoperiod, irritants such as smoking, and so on.
3. Remove any metallic objects from the cage.
4. Consider environmental enrichment techniques (more/different toys; companion of same species if no risk of infection, etc). If left alone for long periods, consider leaving radio or TV on. Birds naturally inhabit noisy environments—silence usually means there is a predator about. Environmental enrichment (including provision of a conspecific companion) has been found to be beneficial in birds displaying both self-mutilation (van Hoek and King 1997) and stereotypies (Meehan et al 2003b, Meehan et al 2004).
5. If pruritic, consider analgesia—meloxicam at 0.2 mg/kg PO, IM body weight once daily.
6. Attend to any obvious wounds. Application of topical amorphous hydrogel dressings (e.g., IntraSite Gel, Smith and Nephew Healthcare Ltd) encourages secondary healing.
7. Where there is significant feather loss, consider supplementary heating to counter loss of insulation.
8. Undertake specific treatment regimens as results of tests dictate.
9. Avoid the use of collars unless absolutely necessary. May stress bird and interfere with normal behavior, including feeding and crop function.
10. Basic training—"Step up," "Step down," "No," and "Stay"—can be useful in both interacting with the bird in a controlled manner and filling in valuable time. The ideal is to establish a parent–child or leader–follower relationship rather than a partner–partner one.
11. Do not forget the owners. They are likely to be embarrassed at the state of the bird and feel guilty if they have been feeding their bird the wrong food or if some other managemental deficit is identified, but you need them on board for what is liable to be a prolonged haul. They must be encouraged not to lose heart, as improvement may take some time.

Upper respiratory tract disorders

Nasal tract

Cere color in budgerigars is a secondary sexual characteristic; in most sexually mature males it is a smooth, bright blue structure, while in most females it has a rougher texture and is brown in color. Young female light blue birds may have a pastel blue cere, leading to incorrect sexing; these darken to a more normal female-type cere with maturity. Gonadal tumors may secrete inappropriate sex hormones that can lead to a change in cere color of adult birds.

Rhinitis

Viral

- Paramyxovirus (see *Lower Respiratory Tract Disorders*)
- Influenza A (orthomyxovirus—see *Lower Respiratory Tract Disorders*)

Bacterial

- Chlamydophilosis
- Mycoplasmosis
- Other bacteria

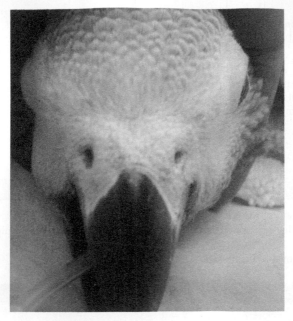

Fig. 8-11. Blocked nares in an African grey parrot.

Fungal

- *Aspergillus*
- *Candida* (see "Treatment" in *Lower Respiratory Tract Disorders*)

Dietary

- Hypovitaminosis A (see *Nutritional Disorders*)

Neoplasia

Other noninfectious problems

- Choanal atresia
- Allergies
- Rhinoliths—require surgical removal followed by antibiotic cover; often linked to hypovitaminosis A (Fig. 8-11)

Investigations

1. Radiography
2. Rhinogram
3. Routine hematology and biochemistry
4. Culture and sensitivity
5. Endoscopy of choana
6. Biopsy

Sinusitis

- Typically presents as swelling of the infraorbital sinus
- For possible etiologies, see "Rhinitis" above and *Lower Respiratory Tract Disorders.*

- Bacterial
- *Mycobacterium* spp.
- Mycoplasmal
- Fungal
- Papillomas
- Sunken eye sinusitis: Collapse of the outer delineating skin due to negative pressure in the infraorbital sinus, which results from blockage of normal connecting diverticuli. Should return to normal when sinus problem is resolved.
- Neoplasia
- Teratoma (Diaz-Figueroa et al 2005)
- Thymoma (Diaz-Figueroa et al 2004)

Treatment

- Appropriate antibiosis
- Flushing of the infraorbital sinus, followed by culture and sensitivity plus cytology as appropriate
- Surgical removal of inspissated material

Lower respiratory tract disorders

Viral

- Paramyxovirus
- Avian pox virus (diphtheritic form)
- Amazon tracheitis virus (herpesvirus)
- Orthoreovirus
- Influenza A (orthomyxovirus)
- Adenovirus—interstitial pneumonia
- PDD—secondary aspiration and inhalation pneumonia

Bacterial

- *Mycoplasma* spp.
- Chlamydophilosis—primarily *C. psittaci*, but other serotypes occasionally encountered
- *Escherichia coli*
- *Pseudomonas* spp.
- *Bordetella avium*
- *Mycobacterium avium*
- Others

Fungal

- Aspergillosis
- Cryptococcosis

Protozoal

- *Sarcocystis falculata (Coccidia)*

Parasitic

- Tracheal mites *Sternostoma tracheacolum* (in small parakeets and cockatiels)
- Air sac worms (e.g., filarid nematodes)
- *Cyathostoma* and *Syngamus* spp. (rare)

Dietary

- Hypovitaminosis A
- Squamous metaplasia of the respiratory tract predisposes to respiratory infections.

Neoplasia

- Glottal neoplasia
- Hemangiosarcoma (Hanley et al 2005)
- Hepatic neoplasia or other coelomic mass

Other noninfectious problems

- Tracheal foreign body—seed husk a common finding in cockatiels
- Polytetrafluoroethane (PTFE) toxicity from overheating of Teflon
- Inhalation of other fumes from fires
- Abdominal disease (e.g., neoplasia, hemocoelom, yolk serositis)
- Hypothyroidism (goiter) in budgerigars on a seed-only diet
- Air sac rupture (usually pathological)
- Cigarette smoke
- Creosote
- Anemia
- Allergic, asthmalike conditions
- Chronic pulmonary interstitial fibrosis (CPIF), especially in older Amazon parrots (Zandvliet et al 2001). Preexisting pulmonary damage or allergies may contribute to the etiology of CPIF.
- Cardiovascular disease (see *Cardiovascular and Hematologic Disorders*)

Findings on clinical examination

- Dyspnea and tachypnea—can be very severe
- Open-mouthed breathing
- Change in voice—may cease "talking"
- Sneezing
- Head swinging and neck stretching. Forward-leaning and extended neck strongly suggests tracheal obstruction.
- Coughing occasionally encountered, but is uncommon. Beware parrots that imitate their owner's cough.
- Tail-pumping
- Increased recovery time/exercise intolerance
- Increased inspiratory sounds often associated with upper respiratory tract disease.
- Increased expiratory sounds often associated with lower respiratory tract disease.
- Abdomen may be distended (fluid, neoplasia, hemorrhage).
- Subcutaneous air-filled swelling; may vary in size (ruptured air sac)
- Yellow urates and peracute death common with *Sarcocystis*. Old World parrots are especially susceptible.

Investigations

1. Radiography
   a. Ventrodorsal view is best for detecting abnormalities of the lungs and air sacs.
   b. Distension of abdominal air sacs indicates upper respiratory obstruction (e.g., tracheal fungal granuloma or seed husk).

Table 8-5 Parrots and related species: *Chlamydophila* serology

Result of *Chlamydophila* serology	Interpretation
Negative (no antibodies to *C. psittaci*)	May not have seroconverted. Retest in 7-10 days in acutely ill birds.
Weak positive	Suspicious, but interpretation may depend on species tested and test used. May also reflect previous exposure.
Strong positive	Highly indicative of infection, especially if accompanied by consistent clinical signs.

2. Fluoroscopy
3. Routine hematology and biochemistry
   a. Very high heterophil count (15 to 40×10^9/L) indicative of aspergillosis
   b. High PCV: 0.55 to 0.74 L/L in chronic pulmonary interstitial hyperplasia. Also often have a respiratory acidosis with a pH of 7.16 to 7.3 (normal, 7.35 ± 0.08), hypoxemia: PO_2 of 33.69 to 52.77 (normal, 49.46 ± 7.62), and hypercapnia: PCO_2 of 48.77 to 80.08 (normal, 37.92 ± 4.23) (figures from Zandvliet et al 2001)
   c. High aspartate transaminase (AST) and creatine kinase (CK), often with *Sarcocystis*
4. Serology for *Sarcocystis, Aspergillus,* and *Chlamydophila*—ideally investigate with repeat sampling to assess rising titer, but screening tests may also be useful (Table 8-5)
5. Hemagglutination inhibition tests and ELISAs may be of benefit in detecting influenza A.
6. Culture and sensitivity
   a. Tracheal lavage; needs GA
7. Cytology
8. Endoscopic biopsy
9. Endoscopy
   a. Endoscopic examination of trachea and syrinx
   b. Air sacs and lungs (high-risk procedure)
10. Transillumination of trachea in small psittacines may reveal mites or nematodes (rare).
    a. Mite or nematode eggs may be detected in feces or sputum microscopic examination.
11. Fecal samples
    a. *Chlamydophila* PCR
    b. Modified Ziehl–Neelsen staining of fecal samples or PCR for mycobacteriosis

Management

1. Reduce stress as much as possible. Placing bird in a darkened room may help.
2. Covering broad-spectrum antibiosis; may be given by nebulization
3. Provide oxygen support.
4. Nutritional support
5. Placement of a tube into a caudal air sac to allow normal breathing in cases of tracheal blockage
6. Bronchodilators (e.g., aminophylline 4.0 mg/kg PO or IM b.i.d.)
7. Mucolytics (e.g., bromhexine at 3.0 to 6.0 mg/kg IM or 6.5 mg/L fresh drinking water daily)

Treatment/specific therapy

- Foreign body
  - Remove if possible; may require endoscopy or tracheotomy
- Emphysema
  - Physical tapping and draining of air from emphysematous lesions. May need to be repeated. If necessary, place a stent if it fails to resolve quickly.
- Viral diseases
  - Provide supportive treatment and covering antibiosis.
  - Amazon tracheitis virus: Acyclovir at 10 to 40 mg/kg IV or SC t.i.d.
  - Influenza: Provide covering antibiosis. Potentially a zoonosis and reverse zoonosis, so avoid contact with infected people.
  - Paramyxovirus: Supportive treatment. Paramyxovirus A (Newcastle disease) is notifiable in the UK.
- Chlamydophilosis
  - Enrofloxacin at 5.0 mg/kg IM daily or 12.5 mg into 100 mL drinking water fresh daily
  - Doxycycline
    - Doxycycline hyclate intravenous human preparation given 60 to 100 mg/kg IM every 5 to 7 days for 45 days
    - Doxycycline hyclate as an in-water powdered medication: Use deionized water. However, Flammer et al (2003) found that drinking water with 400 mg of doxycycline/L over a 14-day period failed to maintain therapeutic plasma doxycycline concentrations.
    - In the same study, hulled seed coated with sunflower oil and doxycycline powder to a concentration of 300 mg of doxycycline hyclate/kg maintained therapeutic plasma doxycycline concentrations for 42 days without notable adverse effects.
    - *Note:* Birds may be intermittent excreters, so at least 3 consecutive negative samples should be achieved before ceasing treatment.
- Bacteria: Appropriate antibiosis
- Mycobacteriosis
  - Potential zoonosis. Consider euthanasia.
  - Two suggested treatment regimens (Rupiper et al 2000) are:
    - Ethambutol (200 mg), isoniazid (200 mg), and rifampin (300 mg) all crushed together and mixed with 10 mL of a simple syrup. This is administered daily according to Table 8-6.
    - Combination therapy of ethambutol (10 mg/kg PO b.i.d.), streptomycin (30 mg/kg IM b.i.d.), and rifampin (15 mg/kg PO b.i.d.)

Table 8-6 Parrots and related species: Volumes required for suggested treatment regime of *Mycobacteriosis*

Bird weight (g)	Volume of mixture (mL)
<100	0.1
100-250	0.2
250-500	0.3
500-1000	0.4

- Fungal diseases: Specific antifungal regimens for *Aspergillus* and *Candida*
  - Clotrimazole (including nebulization)
  - Itraconazole at 5 mg/kg PO daily. *Note:* This is potentially toxic to African grey parrots in particular.
  - Voriconazole at 12.5 mg/kg PO b.i.d. Polyuria may be noted (Flammer et al 2008).
  - Miconazole (Daktarin Oral Gel, Jansssen-Cilag) at 0.1 mL per 500 g body weight
  - Terbinafine at 15 mg/kg PO once daily
  - *Note: Aspergillus* can be a serious sequel to prolonged/inappropriate steroid use (Verstappen et al 2005).
- *Sarcocystis*
  - Trimethoprim–sulfadiazine at 60 mg/kg (combined constituents) PO b.i.d. for 3 days, 2 days off, then repeat for 3 days.
- Air sac worms
  - Ivermectin at 0.2 mg/kg SC. Repeat after 2 weeks.
  - *Cyathostoma* and *Syngamus* spp.: Indirect life cycle using earthworms, slugs, and snails. Treat with fenbendazole at 50 mg/kg PO as a one-off dose.
- Hemocoelom: PCR for polyomavirus. Provide supportive care, but bird is unlikely to survive.
- Hypothyroidism in budgerigars: Usually supplementation with iodine or commercially available iodine-impregnated seeds such as Trill (Pedigree Petfoods) will resolve the problem.
- PTFE poisoning: If still alive (most birds die very quickly), remove from source of toxicity. NSAIDs may be useful in the control of the pulmonary inflammation that is caused.
- Fume inhalation: In addition to general therapy, consider NSAIDs (e.g., meloxicam at 0.2 mg/kg body weight PO, IM once daily). Steroids can be counterproductive in some cases.
- Suspected allergic conditions may respond to steroids (beware iatrogenic effects) and bronchodilators (see "Management," above). These may be given by nebulization. Alternatively, try oral meloxicam.

Gastrointestinal tract disorders

The beak

Beak trimming

1. The beak is a highly sensitive organ and should be regarded as such.
2. In some birds just the maxilla overgrows; in others both the maxilla and mandible need attention, usually due to an underlying malocclusion.
3. With large parrots in particular, radiograph the skull to ascertain the extent of the underlying maxillary bone before shortening the beak.
4. Burring and reshaping of the beak with dental burrs while under GA is preferable and less traumatic to the bird than clipping the beak with nail clippers (Fig. 8-12).

Neoplasia

- Squamous cell carcinoma, basal cell carcinoma, and melanoma (all cited in Girling 2004)

Other noninfectious problems

- Maxillary or mandibular fracture
- Lateral deviation of the maxilla (scissor beak)—can be linked to repetitive bar chewing at the same spot. In hand-reared young chicks repeated syringe feeding from the same side by the carer can cause a distortion of the soft cartilaginous beak.

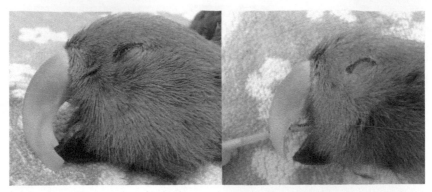

Fig. 8-12. Before and after reshaping of the beak of an eclectus parrot, using a dental burr.

- Damaged area of beak; often marked hemorrhage (fracture)
- Overgrowth of the maxilla or mandible; may be asymmetrical

- Radiography

1. Severe fractures are unlikely to heal. Remove distal part and if the bird is able to use remains of beak to prehend food, then allow to heal.
2. Mild fractures may respond to pinning and cerclage wire plus application of supportive dental acrylics.
3. Provide covering antibiosis.

- Beak abnormalities resulting from fractures will need repeated attention to burr back the abnormal keratin growth that frequently results.
- Scissor beak: In young chicks in which the beak has not calcified, repeated physical repositioning may work. If the beak is too calcified, then an acrylic ramp can be placed on the mandible to try to force the maxilla back into place.

Differential diagnosis for vomiting/regurgitation/dysphagia

Definitions

1. Vomiting—food is refluxed from the proventriculus (i.e., the acid-secreting stomach).
2. Regurgitation—food is brought back from the crop, an outpouching of the esophagus.
3. Dysphagia—abnormality/difficulty in eating, possibly involving prehension or mastication of food while in the mouth.

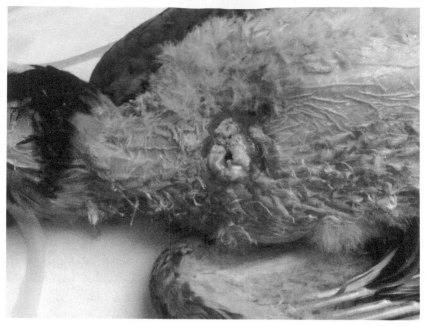

Fig. 8-13. Crop fistula in a blue and gold macaw.

- Normal "mate-feeding" behavior (e.g., some sexually active male budgerigars may regurgitate onto their mirror or even onto their owner)
- Goiter in iodine-unsupplemented budgerigars; hyperplastic thyroid gland partially blocks thoracic inlet.
- Tongue laceration
- Proventriculitis
- *Macrorhabdus ornithogaster* infection (megabacteriosis)
- *Candida*
- Irritation from ingested materials or toxins
- Foreign body
- Neoplasia
  - Squamous cell carcinoma
  - Leiomyosarcoma
- Avian bornavirus (PDD) (see *Gastrointestinal Tract Disorders*)
- Zinc or other heavy-metal poisoning
- Crop fistula in hand-reared psittacines (Fig. 8-13)
- Crop stasis (crop muscle atony) is commonly encountered when hand-rearing psittacines. It results from a physiologic stress.
- Incorrect brooding temperatures
- Incorrect food temperatures
- Hand-rearing formula is too dilute.
- Ingluvoliths—hardened accumulations of material in the crop
- Ingluvitis—inflammation of the crop lining
- Bacterial infection, especially *E. coli, Aeromonas,* and *Pseudomonas* spp.
- Trichomoniasis in crop—very common in budgerigars and cockatiels

- Candidiasis in crop—serious in neonates
  - *Note*: "Sour crop" is fermentation of crop contents subsequent to crop stasis/ingluvitis.
- Temporomandibular rigidity in cockatiel chicks (lockjaw—*Bordetella avium*)
- Systemic disease

Findings on clinical examination

- Undigested seed in vomitus (PDD, megabacteriosis)
- There may be dry, caked-on material around the mouth, cere, and feathering of the face and chin.
- The crop may be swollen.
- Old tongue lacerations may present as a discharging granuloma.
- Weight loss
- Passing of partially digested (megabacteriosis) or undigested food (PDD) in feces

Investigations

- Collection of crop fluid: This is done with a syringe and a reasonably wide crop tube.
- Crop wash/lavage
  - Wet preparation
  - Gram stain
  - Romanowsky stain (Diff-Quik)
- Fecal examination
  - Gram stain (*Macrorhabdus* stains as gram-positive, thick-walled rods; normal gut flora should be predominantly gram-positive)
- Hematology and biochemistry
  - Blood zinc and/or lead levels. Blood levels can be indicative of zinc toxicity, but as with lead, there is no absolute correlation between blood zinc levels and clinical signs. As a general rule, if zinc levels are >32 to 50 µmol/L and there are consistent clinical signs (see also *Neurologic Disorders* and *Gastrointestinal Tract Disorders*), then zinc toxicity should be suspected. Significant levels are often accompanied by an absolute or relative monocytosis.
- Radiography (Figs. 8-14 and 8-15)
  - Standing radiograph for ingested metallic particles
  - Contrast radiography of old, discharging tongue lesions to investigate presence of possible foreign body
  - Ileus may indicate an enteritis, heavy-metal toxicity or PDD (Fig. 8-16)
- Endoscopy
  - Creamy-yellow lesions in the crop and/or esophagus suggest trichomoniasis. Take grab biopsy and look at wet prep under microscope.
- Ultrasonography
- Fluoroscopy

Management

1. Supportive treatment, including fluids (see *Nursing Care*)
2. For proventriculitis, consider:
   a. Metoclopramide at 0.2 to 0.5 mg/kg IM or PO b.i.d.or t.i.d.
   b. Cimetidine at 5 mg/kg PO b.i.d.
   c. Gavage with activated charcoal

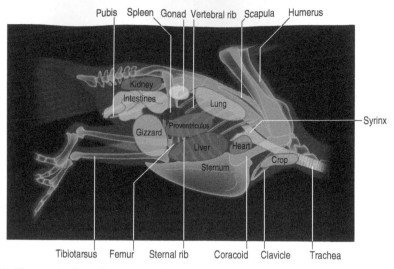

Fig. 8-14. Diagram of radiographic anatomy of a psittacine (lateral view).

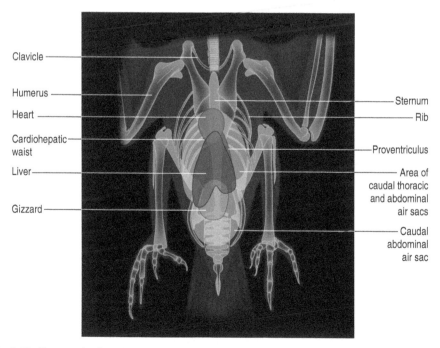

Fig. 8-15. Diagram of radiographic anatomy of a psittacine (ventrodorsal view).

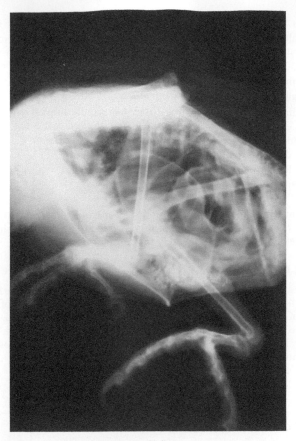

Fig. 8-16. Radiograph of a young African grey parrot with ileus.

Treatment/specific therapy

- *Trichomonas*
  - Metronidazole at 50 mg/kg PO every 12 hours for 3 doses; alternatively 30 mg/kg PO b.i.d. for 5 to 7 days (Girling 2004)
- *Candida*
  - Nystatin at 300,000 IU/kg PO b.i.d. for 10 days
  - Amphoteriin B at 1 mg/kg PO b.i.d.
- Sour crop: Flush with warmed saline solution. May need to be done under GA; consider intubation and packing of the choana prior to flushing.
- Megabacteriosis *(Macrorhabdus ornithogaster)*
  - Amphotericin B at 1 mL/kg PO of 100 mg/mL suspension b.i.d.; for budgerigars 0.5 mg/bird b.i.d. until organism is eliminated.
  - Ketoconazole at 10 mg/kg b.i.d. PO.
- Laceration of the tongue may require suturing.
- Foreign body: Remove either via the oral cavity or surgery (ingluviotomy). If flushing out crop, do so under GA, intubated with head held down and choana packed to reduce risk of aspiration.

- Zinc or other heavy-metal toxicity
  - Sodium calcium edetate at 35 mg/kg IM b.i.d. for 5 days, stop for 3 to 4 days, then repeat. Continue until zinc levels fall.
  - DMSA at 30 mg/kg PO b.i.d. for 10 days or 5 days a week for 3 to 5 weeks
  - Penicillamine at 55 mg/kg PO b.i.d. for 7 to 14 days
- Avian bornavirus (PDD—see *Gastrointestinal Tract Disorders*)
- Crop fistula in hand-reared psittacines: These may require surgical debridement and closure (two layered). Etiology is due to being fed on food that is too hot.
- Crop stasis due to dilute preparation: Increasing the concentration of the food mix to 20% to 30% dry matter will often rectify this problem.
- Ingluvoliths: Removal via the oral route or break down into smaller particles using warmed saline (Girling 2004)
- Goiter
  - Supplement with iodine. A stock solution of 2 mL of strong Lugol's iodine solution in 30 mL water is prepared; 1 drop of this is added to 250 mL drinking water daily for treatment and 2 to 3 times weekly for prevention.

Assessment of droppings

Normally, there are both fecal and urinary portions to a bird dropping. The fecal part should be dark and well formed; the urinary part should contain white crystals of uric acid plus a small amount of liquid urine. However, fecal consistency reflects diet and, therefore, varies according to species, from small, hard droppings in budgerigars to liquid "squirts" in lorikeets. Therefore, birds presenting with diarrhea should have their feces closely examined to differentiate genuine loss of fecal consistency from polyuria.

Assessment of avian droppings

Fecal portion

- The fecal portion may be small or absent if:
  - Bird is anorexic.
  - Cloacoliths or other obstructions are present.
- May be poorly formed—genuine diarrhea (Fig. 8-17)
- May be abnormally colored:
  - Blood may be present.
  - Certain highly pigmented fruits may do this.
- May contain abnormalities such as:
  - Undigested seeds
  - Worm eggs or protozoal cysts (on microscopic examination)

Urinary portion

- May be dry if:
  - Bird is on an all-seed diet (e.g., budgerigar).
- May have a high water content if:
  - Bird is on a high water content diet (e.g., fruit or vegetables).
  - The bird is polydipsic.
  - If the bird is polyuric, always collect a sample and check for glucose, blood, and protein.
- May be abnormally colored:
  - Light to dark green may indicate liver disease due to high biliverdin levels.
  - Greenish to a bronze color may indicate liver disease but can also occur after trauma.

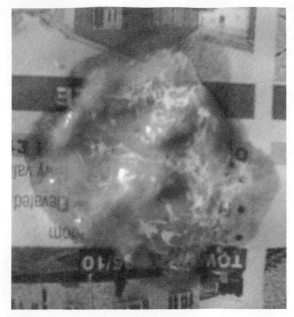

Fig. 8-17. Genuine diarrhea in a parrot. Note the loss of fecal consistency.

Always collect a fresh sample.
- Microscopic examination of a wet preparation will often pick up protozoa and worm eggs.
- Fecal flotation for protozoal oocyst counts
- Gram stain: The normal gut flora of psittacines should be predominantly gram-positive. A Gram stain should highlight changes in the bacterial flora, including yeast overgrowths.
- Swab for bacterial culture and sensitivity if appropriate.

Differential diagnosis for gastrointestinal disorders

Viral
- Avian bornavirus (PDD—formerly known as macaw wasting disease; can affect a variety of psittacines) (Staeheli et al 2010)
- Paramyxovirus
- Chronic paramyxovirus infection can cause cloacal dilatation.
- Papillomatosis (a possible herpesvirus)
- Orthoreovirus and orthoreovirus-like agent (budgerigars)
- Pacheco disease
- Polyomavirus
- Rotavirus
- Picornavirus
- Adenovirus

Bacterial
- Hepatitis, proventriculitis, enteritis due to:
  - *E. coli*
  - *Klebsiella* spp.
  - *Pseudomonas* spp.

- Salmonellosis
- *Yersinia pseudotuberculosis*
- Chlamydophilosis (psittacosis)
- *Mycobacterium avium* (avian tuberculosis)
- Clostridia
  - *Clostridium colinum* and *C. perfringens* in lories (Pizarro et al 2005)
  - Megacolon secondary to *C. tertium*

Fungal

- *Candida*
- Megabacteriosis *(Macrorhabdus ornithogaster)*
- Mucormycosis

Protozoal

- *Giardia*
- *Spironucleus* (Philbey et al 2002)

Parasitic

- Uncommon in psittacines, but ground-feeding Australian parakeets are particularly at risk
- Nematodes
  - Ascarids (especially *Ascaris platycerci* and *Ascaridia hermaphrodita*) and *Porrocaecum* spp.
  - *Capillaria*
  - *Thelazia* and *Oxyspirura* spp.
- Spiruroids: Proventricular worms (e.g., *Geopetitia, Dispharynx, Habronema,* and *Tetrameres* spp.)
- Cestodes (e.g., *Raillietina* spp.)

Dietary

- Dietary indiscretion

Neoplasia

- Gastric carcinoma
- Gastric adenoma
- Papilloma (papillomatosis—see "Viral" above).

Other noninfectious problems

- Calcinosis circumscripta (deep granuloma in tongue)
- Proventricular ulceration
- Proventricular impaction
- Foreign body
- Sloughed koilin due to ventriculitis
- Dysplastic koilin
- Intussusception
- Cloacal prolapse
- Megacloaca
- Cloacal impaction

Findings on clinical examination

- Weight loss
- Vague signs of ill health (e.g., cessation of talking)

- Passing undigested seeds in feces (PDD)
- Melena (ulceration, severe enteritis)
- Hemorrhagic feces (Pacheco disease)
- Neurologic signs (PDD, paramyxovirus)
- Vent soiled with accumulated feces
  - Budgerigars: Usually due to obesity (cannot clean themselves) or herniation of abdominal musculature
  - Central American parrots (e.g., Amazons, macaws, and hawk-headed parrots): Likely to be papillomatosis. This affects the cloaca, but also the oral cavity and proximal gastrointestinal tract.
- Yellow-green diarrhea, wasting, and death (spironucleosis)
- Wide range of clinical signs, including gastrointestinal and respiratory, may be seen with systemic bacterial infections such as *Salmonella* and *Yersinia*. Occasionally neurologic signs may be seen with *Salmonella*.
- Green diarrhea, dyspnea, and sneezing (chlamydophilosis)
- Weight loss *(Mycobacterium avium)*; may also exhibit slow-growing masses
- Cloacal tissue visibly protruding from vent (cloacal prolapse)
- Physiologic enlargement of the cloaca in reproductively active Vasa parrots *(Coracopis vasa)* and lesser Vasa parrot *(C. nigra)*
- Sudden death *(Clostridial* infection); may be linked to stress triggers
- Sudden, mass deaths in budgerigars (orthoreovirus-like agents)

Investigations

1. Routine hematology and biochemistry
2. Serology and PCR (crop swab) for avian bornavirus
3. Samples for culture and sensitivity
   a. Fecal examination
   b. Gram stain
   c. Modified Ziehl-Neelsen staining for mycobacteriosis
   d. Wet preparation/flotation for worm eggs/protozoa (Fig. 8-18)
   e. Abundant motile trophozoites *(Spironucleus)*
4. Proventricular wash for proventricular worm eggs

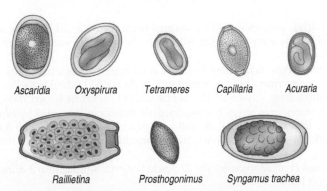

Fig. 8-18. Diagram showing some eggs of intestinal parasites of psittacines (not drawn to scale).

5. Fine-needle aspirate/staining/cytology of any abnormal masses (including staining for mycobacteria)
6. Radiography (including contrast studies)
   a. Dilated crop, proventriculus, gizzard, and gut (PDD, severe enteritis)
   b. Contrast studies for PDD, proventricular ulceration, foreign body
   c. Dilated cloaca (megacloaca)
7. Fluoroscopy
8. *Chlamydophila* PCR; ideally take three samples from each bird: conjunctiva, choana and feces; serology for *Chlamydophila*
9. *Mycobacterium avium* PCR on feces/suspect material
10. PCR for Pacheco disease and polyomavirus
11. ELISA and virus neutralizing tests for orthoretroviral infection: isolation of orthoreovirus from feces, biopsy samples, ascitic fluid, or respiratory secretions
12. Endoscopy
13. Ultrasonography
14. Biopsy
    a. Full-thickness crop wall, including large blood vessel for PPD will allow diagnosis in 75% of cases (Gregory et al 1996). Biopsy of proventriculus is a more difficult operation and carries a higher risk. Biopsy has now been superseded by serologic and PCR testing for avian bornavirus.
15. Postmortem of affected birds
    a. *Yersinia:* a degree of hepatomegaly; patchy discoloration of the liver and in more advanced cases; miliary lesions in liver, kidneys, and spleen

Management

1. Supportive management, including covering antibiosis
2. Fluid therapy

Treatment/specific therapy

- Pacheco disease—see *Hepatic Disorders*
- Orthoreoviral infection: supportive treatment: New World species often respond well, but Old World species carry a poorer prognosis
- Other viral diseases
  - Symptomatic and supportive treatment only
- Parasites
  - Birds in outside aviaries should be wormed twice yearly (avoid breeding season) or have fecal screens every 6 months. All new birds should be wormed during quarantine.
  - Suitable treatments include fenbendazole at 50 mg/kg PO as a once-only dose, or water-soluble avermectins (e.g., moxidectin 0.1% added to drinking water at 20 mg/L for 48 hours). *Note:* Fenbendazole may be toxic to cockatiels (Lloyd 2003).
  - *Capillaria:* Infection is direct, but intermediate stages can be carried by earthworms, so remove fecal material regularly and prevent access to soil. Treat with fenbendazole at 50 mg/kg by crop tube; this may need repeating every 2 weeks until the bird is clear.
  - *Ascaridia* and *Porrocaecum* spp.: The life cycle is direct, although earthworms may act as transport hosts.
  - *Thelazia* and *Oxyspirura* spp.: Carried by intermediate arthropod host

- Proventricular worms (e.g., *Geopetitia, Dispharynx, Habronema,* and *Tetrameres* spp.): Indirect life cycle using insect intermediate hosts
- Cestodes: Single dose of praziquantel at 8 to 10 mg/kg PO
- *Giardia*
  - Metronidazole at 20 mg/kg PO b.i.d.
- *Spironucleus*
  - Metronidazole as above
  - Dimetridazole failed to work (Philbey 2002)
- *Candida* and mucormycosis
  - Nystatin at 300,000 IU/kg PO b.i.d. for 10 days
  - Amphotericin B at 1 mg/kg PO b.i.d.
- Avian bornavirus (PDD): Poor response to treatment but some individuals recover. Treatment should include:
  - Broad-spectrum antibiosis (e.g., enrofloxacin at 5 to 20 mg/kg PO daily, co-trimoxazole at 30 mg/kg PO b.i.d.)
  - Motility modifiers (e.g., cisapride at 1.0 mg/kg PO b.i.d.; metoclopramide 0.5 mg/kg PO, IM, or IV BID-TID)
  - The use of cyclooxygenase-2 (COX-2) inhibitors such as celecoxib (Celebrex, Pfizer) at 10 mg/kg PO daily appears to be beneficial in some cases, but their use should be considered carefully; meloxicam (another COX-2 inhibitor) appeared to exacerbate clinical signs of PDD in experimentally infected cockatiels (Hoppes et al 2013).
  - Keep in-contact birds in strict isolation, although horizontal transmission to immunocompetent, fully fledged birds appears poor (Rubbenstroth et al 2014).
  - Institute good hygiene, ventilation, and other good management.
  - Immediate and thorough investigation of any sick or dead birds
  - Probably an isolation period of 2 to 3 years without any fresh incidence of PDD is needed before declaring an aviary free of the disease (Doneley et al 2007).
- Obesity in budgerigars: Consider supplementing with L-carnitine (1000 mg/kg food).
- Abdominal herniation in budgerigars will often require surgery to remove excess abdominal musculature.
- Papillomatosis: Surgical removal of papillomas from cloaca and oral cavity if causing problems. Infected birds often subsequently develop neoplasia of the pancreas, and bile duct carcinoma has been reported in affected Amazon parrots.
- *Salmonella:* Antibiotics based on culture and sensitivity findings
  - Autogenous vaccination can clear carriers (Harcourt-Brown 1986). Two doses are given 2 weeks apart; each dose consists of 1.0 mL PO and 0.5 mL SC.
- Other bacterial infections: Appropriate antibiosis
- *Yersinia:* Prevent access of wild birds and rodents to aviaries and food stocks.
- Clostridial infections: Metronidazole at 20 mg/kg PO b.i.d.
- *Macrorhabdus ornithogaster*—see "Differential Diagnoses for Vomiting/Regurgitation/Dysphagia"
- *Mycobacterium avium:* Potential zoonosis, so recommend euthanasia. For suggested treatment protocols, see under *Lower Respiratory Tract Disorders.*
- Chlamydophilosis (see *Lower Respiratory Tract Disorders*)
- Proventricular ulceration
  - Cimetidine at 5 mg/kg PO b.i.d.
  - Address underlying factors, including possible secondary bacterial and fungal ulceration.

- Proventricular impaction
  - Flush with warm saline either via mouth or via ingluviotomy incision.
  - If fails may need to undertake a proventriculotomy.
- Cloacal prolapse: Requires cloacopexy
  - A pursestring suture may provide temporary alleviation of the condition, but cloacopexy should give more permanent results.
  - Investigate the possibility of underlying predisposing factors (e.g., cloactitis, etc.).
  - If linked to reproductive activity, see *Reproductive Disorders*.
- Megacloaca: Cloacal reduction surgery (Graham et al 2004)
- Cloacal impaction: Requires manual removal, usually under an anesthetic.
  - Covering antibiotics; investigate and deal with underlying factors

Nutritional disorders

Nutrition

The diet of most psittacine birds is very poor compared with their comparable diet in the wild. Nutritional problems arise by two means:
1. Provision of inappropriate food
2. Selectivity of the bird (Werquin et al 2005)
These apply especially to a sunflower-seed-based diet.

Disorders

- Incorrect protein levels
  - In cockatiels, the optimum protein level for growth and weaning is around 20% crude protein, but:
    - 5% causes severe stunting followed by 100% mortality.
    - 10% to 15% leads to stunting and some mortality.
    - 25% gives good weight gain but also behavioral problems such as aggression.
    - 35% gives paradoxical poor growth and aggression.
- Hypervitaminosis A: Excessively high levels of vitamin A have been associated with cataract formation and bone abnormalities. High levels of carotenoids can cause a yellowing discoloration of skin and fat.
- Hypovitaminosis A: Hyperkeratosis and squamous metaplasia of epithelia, including the pharynx, respiratory tract, and occasionally renal tubules. Often there are sterile white plaques visible in oral mucosa and blunting or loss of the choanal papillae. Rhinitis (and occasionally rhinoliths) and blepharitis are common. Sneezing may occur, and there is a predisposition toward respiratory infections. In severe cases, metaplasia of the renal tubules can result in visceral gout. Hyperkeratosis of the plantar surfaces of the feet is seen.
- Hypervitaminosis D_3: Can result in calcification of viscera, especially the kidneys, triggering a visceral gout
- Metabolic bone disease: This is often a hypovitaminosis D_3 combined with a hypocalcemia and hyperphosphatemia. In particular, African grey parrots appear to have difficulty in mobilizing skeletal calcium reserves. Such birds often present with a hypocalcemic tetany—wings fluttering violently in apparent "fits." Such birds often have high parathormone levels, low 25-hydroxycholecalciferol levels, and low serum ionized and nonionized calcium levels.

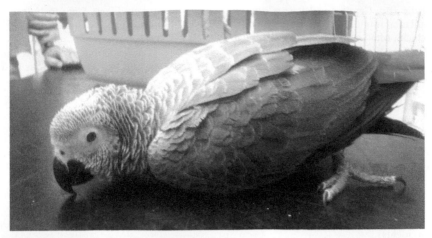

Fig. 8-19. Hypocalcemia in an African grey parrot. Note the three-point stance, using the beak to aid support.

Clinical signs of metabolic bone disease in birds

- General weakness (Fig. 8-19)
- Pathological fractures and/or bending of bones
- Rickets
- Paralysis
- Tetany
- Dystocia
- Low clutch size, thin- or soft-shelled eggs, and low hatchability. (Egg-laying hens may have an episode of acute hypocalcemia that can result in partial paresis and perhaps egg-binding.)
- Polydipsia/polyuria occasionally seen due to increased phosphorus turnover, triggering a diuresis.
- Birds, especially the young, with bone and joint deformities, might be deficient in both calcium and vitamin D_3.

- Hypovitaminosis E: Affected birds may become lethargic and show coordination and equilibrium problems. Complete paralysis can occur. Other signs include white muscle disease. If the gizzard is affected, then undigested seed may be passed. Splayed legs and edema of the neck, wings, and breast may be seen. Reproductive problems can be encountered, including infertility and low hatchability due to weakness in the pipping muscle of the chick.
- Hypovitaminosis K: Can occur with coccidiostats and long-term antibiosis that destroys the normal gut flora. Failure to produce vitamin K leads to blood-clotting problems, which can present as excessive hemorrhage.
- Riboflavin (vitamin B_2): However, adult hens deficient in vitamin B_2 develop fatty livers and elongated flight feathers and have low egg production and low hatchability. In chicks the signs are weakness and diarrhea, inward curling toes, and depigmented feathers (achromatosis) in cockatiels.
- Pantothenic acid: Cockatiels raised on a diet deficient in pantothenic acid fail to grow contour feathers on the chest and back and die at age 3 weeks. Other signs include dermatitis on the face and feet, decreased growth, decreased feathering, and incoordination.
- Biotin: Deficiencies can occur due to ingested mycotoxins in the diet affecting biotin uptake; signs as for pantothenic acid

- Folic acid: Genuine deficiencies can occur with long-term antibiosis. Signs include anemia, immunosuppression, poor egg production, low hatchability, and stunting of chicks, often accompanied by deformation of upper beaks.
- Vitamin B_{12}: Deficiencies are rare but include anemia, poor feathering, reduced growth, reduced food intake, nervous disorders, gizzard erosions, and fatty accumulations in the heart, liver, and kidneys.
- Choline: Deficiencies include poor growth of young birds, fatty liver syndrome in adults, and calcification of soft tissues. Cockatiels on a low-choline diet exhibited unpigmented wing and tail feathers but no calcification.
- Iodine: In budgerigars linked to goiter formation (see "Differential Diagnoses for Vomiting/Regurgitation/Dysphagia" in *Gastrointestinal Tract Disorders*)
- Hypocalcemia: Often combined with hypovitaminosis D_3 (see "Metabolic Bone Disease" above)
- Obesity: Common in Amazon parrots, Galah cockatoos, cockatiels, and budgerigars. Subcutaneous fat deposits may be visible, and there is infiltration of internal organs with fatty tissue. May give rise to atherosclerosis and sequelae (e.g., cerebrovascular accidents)
- Hepatic lipidosis: Obesity; lethargy, depression, and anorexia. Neurologic signs may be seen, consistent with hepatic encephalopathy. Urates may be yellow or green.
- Atherosclerosis (see *Cardiovascular and Hematologic Disorders*)
- Hemochromatosis (iron storage disease): Hepatomegaly is rare.

Investigations

1. Hematology and biochemistry
   a. Hepatic lipidosis may show an increased lactate dehydrogenase, AST, triglycerides, and bile acids.
   b. Blood levels for calcium (including ionized calcium), phosphorus, magnesium (see Table 8-7)
   c. Vitamin D_3 (blood 25-hydroxycholecalciferol levels >50 nmol/L)

Table 8-7 Blood calcium, phosphorus and magnesium levels in two parrots species.

Parameter	Hispaniolan parrot (*Amazona ventralis*)	African grey parrot (*Psittacus erithacus*)
Calcium/mmol/L	2.20-2.60	2.05-5.05
	(2.20-2.58)*	(2.03-2.7)
Ionized calcium/mmol/L		0.96-1.22†
Phosphorus/mmol/L	0.58-1.42	0.81-1.91
	(0.58-1.23)	(0.78-1.71)
Ca: P ratio	2.62-5.39	1.81-3.77
	(2.62-5.39)	(1.67-3.50)
Magnesium/mmol/L	0.74-1.27	0.82-1.4
	(0.82-1.07)	(0.82-1.07)

*Note: Range in parentheses excludes egg-laying females.
†From Shaw 2013.
From de Carvalho 2009.

     d. Vitamin A levels (retinol 0.471 ± 0.209 µg/mL—Torregrossa et al 2005)

     e. Vitamin E levels (α-tocopherol 13.5 ± 6.60 µg/mL)

2. Radiography

     a. Hepatomegaly (hepatic lipidosis, neoplasia)

     b. Hypervitaminosis D_3: Calcification of the kidneys

     c. Skeletal abnormalities: Pathological fractures, healed fractures, bone deformities, osteomalacia (metabolic bone disease)

3. Liver biopsy

4. Dietary analysis

Management

1. Dietary imbalances often predispose to secondary pathogen invasion, so covering antibiosis should be considered. Aim to switch to a more healthy diet, which, depending on the species, should consist of:

     a. Exchanging seed mix for a good proprietary pelleted food (e.g., Harrison's Bird Foods)

     b. Enhancing the diet by increasing the consumption of colored vegetable such as sweet peppers and noncitrus fruits

     c. Using appropriate vitamin and mineral supplements

     d. Sprouting seeds help to convert some of the fat into carbohydrate.

     e. Altering diets can be time consuming. Many parrots are seriously neophobic and are reluctant to eat novel substances.

2. Milk thistle *(Silybum marianum)* is hepatoprotectant. Dose at 4 to 15 mg/kg PO b.i.d. or t.i.d. (Wade 2004).

3. Provide exposure to UVB light—especially important for African grey parrots.

Treatment/specific therapy

- Hepatic lipidosis
  - Poor prognosis
  - Provision of interosseous fluids (Hartmann's), diet high in nutrients (include fructose, biotin, choline, and lactulose), and broad-spectrum antibiotic therapy may be useful.
  - Consider L-carnitine (see "Obesity" below)
- Hypovitaminosis A
  - Injectable vitamin A at 5000 IU/kg once daily for 2 weeks. Then adopt maintenance rate of 5000 IU daily PO or feed colored vegetables such as carrots and peppers.
- Metabolic bone disease
  - Hypocalcemia: Calcium gluconate 10% at 100 to 200 mg/kg (1 to 2 mL/kg) IM daily or 50 to 100 mg/kg by slow IV
  - Supplement with vitamin D_3 at 5000 IU/kg daily, as well as calcium
  - Some cases may need magnesium supplementation (see de Carvalho 2009).
  - Provide access to full-spectrum lighting with an ultraviolet B component (e.g., sunshine or commercially available lighting) to allow natural endogenous vitamin D_3 production.
- Hypervitaminosis D_3
  - In some cases, clinical signs regress when vitamin D_3 levels are returned to normal. Macaws particularly seem to be susceptible to high vitamin D_3 levels, and it is recommended that vitamin D_3 levels should not be higher than 2000 IU/kg of a parrot's diet (with a gross energy diet range of 3200 to 4200 kcal/kg).

- Vitamin E
  - Works synergistically with selenium and can be given as a combined (such as Vitesel, Norbrook (UK)) at 0.01 mL/kg IM every 7 to 14 days
- Other hypovitaminoses: Supplement with appropriate vitamin preparations. Complete revision of diet recommended.
- Iodine: Supplement with iodine (see "Differential Diagnosis for Vomiting/Regurgitation/Dysphagia").
- Hemochromatosis: Select low-iron diet. May be linked to chronic inflammatory conditions.
- Obesity: In budgerigars, L-carnitine at 1000 mg/kg food has been effective in inducing weight loss, along with shrinkage of lipomas.

Hepatic disorders

Note: Psittacines lack a gallbladder.

Viral

- Pacheco disease (herpesvirus)
- Polyomavirus
- Adenovirus

Bacterial

- Bacterial hepatitis
- Chlamydophilosis
- *Yersinia pseudotuberculosis*
- Mycobacteriosis

Fungal

- Aflatoxicosis

Nutritional

- Hemochromatosis
- Hepatic lipidosis

Neoplasia

- Hepatic tumors
- Lymphoma (likely linked to retrovirus infection—see *Cardiovascular and Hematologic Disorders*)

Other noninfectious problems

- Cirrhosis
- Steroid hepatopathy (iatrogenic)
- Amyloidosis

Findings on clinical examination

- Unwell bird, fluffed-up appearance
- Anorexia
- Polydipsia/polyuria
- Very green or yellow appearance of feces
- Ascites (secondary to portal hypertension)

- Respiratory signs (ascites/chlamydophilosis)
- Multifocal follicular and feather pulp hemorrhages (polyomavirus)

Investigations

1. Radiography
   a. Hepatomegaly (Pacheco disease, neoplasia, hemochromatosis)
   b. Ascites
2. Routine hematology and biochemistry
   a. Liver enzymes raised; AST is not liver specific, but raised AST plus bile acid levels indicate liver disease; raised AST plus CK suggests muscle injury. In end-stage liver disease, plasma liver enzyme levels may be normal or low.
3. Culture and sensitivity
4. Coelomic tap (culture and sensitivity, cytology)
5. Fecal or cloacal swab for Pacheco disease PCR
6. Endoscopy
   a. Hepatomegaly, splenomegaly, renal enlargement
7. Ultrasonography
   a. Hepatomegaly (Pacheco disease)
8. Biopsy

Management

1. Supportive therapy, including fluids
2. Lactulose at 0.5 mL/kg PO b.i.d.
3. Milk thistle *(Silybum marianum)* is hepatoprotectant. Dose at 4 to 15 mg/kg PO b.i.d. or t.i.d. (Wade 2004).

Treatment/specific therapy

- Pacheco disease is usually rapidly fatal. Try acyclovir at 80 mg/kg PO t.i.d. for 7 to 10 days or 40 mg/kg IV or SC t.i.d. (cited in Girling 2003)
- Hemochromatosis (see *"Nutritional Disorders"*)
- Hepatic lipidosis (see *"Nutritional Disorders"*)

Splenic disorders

- Chlamydophilosis (see *Lower Respiratory Tract Disorders*)
- Lymphoma (see *Cardiovascular and Hematologic Disorders*)

Cardiovascular and hematologic disorders

Where possible, auscultate tame birds while at rest on a perch or the owner, as stressed birds exhibit such high heart rates that meaningful auscultation is difficult. Any abnormal heart rate or rhythm is likely to be associated with heart disease or a more systemic illness.

Viral

- Polyoma virus—hydropericardium
- Avian bornavirus (PDD)—myocarditis

Bacterial

- Valvular endocarditis—can be thrombotic
- Bacterial infiltration
- Pericarditis
- Chronic systemic lung disease

Fungal

- Pericarditis
- Chronic systemic lung disease

Protozoal

- *Haemoproteus*
- *Leucocytozoon*
- *Akiba* spp.
- *Plasmodium*

Nutritional

- Fat accumulation (lipomatosis cordis)
- Atherosclerosis (especially Amazons and African greys)

Neoplasia

- Lymphoma/lymphosarcoma

Other noninfectious problems

- Chronic pulmonary interstitial fibrosis, especially in older Amazon parrots (Zandvliet et al 2001)—very commonly causes right ventricular enlargement (see *Respiratory Tract Disorders*)
- Right ventricular enlargement also from other causes of systemic lung disease (e.g., chronic mycosis)
- Pericardial effusion with or without ascites
- Ventricular hypertrophy or dilatation
- Myxomatous degeneration of atrioventricular valve (Oglesbee and Lehmkuhl 2001)
- Calcification of the blood vessels
- Lack of exercise (plus poor diet)
- Avocado toxicity—hydropericardium
- Urate deposits in the aorta
- Congenita

Findings on clinical examination

- Exercise intolerance
- Apparent respiratory signs
- Auscultation: Arrhythmias and altered heart sounds (e.g., murmurs)
- Vomiting and wasting (*Leucocytozoon*)
- Concomitant signs such as ascites, pulmonary disease, and air sacculitis
- Neurologic signs—typically cerebrovascular accidents secondary to atherosclerosis

Investigations

1. Radiography
   a. Normal radiographic heart parameters (Table 8-8)
   b. Liver enlargement

Table 8-8 Parrots and related species: Normal radiographic heart parameters

Ratio of cardiac silhouette width to:	(%)
Sternum length (measured on the bird)	35-41
Width of thorax (measured on ventrodorsal radiograph)	51-61
Width of coracoid (measured on ventrodorsal radiograph)	545-672

From Straub et al (2002).

Table 8-9 Parrots and related species: Blood cholesterol levels

Species	Cholesterol (mmol/L)	Triglycerides (mmol/L)		
	Bavelaar et al*	Polo et al[†]	Bavelaar et al*	Polo et al[†]
Palm cockatoo	—	3.6 ± 0.5 (2.8-4.2)	—	1.2 ± 0.5 (0.8-1.9)
Long-billed cockatoo	5.65-6.33	—	0.79-1.78	—
Amazon (yellow-headed Amazon) parrot	7.46-9.65	7.1 ± 2.5 (4.3-10.9)	1.7-2.86	1.6 ± 0.4 (1.1-2.1)
Blue and gold macaw	4.2-4.77	4.2 ± 0.9 (3.1-6.7)	0.35-0.52	1.2 ± 0.7 (0.4-2.5)
Scarlet macaw	5.0-5.3	4.1 ± 1.1 (2.3-6.4)	0.38-0.66	1.0 ± 0.3 (0.5-1.6)
Red fan parrot	4.09-4.54	0.35-0.38	—	—
African grey parrot	—	8.38 ± 2.57 (5.31-18.62)[‡]	—	—

*Values from Bavelaar et al (2005).
[†]Values from Polo et al (1998).
[‡]Bavelaar & Beynen (2003).

2. Routine hematology and biochemistry
   a. Increased blood cholesterol levels are a major risk factor for atherosclerosis (Table 8-9).
3. Cytology (blood smears for hemoparasites)
4. Blood culture and sensitivity
5. ECG
   a. Sinus rhythm normal.
   b. Sinus arrhythmias and second-degree heart block considered physiologic in birds
   c. Partial fusion of P and T waves (P on T phenomenon) can be normal, especially in females.
   d. Isoflurane anesthesia may increase heart rate.
   e. Normal ECG values after Casares et al (2000) and Musulin and Adin (2006) (Table 8-10)
6. Endoscopy
7. Biopsy (liver, kidney, pectoral muscles)
8. Ultrasonography
9. Echocardiography/Doppler

Table 8-10 Parrots and related species: Normal lead II ECGs

Variable	Hyacinth macaw	Green wing macaw	African grey parrot
Body weight (g)	1331 ± 149	1214 ± 173	—
Heart rate (beats/min)	283 ± 65	280 ± 97	—
Electrical axis (degrees)	−101 (81-109)	−98 (86-131)	—
P duration (sec)	0.02 (0.015-0.025)	0.018 (0.015-0.025)	0.012-0.018
P amplitude (mV)	0.3 (0.19-0.4)	0.2 (0.075-0.3)	0.25-0.55
QRS duration (sec)	0.02 (0.015-0.025)	0.02 (0.013-0.025)	0.010-0.016
QRS amplitude (mV)	0.65 (0.35-1.0)	0.5 (0.35-0.85)	—
R amplitude (mV)	0.045 (0.04-0.08)	0.05 (0.02-0.2)	0.0-0.2
T duration (sec)	0.05 (0.035-0.075)	0.045 (0.035-0.05)	—
T amplitude (mV)	0.3 (0.1-0.7)	0.25 (0.1-0.45)	0.18-0.60
PR interval (sec)	0.055 (0.05-0.075)	0.05 (0.04-0.07)	0.040-0.055
QT interval (sec)	0.085 (0.08-0.1)	0.09 (0.08-0.11)	0.048-0.070
ST segment amplitude (mV)	0.1 (0.05-0.15)	0.1 (0.05-0.15)	0.90-0.20

Table 8-11 Normal values of some psittacine cardiac anatomy

Values for myocardium of left free wall	Sternal length (%)
Mean apical myocardium	2.3-2.85
Mean middle left myocardium	8.3-8.7
Mean basal myocardium thickness	7.9-9.0

From Krautwald-Junghanns et al (2004).

Management

1. Reduce stress as much as possible (e.g., remove affected birds from breeding programs).
2. Identify and treat underlying problems (e.g., chronic lung disease).
3. Improve diet.

Treatment/specific therapy

- NSAIDs (e.g., meloxicam at 0.2 mg/kg PO, IM body weight once daily) may be useful for chronic pulmonary interstitial fibrosis.
- Heart disease: Once a diagnosis is achieved, drug regimens may be adapted from mammalian treatments. Examples would be:
  - Enalapril at 1.0 to 2.5 mg/kg PO daily or b.i.d. (Pees et al 2006)
  - Furosemide at 0.15 mg/kg IM daily
  - Digoxin at 0.05 mg/kg PO daily
- *Haemoproteus:* Often considered asymptomatic and self-limiting, but can be a contributing factor to anemia if present. Treat with chloroquine at 250 mg per 120 mL drinking water for 14 days. Avoid ceratopogonid vectors.

- *Plasmodium*
  - Primaquine at 0.75 to 1.0 mg/kg PO once only, combined with an initial loading dose of chloroquine at 25 mg/kg, reducing this to 15 mg/kg at 12, 24, and 48 hours
- *Leukocytozoon*: May be asymptomatic, but can be fatal, with acute hepatitis, renal tubular necrosis, and myocardial hemorrhage. Chronic cases may present with wasting and vomiting. Treat as for *Plasmodium*. Avoid exposure to vectors such as blackflies (*Simulium* spp.) or *Culicoides*/hippoboscids.
- Lymphoma/lymphosarcoma
  - Treatment is speculative and more modern regimens may be more appropriate. However, the following chemotherapeutic drugs have been used in cockatoos (France 1993):
    - Prednisolone at 25 mg/m^2 PO daily
    - Asparaginase at 400 IU/kg IM every 7 days. Premedicate with diphenhydramine at 2 mg/kg IO once only.
    - Cyclophosphamide at 200 mg/m^2 IO every 7 days
    - Doxorubicin at 30 mg/m^2 IO every 2 days. Premedicate with diphenhydramine at 2 mg/kg IO once only.
    - Vincristine sulfate at 0.75 mg/m^2 IO every 7 days for 3 weeks
- Atherosclerosis
  - Treat symptomatically.
  - Linked to deficiency of n-3 polyunsaturated fatty acids, especially α-linolenic acid (Bavelaar et al 2005); supplement by feeding commercial diets and small seeds (e.g., flax seeds).

Musculoskeletal disorders
• •

Viral
- PBFD
- Retroviral infection (renal/gonadal tumors)

Bacterial
- Renal infections can spread to the adjacent lumbosacral plexus.
- Septic arthritis
- Osteomyelitis

Nutritional
- Metabolic bone disease (see *Nutritional Disorders*)

Neoplasia
- Renal tumor (possibly due to retroviral infection)
- Gonadal tumor (especially budgerigars; possibly due to retroviral infection)
- Osteosarcoma

Other noninfectious problems
- Articular gout
- Limb bone fracture—tibiotarsal fractures are particularly common
- Spinal trauma
- Identification ring too tight (especially closed rings)
- Developmental problems of chicks

- Juvenile osteodystrophy
- Metabolic or systemic problems (e.g., cardiovascular disease, hypoglycemia, hypocalcemia, and anemia)

Findings on clinical examination

- Weakness, ataxia
- Unwillingness or inability to move
- Leg paralysis—may be unilateral or bilateral
- Limb deformities, including rotation around joints
- Flight disorders—see "Differential Diagnoses for Loss of Flight"

Investigations

1. Radiography
   a. Radiograph not only the affected limb, but also the whole body, especially if there is obvious muscle wastage.
   b. Contrast studies (e.g., with barium) to assess for displacement of gut by intracoelomic masses. *Note:* Reproductively active females store excess calcium as deposits at the femur. These should not be mistaken for pathological exostoses.
2. Routine hematology and biochemistry
   a. Will need to differentiate from systemic or metabolic disorders
3. Culture and sensitivity
4. Endoscopy
5. Ultrasonography

Management

1. Supportive treatment, including covering antibiosis
2. Hospitalizing weakened birds on soft surfaces (e.g., towels) to reduce the risk of trauma

Treatment/specific therapy

- Renal infection: Appropriate antibiosis
- Fractures: Stabilization by external or internal fixation (Fig. 8-20). In small psittacines conservative management, including analgesia, may be more appropriate for femoral fractures.
- Identification ring too tight: Remove under GA.
- Neoplasia: Treatment rarely viable
  - Osteosarcoma: Treatment has been attempted with doxorubicin at 60 mg/m^2 IV diluted with saline every 30 days (Doolan 1994).
- Juvenile osteodystrophy
  - In very young chicks, developmental problems such as valgus deformities (splay leg) can be corrected by hobbling the legs together before the skeleton becomes reasonably calcified. This should be done at no more than age 5 days. Older chicks may require surgical correction once the bones have sufficiently calcified to withstand such surgery.
  - Reassess hand-rearing conditions, as these often reflect a poor rearing environment. Harcourt-Brown (2004) finds that dusky parrot chicks (*Pionus fuscus*) remain in the

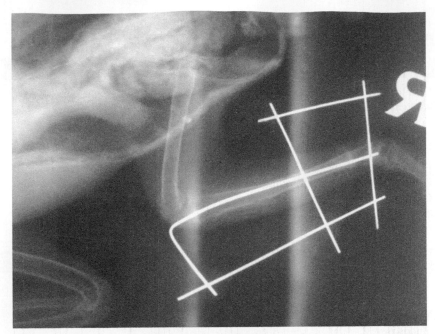

Fig. 8-20. Combined internal and external fixation repair of a fractured tibiotarsus.

nest until day 53; the presence of several chicks in such a combined space may mutually support their growing skeletons, and premature exercise may lead to pathological deformity of the long bones.

Differential diagnoses for loss of flight

Viral

- Polyomavirus
- PBFD

Bacterial

- Pathological fracture (from osteomyelitis)

Fungal

- Pathological fracture (from osteomyelitis)

Neoplasia

- Pathological fracture

Other noninfectious problems

- Cardiovascular disease
- Respiratory disease
- Neurologic disease
- Systemic disease (weakness)
- Fractured coracoid bone
- Other flight bone fractures (e.g., humerus)
- Damage to the leading edge of the wing (propatagium)

- Prepatagial cutaneous ulcerative disease—commonly seen in chronic self-mutilating African greys; too painful to extend wings (see *Skin Disorders*)

Findings on clinical examination

- Unable to fly
  - Flight feathers absent or abnormal
    - Young budgerigars—polyomavirus
    - Older psittacines—PBFD
    - Self-mutilation
  - Flight feathers normal—consider traumatic injuries, etc.
- One wing may be held lower than the other.
- Obvious traumatic injury (i.e., swelling, compound fracture). Check especially the wing tips.
- Nonpainful, immobile swelling (i.e., old, healed fracture)

Investigations

1. Radiography
2. Routine hematology and biochemistry
3. Culture and sensitivity
4. Endoscopy
5. Ultrasonography

Treatment/specific therapy

- Propatagial damage: Make sure that the tendon that supports the leading edge of the propatagium—the tendon of musculis tensor propatagialis longa—is repaired if severed.
- Prepatagial CUD—see *Skin Disorders*
- Fracture repair where feasible.

Systemic disorders

• •

Some conditions present with a variety of clinical signs that may be quite nonspecific. In some cases, this results from immunosuppression, leading to secondary invasion of a variety of pathogens or because of multiorgan involvement.

Viral

- PBFD—especially young African grey parrots
- Retrovirus (leukosis/sarcoma viruses)

Bacterial

- *Staphylococcus aureus* (Hermans et al 2000)
- Chlamydophilosis

Fungal

- *Aspergillosis* (see *Lower Respiratory Tract Disorders*)
- Penicillinosis (Lanteri et al 2011)

Protozoal

- *Sarcocystis*

Nutritional

- See *Nutritional Disorders*

Neoplasia

- Infiltrative neoplasia secondary to retrovirus infection; any organ can be affected (Girling 2003)

Other noninfectious problems

- Amyloidosis
- Iatrogenic steroid prescription

Findings on clinical examination

- Generalized ill health
- Nonspecific clinical signs
- Weight loss
- Anorexia
- Sudden death
- Obvious neoplasia

Investigations

1. Radiography
2. Routine hematology and biochemistry
   a. Young birds with PDFD often profoundly leukopenic
3. Serology *(Sarcocystis, Chlamydophila)*
4. Cytology
5. Culture and sensitivity
6. *Chlamydophila* PCR
7. Endoscopy
8. Ultrasonography
9. Biopsy

Treatment/specific therapy

- PBFD
  - Experimentally, avian interferon has been used to aid elimination of PBFD in viremic, young African grey parrots (Stanford 2003). The dose used was 1,000,000 units of avian γ-interferon IM daily for 90 days. Mammalian (feline) interferon was found to be unsatisfactory.
  - *Note:* PBFD infection is oral, with virus entering via the bursa of Fabricius, which in psittacines can take over 18 to 20 months for normal involution to occur (Schmidt 1997). Any bird testing positive should be immediately quarantined and retested 60 to 90 days later to assess degree of immunity (Girling 2003). Immune birds will not be viremic and so will test negative.
- Steroids: Gradually wean off steroids. Always use antibiotic and antifungal medications in conjunction with steroids to counter the marked immunosuppressive effects of exogenous steroids.
- Penicillinosis—as for aspergillosis
- *Sarcocystis* (see *Lower Respiratory Tract Disorders*)

Neurologic disorders

Viral
- Paramyxovirus
- Avian bornavirus (PDD)
- Pacheco disease
- Adenovirus—budgerigars
- West Nile virus (flavivirus)

Bacterial
- Chlamydophilosis
- Bacterial meningitis

Fungal
- Fungal meningitis

Protozoal
- *Sarcocystis*

Parasitic
- Cerebrospinal angiostrongyliasis due to nematode larvae of *Angiostrongylus cantonensis* (Monks et al 2005)

Dietary
- Hypocalcemia/hypovitaminosis D_3 (African grey parrots especially)
- Hypoglycemia

Neoplasia
Other noninfectious problems
- Zinc toxicity
- Other heavy-metal poisoning (e.g., lead)
- Other toxicities
- Fractures
- Renal disease, including neoplasia (see "Differential Diagnosis of Polydipsia/Polyuria" in *Endocrine Disorders*)
- Other neoplasia
- Idiopathic epilepsy
- Hepatic encephalopathy (severe liver disease)
- Cerebrovascular accidents (atherosclerosis)
- Head trauma (e.g., flying into windows)

Findings on clinical examination

- Weight loss
- Depression
- Torticollis and head tilt
- Ataxia; unable to balance or support itself; may continually hang onto cage bars with beak for support
- Collapse

- Tremors and seizures
- Gastrointestinal signs (undigested seeds, loose droppings) suggestive of paramyxovirus

Investigations

1. Radiography
   a. Standing radiographs in the conscious bird for detection of ingested heavy metals
2. Routine hematology and biochemistry
   a. Serum calcium, zinc, and lead. Alternatively, hepatic lead and zinc concentrations can be assessed from biopsy; these are thought to be much more reliable.
   b. Blood levels can be indicative of zinc toxicity, but as with lead, there is no absolute correlation between blood zinc levels and clinical signs. As a general rule, if zinc levels are >32 to 50 μmol/L and there are consistent clinical signs (see *Neurologic Disorders* and *Gastrointestinal Tract Disorders*), then zinc toxicity should be suspected.
   c. Blood lead levels <9.6 μmol/L
   d. Significant levels often accompanied by an absolute or relative monocytosis
   e. Blood glucose levels; also check out other biochemical parameters as they can be linked with liver disease, infection, and endocrinologic disorders.
3. Serology for paromyxovirus (paired samples)
4. Serology for West Nile virus (paired samples)
5. PCR for Pacheco disease
6. Culture and sensitivity
7. Endoscopy
8. Ultrasonography
9. Biopsy

Management

- Supportive treatment
- Fluids may be best given initially per cloaca rather than by crop tube in case of ataxic/seizuring birds due to high risk of regurgitation and aspiration pneumonia.
- Management of seizures
  - Diazepam 0.5 to 1.0 mg/kg IV or IO every 1 to 4 hours
  - Remove all perches and toys. Food and water dishes may need to be positioned on the floor; food can be scattered loose on the floor.
  - Monitor closely.
  - Investigate underlying causes.
  - Long-term management: Phenobarbital at 1 to 10 mg/kg PO b.i.d.

Treatment/specific therapy

- Zinc/lead poisoning
  - Flushing out of the proventriculus and gizzard
  - Performed under GA with the bird intubated and head held down so as to prevent aspiration of stomach contents
  - Surgical removal of ingested metals
  - Sodium calcium edetate at 35 mg/kg IM b.i.d. for 5 days, stop for 3 to 4 days, then repeat. Continue until zinc levels fall.

- DMSA at 30 mg/kg PO b.i.d. for 10 days or 5 days/week for 3 to 5 weeks
- Penicillamine at 55 mg/kg PO b.i.d. for 7 to 14 days
- Paromyxovirus: Not direct treatment; supportive therapy only. Paramyxovirus A (Newcastle disease) is notifiable in the UK.
- West Nile virus: Supportive treatment only
- *Sarcocystis* (see *Lower Respiratory Tract Disorders*)
- Cerebrospinal angiostrongyliasis due to nematode larvae of *Angiostrongylus cantonensis*. Supportive treatment plus consider ivermectin 0.2 mg/kg PO, SC, or IM or fenbendazole at 50 mg/kg PO
  - Guarded prognosis
- Head trauma
  - Dexamethasone sodium phosphate at 2mg/kg IM once only.
  - Prednisolone sodium succinate at 0.5-1.0mg/kg IM once only
  - Avoid steroids if underlying fungal infection likely.
  - Attend to any haemorrhage.
  - Assess for fractures.
  - Rest in a darkened area.

Ophthalmic disorders

Sclerocorneal (ciliary) muscles along with the sphincter and dilator muscles of the iris are striated muscles that are under voluntary control. Movement of the pupil can be extensive and rapid and is used in intraspecies displays. Such irides appear unresponsive to light, so the lack of pupillary response should not be misinterpreted.

Conjunctivitis can appear as part a "syndrome" of upper respiratory tract signs (e.g., periorbital swelling, conjunctivitis, or intraocular disease) because of interconnectedness of local structures; the infraorbital sinus connects with the caudal nasal concha, the nasal cavity, and the cervicocephalic air sac that covers the head and neck caudally and dorsally. It also has diverticulae extending dorsal, ventral, and caudal to the eye, as well as into the maxillary bill and mandible.

Viral

- Cutaneous papillomatosis
- Avian pox
- Ulceration and crusting of the eyelid margin, especially Amazon parrots
- Conjunctivitis in lovebirds
- Adenovirus (lovebirds)

Bacterial

- Bacterial conjunctivitis
- Chlamydophilosis
- Mycoplasmosis
- Infraorbital sinusitis (see under *Sinusitis*)

Fungal

- Sinusitis

Protozoal

- *Encephalitozoon hellem* (Phalen et al 2006)

Nutritional

- Hypovitaminosis A

Neoplasia
- Space-occupying lesions, especially pituitary adenomas
- Ocular neoplasia

Other noninfectious problems
- Congenital atresia of the eyelids
- Cataracts
- Dermoids (Leber and Bürge 1999)
- Trauma
- Vascular accidents or ischemic necrosis—especially budgerigars
- Heavy-metal poisoning
- Hepatic encephalopathy

Findings on clinical examination

- May be unilateral or bilateral
- Keratoconjunctivitis
- Crusty skin lesions on the eyelids
- Corneal ulceration
- Cataracts—can be normal in an aged macaw (35 to 45 years old)
- Periocular and cutaneous pox lesions suggest avian pox; may also see respiratory signs
- Intraocular hemorrhage (usually linked to head trauma)
- Loss of vision
- Ptosis: Horner syndrome secondary to presumed trauma has been described (Gancz et al 2005).

Investigations

1. Standard ophthalmic examination
2. Topical fluorescein to assess for corneal damage
3. Routine hematology and biochemistry
4. Culture and sensitivity
5. Application of topical sympathomimetic agents (e.g., phenylephrine); if it ameliorates ptosis, this indicates Horner syndrome.
6. Biopsy
   a. Eyelid margin
   b. Conjunctiva
7. Ultrasonography

Management

1. Covering topical and systemic antibiosis
2. Vitamin A supplementation at 10,000 to 25,000 IU/300 g PO every 7 days

Treatment/specific therapy

- Bacterial conjunctivitis: Topical and systemic antibiosis
- Chlamydophilosis: Systemic enrofloxacin or doxycycline

- Mycoplasmosis: Tylosin at 1 mg/mL drinking water for a minimum of 21 days
  - Enrofloxacin at 5 to 10 mg/kg IM daily
  - Topical ofloxacin eyedrops
  - Tetracyclines
- Congenital atresia: Attempt surgical repair, but poorly responsive; long-term steroids may slow healing closure of the defect.
- Corneal ulceration of third eyelid flap: The course of the nictitans is laterodorsally, as opposed to lateroventrally in small mammals. This is of limited use because the nictitans is constantly in motion and sutures tend to tear through eventually.
  - Tarsorrhaphy for 2 to 4 weeks
  - Topical antibiosis and ophthalmic anesthesia if analgesia required
- Cataract: Surgical removal, ideally phacoemulsification. Hypermature cataracts can degenerate, triggering a phacolytic uveitis.
- *Encephalitozoon hellem*
  - Co-trimoxazole at 30 mg/kg PO b.i.d. for at least 3 weeks
  - Albendazole at 10 mg/kg PO s.i.d. for 6 weeks
  - Fenbendazole at 10 mg/kg PO s.i.d. for 1 month

Endocrine disorders

Neoplasia

- Pituitary gland adenoma—especially budgerigars and cockatiels

Other noninfectious problems

- Hypothyroidism
- Adrenal disease

Findings on clinical examination

- Polydipsia/polyuria (pituitary gland adenoma)

Investigations

1. Radiography
2. Routine hematology and biochemistry
   a. Adrenal disease not reported in psittacines
   b. Corticosterone, not cortisol, is responsive to ACTH stimulation.
   c. Experimental ACTH stimulation gave the results shown in Table 8-12 (Zenoble et al 1985).
   d. Serum thyroid hormone levels (nonmolting birds—see Table 8-13)

Table 8-12 Parrots and related species: Experimental ACTH stimulation

	Corticosterone concentrations (mg/dL) before ACTH administration	Corticosterone concentrations (mg/dL) 90 min after ACTH administration
Red-lored Amazon	1.06	4.86
Blue-fronted Amazon	2.09	10.58
African grey parrot	2.33	4.69

Table 8-13 Parrots and related species: Serum thyroid hormone levels (nonmolting birds)

Species	T$_4$ concentration			
	nmol/L		μg/dL	
	Range	Mean	Range	Mean
African grey parrot *(Psittacus erithacus)*	2.02-5.06	3.18	0.16-0.39	0.25
Moluccan cockatoos *(Cacatua moluccensis)*	2.04-6.29	4.66	0.16-0.49	0.36
Blue and gold macaws *(Ara ararauna)*	2.02-4.85	3.36	0.16-0.38	0.26
Umbrella cockatoos *(Cacatua alba)*	2.86-5.96	4.61	0.22-0.46	0.36
Yellow-headed Amazon *(Amazona oratrix)*	2.49-7.68	5.05	0.19-0.60	0.39
Blue-fronted Amazon *(Amazona aestiva)*	3.17-142	23.8	0.25-11.0	1.85
Lovebirds *(Agapornis* spp.)	—	—	0.2-4.3	—

Adapted from Greenacre et al (2001).

3. Culture and sensitivity
4. Endoscopy
5. Biopsy/necropsy
6. Ultrasonography

Treatment/specific therapy

- Hypothyroidism: L-thyroxine at 0.02 mg/kg PO daily or b.i.d.
- Goiter in budgerigars: See *Respiratory Tract Disorders*

Differential diagnosis of polydipsia/polyuria

Viral
- Paramyxovirus
- Avian influenza
- Adenovirus
- Herpesvirus

Bacterial
- Pancreatitis
- Pyelonephritis

Fungal
Protozoal
- *Encephalitozoon hellem*

Nutritional
- Hypovitaminosis A
- Hypocalcemia

Neoplasia
- Renal tubules

Other noninfectious problems

- Renal disease/gout
- Diabetes mellitus
- Hepatitis
- Heavy-metal poisoning, especially zinc
- Amyloidosis (renal; hepatic)
- Trauma
- Physiologic—egg laying

Findings on clinical examination

(See also "Assessment of Droppings" in *Gastrointestinal Tract Disorders*)
- Weight loss
- Weakness
- Polydipsia and accompanying polyuria
- Marked wetting of the bottom of the cage
- Hematuria (especially with heavy metal poisoning)
- Urate fraction may have a strong "fishy" smell common in the white cockatoos with renal disease (Stockdale 2004).
- Large, pale-colored droppings suggest pancreatic damage.
- Unilateral or bilateral lameness caused by pressure of renal tumors on adjacent lumbosacral plexus
- White uric acid tophi may be visible under the skin of the legs and feet. Joints may be swollen (articular gout).
- Neurologic signs (e.g., ataxia, generalized tremors)

Investigations

1. Hematology and biochemistry
   a. Uric acid is secreted by the proximal tubule of the avian kidney and so is not dependent on glomerular filtration rate, so blood uric acids levels may only rise in chronic renal disease. It may also crystallize out as gout tophi in the kidneys (renal gout) or other organs (visceral gout), which again may limit otherwise high blood uric acid levels. Most waste nitrogen is excreted as uric acid, not urea, so urea levels tend to be low. There may be a rise in phosphorus and a change in the calcium to phosphorus ratio (see Table 8-7); therefore, need to assess multiple values (i.e., uric acid, urea, creatinine, calcium, and phosphorus) to assess renal disease
   b. Biochemistry for hepatic disease
   c. Blood glucose: Normal range cockatiel, 12.76 to 24.4 mmol/L; diabetic birds, >55.5 mmol/L
   d. Plasma glucagon to insulin ratio 5 to 10 times higher than in mammals.
2. Urinalysis
   a. Glycosuria and/or ketonuria suggestive of diabetes mellitus but may indicate mixing of feces with urine.
   b. Microscopy: WBCs or renal casts suggest urinary tract disease.
3. Radiography
   a. Plain and contrast (IV pyelogram with iohexol)
4. Endoscopy and biopsy
   a. On endoscopy (or postmortem) uric acid may be seen deposited on certain viscera such as the pericardium or the serosal surface of the liver.

5. Cloacal swabs
   a. Bacteriology: Culture and sensitivity
   b. *Encephalitozoon hellem* (special staining required)

Management

- Supportive treatment, including fluid therapy (see "Differential Diagnosis of Gastrointestinal Disorders")

Treatment/specific therapy

- Anabolic steroids (e.g., nandrolone 1 mg/kg SC) may be of some benefit. *Note:* Some birds react badly to such oily injections.
- Benazepril at <0.1 mg/kg PO daily. *Note:* Some birds may be susceptible to the hypotensive side effects of benazepril.
- Gout: Allopurinol at 10 mg/kg PO or given in drinking water. A stock solution is made from a 100-mg tablet crushed in 10 mL water; 1 mL (10 mg) of this solution is added to 30 mL of fresh drinking water daily. Long-term use may trigger xanthine deposition.
- Diabetes mellitus: Exogenous commercially available insulin rarely of use (disease due to excess glucagon? Failure to respond to mammalian insulin?). A small number of cases may respond to insulin therapy (consider short-acting preparations) at 0.1 to 2 IU/kg IM b.i.d. (Rees Davies 2001).
- Where possible, change the diet to a low-fat, low-carbohydrate, high-fat pelleted diet.
- *Encephalitozoon hellem* treatment protocols include:
  - Co-trimoxazole at 30 mg/kg PO b.i.d. for at least 3 weeks
  - Albendazole at 10 mg/kg PO s.i.d. for 6 weeks
  - Fenbendazole at 10 mg/kg PO s.i.d. for 1 month
  - Also consider anticoccidials (e.g., toltrazuril).
- Many birds are asymptomatic excreters. Often linked with immunosuppressive disorders such as PBFD (Barton et al 2003). Potentially zoonotic
- Hypocalcemia—see "Nutritional Disorders"
- Hypovitaminosis A—see "Nutritional Disorders"

Reproductive disorders

A female parrot will lay an egg every 48 hours. The egg spends around 80% of this time in the shell gland, where it is palpable. Therefore, it useful to know both the normal clutch size for that species and the interval since the last egg was laid.

Bacterial
- Egg peritonitis (coelomitis)

Nutritional
- Hypocalcemia (see *Nutritional Disorders*)

Neoplasia
- Oviductal adenocarcinoma

Other noninfectious problems
- Dystocia (egg-binding)
- Cloacal prolapse (see *Gastrointestinal Tract Disorders*)

- Intracoelomic mass
- Skeletal abnormality
- Oviductal torsion
- Superovulation/excessive egg production—especially cockatiels
- Egg peritonitis (sterile)

Findings on clinical examination

- Bird may be depressed, slightly dyspneic.
- A coelomic mass may be palpable.
- Partial leg paralysis
- History of multiple egg production
- Distended, fluid-filled coelom; dyspnea (egg serositis)

Investigations

1. Hematology and biochemistry: Serum calcium (including ionized calcium)
2. Radiography
3. Ultrasonography
4. Examination under GA
5. Coelomic tap and aspiration (midline)
   a. Cytology
   b. Culture and sensitivity
6. Endoscopy

Management

1. Place bird somewhere darkened, warm, and of high humidity.
2. Give calcium and/or vitamin D_3 supplementation.
3. Deslorelin implants (a GnRH agonist) will give temporary ovarian shutdown for up to 6 months, although times and efficacy may vary between species.

Treatment/specific therapy

- Dystocia (egg-binding)
  - Calcium supplementation: 100 to 500 mg of calcium PO in cases of hypocalcemia
  - Oxytocin 1 to 5 IU/kg IM. Use judiciously as this can have a marked effect on blood pressure.
  - Dinoprost (Lutalyse) 20 to 100 µg/kg IM as a single dose
  - Apply prostaglandin E_2 gel to the cloaca to stimulate contractions.
  - Under GA, the egg may be manipulated out.
  - If the egg is thin-shelled, aspiration of the contents through the abdominal wall with a syringe and hypodermic needle will allow collapse of the egg and its subsequent delivery.
- Superovulation
  - Medroxyprogesterone acetate to inhibit ovulation at 10 mg/kg IM; titrate dose as precisely as possible because overdose likely to trigger severe polydipsia/polyuria
  - Leuprolide, as a single injection, to give a dose of 52 to 156 µg/kg; reversibly inhibits egg-laying in cockatiels for up to 31 days
  - Surgical ovariectomy

- Egg serositis
  - Abdominocentesis to alleviate dyspnea
  - Antibiotics and NSAIDs to reduce inflammation
  - Surgery for abdominal lavage

Growth and weaning

• •

Psittacines (and many passerines) have altricial young and display a characteristic growth curve. This curve rises rapidly to a peak body weight just before the time of weaning and then falls slightly to the weaning weight before continuing up to the eventual adult weight.

Cockatiels younger than 1 week are unable to mobilize body tissues in the face of deficiencies, and cockatiel chicks subjected to a low-protein diet fail to lose weight, maintaining their weight until death. Because of the expected growth curve, and this failure to lose weight in spite of nutritional problems, daily weighing is strongly recommended to monitor the chick's condition. Chicks should typically gain about 17% body weight daily in the first 7 days; all chicks should have doubled their body weight by day 7.

Psittacine chicks are ectothermic on hatching. Correct environmental temperatures are as follows:

Correct environmental temperatures for chicks

1. Newly hatched: 33.3° to 34.4° C
2. Unfeathered: 32.2° to 33.3° C
3. Partially feathered: 29.4° to 32.2° C
4. Fully feathered: 23.9° to 26.7° C
5. Weaned: 20.0° to 23.9° C

- Retained yolk sac
  - Often accompanies umbilical infection
  - Debridement of infected material and antibiosis
  - Aspiration of yolk sac material
  - Surgical resection of yolk sac
- Failure to gain weight—many possible problems, but likely to be bacterial or fungal (*Candida*) infection
  - Start on nystatin at 300,000 IU/kg PO b.i.d. for 10 days and a broad-spectrum antibiotic
  - May need crop tubing; switch from normal hand-rearing formula to a rehydrating/critical care formulation. This will need to be given more frequently to maintain the energy input that the chick requires. After 24 hours, begin to introduce the hand-rearing formula back into the diet over a period or 2 to 3 days.
  - Reassess environmental conditions.
- Crop diseases of chicks (see "Differential Diagnosis for Vomiting/Regurgitation/Dysphagia" in *Gastrointestinal Tract Disorders*)
- Hepatic lipidosis—chicks fed on a too high-fat diet
  - Respiratory distress
  - Hepatomegaly
  - Reduce intake of food; reduce fat content of food; add lactulose to diet
  - Parenteral fluid administration
- Hepatic hematoma
  - Usually following trauma (e.g., dropping the chick)
  - Often hepatic lipidosis concurrent (enlarged, friable liver)
  - Supportive treatment; poor prognosis

Songbirds and softbills

The passerines (songbirds) and softbills are the other major groups of birds kept for ornamental purposes apart from psittacines, rather than utility species such as pigeons and birds of prey. There is inevitably an overlap between the disorders that occur in psittacines and those that occur in the passerines and softbills. This chapter deals with those diseases and disorders specific to various passerines and softbills, but diagnostic options should be considered in conjunction with the appropriate psittacine section, in Chapter 8.

Commonly kept species include:

- Mynahs, including the greater Indian hill mynah *(Gracula religiosa intermedia)*, the lesser Indian hill mynah *(Gracula religiosa indica)*, and the Bali or Rothschild mynah *(Leucopsar rothschildi)*
- Canaries *(Serinus* spp.)
- Estrildidae finches, including the waxbills (including the zebra finch *Taeniopygia guttata)*, parrotfinches *(Erythrura* spp. and *Chloebia* spp.), and mannikins *(Lonchura* spp.)
- Toucans (e.g., the Toco toucan *Ramphastos toco)* and other Ramphastides.

Commonly encountered species are listed in Table 9-1.

Table 9-1	Commonly encountered songbirds and softbills: key facts			
	Canary	**Greater Indian hill mynah**	**Zebra finch**	**Toco toucan**
Average life span (years)	5-15	12+	<17	6+
Weight (g)	18-30	210-270	10-16	450-500
Sexing	Young males will begin singing (sub-songs) at some point between weaning and first molt	Female wattles are smaller than those of the male	The beak is darker red in the male; large orange cheek spots	DNA; surgical sexing
Estimating age		<6- to 8-month-old young have dull feathering plus poorly developed head wattles. The wattles take up to 12 months to develop	Young birds (<6 weeks) have black beaks and pronounced black "tear line" running down from the eye (loses a first molt at 12 weeks old). The white variety lacks this pattern	
Normal clutch size	4-5	3-4	4-6	2-4
Incubation (days)	13-14	14	12.5-16	15-16

Nursing care

(See Chapter 8.)

Analgesia and anesthesia

(See Chapter 8.)

Skin disorders

Pruritus

- Ectoparasites (see below)

Alopecia

- Feather loss around head (toxoplasmosis)
- Feather picking—rarely self-mutilation; usually by other birds, especially zebra finches. May indicate iron storage disease in toucans
- Lice (canaries)
- Dermatomycosis (*Trichophyton* spp. and *Microsporum* spp.)

Scaling and crusting

- Dermatomycosis (*Trichophyton* spp. and *Microsporum* spp.)
- Hyperkeratosis (canaries)

Nodules and nonhealing wounds

- Feather cysts (especially canaries)
- Intracutaneous keratinizing epithelioma has been described in the mynah bird (Rodríguez et al 2006).
- Papillomavirus—wartlike growths of the skin on the feet and legs of European finches
- Abscessation—typically due to *Staphylococci* and *Streptococci*
- Bumblefoot—typically chronic infection and abscessation of the feet, especially the plantar surfaces
- Head and beak lesions in toucans are often the result of intraspecific aggression.
- Constriction of the extremities, especially the toes of canaries and small finches, often due to entanglement with thin foreign bodies such as human hairs

Changes in pigmentation

- Erysipelothrix (see "Skin Disorders in Psittacines")
- Altered feather coloring
  - Nutritional
  - Hepatic disease

Ectoparasites

- Flies: Hippoboscids (flat flies/louse flies) occasionally encountered, especially with aviary birds. Can transmit hemoparasites such as *Haemoproteus* and *Leukocytozoon*, as well as transfer mites and lice, between individuals
- Lice: Can reach significant numbers on debilitated birds; particularly induce baldness in canaries secondary to irritation
- Ticks: Occasionally on new imports. Sudden death associated with tick attachment to head. Suggested etiologies include hypersensitivity reactions, toxin injection, or a tickborne infection. Can also transmit other diseases such as hemoprotozoa, *Borrelia* spp., and louping ill
- Red mite *Dermanyssus avium* and other species

- Northern fowl mite *Ornithonyssus sylviarum*
- Feather mites: Found between the barbs on the ventral surfaces of feathers; often niche specific
- Quill mites such as *Syringophilus, Dermoglyphus,* and *Picobia* spp.; found inside quills. *Harpirhynchus* mites may induce hyperkeratotic epidermal cysts.
- Skin mites
- Knemidocoptid mites; common one encountered is *Knemidocoptes pilae* (scaly face/scaly leg)

Dermatitis

- Commensal bacterial numbers on the skin of birds are considered to be lower than those found on mammals.
- Bacterial
  - Staphylococci
  - Streptococci
- Fungal
  - *Candida*

Burns

Neoplasia

- Neoplastic-like lesions described in masked bullfinch *(Pyrrhula erythaca)* due to pox virus (Dorrestein et al 1993).

Noncutaneous findings on clinical examination

- Respiratory distress, PCV <30% (red mites)

Investigations

1. Aseptic collection of samples for bacteriology/mycology
2. Cytology
3. Radiography. A standing view using horizontal beam is useful for detecting metallic foreign bodies in the conscious bird; otherwise lateral and ventrodorsal (VD) views, under general anesthesia (GA), are required for meaningful radiography.
4. Endoscopy
5. Serology for *Aspergillus* antigen and *Chlamydophila* antigen
6. Fresh fecal samples for parasitic examination (*Giardia*, nematode eggs)
   a. Smears can be dried and stained (Gram stain for bacterial assessment, Romanowsky stains for cytology)
7. Bulk fecal samples (collected over 3 to 5 days) can be submitted for *Chlamydophila* polymerase chain reaction (PCR)
8. Diagnostic imaging, including radiography and endoscopy
9. Biopsy

Management

1. Optimize diet, including the use of multivitamin supplements, reducing seed intake and increasing fruit and/or insect consumption where appropriate for the species.
2. Where there is significant feather loss, consider supplementary heating to counter loss of insulation.

3. Covering broad-spectrum antibiotics may be useful if there are obvious skin lesions.
4. If pruritic consider analgesia—meloxicam (Metacam oral suspension) at 0.1 mg/kg PO body weight b.i.d. Do not use steroids.
5. Avoid the use of collars except in extreme situations; these can be extremely stressful to the bird and can interfere with many normal behaviors, including feeding, flight, and climbing.

- Ticks
  - Ivermectin or fipronil. Remove ticks manually where possible.
- Red mite and other species
  - Ivermectin at 0.2 mg/kg PO, SC or IM. Light dusting with pyrethrin powder. Treat environment in case of red mite; painting woodwork may "seal in" mites. *Note:* Some Estrildid finches appear hypersensitive to pyrethrin.
- Quill mites
  - Apply topical cis-permethrin (e.g., Johnson's Bird Antimite Spray) or fipronil (Frontline) spray (applied to cotton wool and wiped onto bird). Beware hypothermia in small birds due to evaporation of carrier.
- Knemidocoptid mites (e.g., *Knemidocoptes pilae*)
  - Ivermectin at 0.2 mg/kg PO, SC, or IM. A small drop may be applied topically over the jugular vein or onto the back of the neck and seems to work well. Injection is not recommended in birds weighing <500 g due to problems with toxicity. Treat Harpirhynchid, Epidermoptid, and Cheyletiellid mites as for Knemidocoptid mites.
- Feather cysts
  - Manual expression with appropriate analgesia provides only temporary relief; they ideally require surgical removal.
- Abscesses
  - Surgical removal
- Bumblefoot
  - Usually requires surgical intervention; bird may need supportive dressing on affected foot to prevent reinfection of surgical site. If the condition is unilateral, be aware of pressure sores and other sequelae affecting the good leg due to bird shifting weight onto it.
- Candidiasis
  - Amphotericin B at 1.5 mg/kg IV b.i.d. for 3 to 7 days, plus a topical antimycotic (e.g., clotrimazole)
- Dermatomycosis (*Trichophyton* spp. and *Microsporum* spp.)
  - Topical ketoconazole preparation and systemic antimycotic (e.g., itraconazole at 5 mg/kg PO s.i.d.)
- Hyperkeratosis
  - Soften keratin nodules and remove.
  - May be genetic, poor nutrition, an aging change or endocrinologic in origin
- Burns
  - Treat as for other species: Keep moist; may help to apply topical amorphous hydrogel dressings (IntraSite Gel, Smith and Nephew Healthcare Ltd.); to encourage secondary healing; covering antibiosis; fluid therapy.
- Constriction of the extremities
  - Investigate and remove material acting as tourniquet. May result in or require distal amputation of digit

Systemic disorders

Bacterial
- Septicemia

Fungal
- Aspergillosis

Neoplasia

Other noninfectious problems
- Carbon monoxide poisoning
- Polytetrafluoroethane (PTFE) toxicity from overheating of Teflon
- Heavy metal poisoning

Findings on clinical examination

- Nonspecific signs (see *Consultation and Handling* in Chapter 8)
- Severe respiratory signs (carbon monoxide toxicity, PTFE toxicity)
- Vomiting, polyuria, possible CNS signs (heavy metal poisoning)

Investigations

1. Hematology and biochemistry
   a. Blood zinc or lead levels; liver heavy metal levels (biopsy or postmortem)
2. Postmortem
   a. Hemorrhagic, edematous lungs (PTFE poisoning)

Treatment/specific therapy

- PTFE poisoning
  - If still alive (most birds die very quickly), remove from source of toxicity. NSAIDs (e.g., meloxicam) may be useful in control of the pulmonary inflammation that is caused.
- Zinc/lead poisoning
  - Sodium calcium edetate at 20 to 50 mg/kg IM, IV b.i.d. given daily for 7 days, stopped for 7 days, then repeated. This continues until blood levels fall to normal.

Respiratory tract disorders

Nasal tract

Rhinitis (see also "Rhinitis" in Chapter 8).

Viral
- Avian pox (see below)

Differential diagnoses for respiratory disorders

Viral
- Avian pox (septicemic form, especially canaries and other *Serinus* species)
- Coronavirus (tracheitis in canaries)
- Influenza virus A

Bacterial

- *Pasteurella multocida*
- Staphylococci
- Streptococci
- Salmonellosis
- *Klebsiella pneumoniae*
- *Yersinia pseudotuberculosis* (especially toucans and mynahs)
- *Aeromonas* spp. and *Pseudomonas* spp.
- Mycobacteriosis

Fungal

- *Aspergillosis* (especially mynahs)
- *Enterococcus faecalis*
- *Candida*
- Mucormycosis

Protozoal

- Toxoplasmosis
- *Trichomonas*
- Sarcocystis

Parasitic

- Blood-sucking mites (anemia)
- *Sternostoma tracheacolum* (air sac mites—especially Australian finches)
- *Cytodites nudus* mites (also in respiratory tract); rare
- Syngamus trachea (especially mynahs and starlings)

Nutritional

- Hypovitaminosis A (see *Nutritional Disorders*)

Neoplasia

- Coelomic neoplasia (e.g., hepatic)

Other noninfectious problems

- Egg coelomitis
- Anemia (see *Cardiovascular and Hematologic Disorders*)
- Ruptured air sac

Findings on clinical examination

- Dyspnea
- Tachypnea
- Head swinging and neck stretching. Forward-leaning and extended neck strongly suggest tracheal obstruction.
- Coughing is occasionally encountered, but it is uncommon.
- Tail pumping
- Increased recovery time/exercise intolerance
- Increased inspiratory sounds often associated with upper respiratory tract disease
- Increased expiratory sounds often associated with lower respiratory tract disease
- Abdomen may be distended (fluid, neoplasia, hemorrhage).

- Subcutaneous air-filled swelling; may vary in size (ruptured air sac)
- Scabs and pox lesions on eyelids; commissure of mouth and skin; diphtheritic lesions (avian pox)
- CNS signs, iridocyclitis and other ocular signs (toxoplasmosis)
- Loss of voice; abnormal squeaking or wheezing sounds (sternostomosis, aspergillosis)
- Other, nonrespiratory signs
  - Regurgitation (trichomoniasis)
  - Debilitation and death. High mortality of 20% to 100%. Usually due to septicemia (avian pox), *Yersinia pseudotuberculosis* (canaries and finches), pasteurellosis (mynahs)

Investigations

1. Transillumination of trachea (air sac mites)
2. Routine hematology and biochemistry
   a. Anemia (blood sucking mites, anemia of chronic illness)
3. Serology for *Chlamydophila* and aspergillosis
4. Radiography
5. Endoscopy
   a. Culture of aseptically collected samples
6. Nasal discharge
   a. Tracheal wash
   b. Cytology of above samples
7. Fecal samples
   a. Modified Ziehl-Neelsen staining or PCR for mycobacteriosis
8. *Chlamydophila* PCR (collect bulk fecal samples over 5 days to identify intermittent excreters)
9. Biopsy
10. Postmortem
    a. Pneumonia
    b. Hepatomegaly with miliary abscessation; splenomegaly (*Yersinia pseudotuberculosis,* salmonellosis)

Management

1. Improve hygiene. Aeromonad and pseudomonad air sac infections have been associated with infected sprays or misters.
2. General supportive care
3. Milk thistle *(Silybum marianum)* is hepatoprotectant. Dose at 4 to 15 mg/kg PO b.i.d. or t.i.d.

Treatment/specific therapy

- Avian pox: Supportive care. Avoid access to blood-sucking insects (carriers). May also be spread by contact with infected blood, rarely in contaminated food and drinking water. Vaccination
- *Enterococcus faecalis:* Appropriate antibiosis. Infected birds may not recover completely.
- Yersiniosis: Appropriate antibiotics. Source of infection is often fecal contamination from wild birds and rodents.

- Salmonellosis: Treatment as for *Yersinia*; zoonotic potential
- Mycobacteriosis: Significant potential zoonosis, so treatment rarely undertaken
- Aspergillosis (see *Lower Respiratory Tract Disorders* in Chapter 8)
- *Sarcocystis*
  - Treat with trimethoprim-sulfadiazine (30 mg/kg PO s.i.d.) plus pyrimethamine 0.5 to 1.0 mg/kg PO b.i.d. for 30 days. May need to supplement with folic acid
  - The Virginia opossum is the primary host; cockroaches can act as paratenic hosts.
- *Syngamus* spp.: Indirect life cycle using earthworms, slugs, and snails. Treat with fenbendazole at 50 mg/kg PO as a single dose.
- *Sternostoma tracheacolum* (air sac mites)
  - Ivermectin 0.1% in propylene glycol applied as 1 drop to skin over pectoral musculature or lateral to thoracic inlet
- Ruptured air sac: Puncture air sac aseptically to deflate. Address any underlying issues. Will often heal spontaneously, but risk of recurrence is high

Cardiovascular and hematologic disorders

Viral
- Avian polyomavirus (AVP) (finches)

Bacterial
- Endocarditis

Fungal
- Endocarditis

Protozoal
- *Plasmodium* spp.
- *Haemoproteus* spp.
- *Leukocytozoon* spp.
- *Trypanosoma* spp.

Parasitic
- *Schistosoma* spp.
- Blood-sucking mites

Neoplasia
Other noninfectious problems
- Congestive heart failure
- Atherosclerosis
- Endocardiosis

Findings on clinical examination

- Pale mucous membranes (anemia—if severe, may present similar to respiratory disease)
- Exercise intolerance
- Weight loss
- Vague signs of ill health

Investigations

1. Auscultation
   a. Abnormal heart sounds
   b. Abnormal cardiac rhythms
2. Routine hematology and biochemistry
   a. Demonstration of parasites on stained smear
   b. Anemia (*Plasmodium*, blood-sucking mites)
3. Radiography
   a. Hepatomegaly
4. Endoscopy
5. Ultrasonography and Doppler ultrasound
6. Electrocardiogram
7. Postmortem
   a. Myocarditis along with liver abnormalities (AVP)
   b. Splenomegaly *(Plasmodium)*
   c. Lung congestion *(Plasmodium)*

Management

1. Reduce stress.
2. Remove high perches.
3. Supply oxygen.

Treatment/specific therapy

- *Plasmodium, Haemoproteus*
  - Chloroquine at 250 mg/120 mL fresh drinking water, daily for 14 days
  - Pyrimethamine 0.5 mg/kg. PO b.i.d or in feed at 100 mg/kg of food. May need to supplement with folic acid.
  - Control of vectors: mosquitoes *(Plasmodium)*; hippoboscid flies, biting midges, or tabanids *(Haemoproteus)*
- *Leukocytozoon*
  - May be asymptomatic but can be fatal with acute hepatitis, renal tubular necrosis, and myocardial hemorrhage
  - Chronic cases may present with wasting and vomiting.
  - Pyrimethamine 0.5 mg/kg PO b.i.d. or in feed at 100 mg/kg of food may be effective. May need to supplement with folic acid
  - Avoid exposure to vectors such as blackflies (*Simulium* spp.) or *Culicoides*/hippoboscids.
- *Trypanosoma* spp.
  - Treatment usually not required. Avoid exposure to vectors such as hippoboscid flies, red mites, blackflies (*Simulium* spp.), and mosquitoes.
- *Schistosoma* spp.
  - Praziquantel at 10 mg/kg PO once only. Repeat after 1 month if necessary.
- Congestive heart failure: Attempt treatment as for other species:
  - Furosemide at 0.5 to 2.0 mg/kg IM or SC b.i.d. or 5 mg/100 mL drinking water, fresh daily
  - Digoxin 0.02 mg/kg PO s.i.d.
  - Aminophylline 4.0 mg/kg PO or IM b.i.d.

Neurological disorders

Viral

- Paramyxovirus
- Adenolike virus infection (canaries)

Bacterial

- Mycobacteriosis

Fungal

- Mucormycosis

Protozoal

- Atoxoplasmosis *(Isospora serini)* in young canaries 2 to 9 months old

Neoplasia

Other noninfectious problems

- Middle ear disease
- Heavy metal poisoning, especially from zinc in galvanized caging, baths, or drinking receptacles
- Hemochromatosis
- Convulsions similar to epileptic seizures (mynahs)

Findings on clinical examination

- CNS signs such as torticollis and opisthotonos
- Rhythmic nystagmus-like rotations of the head (middle ear disease)
- Collapse
- Depression
- Anorexia
- Weight loss
- Green diarrhea (paramyxovirus)
- Dark spot visible in "abdominal" body wall (hepatomegaly due to a toxoplasmosis)
- Sudden death (paramyxovirus)

Investigations

1. Routine hematology and biochemistry
2. Radiography
3. Postmortem examination
4. Gram stain contents of any lesions
5. Modified Ziehl-Neelsen staining or PCR for mycobacteriosis
6. Histopathology

Management

- Keep in quiet, darkened environment. Fluids may be given per cloaca if there is a risk of aspiration.

Treatment/specific therapy

- Zinc/lead poisoning
  - Sodium calcium edetate at 20 to 50 mg/kg IM b.i.d. given daily for 7 days, stopped for 7 days, then repeated. This continues until blood levels fall to normal.
- Viral infections
  - Supportive treatment only. Give warmth, covering antibiotics, and fluids if necessary.
  - Mynahs infected with Newcastle disease excrete virus for 12 to 119 days post infection (Panigrahy & Senne 1991).
- Mycobacteriosis
  - Potential zoonosis. Consider euthanasia.
  - Two suggested treatment regimens (Rupiper et al 2000) are:
    - Ethambutol (200 mg), isoniazid (200 mg), and rifampin (300 mg) all crushed together and mixed with 10 mL of a simple syrup. This is administered by mouth s.i.d. according to Table 9-2.

Table 9-2 Volumes required for suggested treatment regimen for mycobacteriosis

Bird weight (g)	Volume of mixture (mL)
<100	0.1
100-250	0.2
250-500	0.3
500-1000	0.4

    - Combination therapy of:
      * Ethambutol (10 mg/kg PO b.i.d.)
      * Streptomycin (30 mg/kg IM b.i.d.)
      * Rifampin (15 mg/kg PO b.i.d.)
- Mucormycosis. Usually diagnosed on postmortem. Linked to feeding damp, germinated seeds
- Atoxoplasmosis
  - Toltrazuril at 5.0 mg in 100 mL drinking water for 2 days. Repeat after 12 days.
  - Prevention of re-infection by removing access to droppings. Clean flights regularly. Consider a false wire bottom to the flight.
- Convulsions
  - Consider treatment initially with diazepam 0.5 to 1.0 mg/kg IV or IM.
  - Phenobarbital 1.0 to 5.0 mg/kg PO, IM, or IV b.i.d.

Ophthalmic disorders

Conjunctivitis can appear as part of a "syndrome" of upper respiratory signs (e.g., periorbital swelling, conjunctivitis, or intraocular disease) because of the interconnectedness of local structures; the infraorbital sinus connects with the caudal nasal concha, the nasal cavity, and the cervicocephalic air sac that covers the head and neck caudally and dorsally. It also has diverticulae extending dorsal, ventral, and caudal to the eye, as well as into the maxillary bill and mandible.

Viral
- Pox virus (mynahs)
- Herpesvirus (cytomegaloviruses), especially in Australian and African finches

Bacterial
- Mycoplasmosis
- Chlamydophilosis
- *Nocardia*

Fungal
- *Candida*

Protozoal
- Toxoplasmosis (Gibbens et al 1997)

Dietary
- Hypovitaminosis A (see *Nutritional Disorders*)

Neoplasia
Other noninfectious problems
- Trauma

Findings on clinical examination

- Periocular and cutaneous pox lesions suggest avian pox. May also see respiratory signs
- Keratitis, conjunctivitis, distortion and depigmentation of eyelids (poxvirus in young mynahs)
- May be unilateral or bilateral
- Keratoconjunctivitis
- Crusty skin lesions on the eyelids
- Corneal ulceration (*Candida* keratitis in toucans, trauma)
- Cataracts
- Intraocular hemorrhage (usually linked to head trauma)
- Loss of vision
- Sunken eyes—can be unilateral or bilateral (toxoplasmosis). There may be feather loss around the head.

Investigations

1. Topical fluorescein to assess for corneal damage
2. Routine hematology and biochemistry
3. Serology (*Toxoplasma*)
4. Culture and sensitivity
5. Cytology
6. PCR for *Chlamydophila*
7. Biopsy
   a. Eyelid margin
   b. Conjunctiva
8. Ultrasonography
9. Necropsy and histopathology

Treatment/specific therapy

- Toxoplasmosis
  - Potentiated sulfonamides
- Chlamydophilosis
  - Enrofloxacin (5.0 mg/kg PO or IM)
  - Doxycycline (25 to 50 mg/kg PO s.i.d.) or 1.0 g/kg soft feed
- Mycoplasmosis
  - Tylosin at 1 mg/mL drinking water for a minimum of 21 days
  - Enrofloxacin 5.0 mg/kg PO or IM
  - Topical ofloxacin ophthalmic drops
  - Tetracyclines
  - Doxycycline (as above)
- Nocardiosis. Blindness and lameness described in mynahs (Panigrahy & Senne 1991), along with postmortem signs of bacteremic spread
- Candidiasis
  - Amphotericin B at 1.5 mg/kg IV b.i.d. for 3 to 7 days, plus a topical antimycotic, e.g., clotrimazole
- Trauma
  - As for other species

Gastrointestinal tract disorders

Bacterial

- *Escherichia coli* (normal cloacal inhabitant of toucans; sweating disease)
- *Citrobacter* spp. (especially weaver finches and waxbills)
- *Salmonella* spp.
- *Campylobacter*
- *Erysipelothrix insidiosa* (erysipelas)
- Chlamydophilosis
- Macrorhabdosis/megabacteriosis *(Macrorhabdus ornithogaster)*
- Mycobacteriosis
- *Yersinia pseudotuberculosis*
- *Pseudomonas aeruginosa*

Fungal

- Candidiasis (especially toucans and finches)

Protozoal

- Atoxoplasmosis *(Isospora serini)* in young canaries
- Coccidiosis (*Isospora* spp., *Eimeria* spp., *Dorisella* spp., and *Wendyonela* spp.)
- Cryptosporidiosis
- *Giardia*
- Trichomoniasis
- Cochleostoma (society finches)

Parasitic

- Nematodes
  - *Ascaridia* (direct life cycle)
  - *Porrocaecum* (indirect; needs invertebrate intermediate hosts, such as earthworms)

- *Capillaria* (direct or use earthworms as paratenic hosts)
- Spiruroids: Proventricular worm *(Geopetitia aspiculata)*
- Acuaria skrjabini (gizzard worm)
- Trematodes: *Prosthogonimus* spp. (snails and dragonflies are intermediate hosts)

Dietary

Neoplasia

Other noninfectious problems

- Hemorrhagic diathesis (linked to starvation—Dorrestein 2000)
- Liver disease

Findings on clinical examination

- Lethargy
- Weight loss
- Regurgitation, passing of whole or partially undigested seeds (megabacteriosis)
- Thickened crop wall with whitish lining, regurgitation, diarrhea, molting abnormalities
- Diarrhea (see "Assessment of Droppings" in Chapter 8)
- Yellow droppings (especially Estrildid finches with *Campylobacter*)
- Birds stained ventrally with dirty, yellowish material: diarrhea, dehydration. Nests soiled with wet, yellow material. Chick die-offs (sweating disease—*E. coli*)
- Greenish droppings (liver disease, *Erysipelas* in mynahs)
- Dark patch in abdomen of canary chicks (black spot disease) due to hepatomegaly (atoxoplasmosis)
- Mortalities (usually resulting from septicemia)

Investigations

1. Crop wash
2. Proventricular wash
3. Fecal examination
   a. Culture and sensitivity
   b. Parasitic examination
      i. Wet preparation
      ii. Flotation: *Note: Isospora* carriers shed intermittently, so negative results do not rule out infection (Table 9-3).
   c. Gram stain
   d. Modified Ziehl-Neelsen staining or PCR for mycobacteriosis
4. Cytology
5. PCR for *Chlamydophila*
6. Radiography

Table 9-3 Key to fecal coccidiosis

Isospora spp.	2 sporocysts and 4 sporozoites
Eimeria spp.	4 sporocysts and 2 sporozoites
Dorisella spp.	2 sporocysts and 8 sporozoites
Wendyonela spp.	4 sporocysts and 4 sporozoites

7. Endoscopy
8. Ultrasonography
9. Postmortem
    a. Hemorrhagic enteritis (severe bacterial disease, protozoal). On postmortem, differentiate from hemorrhagic diathesis.
    b. Yellow gut contents, often with undigested seed *(Campylobacter)*
    c. Catarrhal enteritis (mycobacteriosis)

Management

- See "Management" in *Gastrointestinal Tract Disorders* in Chapter 8.

Treatment/specific therapy

- Bacterial diseases: Appropriate antibiosis, good hygiene
- *Campylobacter:* Antibiotics and improvements with hygiene
- *E. coli* (sweating disease): Appropriate antibiosis, hygiene
- Mycobacteriosis: Potential zoonosis. Treatment is rarely attempted.
- Chlamydophilosis
    - Enrofloxacin at 5.0 mg/kg PO or IM s.i.d.
    - Doxycycline
        - Doxycycline hyclate intravenous human preparation given at 60 to 100 mg/kg IM every 5 to 7 days for 45 days
        - Doxycycline hyclate as an in-water powdered medication. Use de-ionized water.
        - *Note:* Birds may be intermittent excreters, so at least three consecutive negative samples should achieved before ceasing treatment.
- Macrorhabdosis/megabacteriosis *(Macrorhabdus ornithogaster)*
    - Amphotericin B at 1-5 mL/kg PO of 100 mg/mL suspension b.i.d. until organism is eliminated
    - Alternatively, ketoconazole at 10 mg/kg PO b.i.d.
    - Nystatin
        - 300,000 IU/kg PO b.i.d.
        - 100,000 IU/L drinking water
        - 200,000 IU/kg soft food
- Atoxoplasmosis: 5 mg toltazuril in 100 mL drinking water for 2 days. Repeat after 12 days.
    - Prevention of re-infection by removing access to their droppings
    - Clean flights regularly. Consider a false wire bottom to the flight.
- Coccidiosis: Potentiated sulfonamides or as for atoxoplasmosis
- *Cryptosporidium:* Good hygiene; no effective treatment
- Cochlosomosis, trichomoniasis, and *Giardia*
    - Ronidazole at 400 mg/kg in soft food and 400 mg/L in fresh drinking water daily for 5 days. Stop for 2 days and then repeat.
    - Metronidazole is reportedly toxic in some finches.
- Parasites
    - Birds in outside aviaries should be wormed twice yearly (avoid breeding season) or have fecal screens every 6 months. All new birds should be wormed during quarantine.
    - Suitable treatments for nematodes, proventricular worms, and gizzard worms include fenbendazole at 50 mg/kg PO as a once only dose, or water-soluble avermectins (e.g., moxidectin 0.1% added to drinking water at 20 mg/L for 48 hours).

- *Capillaria:* Infection is direct, but intermediate stages can be carried by earthworms so remove fecal material regularly and prevent access to soil. Treat with fenbendazole at 50 mg/kg by crop tube; this may need repeating every 2 weeks until the bird is clear.
- *Ascaridia* and *Porrocaecum* spp.: The life cycle is direct, although earthworms may act as transport hosts.
- Proventricular worms *(Geopetitia):* Indirect life cycle using insect intermediate hosts
  - Levamisole at 20 to 40 mg/kg PO once only or 1 to 2 g/4.5 L drinking water over 1 to 3 days. *Note:* Toxicities may be seen.
- *Acuaria skrjabini* (gizzard worm)
  - Levamisole at 20 to 40 mg/kg PO once only or 1 to 2 g/4.5 L drinking water over 1 to 3 days. *Note:* Toxicities may be seen.
- Cestodes and trematodes: Single dose of praziquantel at 8 to 10 mg/kg PO

Hepatic disorders

Viral
- AVP (finches)
- Circovirus
- Herpesvirus
- Avian leukosis

Bacterial
- *Pasteurella multocida*
- *Salmonella* spp.
- *E. coli*
- *Erysipelothrix insidiosa* (erysipelas)
- *Y. pseudotuberculosis*
- Chlamydophilosis

Fungal
Protozoal
- Atoxoplasmosis
- Toxoplasmosis

Dietary
- Hepatic lipidosis
- Hemochromatosis (iron storage disease)

Neoplasia
- Hepatocellular carcinoma
- Hepatoma
- Lymphosarcoma
- Pancreatic adenocarcinoma (possible metastatic spread)

Other noninfectious problems
- Lipogranulomata (canaries)
- Congestive heart failure

Findings on clinical examination

- General malaise
- Poor appetite
- Loss of condition
- Ascites
- Yellow or green feces
- "Black spot" visible in nestling canary abdomen (atoxoplasmosis, circovirus)
- Nestling mortalities; beak deformities (APV)
- Respiratory distress (secondary to hepatomegaly)

Investigations

1. Hematology and biochemistry
   a. Raised liver enzymes
2. Radiography
   a. Hepatomegaly
   b. Ascites
3. Endoscopy
4. Biopsy
5. Ultrasonography
6. Postmortem
   a. Splenomegaly and hepatomegaly (chlamydophilosis, AVP, avian leukosis)
   b. Hepatomegaly with definite bronze to bluish appearance (hemachromatosis)
   c. Hepatomegaly with miliary abscessation; splenomegaly *(Y. pseudotuberculosis)*
   d. Hepatomegaly, mottled and multiple white foci (toxoplasmosis)
   e. Hepatomegaly, splenomegaly, yellowish discoloration of myocardium. In advanced cases there are pinpoint foci throughout these organs (atoxoplasmosis).
   f. Petechiae and ecchymotic hemorrhages of liver and other organs suggest septicemia/bacteremia (*Pasteurella, Salmonella, E. coli,* erysipelas).
   g. Abdominal enlargement, congested gallbladder (visible as "black spot") (circovirus)

Management

1. Diuretics such as furosemide at 0.1 to 2.0 mg/kg IM or SC b.i.d. may be useful in controlling ascites.
2. Milk thistle *(Silybum marianum)* is hepatoprotectant. Dose at 4 to 15 mg/kg PO b.i.d. or t.i.d. (Wade 2004).

Treatment/specific therapy

- Viral infections
  - Supportive treatment only
- Bacterial diseases
  - Appropriate antibiosis and supportive care
- Lipogranulomata are usually incidental findings on postmortem.
- Yersiniosis
  - Appropriate antibiotics. Source of infection is often fecal contamination from wild birds and rodents.

Renal disorders

See also "Differential Diagnosis of Polydipsia/Polyuria" in Chapter 8.

Bacterial
- Nephritis

Fungal
- Nephritis

Neoplasia

Other noninfectious problems
- Amyloidosis (especially Gouldian finches)

Findings on clinical examination

- Weight loss
- Polydipsia and accompanying polyuria
- Marked wetting of the bottom of the cage
- Hematuria (especially with heavy metal poisoning)
- Unilateral or bilateral lameness (caused by pressure of renal tumors on adjacent lumbosacral plexus
- White uric acid tophi may be visible under the skin of the legs and feet. Joints may be swollen (articular gout).
- Neurologic signs (e.g., ataxia, generalized tremors)

Investigations

1. Hematology and biochemistry
   a. Renal parameters can be difficult to interpret. Uric acid levels may only rise in chronic renal disease. Urea levels tend to be low. There may be a rise in phosphorus and a change in the calcium/phosphorus ratio. Therefore, need to assess multiple values (i.e., uric acid, urea, creatinine, calcium, and phosphorus) to assess renal disease.
2. Urinalysis
   a. Microscopy: White blood cells or renal casts suggest urinary tract disease.
3. Radiography
   a. Plain and contrast (IV pyelogram with iohexol)
4. Endoscopy and biopsy
   a. On endoscopy (or postmortem) uric acid may be seen deposited on certain viscera, such as the pericardium or the serosal surface of the liver.
5. Cloacal swabs
6. Bacteriology: Culture and sensitivity.

Management

- Fluid therapy important.

Treatment/specific therapy

- Bacterial nephritis
  - Appropriate antibiotics

- Fungal nephritis
  - Appropriate antimycotics
- Amyloidosis
  - No specific treatment
  - Investigate possible underlying predisposition (e.g., chronic inflammatory disease such as bumblefoot).

Endocrine disorders

- Diabetes mellitus (toucans)

Findings on clinical examination

- Weight loss, polydipsia/polyuria (diabetes mellitus)
- Anorexia

Investigations

1. Routine hematology and biochemistry
   a. Hyperglycemia (>55.1 mmol/L; toucan normal: 11.0 to 19.3 mmol/L)
2. Urinalysis
   a. Glycosuria

Treatment/specific therapy

- Diabetes mellitus
  - Exogenous commercially available insulin rarely of use, possibly due to an excess of glucagon or a failure to respond to mammalian insulin
  - A small number of cases may respond to insulin (consider regular insulin) therapy at 0.1 to 0.5 IU/kg IM, SC b.i.d. (Worell 1997).

Reproductive disorders

See *Reproductive Disorders* in Chapter 8.

Nutritional disorders

Malnutrition is a common underlying factor in disease occurrence in softbills. Those softbills that are granivorous (canaries, finches) do require supplementation with commercial "softbill diets."

- Hypovitaminosis A
  - General ill health
  - Secondary bacterial and fungal infections
  - Genetic disease in recessive white canaries (unable to absorb precursor carotenoids)
  - Supplement with high dietary vitamin A levels (12,000 IU/kg food)
- Hypovitaminosis C
  - Some passerines (e.g., shrikes and bulbuls) require dietary vitamin C.
  - Lethargy, feather loss, intra-articular hemorrhage

- Metabolic bone disease
  - Can be a marginal problem in aviary birds and only during egg production
  - Often a hypovitaminosis D_3 combined with a hypocalcemia and hyperphosphatemia

---

Clinical signs of metabolic bone disease in birds

- General weakness
- Pathological fractures and/or bending of bones
- Rickets
- Paralysis
- Tetany
- Dystocia
- Low clutch size, thin- or soft-shelled eggs, and low hatchability. (Egg laying hens may have an episode of acute hypocalcemia that can result in partial paresis and perhaps egg binding.)
- Polydipsia/polyuria occasionally seen due to increased phosphorus turnover, triggering a diuresis
- Birds, especially the young, with bone and joint deformities might be deficient in both calcium and vitamin D_3.
- Young Ramphastides may present with folding fracture-like lesions of the beak.
- Can occur in breeding females with concurrent tetracycline administration

---

- Hemochromatosis (iron storage disease)
  - Common, especially in mynahs and toucans
  - Weight loss, dyspnea, ascites, and weakness
- Hepatic lipidosis
  - Can occur in Estrildid finches (e.g., zebra finch)

Noninfectious problems

- Starvation, often the result of mistaking seed husks in feed dishes as uneaten seed
- Avocado poisoning
- Green almond poisoning (cyanide)
- Ethanol toxicity (eating thawed frozen fruits—yeasts ferment sugars into ethanol)

Findings on clinical examination

- Check seed pots for husks mistaken for seed (and, therefore, not replenished).
- Dyspnea, swollen abdomen from ascites (hemochromatosis)
- Postmortem
  - Swollen liver, yellow or beige in color; floats in formal saline (hepatic lipidosis)
  - Hemorrhagic diathesis (see *Gastrointestinal Tract Disorders*), apparent renal gout, lack of food in gut (starvation)
  - Lethargy, ataxia, and incoordination (ethanol toxicity)

Investigations

1. Routine hematology and biochemistry
   a. Hypoproteinemia, raised liver enzymes; serum iron levels (hemochromatosis)
   b. Serum iron levels (toucan normal values <6.27 μmol/L)
2. Analysis of crop contents
3. Radiography
   a. Hepatomegaly, ascites (hemochromatosis)

4. Biopsy
   a. Hepatic iron levels (hemochromatosis)
5. Postmortem
   a. Hydropericardium; subcutaneous edema, especially in region of pectoral muscle (avocado poisoning)

Management

- Provide supportive care.

Treatment/specific therapy

- Hypovitaminosis A
  - Supplement with vitamin A
  - For recessive white canaries, switch to canary foods high with dietary vitamin A levels (12,000 IU/kg food)
- Hypovitaminosis C
  - Supplement with vitamin C 50 to 150 mg/kg dry matter of food.
- Metabolic bone disease
  - Supplement with calcium and vitamin D_3.
  - Consider provision of UV light.
  - Stop tetracycline administration.
- Hemochromatosis
  - Low iron diet (<50 ppm)
  - Avoid citrus fruits and other sources of ascorbic acid—these may enhance iron uptake.
  - Offer cold tea as water source—tannins bind strongly to iron and may reduce dietary uptake.
  - Weekly phlebotomies equal to 1% body weight until iron levels are normalized
  - Alternatively deferoxamine at 100 mg/kg SC s.i.d. until liver levels are normalized (Cornelissen et al 1995). *Note:* Serum iron levels do not always reflect liver storage levels.

Lizards

. . . .

A wide variety of lizards are available in the pet trade. The most common species encountered are described in Table 10-1. The internal anatomy of a lizard is shown in Figure 10-1.

The long-term welfare of lizards is, more so than the majority of snakes, dependent upon correct environmental conditions.

Temperature

Many lizards are "exercised" outside of their vivarium by well-meaning owners. This can lead to prolonged periods of the lizard being exposed to suboptimal temperatures, producing immunosuppression and increased susceptibility to disease. Inside the vivarium, aggression between its inhabitants can mean some individuals are deprived of suitable basking opportunities, leading to immunosuppression. Some lizards require exceptionally high daytime temperatures. Bearded dragons, for example, need a basking spot set at around 35 to 38° C during the day; however, a nighttime temperature drop is no problem.

Ultraviolet exposure

Most diurnal lizards require exposure to ultraviolet B lighting (290 to 315 nm) for endogenous vitamin D_3 synthesis. Dietary supplementation alone is not sufficient for many species, including iguanas, bearded dragons, monitor lizards (*Varanus* spp.), and chameleons, so ultraviolet exposure is achieved by installing a full-spectrum light with a specified UVB output (e.g., 2%, 5%, or 8%).

Common mistakes include:
1. Failure to provide full-spectrum lighting at all
2. Relying upon placing the reptile close to a sunny window (glass filters out UV light)
3. Use of an incorrect bulb (because glass filters UV light, the bulbs should be made from quartz)
4. Failure to replace full-spectrum lights (UV output declines over time but we cannot see this, so replace every 6 to 8 months or according to manufacturer's instructions)
5. Allowing intraspecies and interspecies aggression that prevents one or more lizards from gaining a suitable spot to bask beneath the full-spectrum light

Nutritional supplementation

Crickets, locusts, waxworms, and mealworms are commonly fed to lizards not because they are nutritionally good, but because they are easy to farm commercially and they trigger normal feeding in insectivorous species. Insects are inherently low in calcium, and so this must be balanced with commercial calcium supplements. These are applied to the insects either by dusting a calcium-rich powder onto the prey, or feeding a calcium-rich food. *Note:* Many commercial calcium supplements also contain vitamins, including vitamin D_3, as well as amino acids.

Consultation and handling
. . . .

Small lizards such as leopard geckos can be examined relatively easily. Larger lizards may require a more managed technique involving assistance—iguanas and monitor lizards rarely

Table 10-1 Species of lizard most likely to be encountered: Key facts

Species	Notes	Common disorders
Bearded dragons (Pogona vitticeps)	Medium-sized, characterful lizards. They do like it warm, and the hot spot should be up to 38° C during the day.	Metabolic bone disease, Isospora, and foreign body ingestion. Secondary infections often are the result of inadequate temperatures. Brumation
Leopard gecko (Eublepharis macularius)	An ideal beginner's lizard. Feeds well on supplemented insect prey including mealworms. Available in a wide variety of color morphs, some of which carry very high prices.	Cryptosporidiosis and foreign body ingestion
Crested gecko (Rhacodactylus ciliatus)	Popular because of its looks and wide natural color variations, this gecko's wild diet is rich in fruits and so it can be kept using commercially available foods rather than live foods.	Metabolic bone disease is occasionally seen, as is a muscular-dystrophy-like disease often mistaken for metabolic bone disease
Green iguana (Iguana iguana)	A large stunning lizard as an adult, its vegetarian diet makes it prone to calcium deficiencies.	Metabolic bone disease, abscessation (secondary to prolonged low environmental temperatures), and aggression-related behavioral problems
Veiled chameleon (Chamaelo calyptratus)	Chameleons are generally not good starter lizards, but the veiled chameleon, providing it is offered water via a spray and given supplemented foods, will often do well.	Metabolic bone disease and dystocia

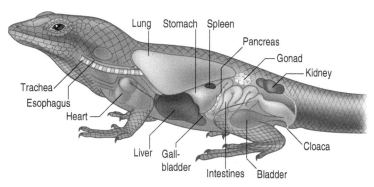

Fig 10-1. Internal anatomy of a lizard (lateral). (Coelomic fat pads removed for clarity)

bite, however (*note:* this does not mean that they do not bite) and, in preference, will attempt to fend you off by whipping with their tail.

Restraint involves grasping the animal from behind across the shoulders and across the pelvis, the handler holding the reptile away from the body. If a large lizard, such as an iguana, is especially aggressive, then placing a damp towel over its head is often sufficient to disorientate it and allow you to gain a hold (N. Highfield, *personal communication*).

Many lizards, such as Chinese water dragons and young iguanas, can be temporarily immobilized by applying digital pressure to both eyes simultaneously. This technique, plus gentle handling, will allow many feisty lizards to be weighed and examined in a controlled fashion,

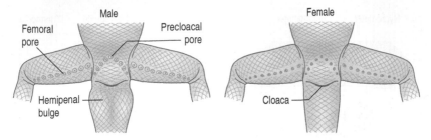

Fig 10-2. Sexing lizards.

before gentle stimulation (such as rerighting the reptile) returns it to a normal state of awareness. This may be a manifestation of the oculocardiac reflex.

In those lizards with hypocalcemia/metabolic bone disease, the bones may be so fragile that fractures of the long bones, especially the femurs, can occur if excessive force is applied. A lizard that is presented as flaccid with little or no muscle tone is likely to be hypocalcemic. Other causes can include septicemia or poisoning, but these are much less likely. In such cases, IV calcium is strongly recommended as soon as possible.

When beginning an examination, examine the head first. Most lizards can be induced to open their mouths even if it is in an attempt to bite you. With iguanas, firm traction on the dewlap will often induce them to open up.

Some lizards will shed their tails naturally if stressed or poorly handled (autotomy). These include iguanids, lacertids, geckos, and some skinks. In these species, the tail will regrow but usually has a different shape and/or markings. *Note:* The crested gecko *(Rhacodactylus ciliatus)* is an exception—unlike the other geckos in the *Rhacodactylus* genus, the tails do not regrow once shed.

Microchipping

- Left quadriceps muscle, or subcutaneously in this area (all species)
- In very small species, subcutaneously on the left side of the body
- Skin closure is achieved either by suture or with tissue glue.

Sexing

Many lizards are sexually dimorphic as adults and can be readily distinguished, typically by the presence of pronounced pores cranial to the cloaca (precloacal pores) or medial thigh (femoral pores), combined with the presence of hemipenile bulges caudal to the cloaca (Fig. 10-2). Male veiled chameleons have a caudal spur on each hind foot, present from birth.

Nursing care

Provide the appropriate environment, including provision of:
1. Optimal temperature (e.g., basking lights, heat mats to allow thermoregulation). Use of max-min thermometers will assist in monitoring temperature ranges incumbent reptiles are exposed to
2. Full-spectrum lighting (provision of UVA and UVB)
3. Humidity
4. Ventilation
5. Easily cleaned accommodation; use paper substrate and disposable/sterilizable hides and other vivarium furniture (Fig. 10-3).
6. Keep individually to minimize intraspecies stress and competition for resources.

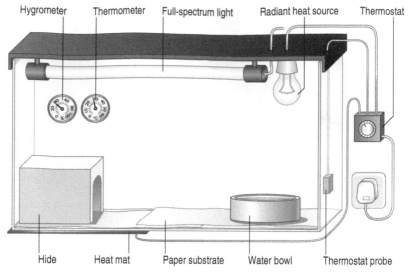

Hygrometer   Thermometer   Full-spectrum light   Radiant heat source   Thermostat

Hide   Heat mat   Paper substrate   Water bowl   Thermostat probe

Fig 10-3. A clinical vivarium setup for lizards and *Chelonia*.

Fluid therapy

Reptiles lack the loop of Henle and are, therefore, unable to produce hyperosmotic urine. Uric acid is excreted instead of ammonia; this is sparingly soluble and can be excreted at high concentration with minimal water loss as a sludge or paste.

The assessment of dehydration in reptiles can be difficult visually. Typically, signs of dehydration are sunken eyes, extensive skin folding, and tenting.

Selection of fluids for reptiles

1. Isotonic fluids for blood loss, surgery, and diarrhea
2. Hypotonic in cases of prolonged anorexia
3. Hypertonic: There is little indication except in exceptionally large reptiles.
4. Blood transfusions can be undertaken using blood from a lizard of the same species or closely related (same genus). Blood can be given IO or IV.
5. Oxyglobin
6. Overhydrating reptiles with compromised renal function can lead to vascular overload, heart failure, and death.

Fluid replacement

1. Plasma volume in reptiles is around 6.0 mL/100 g.
2. Fluid replacement rates are suggested as:
   a. 0.5 to 1.0 mL/100 g/hour, averaging around 1.5 to 3.0 mL/100 g/day
   b. Administer up to 0.5% to 2% body weight maximum of an isotonic replacement fluid, such as Hartmann's solution (i.e., 5 to 20 mL/kg), reducing this once the hydration status becomes normal.
3. Daily bathing in shallow, warm water is often beneficial; it encourages many lizards to drink as well as defecate and urinate.

Fluids administration

1. Stomach tubing is relatively straightforward in smaller lizards.
2. Esophagostomy tubes can be used in some cases.
3. All parenteral fluids should be warmed to around 26° C.
4. The easiest vein to access is the ventral tail vein. If attempting to use this vein in male lizards, always allow a gap caudal to the cloaca for the hemipenes.
5. Alternatively, a surgical cutdown onto the cephalic vein will allow catheterization.
6. For IO fluids the tibial cavity (via the tibial crest) is suggested.
7. Intracoelomic fluids should be used with caution:
   a. There is a large ventral midline abdominal vein that is likely to be pierced if one attempts to give fluids via the linea alba. Place the needle into a paramedian position—this should also avoid the dorsally positioned lungs.
   b. There is no separation of the coelom into an abdomen and thorax, so excessive fluid build-up can compress the lungs.

Nutritional support

Liquidized normal diet or proprietary support diets can be used, given either by stomach tube or by esophagostomy tube.

Analgesia

Table 10-2 Lizards: Analgesic doses

Analgesic	Dose
Buprenorphine	0.01-0.2 mg/kg IM every 24-48 hours
Butorphanol	0.4-2.0 mg/kg SC or IM b.i.d.
Carprofen	1.0-4.0 mg/kg SC or PO every 24-72 hours
Ketoprofen	2.0-4.0 mg/kg SC or IM every 24-48 hours
Meloxicam	0.1-0.5 mg/kg SC or PO every 24-48 hours
Morphine	5-20 mg/kg IC every 6-8 hours
Meperidine/pethidine	2-4 mg/kg IC every 6-8 hours

Anesthesia

All reptiles should be at their optimum temperature. Gaseous anesthetics can be of limited use as induction agents due to intracardiac shunting, tolerance of hypoxia, and physiologic diving reflexes (depending on the species). Chameleons respond relatively quickly, whereas semiaquatic species may take some time.

Standard anesthetic protocol

1. Pre-medication
   a. Atropine sulfate at 0.01 to 0.04 mg/kg IM or IC given 10 to 15 minutes prior to induction may help prevent intracardiac shunting.
   Several anesthetic protocols have been documented. The author has found the following the most useful:

2. Induction
   a. Propofol at 10 mg/kg IV delivered into ventral coccygeal (tail) vein (for alternative dose rates, see Chapters 11 and 12)
3. Intubate and maintain with isoflurane.
4. Most reptiles cease to breathe during anesthesia; therefore, adopt intermittent positive-pressure ventilation (IPPV) every 30 seconds, because high P_{O_2} inhibits ventilation.
5. In larger lizards such as iguanas and water dragons a jugular pulse can be seen sometimes; otherwise the use of pulse oximeters, ultrasound, and/or ECG is required for monitoring.
6. For optimum anesthesia, it can be of benefit to infiltrate the surgical site with local anesthetic.

Parenteral anesthesia

1. Ketamine at 5.0 mg/kg IM plus medetomidine 100 to 150 µg/kg IM
2. Reverse with atipamezole at 5 times medetomidine dose (can take 25 to 90 minutes to take effect).

Recovery

1. Continue with IPPV until spontaneous respiration is resumed.
2. If using oxygen alone, switch to manual ventilation with air if possible.
3. Lizards are tolerant of anoxia; therefore, continue with IPPV even if there is no obvious response.
4. Doxapram at 5 to 10 mg/kg IV, IO, or onto lingual mucosa may be beneficial.

Skin disorders

The epidermis of both lizards and snakes consists of two layers:
1. The stratum corneum, which consists of:
   a. Oberhautchen layer
   b. β-keratin layer
   c. α-keratin layer
   d. Thickened plates of stratum corneum form the scales. This layer also contains a complex mixture of neutral and polar lipids designed to reduce water loss across the skin.
2. Stratum germinativum

The dermis is mainly connective tissue; it may contain bony plates termed *osteoderms*.

Most lizards shed their skin piecemeal and uncoordinated—cellular proliferation and keratinization are continuous; however, geckos normally shed their skin simultaneously over the whole of the body surface. Many lizards, such as leopard geckos (*Eublepharis macularis*), will eat their shed skin.

Differential diagnoses of skin disorders

Shedding difficulties (dysecdysis)

- Humidity too low
- Other environmental problems (e.g., incorrect photoperiod, temperature, nutrition)
- Lack of cage furniture to allow initiation of shedding
- Ectoparasites (e.g., *Hirstiella* spp.; snake mites, or *Ophionyssus natracis*)
- Scarring or other underlying dermal disease
- Hypovitaminosis A
- Hypothyroidism and possibly other endocrinopathies
- Secondary bacterial and fungal infections common

Pruritus
* Ectoparasites

Scaling and crusting
* Dysecdysis (see above)
* Bacterial dermatitis (*Aeromonas* spp., *Pseudomonas* spp., *Serratia* spp.)
* Dermatophilosis
* Burns
* Hypovitaminosis A

Erosions and ulceration
* Behavioral interactions with transparent barriers (ITB). Rostral nares and intermandibular joint often affected.
* Lesions from hungry, uneaten crickets and other invertebrate prey
* Bites from conspecifics, especially during mating—these are typically over the shoulders and back of the neck.

Nodules and nonhealing wounds
* Abscess
* Filarial nematodes (see also *Systemic Disorders*), especially chameleons and day geckos
* Granulomas (mycobacterial—see also *Systemic Disorders*; fungal—e.g., *Chrysosporium* anamorph of *Nannizziopsis vriesii*, or CANV, *Trichophyton* spp., *Aspergillus* spp., *Geotrichium candidum, Cryptococcus neoformans*)
* Poxvirus
* Viral papillomas (green lizard *Lacerta viridis* and occasionally other lacertids); often very dark to black, and proliferative
* *Trichomonas* spp. (subcutaneous abscesses in leopard gecko)
* Sebaceous cysts (green iguana)
* Pseudoaneurysm, especially on the head (bearded dragon)
* Calcinosis cutis and calcinosis circumscripta
* Endolymphatic glands in certain geckos, such as day geckos (*Phelsuma* spp.)

Changes in pigmentation
* Scarring
* Yellowing of skin patches in bearded dragons (*Pogona* spp.); common following skin disease (e.g., burns, dysecdysis, infections) but also linked to yellow fungus disease
* Yellow fungus disease of bearded dragons
* Dermatomycosis: *Trichophyton*, CANV

Ectoparasites
* Arthropods
* Ticks (*Aponomma exornatum, A. varanensis, A. fuscolineatus*, see Kenny et al 2004)
* Lizard mites (*Hirstiella trombidiiformis, Geckobiella* spp., *Pterygosoma* spp.)
* Snake mite (*Ophionyssus natracis*—Walter and Shaw 2002)

Burns
Neoplasia
* Fibrosarcoma
* Squamous cell carcinoma
* Liposarcoma
* Chromatophoroma (malignant)

Findings on clinical examination

- Distinct single or multiple swellings palpable in the skin
- Dysecdysis: Patches of dull, thickened skin may indicate areas where several layers of skin have built up over successive dysecdysis episodes. Rings of unshed skin may form bands around the tips of extremities such as toes and tail tips. These may constrict as they dry, acting as tourniquets and compromising blood flow to the extremities. Lizards that have had previous problems may lack one or more digits.
- Thickened or hyperkeratotic skin. History of high-protein diet (e.g., rodents with no vegetable or vitamin supplementation fed long term to known omnivorous lizards, such as monitors), tegus (hypovitaminosis A)
- Damage to rostral nares and intermandibular joint, linked to repetitive trauma against transparent barriers such as glass doors and sides. Particularly common in water dragons (*Physignathus* spp.), which consistently attempt to leap through the barrier (ITB)
- Anemia (heavy ectoparasitic infestations)
- Pseudoaneurysm—large fluctuant swelling on neck
- Burns
- Bilateral swellings on the neck of certain gecko species such as day geckos (*Phelsuma* spp.). These are normal calcium storage sites and can be quite pronounced in healthy breeding females.

Investigations

1. Radiography
2. Routine hematology and biochemistry
3. Thyroid levels (Table 10-3)
4. Culture and sensitivity
5. Cytology
   a. Fine needle aspirate
   b. Aspiration—whole blood (pseudoaneurysm)
6. Endoscopy
7. Biopsy/necropsy
   a. Circulating microfilaria (Orós et al 2002)
8. Ultrasonography

Table 10-3 Lizards: Thyroid levels		
Species	**Total T$_4$ nM/L**	**Total T$_3$ nM/L (Free T$_3$ pM/L)**
Sceloporus undulatus Adult	11.1-13.1	3.1-3.2
Ameiva undulata Adult	8.2	—
Dipsosaurus dorsalis Adult	3.2-14.5	—
Dipsosaurus dorsalis Hibernating adult	1.3	—
Dipsosaurus dorsalis Adult (spring)	13.0	0.5
Trachydosaurus rugosus Adult	3.0	0.3
Podarcis sicula Adult	—	0.15 (1.7)
From Hulbert (2000).		

Treatment/specific therapy

- Dysecdysis
  - Moisten the affected areas to loosen the retained skin from the underlying epidermis.
  - Retained spectacular scales in geckos are best removed using a damp cotton bud.
  - Injection of vitamin A at 1000 to 5000 IU/kg IM will often trigger a further shed, allowing a closer management of the sloughing procedure such that both the old shed and the new are removed.
  - Supplementation with thyroxine will often help with lizards showing dysecdysis. Serum thyroid levels may be useful, but normal ranges for comparison may not be available for your target species.
- Abscess
  - Requires surgical removal if possible
- ITB
  - Treat lesions topically or systemically as required. May require removal of devitalized bone with associated teeth.
  - Alter environment—attempt to remove to a larger, more naturalistic environment without transparent boundaries (Scott and Warwick 2002).
- Poxvirus: No treatment
- Viral papillomas
  - Usually self-limiting; may require surgical resection if present at a sensitive site (e.g., mouth, where they may interfere with normal feeding)
- Fungal dermatitis, granulomas, yellow fungus disease
  - Ketoconazole at 10 to 30 mg/kg PO s.i.d.
  - Topical ketoconazole cream
  - Itraconazole 5 mg/kg PO every other day
  - Topical chlorhexidine solution
  - Topical iodine solution
    - *Note:* CANV can act as a primary reptile pathogen.
- Filarial nematodes
  - Surgical resection where feasible
  - Ivermectin at 200 μg/kg SC. Repeat after 4 weeks if necessary. (care with Solomon Island skinks, *Corucia zebrata*)
- Ticks
  - Individual removal of ticks
  - Ivermectin at 200 μg/kg SC. Repeat after 4 weeks if necessary (care with Solomon Island skinks, *Corucia zebrata*)
    - *Note:* Ticks are vectors for *Babesia/Hepatozoon* and *Ehrlichia*-like organisms.
- Snake and lizard mites
  - Snake mites are parthenogenetic, so numbers can rapidly build up in vivaria; treatment must include thorough cleaning of all affected vivaria. What cannot be sterilized with a mild bleach solution (5 mL/gallon) must be disposed of.
  - Replace usual substrate with paper (changed daily)
  - Repeated washing with warm water will physically remove any mites.
  - Application of topical fipronil spray once weekly for at least 4 weeks. This is best first applied to a cloth and rubbed over the entire surface of the lizard. Fipronil spray can also be used to treat the environment.
  - Injection of ivermectin at 200 μg/kg SC (*note:* toxic to indigo snakes and chelonia) every 2 weeks will kill those that feed on the lizard.

- Commercial imidacloprid (100 g/L) plus moxidectin (25 g/L) (Advocate Dog (UK), Advantage Multi (USA), Bayer) applied at double (32 mg/kg imidacloprid + 8.0 mg/kg moxidectin) to 10-fold dosages (160 mg/kg imidacloprid + 40 mg/kg moxidectin) according to thickness of skin (care with lacertids, especially the six-striped grass lizard *Takydromus sexlineatus*) (Mehlhorn et al 2005a)
  - Cultures of predatory mites *(Hypoaspis miles)* are commercially available for use in vivaria.
- Pseudoaneurysm
  - Surgical repair
- Hypothyroidism
  - Supplement with levothyroxine at 0.02 mg/kg PO every other day.
- Calcinosis circumscripta and calcinosis cutis
  - Consider surgical resection if viable.
  - May be linked with renal disease
- Neoplasia
  - Surgical resection
  - Chemotherapy in reptiles is in its infancy. Accessible cutaneous tumors can be treated by injecting cisplatin directly into the tissue mass on a weekly basis as a debulking exercise.
  - Radiation has been used to treat an acute lymphoblastic leukemia in a sungazer lizard *(Cordylus giganteus)*, while surgical laser has been used in the treatment of a dermal melanoma in a green iguana.
  - Chromatophoromas carry a poor prognosis with early metastasis.

Respiratory tract disorders

Viral
- Ophidian paramyxovirus (OPMV)

Bacterial
- Mycobacterial (see also *Systemic Disorders*)
- Bacterial pneumonia (especially water dragons)

Fungal
- Mycotic pneumonia
- Mycotic pleuritis

Parasitic
- Lungworms (*Entomelas* spp.; verminous pneumonia)
- Pentastomids (e.g., *Raillietiella*, especially monitor lizards—*Varanus* spp.)

Neoplasia
- Metastases

Other noninfectious problems
- Sneezing in iguanas—normal removal of salts from nasal salt glands
- Firefly (*Photonis* spp.) intoxication (see also *Systemic Disorders* and *Cardiovascular and Hematologic Disorders*)
- Aspiration pneumonia (following oral administration of food or fluids; regurgitation after stomach tubing)
- Glottal foreign bodies
- Cardiovascular disease (see *Cardiovascular and Hematologic Disorders*)

- Epistaxis (metastatic mineralization of nasal vasculature, trauma, infection, liver disease)
- Anemia (various causes)

Findings on clinical examination

- Dyspnea
- Tachypnea
- Open-mouthed breathing and respiratory distress
- Oral and/or nasal discharge
- Unusual respiratory noises
- Altered color of respiratory membranes (cyanosis, pallor)
- Neck extension
- Epistaxis
- Anorexia
- Depression
- Muscle wastage
- Sudden death

Investigations

1. Microscopy
   a. Sputum examination (either from mouth, pulmonary lavage, or endoscopic collection)
   b. Staining for cytology
   c. Gram stain
   d. Lungworm eggs and larvae
   e. Pentastomid eggs
2. Fecal examination
   a. Pentastomid eggs
   b. *Entomelas* eggs (swallowed from trachea)
3. Radiography
   a. Pneumonia—areas of increased opacity in the lung fields
4. Routine hematology and biochemistry
5. Serology for OPMV
6. Culture and sensitivity
7. Endoscopy
   a. Adult pentastomes present in lung
8. Biopsy/necropsy
9. Proliferative interstitial pneumonia (OPMV)
10. Ultrasonography

Management

- If very cyanosed, provide oxygen; otherwise normal supportive care (see *Nursing Care*)

Treatment/specific therapy

- OPMV
  - No direct treatment
  - Supportive treatment only
  - Often asymptomatic—frequently diagnosed and monitored serologically

- Lungworm
  - Fenbendazole at 50 to 100 mg/kg PO. Repeat every 2 weeks if necessary. *Note:* Fenbendazole is metabolized to oxfendazole by the liver.
  - Oxfendazole at 68 mg/kg PO. Repeat every 2 weeks if necessary.
  - Ivermectin at 0.2 mg IM, SC repeated every 2 weeks for 3 treatments (care with Solomon Island skinks, *Corucia zebrata*)
  - Lungworms have a direct life cycle; infective larvae can penetrate the skin or infect via contaminated food and water.
- Pentastomids
  - Ivermectin at 0.2 mg IM repeated every 2 weeks for 3 treatments (care with Solomon Island skinks, *Corucia zebrata*)
- Foreign body
  - Attempt surgical removal. Likely to need tracheotomy
- Epistaxis
  - Investigate possible causes.
- Anemia
  - Investigate causes (e.g., hemorrhage, high ectoparasite load, gastrointestinal disease, renal disease).

Gastrointestinal tract disorders

Disorders of the oral cavity

In crested geckos, calcium is stored in bilaterally symmetrical endolymphatic glands dorsally at the back of the pharynx. In breeding females on a good calcium intake these can appear as quite pronounced whitish to grayish swellings and should not be mistaken for pathological lesions.

- Periodontal disease
  - Especially affects acrodont lizards (agamids—including bearded dragons, water dragons, and chameleons)
  - May be related to feeding soft insects, such as crickets, waxworms
  - Discoloration, loss of tissue and teeth, osteomyelitis
  - Radiography to assess underlying osteomyelitis
  - Culture of lesions
  - Appropriate antibiosis
  - Ultrasonic and instrument scaling
  - Regular cleaning with oral cleansing product as control measure
- Metabolic bone disease
  - Softening or pathological fractures of the mandibles
  - The weakened bone is unable to support orthopedic techniques; in some cases supporting the jaw closed with strong adhesive plaster (taking care to leave the nares open) accompanied by placement of an esophagostomy tube may allow healing to occur.
- Ossifying fibroma
  - Usually unilateral; typically affects mandibles
  - Occasionally seen in iguanas
  - Surgical debulking and/or cryosurgery
  - Usually self-limiting
- Other neoplasia (Fig. 10-4)

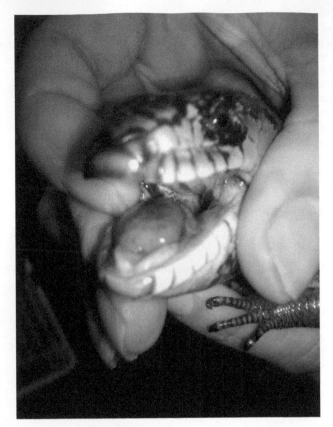

Fig 10-4. Oral mass in a pink-tongued skink.

- Fungal mandibular periodontal osteomyelitis
  - Attempt systemic antimycotics such as:
    - Ketoconazole at 10 to 30 mg/kg PO s.i.d.
    - Topical ketoconazole cream
    - Itraconazole 5 mg/kg PO every other day
- Stomatitis
  - Uncommon. Often linked with respiratory or gastrointestinal diseases (see *Gastrointestinal Tract Disorders*). See Chapter 11 for further advice on treatment of stomatitis.
    - Mycotic (*Emmonsia* spp.)
    - Herpesvirus (Wellehan et al 2003c)
    - Infection of the temporal glands on chameleons
- Swellings dorsolateral to the angle of the jaw: Require debridement under general anesthesia (GA) and appropriate antibiosis
- Pharyngeal edema
  - Renal disease
  - Cardiovascular disease
- Icterus (see *Hepatic Disorders* and *Cardiovascular and Hematologic Disorders*). Adult bearded dragons naturally have very yellow mucous membranes.

- Cyanosis (see *Respiratory Tract Disorders*)
- Disorders of the tongue
  - In many lizards including the green iguana the rostral tip of the tongue bears a symmetrical darker patch that may be mistaken for an ulcer or inflammatory condition.
  - Chameleons and monitor lizards have long tongues that are vital for food location and prehension.
  - Lingual sheath may become infected and adhesions may result. Debride under GA and instigate appropriate antibiosis.
  - Hypocalcemia/metabolic bone disease in chameleons may present as partial or complete paralysis of the tongue.
  - In some old chameleons there is a failure of the tongue-protruding mechanism. These must be hand-fed.

Differential diagnoses for gastrointestinal disorders

Viral

- Reovirus (Drury et al 2002)
- Adenovirus (fat-tailed gecko *Hemitheconyx caudicinctus*—Wellehan et al 2003b)

Bacterial

- *Salmonella* spp.
- *Escherichia coli*
- Other bacteria

Fungal

- Mycotic enteritis (especially chameleons)
- Yeast infections (in some cases may be linked with long-term antibiosis)

Protozoal

- *Cryptosporidium* spp.
- Flagellates (e.g., *Trichomonas*)
- *Giardia*
- *Isospora* (especially *I. amphiboluri* in bearded dragons)
- *Eimeria* spp.
- Cilates (e.g., *Nyctotherus,* green iguana, and *Clevelandellida* spp.)

Parasitic

- Hookworms: *Oswalsocruzia* spp.
- Spirurids (stomach worms), such as *Abbreviata* spp., *Physaloptera* spp. (in ant-eating lizards, such as the horned lizard *Phrynosoma*)
- Pinworms
- Oxyurids (e.g., *Pharyngodon* spp).
- *Capillaria*
- *Strongyloides*
- Trematodes, especially molluscivores (e.g., pink-tongued skinks)

Nutritional

- Metabolic bone disease
- Intestinal tympany secondary to excessive fermentable carbohydrate intake in folivorous lizards

Neoplasia

- Colonic adenocarcinoma (Patterson-Kane and Redrobe 2005)

Other noninfectious problems

- Foreign body/impaction (especially large/inappropriate pieces of substrate)
- Cloacal prolapse

Findings on clinical examination

- Progressive weight loss (tail shrinkage in leopard geckos and related fat-tailed geckos)
- Inappetence
- Very wet or fluidy feces (flagellates, *Strongyloides*)
- Lack of feces
- Hemorrhagic and/or mucusy feces (hookworms)
- Chronic wasting, mortalities, high parasitism levels (possible reovirus—see Drury et al 2002)
- Gastrointestinal stasis and bloating may occur as part of metabolic bone disease, often accompanied by more typical signs (see *Nutritional Disorders*).
- Vomition (uncommon)
- Cloacal prolapse
  - Cloacitis
  - Cloacoliths
  - Intestinal foreign body
  - Intussusception
  - Extraintestinal mass (e.g., renal neoplasm)
  - Dystocia
  - Hypocalcemia/metabolic bone disease
  - Parasitism

Investigations

1. Fecal examination
   a. Wet prep
      i. Worm eggs (Fig. 10-5)
         (1) Ascarid eggs
         (2) *Capillaria* (vase-shaped eggs with two poles)
         (3) Hookworm eggs (thin-walled, oval eggs)
         (4) Oxyurid eggs; note that rodent pinworm eggs may be seen in lizards fed on infested prey rodents
         (5) Spiruroid eggs (medium walled; contain larvae)
         (6) *Strongyloides* (larvae in fresh fecal samples; eggs are thin-walled and similar to *Entomelas*)
         (7) Flagellates (seen as motile protozoa)
         (8) Pentastomid eggs (see *Respiratory Tract Disorders*)
         (9) Trematode eggs
         (10) Protozoal cysts (Table 10-4)
   b. Gram stain

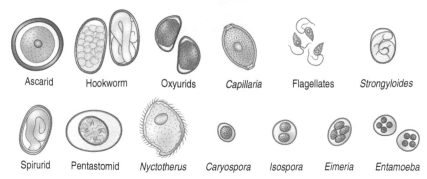

Ascarid   Hookworm   Oxyurids   *Capillaria*   Flagellates   *Strongyloides*

Spirurid   Pentastomid   *Nyctotherus*   *Caryospora*   *Isospora*   *Eimeria*   *Entamoeba*

Fig 10-5. Common gastrointestinal parasites of lizards (not drawn to scale).

Table 10-4 Lizards: Protozoal cysts	
Protozoa	**Description**
Eimeria	4 sporocysts each containing 2 sporozoites
Isospora	2 sporocysts containing 4 sporozoites
Caryospora	1 sporocyst
Cryptosporidium	Very small (2.5-6.0 μm). Identify using special stain, e.g., MZN
1 *Giardia*	Double anterior nuclei (resemble eyes)
2 *Entamoeba invadens*	Circular cyst containing 1-4 nuclei

Table 10-5 Radiographic contrast studies with 25 mL/kg of 25% barium sulfate in the green iguana *(Iguana iguana)*		
Position of barium sulfate	**Iguanas at 29.4° C**	**Iguanas at 24° C**
Complete gastric emptying (hr)	6-12	24
Small intestinal transit time (hr)	4-6	7
Complete small intestine emptying (hr)	16	23-29
Colon transit time (hr)	3-27	18-40
Complete colon emptying (hr)	33-68	112-147
Adapted from Smith et al (2001).		

2. Radiography
   a. Contrast studies with 25 mL/kg of 25% barium sulfate in the green iguana *(Iguana iguana)* (Table 10-5)
   b. Recommended timing for serial radiographs in iguanas is 0, 1, 2, 3, 4, 5, and 6 hours postgavage, then every 12 hours until barium is present within the distal descending small colon. *Note:* The total gut transit time for carnivorous lizards will be significantly shorter than for a herbivorous lizard such as the green iguana.
   c. Herbivorous lizards (e.g., green iguana) have a large sacculated colon adapted as a fermentative vat, which may normally appear as a large, gas-filled viscus on radiography.

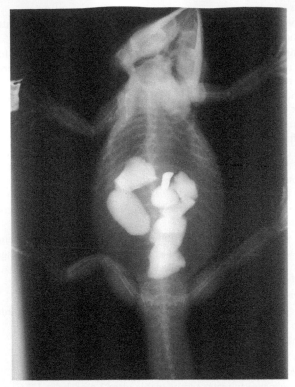

Fig 10-6. Radiograph of a bearded dragon following ingestion of large pieces of gravel.

    d. Enteritis: Gas-filled intestine especially obvious in carnivorous (i.e., simple gut) lizards.

    e. Radiodense foreign bodies (e.g., stones, gravel, and sand impactions; Fig. 10-6)

    f. Radiolucent foreign bodies (e.g., bark chippings) may require contrast studies to identify.

3. Routine hematology and biochemistry
4. Culture and sensitivity
5. Endoscopy
6. Biopsy/necropsy
    a. *Cryptosporidium*—especially the large intestine/colon
7. Ultrasonography

Management

- Good nursing care including fluid therapy (see *Nursing Care*)

Treatment/specific therapy

- Adenovirus
  - No treatment. Supportive therapy only
- Reovirus
  - No treatment. Supportive therapy only

- Salmonellosis
  - Probably best considered as a normal constituent of lizard cloacal/gut microflora
  - Rarely pathogenic to lizards
  - Excretion likely to increase during times of stress (e.g., movement, illness)
  - Treatment usually not appropriate, as unlikely to be effective long term and may encourage resistance
  - Recommendations for prevention of salmonellosis from captive reptiles issued by the Centers for Disease Control and Prevention include:
    - Pregnant women, children <5 years of age, and persons with impaired immune system function (e.g., AIDS) should not have contact with reptiles.
    - Because of the risk of becoming infected with *Salmonella* from a reptile, even without direct contact, households with pregnant women, children <5 years of age, or persons with impaired immune system function should not keep reptiles. Reptiles are not appropriate pets for childcare centers.
    - All persons should wash hands with soap immediately after any contact with a reptile or reptile cage.
    - Reptiles should be kept out of food preparation areas such as kitchens.
    - Kitchen sinks should not be used to wash food or water bowls, cages or vivaria used for reptiles, or to bathe reptiles. Any sink used for these purposes should be disinfected after use.
- *Cryptosporidium*
  - Direct life cycle; infection by exposure to water or feces containing infective oocysts
  - There is no recognized effective treatment.
  - Try metronidazole at 100 to 275 mg/kg PO once only.
  - Nitazoxanide at 5 mg/kg PO s.i.d.
  - Paromomycin at 300 to 800 mg/kg PO s.i.d. for 10 days
  - Oocysts *(C. parvum)* in water can be viable after 7 months at 15° C.
  - Disinfect by exposing to water above 64° C for >2 minutes.
  - *Cryptosporidium* oocysts are very resistant to chlorine or iodine.
- *Isospora* and *Eimeria* spp.
  - Direct life cycle
  - Sulfadimethoxine at 90 mg/kg PO (loading dose), then 45 mg/kg PO s.i.d. for 7 days plus thorough cage cleaning (Stahl 2000)
  - Trimethoprim-sulfa at 30 mg/kg PO daily for 5 days then every other day until elimination
  - Prey insects not eaten within 24 hours should be discarded and not recycled.
  - Treatment may be needed for several (2 to 6) weeks.
  - Quarantine all new introductions and undertake repeat fecal examinations.
- Flagellates and ciliates
  - Metronidazole
    - 100 to 257 mg/kg PO body weight once only. Repeat after 2 weeks if necessary.
    - 50 mg/kg PO every 5 to 7 days as necessary
  - Fenbendazole at 50 mg/kg PO daily for 5 days
  - *Note:* This may occur simultaneously with *Cryptosporidium* (Taylor et al 1999).
- *Giardia*
  - Metronidazole at 125 to 250 mg/kg PO every 48 to 72 hours for 7 to 14 days
  - Potential zoonosis
- Ascarids, hookworms, stomach worms, and oxyurids
  - Fenbendazole at 50 mg/kg PO weekly for 3 weeks. *Note:* Fenbendazole is metabolized to oxfendazole by the liver.
  - Oxfendazole at 68 mg/kg PO. Repeat every 2 weeks if necessary.

- Ivermectin at 200 μg/kg SC (care with Solomon Island skinks, *Corucia zebrata*)
- Topical emodepside plus praziquantel preparations (Profender, Bayer) at 56 μL/100 g body weight (Mehlhorn et al 2005b)
- *Note: Oxyuris* worms usually have a direct life cycle.
- Hookworms have a direct life cycle; infective larvae can penetrate the skin or infect via contaminated food and water.
- Trematodes
  - Praziquantel at 10 mg/kg PO; repeat after 2 weeks.
- Intestinal tympany
  - Pass stomach tube to release gas from stomach if present.
  - Administer activated charcoal or simethicone through stomach tube.
  - Typically linked to an excess intake of fermentable carbohydrate; may be linked with abnormal gut motility or obstruction
- Cloacal prolapse
  - Purse-string suture around cloaca for several weeks
  - Limit feeding to reduce straining during defecation.
  - If repeated prolapses, consider cloacopexy
- Foreign body
  - Surgical removal

Nutritional disorders

- Obesity (see also "Hepatic Lipidosis" in *Hepatic Disorders*)—especially bearded dragons, monitor lizards
- Metabolic bone disease (see *Musculoskeletal Disorders*)
- White muscle disease (especially in herbivorous reptiles)—vitamin E and selenium deficiency
- Hypovitaminosis A (see *Skin Disorders*)
- Biotin deficiency (see *Neurologic Disorders*)

Findings on clinical examination

- Gross enlargement of the coelom
- Anorexia
- Constipation (due to compression of gut by fat pads)
- Weakness
- Swollen long bones; mandibles, weakness, knuckling, inability to lift body, fractures (metabolic bone disease)

Investigations

1. Radiography
   a. Enlarged abdominal fat pads
   b. Assess skeletal integrity and bone density.
2. Routine hematology and biochemistry
   a. Obesity: Aspartate transaminase (AST) and bile acids may be elevated.
   b. Serum ionized and nonionized calcium, blood vitamin D_3 (25-hydroxycholecalciferol) levels
3. Culture and sensitivity

4. Endoscopy
5. Biopsy/necropsy
6. Ultrasonography
   a. Hepatic enlargement
   b. Ascites

Treatment/specific therapy

- Obesity
  - Fluid therapy and nutritional support
  - Attempt to reduce calorific intake if still feeding
  - Vitamin E supplementation to reduce risk of steatitis

Hepatic disorders

Viral

- Adenovirus (especially bearded dragons *Pogona* spp., water dragons *Physignathus* spp.—see *Systemic Disorders*)
- Herpesvirus (chuckwalla: *Sauromalus varius*—Wellehan et al 2003a)

Bacterial

- Mycobacteriosis (granulomas—may be multifocal)

Fungal

Protozoal

- Microsporidae (see *Systemic Disorders*)

Nutritional

- Hepatic lipidosis

Neoplasia

- Cholangiocarcinoma
- Spindle-cell sarcoma (Martorell et al 2002)
- Hepatoma

Other noninfectious problems

- Biliary hyperplasia (Wilson et al 2004)
- Melanomacrophage hyperplasia
- Amyloidosis

Findings on clinical examination

- Lethargy
- Anorexia
- Vomiting
- Coelomic distension (there may be an associated dyspnea—see also *Swollen/Distended Body Cavity*)
- Edematous swelling at back of pharynx
- Jaundice (icterus). *Note:* Bearded dragons (*Pogona* spp.) naturally have yellow-pigmented oral mucous membranes.

- Yellow urates
- Neurologic signs
- Petechial to ecchymotic hemorrhages (adenovirus)
- Severe postoperative hemorrhage (loss of clotting factors)

Investigations

1. Radiography
   a. Hepatomegaly (will often displace lungs and intestines dorsally)
2. Transillumination
   a. Useful in small, lightly pigmented lizards such as leopard geckos
   b. Direct a small bright light (e.g., from otoscope) through the body so as to view the underside of the lizard. The liver is usually readily identified and its relative size assessed.
3. Routine hematology and biochemistry
   a. Bile acids (fasting) <60 μmol/L

Bile acid stimulation test in the green iguana *(Iguana iguana)*

- 48-hour fast
- Initial blood sample taken
- Gavage with 4 mL of enteric herbivore diet (257 mg fat)
- Blood sample taken at 3 hours (emergence of food from pylorus)
- Blood sample taken at 8 hours (complete emptying of stomach)
- Results: Average bile acids (μmol/L) (*n* = 11). 0 h, 7.5 μmol/L; 3 h, 33.3 μmol/L; 8 h, 32.5 μmol/L.

From McBride et al (2004), undertaken on iguanas weighing between 356 g and 496 g.

---

4. Coelomic tap and cytology
   a. Avoid midline as likely to puncture ventral vena cava.
5. Culture and sensitivity
6. Endoscopy
7. Biopsy/necropsy
   a. Pale-colored liver (hepatic lipidosis)
   b. Hepatomegaly (Fig. 10-7)
8. Ultrasonography
   a. Hepatomegaly
   b. Ascites

Management

- Milk thistle *(Silybum marianum)* is a hepatoprotectant. Dose at 4 to 15 mg/kg PO b.i.d. or t.i.d.
- For ascites try furosemide at 2 to 5 mg/kg PO, SC, IM s.i.d. if ascitic.
- Lactulose 0.05 mL/100 g PO s.i.d.

Treatment/specific therapy

- Adenovirus
  - Supportive therapy only

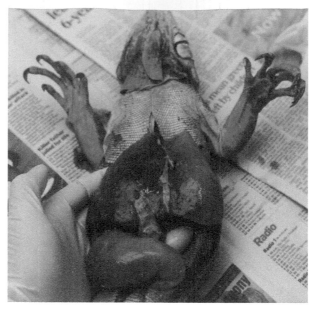

Fig 10-7. Hepatomegaly in a green iguana (postmortem).

- Herpesvirus
  - Attempt treatment with acyclovir at 80 mg/kg PO s.i.d. Very guarded prognosis
- Mycobacteriosis
  - Potential zoonosis. Consider euthanasia.
  - No successful treatment for mycobacteriosis in reptiles reported
- Hepatic lipidosis
  - Fluid therapy and nutritional support
  - Covering antibiotics
  - Lactulose 0.05 mL/100 g PO s.i.d.
  - Esophagostomy tube may be appropriate in some cases.
- Neoplasia: Treatment unlikely
- Amyloidosis
  - No treatment. Address possible initiating factors (e.g., chronic inflammatory conditions).

Pancreatic disorders

Diabetes mellitus (see *Endocrine Disorders*)

Cardiovascular and hematologic disorders

Viral

- Iguana herpesvirus
- Chameleon erythrocyte virus (iridovirus)

Bacterial

- Vegetative endocarditis (e.g., *Salmonella*, *Streptococcus*)

Fungal

Protozoal

- *Haemogregarina* spp.
- *Haemoproteus* spp.
- *Plasmodium* spp.
- *Shellackia* spp.
- *Sauroplasma* spp.

Parasitic

- Filarial nematodes (especially chameleons)

Nutritional

- Calcification of major vessels, including the aorta

Neoplasia

- Lymphoproliferative disorders (e.g., lymphoid and monocyte leukemia—see *Systemic Disorders*)

Other noninfectious problems

- Endocardiosis
- Myocardiosis
- Cardiomyopathy
- Myocardial infarction
- Metastatic calcification, especially of aorta
- Visceral gout (uric acid in pericardial sac—see *Renal Disorders*)
- Firefly (*Photonis* spp.) intoxication, especially in bearded dragons (see also *Systemic Disorders* and *Respiratory Tract Disorders*)
- Autoimmune hemolytic anemia (Boyer 2002)

Findings on clinical examination

- Lethargy
- Anorexia
- Edema, especially in back of pharynx
- Pale mucous membranes
- Exophthalmia (see also *Ophthalmic Disorders*)
- History of exposure to fireflies, linked with clinical signs of gaping, head shaking, blackened coloration, breathing difficulties, and death
- Swollen pharynx, hepatomegaly, depression, anorexia
- Murmurs may be heard in cases with marked heart disease (e.g., endocarditis). In most reptiles nothing will be heard.
- Necrosis of the extremities secondary to septicemic thrombi (often resulting from vegetative endocarditis—see *Systemic Disorders*; Fig. 10-8)

Investigations

1. Auscultation
   a. For many lizard species no heartbeat is audible with standard stethoscopes, except in cases of severe cardiac disease such as endocarditis. However, larger lizards such as bearded dragons can often be auscultated.

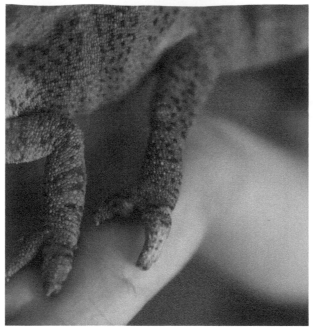

Fig 10-8. Necrosis of the digits in a Parson's chameleon secondary to septicemic thrombi.

   b. Frequency (HBF) per minute in reptiles can be estimated at:

     HBF = 33.4 $\left(\text{Weight}_{\text{kg}}^{-0.25}\right)$ assuming the reptile is at its correct body temperature

2. Radiography
   a. In many lizards the heart lies in the thoracic girdle and is, therefore, obscured somewhat radiographically.
   b. Mineralization of the aorta and intrapulmonary airways (metastatic calcification)
3. Ultrasonography and Doppler blood-flow detectors
4. Electrocardiogram
   a. ECG values recorded from lacertid lizard (*Gallotia bravoana*—Table 10-6)
   b. In this study higher temperatures increased the P segment and decreased the ST duration, RR duration, and cardiac axis.
5. Routine hematology and biochemistry
6. Cytology: May find filarial worms on blood smear
   a. Iguana blood: Clear spherical intracytoplasmic lesions (iguana herpesvirus)
   b. Chameleon blood: Intracytoplasmic inclusions (iridovirus)
7. Autoagglutination, Rouleaux formation, anisocytosis (autoimmune hemolytic anemia)
8. Culture and sensitivity
   a. Blood culture
9. Endoscopy
10. Biopsy/necropsy

Table 10-6 ECG values recorded from lacertid lizard (*Gallotia bravoana*)

	Mean	Range	SD
Weight (g)	166	105-244	53
Ambient temperature (°C)	20	20-21	0
Internal temperature (°C)	21	18-24	3
Heart rate (beats/min)	44	35-60	9
R-R interval (s)	1.43	1.05-1.78	0.3
P duration (s)	0.09	0.08-0.1	0.01
P amplitude (mV)	0.08	0.05-0.1	0.3
P-R interval (s)	0.15	0.1-0.18	0.03
R amplitude (mV)	0.15	0.1-0.18	0.03
QRS duration (s)	0.08	0.05-0.1	0.02
Q-T interval (s)	0.21	0.1-0.32	0.09
S-T interval (s)	0.14	0.02-0.2	0.07
S amplitude (mV)	0.03	0.02-0.05	0.01
T duration (s)	0.12	0.1-0.15	0.03
T amplitude (mV)	0.07	0.03-0.14	0.04
SV amplitude (mV)	0.12	0.04-0.2	0.05
SV duration (s)	0.13	0.08-0.2	0.05
Mean electrical axis (degrees)	80	45-135	44
QT:RR ratio	0.15	0.06-0.26	0.07
PR:RR ratio	0.1	0.09-0.13	0.02

From Martinez-Silvestre et al (2003).

Treatment/specific therapy

- Iguana herpesvirus
  - Acyclovir 80 mg/kg s.i.d. for 6 weeks
  - Often associated with severe hepatic fibrosis and interstitial nephritis
- Chameleon erythrocyte virus: No treatment
- Filarial nematodes—see *Skin Disorders*
- Firefly (*Photonis* spp.) intoxication
  - Fireflies contain cardiac glycoside-like cardenolides that suppress heart rate.
  - Supportive treatment, including gavage with activated charcoal
- Hemoparasites
  - Loading dose of chloroquine phosphate (5 mg/kg PO) and primaquine phosphate (0.5 mg/kg PO)
  - Continue with chloroquine at 2.5 mg/kg PO once weekly and primaquine at 0.5 mg/kg PO once weekly for 12 to 16 weeks
- *Shelackia* spp.: Rarely pathogenic—may indicate immunosuppression consistent with concurrent disease or poor environmental conditions
- Leukemia
  - Treatment potentially difficult and untried
  - Radiation therapy was used by Martin et al (2003). Single low-dose whole-body radiation treatment of 1 gray. A reduction in WBC count was noted after 1 month and was normal, with normal differential by 3 months.

- Autoimmune hemolytic anemia
  - Prednisolone at 0.5 mg/kg PO s.i.d. for 2 weeks and then every other day until packed cell volume (PCV) stable
  - Cimetidine 4 mg/kg PO s.i.d. if evidence of gastric hemorrhage
  - Covering antibiosis
  - Blood transfusion
- Cardiomyopathies and other cardiac disorders
  - Furosemide at 2 to 5 mg IM, IV, or PO s.i.d. or b.i.d.
  - Pimobendan at 0.2 mg/kg PO s.i.d.
- Metastatic calcification
  - See *Musculoskeletal Disorders.*

Systemic disorders

Brumation

Brumation is a naturally occurring period of reduced activity that in the wild is associated with adverse environmental conditions such as low temperatures, aridness, or inadequate food supplies. It can be incorrectly referred to as hibernation.

Brumation is commonly seen in bearded dragons but may be seen in other species from high-latitude areas or climates that experience adverse seasons such as leopard geckos. Normal brumation behavior involves the lizard going off its food, basking less, and hiding away more. This change in behavior can be quite rapid and alarming if not expecting it. If unsure, check these pointers:

1. Weigh the lizard every 3 to 4 days. Brumating reptiles lose little or no weight during brumation, typically no more than around 1% to 2% per month.
2. Assess the lizards. A sick lizard will show fairly rapid signs of loss of condition, closed eyes, and loss of muscle tone and may gape, whereas a brumating reptile will appear otherwise normal and healthy with bright eyes and an alert appearance when disturbed.
3. Has this happened before? With older reptiles there may be a history of its happening around the same time the previous year.

If you are confident that your bearded dragon is brumating, then reduce the ambient temperature by a few degrees and alter the day-length settings to around 8 to 10 hours and monitor. Do not offer food during brumation unless the lizard appears hungry. Typically brumation will last for around 6 to 8 weeks, although it can extend up to 5 months.

Viral

- Adenovirus (inland bearded dragon *Pogona vitticeps* and Rankin's dragon *P. henrylawsonii*)
- Iguana herpesvirus (see *Cardiovascular and Hematologic Disorders*)
- Iridovirus

Bacterial

- Septicemia/bacteremia
- *Chlamydophila* and *Chlamydophila*-like organisms
- Mycobacteriosis (see also *Respiratory Disorders* and *Skin Disorders*)
- Streptococci (bacteremia)
- *Salmonella arizona*
- *Listeria monocytogenes* (Girling and Fraser 2004)

Fungal

Protozoal

- Intranuclear coccidiosis
- Microsporidae (see also *Hepatic Disorders*), especially bearded dragons

Parasitic

- Filarial nematodes (see also *Skin Disorders* and *Cardiovascular and Hematologic Disorders*)

Neoplasia

- Lymphoma and leukemia
- Mesothelioma
- Hemangiosarcoma

Other noninfectious problems

- Cardiac disease (see *Cardiovascular and Hematologic Disorders*)
- Intracoelomic hemorrhage
- Firefly (*Photonis* spp.) intoxication (see also *Cardiovascular and Hematologic Disorders* and *Respiratory Tract Disorders*)
- Gout (visceral, articular, and renal—see *Renal Disorders*)
- Amyloidosis

Findings on clinical examination

- Lethargy
- Anorexia (see *Anorexia* notes in Chapter 11 for a differential list)
- Edema
- Sudden mortalities
- Neurologic signs
- Anorexia, lethargy, and death, especially in bearded dragons (adenovirus). Petechial to ecchymotic hemorrhages may occur.
- Necrosis of the extremities secondary to septicemic thrombi (often resulting from vegetative endocarditis—see *Cardiovascular and Hematologic Disorders*)

Investigations

1. Radiography
2. Routine hematology and biochemistry
3. Cytology: May find filarial worms on blood smear
4. Culture and sensitivity
   a. Blood culture
5. Ziehl-Neelsen staining and polymerase chain reaction (PCR) for mycobacteria
6. Immunohistochemistry and PCR for *Chlamydophila* and *Chlamydia*-like organisms (Soldati et al 2004)
7. Endoscopy
8. Biopsy/necropsy
   a. Single or multiple granulomas (mycobacteria, fungi, *Chlamydophila pneumoniae*, *Chlamydia*-like organisms)
   b. Microsporida (gram-positive, acid fast) found in liver, kidneys, lung, gonads, and CNS
   c. Adenovirus
   d. Neoplasia
9. Ultrasonography

Treatment/specific therapy

- Adenovirus
  - Symptomatic treatment only
  - Exclude parents and siblings from breeding groups to eliminate potential carriers.
- Iridovirus
  - Symptomatic treatment only
  - Some may actually be invertebrate iridoviruses, originating from infected crickets.
- Bacterial infections
  - Appropriate antibiosis
  - Supportive therapy
  - Symptomatic management of necrotic extremities; may require surgical amputation
- Listeriosis
  - Not normally a part of reptile gut flora
  - Case described in Girling and Fraser (2004) linked to feeding contaminated mouse pups that had been frozen and defrosted
- Mycobacteriosis
  - Potential zoonosis. Consider euthanasia.
  - No successful treatment for mycobacteriosis in reptiles reported
- Microsporidae
  - No effective treatment
  - Albendazole at 10 mg/kg PO s.i.d. may prevent replication.
  - Fenbendazole at 10 to 20 mg/kg PO s.i.d.
- Intranuclear coccidiosis
  - Potentiated sulfonamides at 30 mg/kg PO s.i.d.
- Filarial nematodes
  - Ivermectin at 200 µg/kg SC (care with Solomon Island skinks, *Corucia zebrata*)
  - Surgical resection of associated skin granulomas
- Neoplasia
  - Surgical resection if feasible
- Lymphoma and leukemia (see *Cardiovascular and Hematologic Disorders*)

Swollen/distended body cavity

Infections may cause organopathies that in turn result in a swollen or distended coelom.

Neoplasia
- Hepatic neoplasia
- Renal neoplasia

Other noninfectious problems
- Obesity (enlarged coelomic fat pads)
- Distension of the gastrointestinal tract (e.g., secondary to foreign body obstruction, intussusception, or hypocalcemia—intestinal atony)
- Distension of the bladder (bladder calculi, bladder atony, CNS lesions)
- Hepatomegaly
- Ascites
- Liver disease
- Hypoproteinemia

- Cardiovascular disease
- Septicemia
- Renomegaly

Reproductive causes

- Gravid
- Dystocia (see *Reproductive Disorders*)

Findings on clinical examination

- Swollen coelom
- Constipation (secondary to external compression of the gut by enlarged fat pads)
- Dyspnea
- Other clinical signs may be present depending on the underlying cause.

Investigations

1. Radiography
   a. Distended viscus
   b. Bladder calculi
   c. Foreign bodies (e.g., sand or stone impactions)
2. Routine hematology and biochemistry
3. Coelomic tap
4. Culture and sensitivity
5. Endoscopy
6. Biopsy/necropsy
7. Ultrasonography
   a. Coelomic fluid
   b. Distended viscus

Management

- Fluid can be drawn from the coelom to relieve the distension, but this may interfere with the fluid balance of the lizard.
- Furosemide at 2 to 5 mg IM, IV, or PO s.i.d. or b.i.d.

Treatment/specific therapy

- See individual headings.

Musculoskeletal disorders

Bacterial

- Septic arthritis
- Osteomyelitis
- Cellulitis
- Myositis

Fungal
Parasitic

- Heavy parasite burden, especially hemoparasites (anemia) or gastrointestinal parasites (protozoa, helminths)

Nutritional

- Metabolic bone disease
- Nutritional secondary hyperparathyroidism from dietary calcium deficiency, dietary calcium/phosphorus imbalance, hypovitaminosis D_3 (lack of exposure to ultraviolet light, lack of dietary vitamin D_3, protein deficiency—see also "Noninfectious Problems")
- Metastatic calcification of smooth muscle of various organs, including cardiovascular system, pulmonary system, gut, and urogenital system. Typically linked to excess dietary vitamin D_3 intake (e.g., oversupplementation, feeding with dog and cat food). Especially problematic in herbivorous reptiles, such as iguanas (but see "Treatment")
- Hypovitaminosis E (often combined with selenium deficiency)

Neoplasia

- Fibromas (especially mandibles in green iguana)
- Liposarcoma
- Myeloma
- Osteosarcoma

Other noninfectious problems

- Metabolic bone disease
- Renal secondary hyperparathyroidism
- Also liver and intestinal disease—see also "Nutritional" above
- Autotomy (geckos, iguanids, lacertids, and some skinks)
- Fractures (traumatic), especially long-toed lizards such as green iguanas and water dragons
- Spondylosis/spondylitis
- Hypertrophic osteopathy (also known as hypertrophic pulmonary osteoarthropathy, HPOA)
- Osteopetrosis
- Kyphosis/scoliosis: Genetic; disease of the associated musculature (myopathies); nutritional disorders
- Floppy-tail—a particular form of kyphosis associated with small arboreal lizards, especially day geckos and crested geckos
- Dysecdysis with resultant sloughing of distal extremities, such as toes and tail-tip (see *Skin Disorders*)
- Avascular necrosis of the distal tail
- Swelling at tail base in males (seminal plugs—see *Reproductive Disorders*)
- Congenital defects—typically abnormal incubation environment

Findings on clinical examination

- Any limb or spinal swelling, fracture, or paralysis should be considered as a possible sign of a pathological fracture (Fig. 10-9).
- Soft mandibles, foreshortening of the maxillae, swollen midshaft of long bones, kyphosis/scoliosis, weakness, inability to support own body weight (metabolic bone disease)
- Muscle weakness, inability to support body or hunt/locate food (Fig. 10-10)

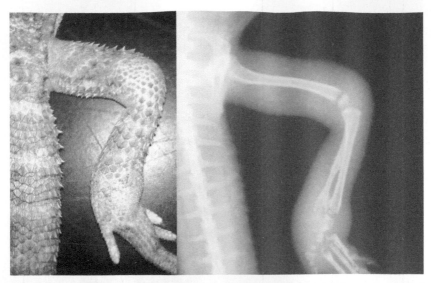

Fig 10-9. Swollen tarsus with osteolysis arising from a septic arthritis in the bearded dragon above. Note the pathological fracture in the distal femur.

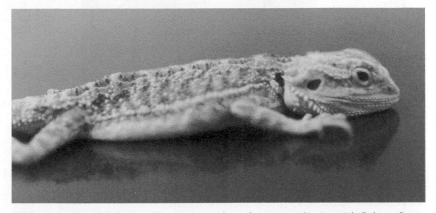

Fig 10-10. A young bearded dragon with extreme muscle weakness secondary to metabolic bone disease.

- Muscle fasciculations and other neurologic signs
- Withering and fracture of distal tail
- Loss of digits
- Scoliosis in crested geckos, often accompanied by kinking of the tail
- In arboreal geckos the tail hangs either to the side or over the back when resting in a head-down position (floppy-tail).

Investigations

1. Husbandry
   a. Discuss access to full-spectrum lighting, frequency of lightbulb changing, provision of calcium/provision in suitable form, intraspecies or interspecies interactions that may influence access to basking sites and/or food/calcium sources.

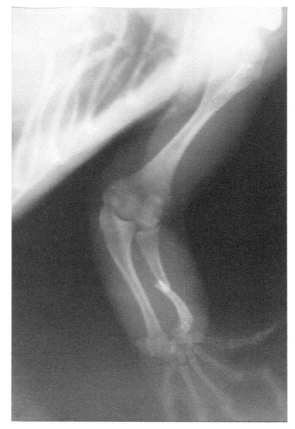

Fig 10-11. Traumatic fracture of the radius in a green iguana.

2. Radiography
   a. Pathologic (metabolic bone disease, neoplasia) or traumatic fractures (Fig. 10-11)
   b. Osteolysis (osteomyelitis, myeloma, osteosarcoma)
   c. Fibrous osteodystrophy (metabolic bone disease)
3. Other signs of metabolic bone disease: Loss of bone density and cortical bone thinning
   a. Fibromas and other neoplasias
   b. Hypertrophic osteopathy
   c. Osteopetrosis—excessive thickening of the bones
   d. Septic arthritis
   e. Gout: Radiolucent uric acid accumulation
4. Routine hematology and biochemistry
   a. Blood vitamin D_3 (25-hydroxycholecalciferol) levels: normal plasma levels for Pogonids = 105 nmol/L; for green iguana (*Iguana iguana*) = 265 nmol/L
   b. Total calcium, ionized calcium, phosphate
   c. Hyperphosphatemia (renal secondary hyperparathyroidism)
5. Culture and sensitivity
6. Spondylitis, osteomyelitis

7. Cytology (fine-needle aspiration)
8. Endoscopy
9. Biopsy
10. Ultrasonography

Treatment/specific therapy

- Autotomy
  - For those species that naturally autotomize, then no treatment beyond minimizing blood loss is necessary; suturing will prevent normal tail regeneration. *Note:* The crested gecko *(Rhacodactylus ciliatus)* is an exception—unlike the other geckos in the *Rhacodactylus* genus the tails do not regrow once shed. For other species with traumatic or surgical tail amputation, skin closure is necessary.
- Metabolic bone disease
  - Usually due to secondary nutritional hyperparathyroidism linked with either failure to provide sufficient calcium supplementation or exposure to UVB
  - Parenteral calcium gluconate or lactate at 1.0 to 2.5 mg/kg daily
  - Oral vitamin D_3 at 200 IU/kg every 7 days PO, IM
  - Dietary calcium supplementation
  - Exposure to full-spectrum lighting as a UVB source
  - Calcitonin at 1.5 IU/kg SC s.i.d. if normocalcemic
- Metastatic calcification
  - No effective treatment
  - Reduce hypercalcemia by
    - Calcitonin at 1.5 IU/kg SC s.i.d.
    - Fluid therapy at 15 mL/kg Hartmann's solution intracoelomic until normocalcaemic
  - Although often linked to excessive vitamin D_3 supplementation, many cases may be due to low levels of calcitrol, commonly secondary to renal disease. This leads to toxic levels of parathormone production with associated abnormal tissue mineralization and further renal damage.
- Osteopetrosis
  - Hereditary disorder. Symptomatic treatment
- Hypertrophic osteopathy
  - Symptomatic treatment
  - Usually terminal
- Heavy parasite burden
  - Treat as described under relevant sections.
- Septic arthritis
  - Surgical investigation and treatment. May require partial or complete amputation. Consider underlying possibility of vegetative endocarditis (see *Cardiovascular and Hematologic Disorders*).
- Abscessation and osteomyelitis, myositis
  - Appropriate antibiosis
  - Consider amputation if damage is extensive.
- Spondylosis: No treatment
- Spondylitis
  - Appropriate antibiosis
  - Consider NSAIDs (e.g., meloxicam at 0.2 mg/kg once daily or every other day); in the green iguana, see Hernandez-Divers 2006b

- Kyphosis/scoliosis/ floppy-tail
  - No specific treatment
  - Assess for underlying metabolic bone disease (see above).
  - Can occur in crested geckos without obvious metabolic bone disease. May be a muscular dystrophy–like disorder
  - Floppy-tail is an acquired disorder seen in certain arboreal lizards and is related to excessive time resting head-down on completely vertical surfaces (e.g., vivarium sides). It is not always associated with metabolic bone disease but is associated with pelvic and sacral abnormalities, which are presumed to be linked to the mechanical stress of the weight of the tail on the tail base musculature and underlying skeleton.
- Hypertrophic pulmonary osteopathy
  - Likely linked to multiple organ disorders. Very guarded prognosis
- Neoplasia
  - Surgical resection if possible (e.g., amputation of distal extremities)

Neurologic disorders

Viral
- Paramyxovirus
- Adenovirus (rare)

Bacterial
- Septicemia
- CNS granuloma

Fungal
- CNS granuloma

Protozoal
- Microsporidae (see *Systemic Disorders*), especially bearded dragons
- *Acanthamoeba*
- *Toxoplasma*

Parasitic
- Larval migrans

Nutritional
- Biotin deficiency
- Hypovitaminosis E (often combined with selenium deficiency—see *Musculoskeletal Disorders*)
- Hypocalcemia (see "Metabolic Bone Disease" in *Musculoskeletal Disorders*)
- Hypoglycemia

Neoplasia
- Schwannoma

Other noninfectious problems
- Hepatic disease (see *Hepatic Disorders*)
- Toxins
- Iatrogenic (e.g., aminoglycosides, ivermectin, metronidazole)

- Nicotine
- Cedar wood shavings
- Ingestion of toxic plants (e.g., *Diffenbachia*, azaleas)

Findings on clinical examination

- Twitching of toes, occasionally tail tip, muscle fasciculations (hypocalcemic tetany). May be pronounced or complete muscle flaccidity. Often accompanied by other signs of metabolic bone disease (see *Musculoskeletal Disorders*)
- Varied neurologic signs may be seen with paromyxovirus infections in lizards, but infections are often asymptomatic.
- Weakness
- Head tilt (vestibular disease)
- Convulsions
- Death
- History of prolonged intake of raw eggs (biotin deficiency)

Investigations

1. Radiography
2. Routine hematology and biochemistry
   a. Blood vitamin D$_3$ (25-hydroxycholecalciferol) levels; also total calcium, ionized calcium, phosphate
   b. Serology for paromyxovirus
3. Culture and sensitivity
4. Endoscopy
5. Biopsy/necropsy
6. Ultrasonography

Treatment/specific therapy

1. *Acanthamoeba* and *Toxoplasma*
   a. Treatment difficult
   b. Metronidazole at 100 to 275 mg/kg PO once only
   c. Trimethoprim-sulfadiazine at 15 mg/kg PO daily
   d. Potential zoonoses
2. Biotin deficiency
   a. Described in monitor lizards (*Varanus* spp.) fed on raw eggs
   b. Supplement diet.
   c. Treat symptomatically.
3. Hypoglycemia
   a. Uncommon
   b. Parenteral and oral glucose therapy
4. Larval migrans: Treat as for endoparasites. Poor prognosis
5. Toxins
   a. Remove from source of toxin.
   b. For ingested toxins, flush out stomach under GA or perform gastrotomy.
   c. Provide supportive care.

Ophthalmic disorders

Ophthalmic examination

Diurnal lizards have all cone retinae; nocturnal lizards have both rods and cones. Lizards have one or two fovea and a conus papillaris (analogous to the avian pecten). The lacrimal and harderian glands are well developed.

Most lizards have eyelids, but many geckos possess instead a snakelike spectacle (an exception to this is the commonly kept leopard gecko, *Eublepharis macularis*). The eyelids may be fused as in chameleons. These lizards also lack a nictitating membrane.

Examination of the posterior segment of the eye is difficult as the iris muscle fibers are striated and partly under voluntary control. Therefore, parasympatholytics (e.g., atropine) and sympathomimetics (e.g., phenylephrine) will not work. Consider examination by:

1. Using low light levels
2. General anesthesia
3. Nonparasympatholytic mydriatics such as vecuronium. These are inappropriate in lizards that possess a spectacle.

Differential diagnoses for ophthalmic disorders

Bacterial

- *Pseudomonas*
- *Aeromonas*

Fungal

- Keratitis
- Panophthalmitis

Protozoal

- *Trichomonas* spp. (subspectacular abscess)

Nutritional

- Hypovitaminosis A (chameleons)

Neoplasia

Other noninfectious problems

- Trauma
- Photokeratitis
- Foreign body
- Retained spectacle
- Occlusion of nasolacrimal duct
- Congenital absence of nasolacrimal duct
- Stenosis due to or following inflammation
- Cardiovascular disease (bilateral exophthalmos)
- Congenital defects
- Microphthalmia—often associated with head abnormalities
- Some Caribbean iguanas have red sclerae; this should not be mistaken for pathology.

Findings on clinical examination

- Conjunctivitis
- Blepharitis

378

- Blepharospasm (foreign body, ulceration)
- Ocular discharge
- Corneal ulceration
- Deep ulceration followed by perforation and iris collapse
- Hypopyon
- Uveitis
- Keratitis
- Whitish material in eye (hypovitaminosis A, secondary infection)
- Cataracts
- Retinal degeneration
- Exophthalmia
- Distension of the subspectacular space (in species with a spectacle)

Investigations

1. Ophthalmic examination
   a. For those species with a spectacle:
      i. Space beneath spectacle distended with *clear* fluid (occlusion of nasolacrimal duct)
      ii. Subspectacular abscess: The eye appears *opaque* and the spectacle may be bulge due to increased pressure in the corneospectacular space. This condition may be unilateral or bilateral.
2. Radiography
3. Routine hematology and biochemistry
4. Culture and sensitivity
5. Endoscopy
6. Biopsy/necropsy
7. Ultrasonography

Treatment/specific therapy

- Bacterial keratitis
  - Topical ophthalmic antibiotics; may also benefit from systemic antibiotics
- Fungal keratitis
  - Topical ophthalmic antimycotics
- Corneal ulceration
  - Topical antibiosis and lubrication
  - Suturing of eyelids together may be of benefit.
  - Excoriation followed by topical tissue glue may be of use.
  - Deep ulceration followed by perforation and iris collapse
  - Enucleation if ocular penetration and uveitis
- Subspectacular abscess
  - Treatment involves surgical incision into the spectacle to allow an assessment for any corneal lesions.
  - All debris should be flushed from the corneal surface and, if possible, the nasolacrimal duct cannulated and flushed.
  - Topical ophthalmic antibiotic or antimycotic preparations should be used.
  - A new spectacle should form at the next skin shed. To prevent desiccation, consider attempting to suture the contact lens in place.

- Photokeratitis
  - Treat topically as for keratitis in other species.
  - Remove full-spectrum lighting for several days and adjust lighting.
  - Usually associated with incorrect positioning of full-spectrum lights—lights should be above the reptile, not to the side, where horizontal rays of UVB can bypass protective eyebrow ridges and damage the cornea.
- Nasolacrimal duct occlusion
  - Treatment is similar to subspectacular abscess.
- Congenital defects
  - No treatment
  - Consider incubation parameters (temperature, humidity, etc.) as well as genetic factors when considering cause.

Endocrine disorders

Endocrine disorders are poorly investigated in reptiles.
- Hypothyroidism (see *Skin Disorders*)
- Diabetes mellitus

Findings on clinical examination

- Anorexia
- Polydipsia/polyuria
- Weight loss
- Dysecdysis (see *Skin Disorders*)

Investigations

1. Radiography
2. Routine hematology and biochemistry
   a. Hyperglycemia (differentiate from stress hyperglycemia)
   b. Serum insulin
   c. Serum glucagon (may be more important in glucose regulation than insulin)
3. Coelomic tap
4. Culture and sensitivity
5. Endoscopy
6. Biopsy/necropsy
7. Ultrasonography

Treatment/specific therapy

- Diabetes mellitus
  - Symptomatic therapy
  - Start on high-fiber, low-protein diet.
  - Consider use of insulin.

Renal disorders

Impairment of fluid balance, or renal disease, causes pathological crystallization of uric acid crystals, which presents as visceral or articular gout.

Viral

- Iguana herpesvirus (see *Cardiovascular and Hematologic Disorders*)

Bacterial

- Bacterial nephritis

Fungal

- Fungal nephritis

Neoplasia

Other noninfectious problems

- Gout (renal, visceral, and articular)
- Bladder calculi
- Renal failure of middle-aged iguanas
- Iatrogenic (nephrotoxic drugs, such as aminoglycosides)

Findings on clinical examination

- Anorexia
- Lethargy
- Weight loss
- Polydipsia/polyuria (see also "Diabetes Mellitus" in *Pancreatic Disorders*)
- Anuria
- Edema and swellings (Fig. 10-12)
- Hind-limb weakness (see also *Neurologic Disorders*)

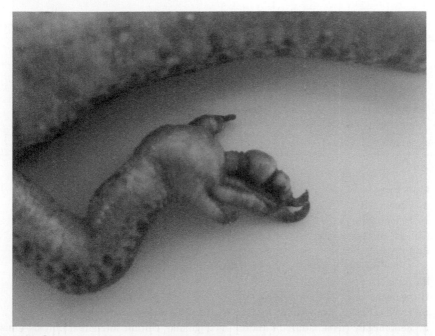

Fig 10-12. Severe gout in the foot of a pink-tongued skink.

- Constipation (swollen kidneys may occlude pelvic canal)
- Pale mucous membranes
- Pharyngeal edema
- Mortalities
- Vague ill health, anorexia in 3- to 8-year-old iguanas (renal failure of middle-aged iguanas)

Investigations

1. Radiography
   a. Renomegaly. The kidneys of many lizards, especially iguanids, are located in the pelvic cavity. Difficult to see normally, they can extend into the coelomic cavity if enlarged.
2. Routine hematology and biochemistry
   a. No good single test
   b. Lizards with renal disease may show hyperuricemia, hyperuremia, hyperphosphatemia, hyperkalemia, hyponatremia, and hyperproteinemia or hypoproteinemia, although none of these is a consistent finding.

Renal failure of middle-aged iguanas

1. High serum phosphorus (normal range 1.0 to 3.0 mmol/L; can be up to 5.7 mmol/L in gravid female iguanas) and $Ca:PO_4 < 1$.
2. Serum urea and creatinine levels usually normal. Uric acid levels only elevated in terminal disease.
3. Creatine kinase and AST often high.
4. May be hypocalcemic or hypercalcemic.

Estimation of renal clearance in the green iguana

1. Fast the reptile for 24 hours (allow normal access to water).
2. Maintain at preferred body temperature.
3. Inject IV iohexol at 75 mg/kg.
4. Collect blood samples (minimum 0.5 mL) at 4 hours, 8 hours, and 24 hours.
5. Centrifuge and submit plasma on ice for analysis.
6. Mean glomerular filtration rate (GFR) for healthy iguanas is 14.8 to 18.3 mL/kg per hour.

(Hernandez-Divers 2006a)

---

3. Urinalysis
   a. Renal casts
   b. Inflammatory cells
4. Culture and sensitivity
5. Endoscopy
   a. Abnormalities in shape, color, or size of kidneys
6. Biopsy/necropsy
7. Ultrasonography
   a. Hyperechoic or hypoechoic, focal or multifocal changes; alteration of size
   b. Renomegaly (renal failure of middle-aged iguanas; chronic interstitial fibrosis—may be associated with iguana herpesvirus; renal gout)

Management

- For fluid therapy, see *Nursing Care.*

Treatment/specific therapy

- Renal failure of middle-aged iguanas
  - Etiology probably dietary (excessive animal protein) and may include chronic mild dehydration
  - Fluid therapy
  - Other renal therapeutic drugs could, with caution, be tried.
- Gout
  - Fluid therapy
  - Allopurinol at 10 mg/kg PO s.i.d. *Note:* This will only prevent subsequent uric acid deposition.
  - Very guarded prognosis
  - May be linked to excess dietary protein, renal disease, chronic dehydration, use of nephrotoxic drugs

Reproductive disorders

Nutritional

- Hypocalcemia (with subsequent oviductal inertia)

Neoplasia

Other noninfectious problems

- Hemorrhage from ovarian artery
- Dystocia
- Preovulatory ovarian stasis (POOS)
- Egg stasis (postovulatory)
- Egg yolk peritonitis
- Ovarian necrosis
- Seminal plugs (caseous debris accumulating in the inverted hemipenes)

Findings on clinical examination

- Inappetence, anorexia
- History of reproductive activity (e.g., mating, burrowing in nesting chamber or other areas of vivarium). Some eggs may have been laid. *Note:* Some healthy females (especially iguanas, water dragons, bearded dragons, veiled chameleons) will spontaneously ovulate without the presence of a male or others of the same species.
- Restlessness
- Obvious swelling of the coelomic cavity (not always obvious)
- Hind-limb weakness
- Signs of metabolic bone disease (see *Systemic Disorders*)
- Dehydration in neglected cases (especially veiled chameleons)
- Swelling caudal to cloaca in males (seminal plugs)
- Sudden death (hemorrhage from ovarian artery)

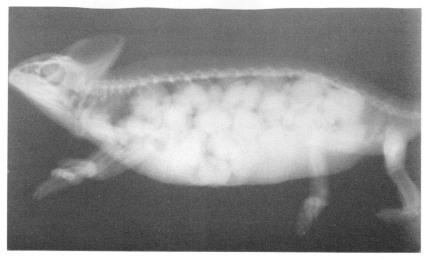

Fig 10-13. Dystocia complicated by superovulation in a veiled chameleon.

Investigations

1. Radiography
   a. The hemipenes are calcified and therefore visible in some lizard species, especially monitor lizards (Varanidae).
   b. Eggs may be reasonably well calcified (many geckos) or poorly calcified (iguanas, water dragons); these latter are visible as circular to oval opacities. Typically these are in the caudal coelom, but because there is no diaphragm, in extreme cases they can occupy much of the coelomic cavity, displacing other organs dorsally. Eggs that are heavily mineralized, excessively large, or irregular in shape are usually abnormal (Fig. 10-13).
   c. Ensures there are no obvious obstructions (e.g., pelvic deformities from metabolic bone disease)
   d. Fetal skeletons may be visible in advanced gestation in live-bearing lizards, such as Solomon Island skinks *(Corucia zebrata)*.
2. Transillumination
   a. Useful in small, lightly pigmented lizards such as leopard geckos
   b. Direct a small bright light (e.g., from an otoscope) through the body so as to view the underside of the lizard. The liver is usually readily identified and its relative size assessed. Eggs, bladder size, and fat pads can all be identified and assessed.
3. Routine hematology and biochemistry
   a. Blood calcium levels
4. Culture and sensitivity
5. Endoscopy
6. Biopsy/necropsy
   a. Hemorrhage in periovarian tissue
7. Ultrasonography
   a. Useful for preovulatory ovarian stasis

Treatment/specific therapy

- Seminal plugs
  - Gentle removal
  - May be linked with hypovitaminosis A
- Dystocia
  - Provision of correct environment, including appropriate temperature, humidity, and nesting chamber, may induce normal egg-laying. Supplement with calcium (e.g., calcium gluconate at 1 mL/kg PO b.i.d.).
  - Medical induction
    - Calcium gluconate at 100 mg/kg IM, SC every 6 to 12 hours
    - Oxytocin 5 to 20 IU/kg IM given 1 hour after last calcium
    - Repeat over 2 to 3 cycles if lizard is otherwise healthy.
    - If some eggs still retained after 48 hours, consider surgery.
    - Argipressin at 0.01 to 1.0 µg/kg IV every 12-24 hr for several treatments (more potent than oxytocin in reptiles)
  - Percutaneous ovocentesis (Hall and Lewbart 2006)
  - Only useful in small lizards with small numbers of eggs
  - Performed under anesthesia with sterile 23G butterfly catheter. Beware of yolk leaking into coelomic cavity, aspiration of the viscera or their contents, both of which will trigger a serositis. Allow lizard to pass collapsed eggs.
  - Salpingotomy
  - Ovariosalpingectomy: Make a paramedian incision. Avoid incising into the ventral midline due to ventral vena cava (visible with transillumination).

Neonatal disorders

See *Neonatal Disorders* in Chapter 11.

Behavioral disorders

- Behavioral ITB (see *Skin Disorders*)
- Aggression in adult male iguanas

Signs

- Heightened aggression; iguanas may attack owner or passersby through the vivarium glass.
- Some male iguanas show heightened aggression at particular times of their female owner's menstrual cycle. Thought to be pheromonal in origin

Treatment/specific therapy

- Behavioral management is difficult due to restricted space available to give each iguana its personal space.
- With sexually motivated behavior, temporary improvement may be achieved with regular injections of delmadinone acetate at 1 mg/kg IM. Repeat as necessary.
- If delmadinone is effective, consider castration.

11

Snakes

Snakes are popular reptile pets, and there has been a resurgence in their popularity with the breeding of a variety of color morphs. A huge number of species are available in the pet trade, but the commonly kept species are listed in Table 11-1.

The internal anatomy of a snake is shown in Figure 11-1 (see also "Radiography" in *Musculoskeletal Disorders*).

Table 11-1 Commonly kept species of snake: Key facts		
Species	**Notes**	**Common disorders**
Royal python (*Python regius*)	This is a small python, growing to 90 to 120 cm. It has a not undeserved reputation for prolonged fasting, probably as a result of poor husbandry and endogenous cycles, although this is less pronounced with the modern captive-bred individuals and color morphs.	Dermatitis, dysecdysis, and pneumonia Anorexia, especially in wild-caught or captive farmed individuals
Burmese python (*Python bivittatus*)	This python is a potentially very large snake; adults can reach up to 5 to 7 m long with a large muscular cross section. Adults are usually reasonably behaved, but hatchlings and youngsters can be aggressive.	Dysecdysis, burns, pneumonia, IBD
Boa constrictor (*Boa constrictor constrictor*)	A large snake up to 1.8 to 3.0 m long. Usually handleable but some individuals can be aggressive. Several color morphs available; there has been some selective breeding to reduce size using naturally occurring dwarf island subspecies.	Snake mites, dysecdysis, IBD
Corn snake (*Elaphe guttata guttata*)	Moderate-sized rodent-eating snake that makes excellent introduction to snake-keeping. This is probably the nearest there is to a domestic snake; it is available in a very wide range of color morphs, grows to a manageable size (around 1.0 m), and readily takes frozen-defrosted prey.	Dysecdysis, *Cryptosporidium*
King snakes (*Lampropeltis* spp.)	King snakes are natural predators of snakes and other reptiles and so are usually kept individually.	Dysecdysis, obesity
Garter snakes (*Thamnophis* spp.)	Small to medium-sized snakes. Can be nervous on handling. Many of these are earthworm, fish, and amphibian predators, although they can be readily converted onto mammalian prey.	Septicemia, thiamine deficiency
IBD, *inclusion body disease.*		

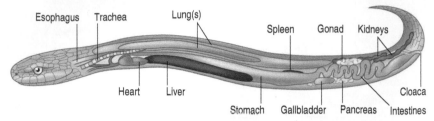

Fig 11-1. Internal anatomy of a snake (lateral).

Consultation and handling

A healthy snake should be reasonably alert and responsive to touch. If it is flaccid or exhibiting CNS signs, such as "star-gazing," it is likely to be suffering a septicemia, poisoning, or possibly a protozoal infection such as *Acanthamoeba*.

Start the examination at the head and work backward. Larger snakes such as the pythons and boas may require one or more people to hold them while you perform your examination. A gag is usually required to open the mouth—wooden spatulas work reasonably well and are less traumatic than metal equivalents. Do not encourage staff or clients to drape large constricting snakes across the shoulders and around the neck because if the snake feels insecure, it may well tighten its grip unexpectedly.

Venomous snakes require specialist handling equipment and should only be handled by a competent herpetologist or while under an anesthetic.

Microchipping

- Left nape of the neck, subcutaneously placed at twice the length of the head from the tip of the nose
- Skin closure is achieved either by suture or with tissue glue.

Sexing

Many snakes are not obviously sexually dimorphic or dichromatic. The safest and most popular way of sexing monomorphic snakes is by "probe-sexing," in which a small, well-lubricated and blunt-ended rod is gently inserted into the cloaca and then directed caudally to one side of the midline so as to slot into the inverted hemipenes of the male, if present. If female, the probe will only travel a few subcaudal scales, while in a male it will pass a significant distance (Fig. 11-2).

Nursing care

Provide an appropriate environment, including provision of:
1. Optimal temperature (basking lights, heat mats, etc., to allow thermoregulation). Use of max–min thermometers will assist in monitoring temperature ranges incumbent reptiles are exposed to.
2. Full-spectrum lighting appears to be relatively unimportant for snakes with some exceptions (e.g., rough green snake—*Opheodrys aestivus*).
3. Humidity
4. Ventilation
5. Easily cleaned accommodation; use paper substrate and disposable/sterilizable hides and other vivarium furniture (Fig. 11-3).
6. Keep individually to minimize intraspecies stress and competition for resources.

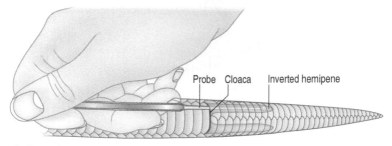

Fig 11-2. Sexing snakes.

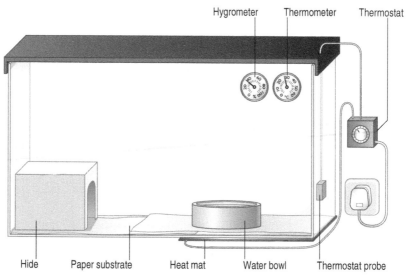

Fig 11-3. Clinical vivarium setup for snakes (lighting is optional—see text).

Fluid therapy

See "Fluid Therapy" under *Nursing Care* in Chapter 10.

Dehydrated snakes typically show an increase in skin tenting and folding, especially longitudinal folding. Daily bathing in shallow, warm water is often beneficial; it encourages many snakes to drink as well as defecate and urinate.

Fluids administration in snakes

1. Stomach tubing is relatively straightforward in snakes as the cardia is relatively weak.
2. Esophagostomy tubes can be used in some cases.
3. Intracoelomic fluids can be given, but try for the ventral tail vein or even the palatine vein.
4. A jugular cutdown can be performed if the snake is anesthetized and a catheter inserted, and small volumes may be administered as a bolus into the ventricle.
5. Small volumes may be given per cloaca.

Liquidized normal diet or proprietary support diets can be used, given either by stomach tube or by esophagostomy tube. Force-feeding of prey species may prove traumatic in inexperienced hands.

Analgesia

See "Analgesia" in Chapter 10.

Anesthesia

1. For general notes, see "Anesthesia" under *Nursing Care* in Chapter 10.
2. Induction: Propofol at 10 mg/kg IV into the ventral tail vein or 1.0 to 2.0 mg/kg intraventricular.
3. Otherwise as for lizards.

Skin disorders
• •

Normal ecdysis in snakes

Shedding in snakes is a cyclical event, with synchronous replacement of the whole epidermis at the same time. Snakes should shed their skin in one continuous sheet, starting rostrally, and any deviation from this should be considered abnormal. Ecdysis is under both environmental and endocrinologic control. Ecdysis in snakes follows the following sequence:
1. Resting phase. There is only one stratum corneum and stratum germinativum.
2. The stratum germinativum undergoes intense proliferation to form a new stratum corneum, but there is no outward visible change in the snake.
3. The new stratum corneum begins to differentiate and keratinize. At this point there is a slight dulling of the skin of the snake, and the spectacle may appear slightly cloudy.
4. A new layer—the stratum intermedium—is now apparent. This lies between the inner and outer layers of strata cornea. The epidermis is thickest now, and so the snake's colors are at their dullest; the spectacle is cloudy.
5. The stratum intermedium is dissolved away by lymph-carrying enzymes—this leaves a cleavage plane between the two strata cornea. The snake's colors will be seen to brighten and the spectacle will clear.
6. Approximately 4 to 7 days after the spectacles clear, the outer stratum corneum is shed.

Differential diagnoses of skin disorders

See also *Skin Disorders* in Chapter 10.

Shedding difficulties (dysecdysis)
• Humidity too low
• Other environmental problems (e.g., incorrect photoperiod, temperature, nutrition)
• Lack of cage furniture to allow initiation of shedding
• Snake mites (*Ophionyssus natracis*)
• Scarring or other underlying dermal disease
• Hyperthyroidism (excessive, repeated skin shedding)
• Secondary bacterial and fungal infections common

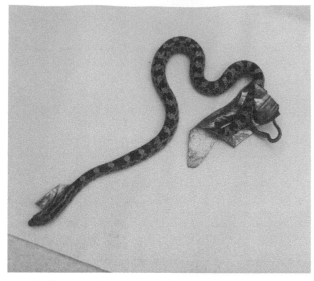

Fig 11-4. A young anerythristic corn snake caught up in duct tape used on the electrics in a home-made vivarium.

Pruritus

- Snake mites
- Irritation; large numbers can be associated with anemia, dysecdysis, depression, and anorexia.

Erosions and ulceration

- Rodent bites
- Adhesive tape (Fig. 11-4)
- Blisters and sores, especially on the ventral scales (ventral dermal necrosis, vesicular dermatitis, blister disease); typically bacterial—*Pseudomonas* spp., *Aeromonas* spp., *Proteus* spp.
- Mycotic dermatitis (e.g., *Chrysosporium* anamorph of *Nannizziopsis vriesii*, or CANV)
- *Kalicephalus* larvae

Nodules and nonhealing wounds

- Granulomas (bacterial, mycobacterial, fungal)
- Dermatophilosis (*Dermatophilus chelonae*)
- Dermatophytosis, include *Penicillium* spp., *Trichophyton mentagrophytes*, *Candida albicans*, *Aspergillus* spp., *Fusarium* spp.
- Filarial worms (*Oswaldofilaria*, *Foleyella*, *Macdonaldius* spp.)
- Pentastomids (especially *Armillifer armillifer*, *Porocephalus* spp., *Kiricephalus* spp.—see also *Respiratory Tract Disorders*)
- Cestodes: *Diphyllobothrium* and *Spirometra* (sparganosis)

Changes in pigmentation

- Petechial hemorrhages: septicemia (see *Systemic Disorders*), *Kalicephalus* spp. (see *Gastrointestinal Tract Disorders*)

Ectoparasites

- Helminths
  - *Kalicephalus* (hookworm) larvae (see *Gastrointestinal Tract Disorders*)
  - Filarial worms (*Oswaldofilaria, Foleyella, Macdonaldius* spp.)
- Cestodes: *Diphyllobothrium* and *Spirometra* (sparganosis)
- Arthropods
  - Ticks (*Aponomma latum* and *Amblyomma* spp.; see Kenny et al 2004)
  - Snake mite *(Ophionyssus natracis)*
  - Pentastomids (e.g., *Raillietiella*)

Burns

- Many snakes are thigmotherms; powerful unprotected heating equipment can cause severe localized burning of the dermis.

Spontaneous rupture of skin

- Hypovitaminosis C

Neoplasia

- Squamous cell carcinoma
- Fibrosarcoma
- Chromatophoroma (malignant)
- Liposarcoma
- Lipoma (especially corn snakes, *Elaphe guttata*)
- Papillomatosis (especially boas)

Findings on clinical examination

- Dysecdysis
  - One or more patches of retained skin. In some areas the skin will appear dull and thickened where several layers of skin have built up over successive dysecdysis episodes. In some cases rings of unshed skin may form bands around the tip the tail. As these dry they constrict, acting as tourniquets and compromising blood flow to the extremity. The spectacles may be retained (see *Ophthalmic Disorders*).
- Small mites found on snakes; tend to accumulate under the scales, the postorbital area, labial pits, and any skinfolds around the mouth or cloaca. Snake may spend much of the time submerged in water bowl (snake mites).
- Large arthropod parasites (ticks)
- Red patches resembling bruising (hemorrhages—septicemia, trauma)
- Anemia (heavy ectoparasitic infestations)
- Swellings (neoplasia, subcutaneous parasites, such as filarial nematodes, but also consider coelomic disorders)

Investigations

1. Cytology (fine-needle aspirate)
   a. Fecal or sputum examination
   b. Pentastomid eggs
2. Routine hematology and biochemistry
   a. Thyroid levels (see *Endocrine Disorders*)
3. Aseptic collection of samples
   a. Culture and sensitivity

4. Endoscopy
   a. Adult pentastomids (look like strange caterpillars)
5. Radiography
6. Biopsy
7. Ultrasonography

Treatment/specific therapy

- Dysecdysis
  - Moisten the affected areas to loosen the retained skin from the underlying epidermis. If the skin feels firmly attached, leave it and try again after further moistening.
  - Placing the snake in a warm, damp towel, pillowcase, or duvet cover (for large snakes) provides rehydration, lubrication, and soft, slightly abrasive surfaces against which to rub. Enforced bathing in warm water may also help, but beware the possibility of drowning.
  - Retained spectacular scales are best removed using a damp cotton bud (see *Ophthalmic Disorders*).
  - Vitamin A at 1000 to 5000 IU/kg IM will often trigger a further shed, allowing a closer management of the sloughing procedure such that both the old shed and the new are removed.
- Hyperthyroidism
  - Antithyroid drugs (e.g., methimazole at 2 mg/kg PO s.i.d.)
  - Possibly try other antithyroid drugs such as carbimazole.
  - Partial or complete thyroidectomy may also be appropriate depending on the case.
- Ventral dermal necrosis
  - Usually associated with too damp an environment—in semi-aquatic species, it can be initiated by the dermal penetration of hookworm larvae. If left untreated it may progress to a septicemia.
  - Treatment is with topical povidone-iodine plus appropriate systemic antibiosis—successful antibiotics include enrofloxacin, amikacin, or even gentamicin.
  - Parenteral vitamin A at 1000 to 5000 IU will induce ecdysis, helping to remove much of the infected skin and necrotic material.
- Abscess/granuloma
  - Any abnormal swelling should be investigated as a potential abscess or granuloma and may require surgery plus systemic antibiosis.
- Dermatophytosis and fungal mycoses
  - Topical chlorhexidine (0.26 mL/L)
  - Topical antifungals (e.g., miconazole, terbinafine)
  - Ketoconazole at 15 mg/kg PO every 72 hours
  - Griseofulvin at 15 mg/kg PO every 72 hours
- *Kalicephalus*
  - Fenbendazole at 25 mg/kg PO weekly for at least 2-3 weeks)
- Filarial nematodes and pentastomids
  - Ivermectin at 200 μg/kg SC (toxic to indigo snakes)
  - Surgical resection of associated skin granulomas
  - Adult pentastomids usually present in lung following extensive tissue migration
- Cestodes
  - Surgical removal where feasible
  - Praziquantel at 5 mg/kg PO, SC, or IM. Repeat after 2 weeks.

- Adhesive tape entanglement
  - The outer epithelial layers may be removed and owners may tear the skin in their efforts to remove the tape.
  - Use a solvent (such as halothane or isoflurane) to gradually remove the adhesive; an anesthetic may be required, especially if tape is adhered to the spectacle (see *Ophthalmic Disorders*).
  - Repair any skin lesions; small lesions can be sealed with tissue glue, larger may require suturing.
  - Covering antibiosis if necessary
- Burns
  - Debride necrotic material (may require anesthetic) and treat with a topical amorphous hydrogel dressings, such as IntraSite Gel (Smith and Nephew Healthcare Ltd.) and/or povidine-iodine.
  - Covering antibiotic or antifungal medication
  - If the burns are extensive then fluid therapy should be instigated (see *Gastrointestinal Tract Disorders*).
  - Scarring will eventually result, which may lead to localized areas of dysecdysis; extensive scarring can lead to problems.
  - Restrictive scarring may mean that constricting snakes have difficulty completing the behavioral repertoire necessary for normal feeding.
- Spontaneous rupture of skin
  - Clean, debride, and suture edges of lesion.
  - Supplement with ascorbic acid. May be linked to feeding starved and, therefore, vitamin C–deficient rodent prey
- Ticks
  - Individual removal of ticks
  - Ivermectin at 200 μg/kg SC (toxic to indigo snakes). *Note:* Ticks are vectors for *Babesia/Hepatozoon* and *Ehrlichia*-like organisms.
- Snake mites
  - Parthenogenetic, so numbers can rapidly build up in vivaria; treatment must include the thorough cleaning of all affected vivaria. What cannot be sterilized with a mild bleach solution (5 mL per gallon) must be disposed.
  - Replace usual substrate with paper (changed daily).
  - Repeated washing with warm water will physically remove any mites.
  - Application of topical fipronil spray once weekly for at least 4 weeks. This is best first applied to a cloth and rubbed over the entire surface of the snake. Fipronil can also be used to treat the environment.
  - Injection of ivermectin at 200 μg/kg SC (*Note:* Toxic to indigo snakes and chelonia) every 2 weeks will kill those that feed on the snake.
  - Commercial imidacloprid (100 g/L) plus moxidectin (25 g/L) (Advocate Dog (UK), Advantage Multi (US), Bayer) applied topically at double (32 mg/kg imidacloprid + 8.0 mg/kg moxidectin) to 10-fold dosages (160 mg/kg imidacloprid + 40 mg/kg moxidectin) according to thickness of skin (care with garter snakes *Thamnophis* spp.—Mehlhorn et al 2005b)
  - Cultures of predatory mites (*Hypoaspis miles*) are commercially available for use in vivaria.
  - Linked to septicemia and inclusion body disease (IBD) outbreaks (see *Systemic Disorders*) as possible vector
- Neoplasia
  - Surgical resection
  - Chromatophoromas carry a poor prognosis with early metastasis.

- Chemotherapy in reptiles is in its infancy, and most tumors are managed surgically. Accessible cutaneous tumors can be treated by injecting cisplatin directly into the tissue mass on a weekly basis as a debulking exercise.

Respiratory tract disorders

Viral

- Reovirus
- Paramyxovirus 1 and 7
- Ferlavirus (paramyxovirus)
- Ball python nidovirus (Stenglein et al 2014)

Bacterial

- Abscesses
- Granulomas
- Pneumonia/air sacculitis (Fig. 11-5)

Fungal

- Abscesses
- Granulomas
- Pneumonia/air sacculitis
- *Cryptococcus neoformans* (see also *Systemic Disorders* and *Neurologic Disorders*)
- Coccidiomycosis
- *Aspergillus* spp., *A. niger*

Parasitic

- Lungworm; *Rhabdias* spp.

Neoplasia

- Metastases (e.g., from renal carcinomas)
- Chondroma (tracheal)

Other noninfectious problems

- Occluded nostrils

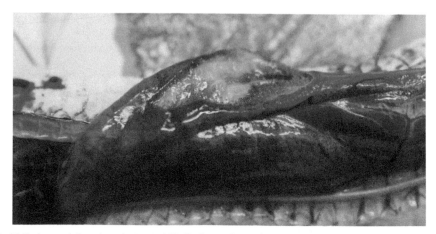

Fig 11-5. Accumulation of purulent material in the lungs of a royal python with pneumonia.

Findings on clinical examination

- Nasal discharge/rhinitis
- Open-mouthed breathing
- "Wet" or unusual respiratory noises
- Discharge around the glottis or inside the proximal trachea. Must differentiate from esophageal discharge (gastritis/enteritis) or secondary to stomatitis. Some conditions may occur concurrently.
- Snake mucus is often thick and tenacious. Mucus may be found as gobbets in the vivarium.
- Snakes have limited ability to cough and the trachea is long so obstructions due to mucus can be serious and may require flushing.
- Occluded nostrils
- Sudden death

Investigations

1. Microscopy
   a. Sputum examination (either from mouth, pulmonary lavage, or endoscopic collection)
   b. Staining for cytology
   c. Gram stain
   d. Lungworm eggs and larvae
2. Radiography
3. Routine hematology and biochemistry
4. Serology for *Cryptococcus* (also consider isolation from lung lavage)
5. Polymerase chain reaction (PCR) and hemagglutination inhibition serology for paramyxovirus 1 and 7 and ferlavirus
6. Culture and sensitivity
7. Endoscopy
8. Biopsy
9. Ultrasonography
10. CT scan
    a. Pees et al (2007) in Table 11-2 offer the measurements for computed tomography (CT) examinations of the lungs of healthy Indian pythons *(Python morulus)* and pythons with respiratory tract disease.
    b. Also the mean (±SD) measurements of attenuation in defined lung areas for CT examinations of healthy pythons and pythons with respiratory tract disease (Table 11-3)

Management

- If respiratory disease is severe provide a high oxygen atmosphere.
- Aminophylline at 2.0 to 4.0 mg/kg IM once only

Treatment/specific therapy

- Viral infections
  - No treatment. Supportive therapy only. Those diagnosed with paramyxovirus or ball python nidovirus should be removed from the collection.

Table 11-2 Measurements for CT examinations of the lungs of healthy Indian pythons (*Python molurus*) and pythons with respiratory tract disease

Pythons	Length (mm) (mean ± SD)		Mean area in cross-section (mm²) (mean ± SD)	Mean thickness value at each location for the dorsal, left, right, and ventral part of the lung (mm) (mean ± SD)		
	Right lung	Left lung		At point 25% of the length of the respiratory tissue	At point 50% of the length of the respiratory tissue	At point 75% of the length of the respiratory tissue
Healthy	222 ± 86 (89-348)	188 ± 69 (89-295)	279 ± 188 (79-594)	5.1 ± 2.1 (2.2-9.4)	4.2 ± 1.2 (2.2-6.0)	2.7 ± 0.8 (2.2-5.6)
Respiratory disease	307 ± 23 (283-336)	244 ± 29 (205-286)	483 ± 133 (347-675)	6.8 ± 1.8 (2.2-6.0)	5.0 ± 1.0 (4.0-6.0)	2.8 ± 0.8 (3.5-6.0)

Pees M C, Kiefer I, Ludewig E W et al 2007 Computed tomography of the lungs of Indian pythons (Python molurus). *Am J Vet Res* 68:428–434.

- Bacterial infections
  - Appropriate antibiosis. Consider nebulizing.
- Fungal infections
  - Ketoconazole at 15 mg/kg PO every 72 hours
  - Griseofulvin at 15 mg/kg PO every 72 hours
- Lungworm
  - Fenbendazole at 50 to 100 mg/kg PO. Repeat every 2 weeks if necessary. *Note:* Fenbendazole is metabolized to oxfendazole by the liver.
  - Oxfendazole at 68 mg/kg PO. Repeat every 2 weeks if necessary.
  - Ivermectin at 0.2 mg SC or PO repeated every 2 weeks for 3 treatments (toxic to indigo snakes)
  - Lungworms have a direct life cycle; infective larvae can penetrate the skin or infect via contaminated food and water.
- Chondroma
  - Surgical debulking/resection
- Occluded nostrils
  - Flush and remove as much debris as possible. May require anesthesia to undertake

Gastrointestinal tract disorders

Disorders of the oral cavity

Note: Mucus may be seen in the mouth as part of respiratory disease and should be differentiated.

Bacterial

- Stomatitis (a variety of gram-negative bacteria, especially *Aeromonas, Pseudomonas, Proteus, Morganella*)

Table 11-3 Mean ± SD measurements of attenuation in defined lung areas for CT examinations of healthy pythons and pythons with respiratory tract disease

Pythons		Entire lung tissues		Dorsal part of lungs		Left part of lung		Right part of lung		Ventral part of lungs	
		Attenuation	Variability of attenuation	Attenuation	Variability of attenuation	Attenuation	Variability of attenuation	Attenuation	Variability of attenuation	Attenuation	Variability of attenuation
Healthy	Mean ± SD	744.4 ± 47.1	94.8 ± 9.7	−761.0 ± 43.1	48.4 ± 8.0	−756.8 ± 53.0	50.6 ± 18.0	−755.4 ± 51.3	54.3 ± 17.0	−761.8 ± 50.0	61.4 ± 6.9
	Range	−805.3-672.0	82.2-111.9	−819.1-693.7	34.8-63.8	−819.9-670.0	28.8-84.1	−831.2-664.0	28.1-85.7	−847.6-706.0	49.9-72.3
Respiratory disease	Mean ± SD	−613.7 ± 176.4	160.9 ± 56.4	−655.5 ± 155.0	99.6 ± 61.6	−624.4 ± 173.9	102.0 ± 65.1	−604.3 ± 193.1	121.4 ± 77.2	−555.9 ± 214.5	165.3 ± 56.9
	Range	−789.0-359.0	98.9-226.2	−808.1-424.9	44.2-192.1	−770.2-350.1	39.9-198.1	−829.7-372.6	44.9-213.2	−771.8-266.7	73.3-211.9

Pees M C, Kiefer I, Ludewig E W et al 2007 Computed tomography of the lungs of Indian pythons (Python molurus). Am J Vet Res 68:428-434.

- Intermandibular cellulitis (*Pseudomonas* and *Aeromonas*)
- Venom gland infection (venomous snakes)

Fungal

- Stomatitis

Parasitic

- Ocheostomid trematodes

Neoplasia

- Undifferentiated sarcoma (Abou-Madi et al 1994—see also *Systemic Disorders*)

Other noninfectious problems

- Fractures (traumatic, pathological)

Findings on clinical examination

- Discharge from the mouth and nares
- Fluid respiratory noises
- Inflammation of the oral and pharyngeal membranes; may progress to ulcerative lesions of the palatine area, the trachea, and the tongue sheath. A diphtheritic membrane may be present (stomatitis).
- Occasionally infection may track up the lachrymal duct, resulting in a subspectacular abscess over one or both corneas (stomatitis—see *Ophthalmic Disorders*).
- Obvious flat helminth-like parasites in oral cavity (trematodes)
- Gross swelling of the lower jaw and intermandibular area (intermandibular cellulitis)
- Permanent apparent dislocation of the mandible/swelling of one or both mandibles (fracture)
- Abnormal coloring of mucous membranes (icterus, cyanosis)
- Unilateral (or occasionally bilateral) swelling on the face, below eye, and/or along maxilla (venom gland infection/abscess)

Investigations

1. Radiography
   a. Stomatitis with possible underlying osteomyelitis
2. Routine hematology and biochemistry
3. Cytology (may need FNA) including Gram staining
4. Culture and sensitivity
5. Endoscopy
6. Biopsy
7. Ultrasonography

Treatment/specific therapy

- Stomatitis
  - Snakes may not feed while suffering from stomatitis, so may require fluid support such as Hartmann's solution at 15 to 25 mL/kg; nutritional support should be given by stomach tube during this time.
  - The stomach tube should be lubricated and coated with appropriate antibiotic to try to prevent iatrogenic spread of infection to the esophagus and further.

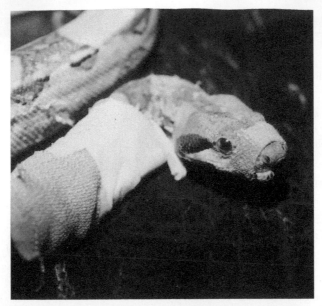

Fig 11-6. Taping the jaw of a young boa constrictor with a fractured mandible. Note the esophagostomy tube in place.

- Topical antibiotics plus topical povidone-iodine daily may be sufficient.
- Surgical debridement of necrotic tissue followed by systemic and topical treatments may be required.
- Intermandibular cellulitis
  - A synergistic infection of both *Pseudomonas fluorescens* and *Aeromonas hydrophila*
  - Supportive treatment
  - Appropriate antibiotics
- Fractured jaw
  - Pathologically weakened bone, or mandibles of small snakes, may be unable to support orthopedic techniques; in some cases taping the jaw closed with strong adhesive plaster (taking care to leave the nares open) accompanied by placement of an esophagostomy tube may allow healing to occur (Fig. 11-6).
- Trematodes
  - Often asymptomatic; may cause snake to gape
  - Praziquantel at 5 mg/kg PO, SC, or IM. Repeat after 2 weeks.
  - Freeze food items (e.g., frogs, fish) for 3 days prior to feeding to eliminate intermediate stages.
- Icterus (see *Hepatic Disorders* and *Cardiovascular and Hematologic Disorders*)
- Cyanosis (see *Respiratory Tract Disorders*)
- Neoplasia (see "Treatment" under *Skin Disorders*)
- Venom gland infection
  - Surgical removal of infected venom gland
  - Covering antibiosis
  - *Note:* Removal of both venom glands renders the snake incapable of taking live prey, may alter the shape of the head, and may affect digestion.

Differential diagnosis for gastrointestinal disorders

Viral
- Reovirus (Reavil et al 2003)

Bacterial
- *Salmonella* spp.
- *Escherichia coli*
- *Chlamydophila* spp. (see also *Systemic Disorders*)

Fungal
- Candidiasis

Protozoal
- *Cryptosporidium serpentis*
- *Entamoeba invadens*
- *Eimeria*
- *Caryospora*
- *Isospora*
- Flagellates e.g., *Trichomonas.*

Parasitic
- Ascarids
- *Ophiascaris*
- *Polydelphis*
- *Hexametra*
- *Ophiostrongylus*
- Hookworms
- *Kalicephalus*
- *Capillaria*
- *Strongyloides*
- Oxyurids
- Tapeworms
- Flukes
- Pentastomids (especially *Armillifer armillifer, Porocephalus* spp., *Kiricephalus* spp.—see also *Skin Disorders*)

Neoplasia
- Adenocarcinomas

Other noninfectious problems
- Foreign body ingestion or impaction
- Constipation
- Dystocia (as a cause of constipation)
- Cloacal prolapse
- Cloacitis
- Cloacoliths
- Intestinal foreign body
- Intussusception
- Extraintestinal mass (e.g., renal neoplasm)
- Dystocia

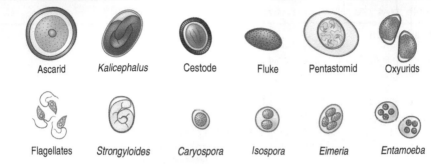

Fig 11-7. Common gastrointestinal parasites of snakes (not drawn to scale).

- Hypocalcemia/metabolic bone disease (see *Nutritional Disorders*)
- Parasitism

Findings on clinical examination

- Vomiting/regurgitation
- Weight loss
- Lethargy
- Chronic regurgitation, extreme weight loss, depression, mucus-laden stools, and an obvious abdominal bulge caused by hypertrophy of the gastric mucosa (cryptosporidiosis)
- Dysentery (mucus-laden, bile stained, and/or showing frank blood), anorexia, dehydration, wasting, and death *(Entamoeba invadens)*
- A coelomic mass may be palpable.
- Petechial skin hemorrhages (*Kalicephalus*—see *Skin Disorders*)
- Cloacal prolapse (differentiate from prolapse of the colon or hemipenes)

Investigations

1. Microscopy
   a. Fresh fecal sample—"wet prep" (Fig. 11-7 and Table 11-4)
2. Radiography
   a. Plain radiographs
   b. Contrast studies (e.g., for hypertrophic gastritis—cryptosporidiosis)

Contrast studies in snakes

1. Barium sulfate suspension given by gavage at 5 mL/kg
2. Double contrast: Immediately follow barium with 45 mL/kg air
3. Take first radiograph after 15 minutes.

---

3. Routine hematology and biochemistry
4. Culture and sensitivity
5. Endoscopy
6. Biopsy/necropsy
7. Electromicroscopy
   a. Reovirus
8. Ultrasonography

Table 11-4 Parasites found in fresh fecal samples

Fecal parasite	Comments
Ascarid eggs (Ophiascaris, Polydelphis)	Typical ascarid eggs
Oxyurid eggs	Rodent pinworm eggs may also be seen in snakes fed on infested prey rodents.
Hookworm eggs	Thin-walled, oval eggs
Strongyloides	Larvae in fresh fecal samples; eggs are thin-walled and similar to Rhabdias
Capillaria	Typical urn shape with operculae at either end (see Hepatic Disorders)
Tapeworm eggs	Thick-walled with several dark hooklets in the center
Fluke eggs	Thin-shelled, often with single operculum. Orange or deep yellow color. Miracidium may be visible.
Flagellates	Numerous motile pear-to-circular-shaped protozoa approximately 8×5 µm
Cryptosporidium	Oocysts may be visible using phase contrast microscopy after floatation. Otherwise consider Modified Ziehl-Neelsen staining.
Isospora oocysts	Circular
Eimeria oocysts	Elongate
Entamoeba	Cysts and ameboid protozoa

Management

- For fluid therapy and general management, see *Nursing Care.*

Treatment/specific therapy

- Reovirus
  - Supportive treatment only
- Salmonellosis
  - Probably best considered as a normal constituent of the snake cloacal/gut microflora
  - Occasionally pathogenic to snakes. May cause erosive gut lesions with subsequent bacteremia/septicemia
  - Excretion likely to increase during times of stress (e.g., movement, illness)
  - Treatment usually not appropriate as unlikely to be effective long term and may encourage resistance
  - Recommendations for prevention of salmonellosis from captive reptiles issued by the Centers for Disease Control and Prevention in the United States include:
    - Pregnant women, children <5 years of age, and persons with impaired immune system function (e.g., AIDS) should not have contact with reptiles.
    - Because of the risk of becoming infected with *Salmonella* from a reptile, even without direct contact, households with pregnant women, children <5 years of age, or persons with impaired immune system function should not keep reptiles. Reptiles are not appropriate pets for childcare centers.
    - All persons should wash hands with soap immediately after any contact with a reptile or reptile cage.
    - Reptiles should be kept out of food preparation areas such as kitchens.

- Kitchen sinks should not be used to wash food or water bowls, cages, or vivaria used for reptiles or to bathe reptiles. Any sink used for these purposes should be disinfected after use.
- *Cryptosporidium serpentis*
  - Direct life cycle; infection by exposure to water containing infective oocysts
  - There is no recognized effective treatment.
  - Metronidazole
    - In general, 100 to 257 mg/kg PO body weight. Repeat after 2 weeks if necessary.
    - For colubrids, 40 mg/kg PO repeated after 2 weeks
    - *Boidae, Elaphidae,* and *Viperidae* 125 to 250 mg/kg PO repeated after 2 weeks
    - Alternatively, 20 mg/kg PO every other day until eradication
  - Nitazoxanide at 5 mg/kg PO s.i.d.
  - Paromomycin at 300 to 800 mg/kg PO s.i.d. for 10 days
  - Oocysts *(C. parvum)* in water can be viable after 7 months at 15° C.
  - Disinfect by exposing to water above 64° C for >2 minutes. *Cryptosporidium* oocysts are very resistant to chlorine or iodine.
- *Isospora, Caryospora,* and *Eimeria*
  - Sulfadimethoxine at 50 mg/kg PO daily for 3 days; stop for 3 days, then repeat 3-day course.
  - Toltrazuril at 7.5 mg/kg PO s.i.d. for 2 days. Repeat after 12 days.
  - Young/stressed snakes more susceptible
  - Rodent prey may be the source of contamination.
- *Entamoeba invadens*
  - Ingestion of feces-contaminated water or food with the infective cysts
  - Often commensally present in gut of herbivorous reptiles (e.g., terrestrial *Chelonia*) so do not keep snakes with such reptiles.
  - Metronidazole (as for *Cryptosporidium* above)
  - Chloroquine
    - 125 mg/kg PO every 48 hours for three treatments
    - 50 mg/kg IM every 7 days for 3 weeks
  - Iodoquinol/diiodohydroxyquin 50 mg/kg PO s.i.d. for 21 days. *Note:* Possibly toxic to black rat snakes
  - Paromomycin
    - 300 to 360 mg/kg PO every other day for 14 days
    - 25 to 100 mg/kg PO daily for 4 weeks
  - Potential zoonosis
- Flagellates
  - Metronidazole (as for *Cryptosporidium* above)
- Ascarids, hookworms, and oxyurids
  - Fenbendazole at 50 to 100 mg/kg PO. Repeat every 2 weeks if necessary. *Note:* Fenbendazole is metabolized to oxfendazole by the liver.
  - Oxfendazole at 68 mg/kg PO. Repeat every 2 weeks if necessary.
  - Ivermectin at 0.2 mg SC or PO repeated every 2 weeks for 3 treatments (toxic to indigo snakes)
  - Topical emodepside plus praziquantel preparations (Profender, Bayer) at 56 µL/100 g body weight (Mehlhorn et al 2005a)
  - *Note: Oxyuris* worms usually have a direct life cycle.
  - Hookworms have a direct life cycle; infective larvae can penetrate the skin or infect via contaminated food and water.
- Tapeworms
  - Praziquantel at 5 mg/kg PO, SC, or IM. Repeat after 2 weeks.

- Foreign body/intussusception
  - Surgical enterotomy/enterectomy
- Fecal impaction (constipation)
  - Investigate for underlying cause (e.g., foreign body, dystocia, neoplasia)
  - Fluid therapy (see *Nursing Care*)
  - Gut motility enhancers (e.g., metoclopramide at 60 µg/kg PO; cisapride at 1.0 mg/kg PO s.i.d.)
  - Enema under general anesthesia
  - Surgical enterotomy
- Cloacal prolapse
  - Pursestring suture around cloaca for a minimum of 14 days
  - Limit feeding to reduce straining during defecation.
  - If repeated prolapses, consider cloacopexy.

Anorexia

Environmental factors

- Inappropriate environment
  - Temperature too high/low
  - Humidity too high/low
  - Failure to provide adequate (size and/or number) of hiding places (insecurity)
  - Excessive handling, especially in the days to weeks after purchase
  - Excessive lighting and/or light duration—at least 10 hours of dark required
  - Excessive disturbance outside the vivarium

Physiologic

- Preparatory to brumation (hibernation) in temperate snakes
- Preparatory to ecdysis

Reproductive

- Prior to egg laying
- Reproductive seasonality in both sexes; note that male snakes exhibiting anorexia linked with reproductive activity may have large numbers of spermatozoa present in their urine.
- For wild royal pythons *(Python regius)*, a reproduction-associated anorexia occurs naturally in the spring, which corresponds to autumn in northern latitudes, so loss of appetite in captive royal pythons at this time may be normal. Males become sexually mature at weights above 650 g, while females are usually over 1000 g.

Stress

- Overcrowding
- Inappropriate species combinations
- Interference from uneaten prey animals

Inappropriate feeding

- Not weaned onto dead food
- Wrong food offered
- Food offered not identified as food (e.g., white mice ignored whereas agouti-colored mice taken). This may depend on previous experience.
- Poorly prepared food (e.g., partly defrosted/refrozen prey offered)
- Offering food at inappropriate time of day (e.g., during day for nocturnal species)

Disease

- See relevant sections.

Findings on clinical examination

- Snakes with physiologic anorexia tend to lose body condition slowly. This applies especially to the large constricting boas and pythons.
- Snakes with disease processes often lose condition comparatively quickly and obviously.
- Loss of muscle mass especially along the epaxial musculature
- Other obvious clinical signs (e.g., masses, stomatitis, ectoparasites)

Treatment/specific therapy

- Weigh regularly and record—once weekly is usually sufficient.
- Reevaluate the snake's environment and husbandry based on research about that particular species' need.
- In physiologic cases no remedial action is necessary; provided the snake maintains reasonable condition it should resume feeding, although this may persist until either endogenous or exogenous stimuli alter. This may take up to 3 to 4 months in some species.
- If the snake is losing condition or if a physiologic cause has been eliminated, then investigate as for other disease problems.
- Force feeding
  - Liquidized diet
  - Lubricated whole prey

Nutritional disorders

- Obesity
- Hepatic lipidosis (see *Hepatic Disorders*)
- Steatitis
- Vitamin B_{12} deficiency
- Metabolic bone disease (uncommon in snakes—see in Chapter 10 if suspected)
- Hypoglycemia (see *Neurologic Disorders*)

Findings on clinical examination

- Gross, swollen appearance to body (obesity); head may appear unnaturally small. In extreme cases fat may appear partially sectioned, giving a "string of doughnuts" appearance.
- Coelomic and subcutaneous fat becomes hard (steatitis).
- CNS signs (vitamin B_{12} deficiency—see *Neurologic Disorders*)

Investigations

1. Fecal examination
   a. *Capillaria* eggs. Typical urn shape with operculae at either end (see "Investigations" in *Gastrointestinal Tract Disorders*)

2. Radiography
   a. Hepatomegaly
   b. Evidence of extreme soft tissue covering
3. Routine hematology and biochemistry
   a. Cholesterol and triglyceride levels
4. Endoscopy
5. Biopsy/necropsy
6. Ultrasonography

Treatment/specific therapy

- Obesity
  - Gradual weight loss
  - Long-term starvation likely to generate a ketoacidosis
  - Supplement with vitamin E to reduce the risk of steatitis.
- Steatitis
  - Secondary to a diet high in saturated fats (e.g., obese rodents)
  - Treat with vitamin E at 50 mg/kg PO or IM.
  - Offer a diet low in saturated fats.

Hepatic disorders

Viral

- Adenovirus (Boidae)
- Reovirus (king snakes—Reavil et al 2003)

Bacterial

- Mycobacteriosis (granulomas—may be multifocal)

Fungal
Protozoal

- *Entamoeba invadens* (see *Gastrointestinal Tract Disorders*)

Parasitic

- *Capillaria* spp. (especially earthworm-fed garter and water snakes)

Nutritional

- Hepatic lipidosis

Neoplasia

- Hepatocellular adenoma (garter snake, *Thamnophis radix*)
- Secondaries from other tumors

Other noninfectious problems

- Biliary cysts

Findings on clinical examination

- Loose feces (see also *Gastrointestinal Tract Disorders*)
- Large swelling midbody (hepatomegaly, biliary cysts)

- Neurologic signs (hepatic encephalopathy—see *Neurologic Disorders*)
- Jaundice (icterus)

Investigations

1. Fecal examination
   a. *Capillaria* eggs: Typical urn shape with operculae at either end (see "Investigations" in *Gastrointestinal Tract Disorders*)
2. Radiography
   a. Hepatomegaly
   b. Hepatic masses
3. Routine hematology and biochemistry
4. Culture and sensitivity
5. Endoscopy
6. Biopsy/necropsy
   a. Adenoviral inclusions
   b. Ziehl-Neelsen staining and PCR for mycobacteria
7. Electromicroscopy
8. Ultrasonography

Management

- Milk thistle (*Silybum marianum*) is hepatoprotectant. Dose at 4 to 15 mg/kg PO b.i.d. or t.i.d.
- For ascites try furosemide at 2 to 5 mg/kg PO, SC s.i.d. if ascitic.

Treatment/specific therapy

- Mycobacteriosis—see *Systemic Disorders*
- *Capillaria*
  - Fenbendazole at 25 mg/kg PO every 2 weeks for 3 treatments
- Biliary cysts
  - Removal of fluid percutaneously
  - Surgical resection
- Hepatic lipidosis
  - Fluid therapy and nutritional support
  - Covering antibiotics
  - Lactulose 0.05 mL/100 g PO s.i.d.

Pancreatic disorders

Viral

- Paramyxovirus

Investigations

1. Radiography
2. Routine hematology and biochemistry

3. Culture and sensitivity
4. PCR and HI testing for paramyxovirus
5. Endoscopy
6. Biopsy/necropsy
   a. Pancreatic ductular lesions (paramyxovirus)
7. Ultrasonography

Treatment/specific therapy

- Paramyxovirus: No specific treatment

Cardiovascular and hematologic disorders

Bacterial
- Vegetative endocarditis
- Granulomatous pericarditis

Protozoal
- *Haemogregarina* spp.
- *Hepatozoon* spp.

Parasitic
- Filarial worms (*Oswaldofilaria, Foleyella, Macdonaldius* spp.—see also *Skin Disorders*)

Nutritional
- Visceral gout (uric acid in pericardial sac—see *Renal Disorders*)
- Neoplasia
  - Leukemia

Other noninfectious problems
- Anemia
- Cardiomyopathy
- Myocardial mineralization
- Thromboembolism
- Myocardial ischemia
- Congestive heart failure
- Developmental abnormalities

Findings on clinical examination

- Lethargy
- Apparent respiratory disease (see also *Respiratory Tract Disorders*)
- Pale mucous membranes
- Edema
- Cardiomegaly—may be visible externally as a mass around 22% to 35% of the snout-vent length. It may be seen to be beating (differentiating the heart from pericardiac masses, such as granulomas). *Note:* Very thin, anorexic snakes may appear to have a large heart secondary to loss of surrounding tissue.
- Avascular necrosis of the tail tip (thromboembolism)

Investigations

1. Radiography
   a. Cardiomegaly
   b. Calcification of blood vessels
2. Ultrasonography and Doppler blood-flow detectors
   a. Cardiomyopathy
   b. Pericardial effusions
   c. Vegetative endocarditis
3. Electrocardiogram
   a. Valentinuzzi et al (1969b) suggest that an ECG can be taken with two leads:
      i. A longitudinal lead that consists of a rostral electrode located at 10% of the body length and a caudal electrode at 50% of the body length; both electrodes are on the ventral surface of the animal.
      ii. Two transverse electrodes are located bilaterally at the level of the heart (approximately 24% of the body length).
      iii. Changes in the position of the heart, either during handling or by artificial respiration, may cause significant changes in the magnitude and orientation of the vectors. During recording of the transverse leads, rotation around the YY axis usually produces large variations in the amplitudes of the ECG waves. Spontaneous changes in T amplitude are relatively common.
   b. ECG of the boa constrictor at rest and at room temperature (Table 11-5)
      i. The ventricular T wave is generally in the same direction as the major deflection R; Q and S are poorly developed. The T wave also varies greatly in amplitude and may become completely inverted without apparent change in the position of the leads relative to the heart.
      ii. There is an SV complex preceding the P wave.
      iii. Valentinuzzi et al (1969a) found experimentally that as the heart deteriorates and dies, the relative and absolute amplitude of the SV complex markedly increases.
4. Routine hematology and biochemistry
   a. Anemia
   b. May be artifactual due to lymph contamination and dilution

Table 11-5 ECG of the boa constrictor, at rest and at room temperature

Variable	Value
Heart rate (beats/min)	24
SV–P (s)	0.50
P-R (s)	0.55
SV–P/SV–SV	0.18
P–R/P–P	0.20
SV (ms)	100
P (ms)	80
QRS (ms)	140
Q-T (s)	1.4

ECG, *electrocardiogram.*
From Valentinuzzi et al (1969c).

5. Cytology: May find filarial worms on blood smear
6. Culture and sensitivity
7. Endoscopy
8. Biopsy/necropsy

Management

- Provide high-oxygen environment.

Treatment/specific therapy

- Hemoparasites
  - Loading dose of chloroquine phosphate (5 mg/kg PO) and primaquine phosphate (0.5 mg/kg PO)
  - Continue with chloroquine at 2.5 mg/kg PO once weekly and primaquine at 0.5 mg/kg PO once weekly for 12 to 16 weeks.
- Filarial nematodes (see *Skin Disorders*)
- Thromboembolism
  - No established treatment. Possibly try NSAIDs
  - Necrotic extremities may require surgical amputation.
  - Investigate underlying factors (e.g., septicemia, low temperatures)
- Cardiomyopathies
  - Furosemide at 2 to 5 mg IM, IV, or PO s.i.d. or b.i.d.
- Leukemia
  - Treatment potentially difficult and untried
  - Radiation therapy has been used with lizards (see Chapter 10) with a single low-dose whole-body radiation treatment of 1 gray.
- Anemia
  - The underlying cause should be investigated.
  - Blood transfusion from a conspecific or possibly a close relative (same genus) could be attempted.
  - Oxyglobin

Systemic disorders

Viral

Bacterial

- Septicemia/bacteremia
- *Salmonella arizona*
- *Chlamydophila pneumoniae*
- *Chlamydophila* spp. (Jacobson et al 2002)
- Mycobacteriosis

Fungal

- *Cryptococcus neoformans*
- *Zygomycete* fungi

Neoplasia

- Sarcoma (Abou-Madi et al 1994)
- Mesothelioma

- Lymphocytic leukemia (Raiti et al 2002)
- Multicentric T-cell lymphoma (Raiti et al 2002)

Other noninfectious problems

- Cardiac disease (see *Cardiovascular and Hematologic Disorders*)
- Gout (see *Renal Disorders*)
- Amyloidosis

Findings on clinical examination

- Anorexia
- Weight loss
- Lethargy
- Altered behavior (e.g., shunning normal basking areas, constantly hiding)
- Inappetence; petechial hemorrhages visible in the skin, especially the ventral scales; may show CNS signs such as incoordination, frantic movements, or loss of the righting reflex (septicemia)
- Swellings (neoplasia)
- Clinical signs may vary with organ system affected.

Investigations

1. Radiography
2. Routine hematology and biochemistry
   a. High actual or relative heterophila (inflammatory)
   b. Multiple abnormal leukocytes (leukemia)
3. Culture and sensitivity
   a. Blood culture (septicemia/bacteremia)
4. Serology for *Cryptococcus*
5. Cytology
   a. Ziehl-Neelsen staining and PCR for mycobacteria
   b. Immunohistochemistry and PCR for *Chlamydophila* and *Chlamydia*-like organisms (Soldati et al 2004)
   c. Tracheal washings or cerebrospinal tap to isolate *Cryptococcus*
6. Endoscopy
7. Biopsy/necropsy
   a. Single or multiple granulomas (mycobacteria, fungi, *Chlamydophila pneumoniae*, *Chlamydia*-like organisms)
8. Ultrasonography

Management

- Fluid therapy—see *Nursing Care*.

Treatment/specific therapy

- Septicemia
  - Supportive treatment
  - Antibiotics

- Mycobacteriosis
  - Potential zoonosis. Consider euthanasia.
  - No successful treatment for mycobacteriosis in reptiles reported
- Cryptococcosis
  - Difficult to treat. Consider using:
    - Ketoconazole at 10 to 30 mg/kg PO s.i.d.
    - Topical ketoconazole cream
    - Itraconazole 5 mg/kg PO every other day
- Lymphoma and leukemia
  - Treatment potentially difficult and untried, but see Chapter 10
- Sarcoma—see *Musculoskeletal Disorders*

Musculoskeletal disorders

Bacterial
- Osteomyelitis
- Abscessation

Fungal
- Granulomata

Protozoal
Parasitic
- Cestodes: *Diphyllobothrium* and *Spirometra* (sparganosis)

Nutritional
- Prolonged anorexia

Neoplasia
- Sarcoma
- Spinal neoplasia
- Fibrosarcoma
- Osteosarcoma

Other noninfectious problems
- Traumatic fractures
- Spondylitis/spondylosis
- Myopathies
- Congenital abnormalities
- Steatitis
- Fecal impaction—see *Gastrointestinal Tract Disorders*
- Congenital deformities due to incorrect incubation temperatures; drug administration while gravid; inbreeding
- Osseous dysplasia (inheritable)
- Muscle wastage secondary to chronic anorexia (see *Anorexia*)

Findings on clinical examination

- Severe kinking of the spine (myopathies, spondylitis/spondylosis, fractures)
- Obvious abnormalities, especially of the skull

- Swellings and/or erosions (neoplasia, osteomyelitis, abscessation, osseous dysplasia)
- Extreme muscle wastage

Investigations

1. Radiography
   a. Approximate body organ position in snakes based on percentage of snout to vent (cloaca) length as measured from the rostral nares (Table 11-6). *Note:* This measurement does not include the tail.
   b. Fractured ribs are a common finding (Hernandez-Divers & Hernandez-Divers 2001) that usually require no treatment.
   c. Steatitis may be indicated by enlargement and greater density of the fat body.
   d. Spondylosis/spondylitis, osseous dysplasia
2. Routine hematology and biochemistry
3. Culture and sensitivity
4. Endoscopy
5. Biopsy/necropsy
6. Ultrasonography

Table 11-6 Approximate body organ position in snakes based upon percentage of snout to vent (cloaca) length as measured from the rostral nares

Organ	(%)
Heart	22-35
Lungs	25-50
Air sac	45-85
Liver	35-60
Stomach	45-65
Spleen, pancreas, and gallbladder	60-70
Small intestine	65-80
Kidneys	65-90
Colon	80-100

Treatment/specific therapy

- *Diphyllobothrium* and *Spirometra* (sparganosis)
  - Surgical removal where feasible
  - Praziquantel at 5 mg/kg PO, SC, or IM. Repeat after 2 weeks.
  - Only feed prey prefrozen for at least 30 days.
  - Complex life cycles
- Sarcoma
  - Attempt surgical resection.
  - Chemotherapy has been attempted (Rosenthal 1994) after surgical reduction.
  - Doxorubicin at 1 mg/kg IV every 7 days for 2 weeks, then once every 2 weeks, then once every 2 weeks for a total of 6 doses of doxorubicin
  - Intravenous access was maintained using a vascular port with the catheter tip into the right atrium.

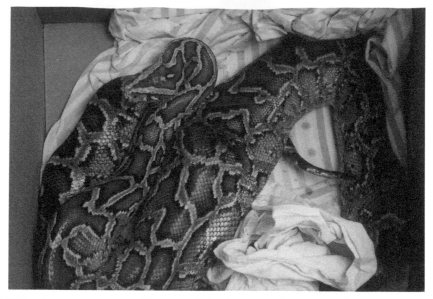

Fig 11-8. A large Burmese python with a severe discharging abscessation of the spinal column. Radiography revealed osteolysis of the underlying vertebrae and a complete loss of continuity of the spinal column and spinal cord. This snake was paralyzed caudal to the lesion.

- Other neoplasia
  - Attempt surgical resection.
  - Cryosurgery
- Spondylitis/spondylosis
  - Some cases may represent a Paget syndrome-like disease.
  - Many cases actually have a spinal infection triggering osteolysis (Fig. 11-8), exostoses, and bony fusion of the vertebrae.
  - Consider use of antibiosis and NSAIDs (e.g., meloxicam at 50 µg/kg PO or IM s.i.d.).
  - Those constricting snakes with extensive fusion of the spine may be unable to prehend and feed properly and so should be considered for euthanasia.
- Osseous dysplasia
  - Inherited condition. No treatment. Avoid use of parents carrying this disorder in breeding programs.
- Myopathies
  - Guarded prognosis
  - Attempt treatment with vitamin E and selenium supplementation.

Neurologic disorders

Viral

- IBD (arenavirus—Stenglein et al 2012)
- Paramyxovirus
- Reovirus
- Lentivirus

Bacterial

- Septicemia
- CNS granuloma
- Encephalitis

Fungal

- CNS granuloma
- *Cryptococcus neoformans* (see also *Systemic Disorders* and *Respiratory Tract Disorders*)

Protozoal

- *Acanthamoeba*
- *Toxoplasma*

Nutritional

- Thiamine deficiency (especially fish-eating snakes such as garter snakes—*Thamnophis* spp.)
- Biotin deficiency
- Hypoglycemia

Neoplasia

- Schwannoma

Other noninfectious problems

- Organophosphate toxicity (e.g., insecticidal aerosols and diffusers)
- Gout (see *Renal Disorders*)
- Liver disease (hepatic encephalopathy)
- Metabolic disease
- Trauma
- Ivermectin overdose
- Cedar shavings
- Spider gene in ball pythons *P. regius*

<hr>

Findings on clinical examination

- Slight to marked head tremor
- Muscle tremors
- Loss of righting reflex
- "Star gazing" (Fig. 11-9)
- Aberrant behavior
- CNS signs and/or regurgitation in pythons and boas (IBD)

<hr>

Investigations

1. Radiography
2. Routine hematology and biochemistry
3. PCR (esophageal swab and blood for IBD)
4. Cytology
   a. Intracytoplasmic inclusion bodies (IBD)
   b. Raised liver enzymes (hepatic encephalopathy)

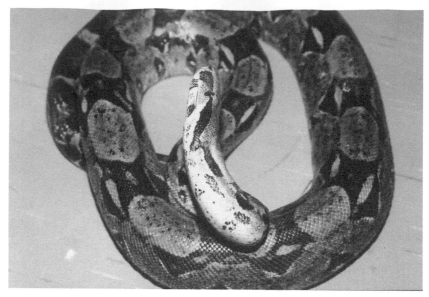

Fig 11-9. A boa constrictor showing classic "star-gazing" behavior.

5. Culture and sensitivity
   a. Blood culture (septicemia)
6. Endoscopy
7. Biopsy
   a. Liver, lung, esophageal tonsil, and other organs (IBD)
8. Ultrasonography

Treatment/specific therapy

- Septicemia
  - Antibiotics
  - Fluid therapy (see *Nursing Care*)
- Thiamine (vitamin B₁) deficiency
  - Due to feeding fresh fish rich in thiaminase (e.g., whitebait)
  - Treatment is with B₁ supplementation, and deficiency is avoided by providing a dietary vitamin B₁ supplement plus boiling of fish before feeding to denature the thiaminase.
- Biotin deficiency
  - Seen in egg-eating snakes
  - Supplement with biotin.
  - Treat symptomatically.
- *Acanthamoeba* and *Toxoplasma*
  - Treatment difficult
  - Metronidazole at 100 to 275 mg/kg PO once only (only 40 mg/kg for king snakes and indigo snakes)
  - Trimethoprim-sulfadiazine at 15 mg/kg PO daily
  - Potential zoonoses

- Organophosphate toxicity
  - Atropine at 0.04 mg/kg IM
  - Supportive treatment
- IBD
  - No effective treatment
  - Supportive therapy
- Spider gene in ball pythons
  - Alters the patterning into a weblike mesh along the body but can give rise to a range of pattern changes
  - Dominant gene
  - Clinical signs can vary from mild head tremor to star gazing and loss of equilibrium.
  - No treatment. The continued breeding of such affected snakes may represent a significant welfare problem.

Ophthalmic disorders

The cornea is protected by a transparent spectacle made from fusion of the upper and lower eyelids. Snakes have rods and cones but lack a fovea; some snakes possess a conus papillaris (analogous to avian pecten).

Snakes have well-developed harderian glands; their secretions lubricate the subspectacular space. A second duct drains this space into the vomeronasal organ.

Examination of the posterior segment of the eye is difficult as the iris muscle fibers are striated and partly under voluntary control and so parasympatholytics (e.g., atropine) and sympathomimetics (e.g., phenylephrine) will not work. In addition the cornea is protected by the spectacle, which prevents absorption of topical nonparasympatholytic mydriatics (such as vecuronium). Consider ophthalmic examination either by using low light levels or GA.

Bacterial

- Subspectacular abscess
- Keratitis
- Panophthalmitis

Fungal

- Subspectacular abscess
- Keratitis
- Panophthalmitis

Neoplasia

Other noninfectious problems

- Trauma
- Retained spectacle
- Avulsion of the spectacle (usually iatrogenic)
- Occlusion of nasolacrimal duct
- Congenital absence of nasolacrimal duct
- Stenosis due to or following inflammation
- Congenital abnormalities
- Cyclopia
- Microphthalmia—often associated with head abnormalities
- Anophthalmia
- Exposure to excessive low temperature during hibernation (cataracts)
- Lenticular cataract

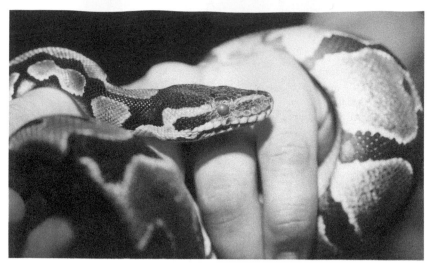

Fig 11-10. Retained spectacle in a young royal python.

Findings on clinical examination

- Permanent opacity of the spectacle due to one or more retained spectacles (Fig. 11-10). Associated retained skin may be visible on the head.
- Space beneath spectacle distended with clear fluid (occlusion of nasolacrimal duct)
- Subspectacular abscess
- The eye appears opaque and the spectacle may be bulge due to increased pressure in the corneospectacular space. This condition may be unilateral or bilateral. This condition can be associated with retained spectacle (dysecdysis—see *Skin Disorders*) or stomatitis (subspectacular abscess—see also *Gastrointestinal Tract Disorders*).
- Hypopyon
- Uveitis
- Cataracts
- Retinal degeneration
- Panophthalmitis

Investigations

1. Ophthalmic examination
   a. Assess whether eye is able to rotate beneath the spectacle during rotation of the head (i.e., that there are no corneospectacular adhesions).
   b. Space beneath spectacle distended with clear fluid (occlusion of nasolacrimal duct)
   c. Subspectacular abscess: The eye appears opaque and the spectacle may bulge due to increased pressure in the corneospectacular space. This condition may be unilateral or bilateral.
2. Radiography
3. Routine hematology and biochemistry
4. Culture and sensitivity
5. Biopsy/necropsy
6. Ultrasonography

Treatment/specific therapy

- Retained spectacle. This is often associated with:
  - Low humidity
  - Anorexia
  - Dermatologic conditions, including snake mites (see *Skin Disorders*)
  - If the spectacle over the cornea is retained, then gentle rubbing while applying slight pressure with a damp cotton bud should eventually cause some ruching of the spectacle and allow its removal.
  - Do not pull with forceps as you risk avulsing the cornea with consequent loss of the use of that eye. If very adherent, the spectacle can be loosened by application of 10% acetylcysteine.
- Subspectacular abscess
  - Treatment involves surgical incision into the spectacle to allow an assessment for any corneal lesions.
  - All debris should be flushed from the corneal surface, and if possible the nasolacrimal duct can be cannulated and flushed.
  - Topical ophthalmic antibiotic or antimycotic preparations should be used (see *Skin Disorders*).
  - Attend to any underlying conditions (e.g., stomatitis).
  - A new spectacle should form at the next skin shed. To prevent dessication, consider attempting to suture a contact lens in place.
- Nasolacrimal duct occlusion
  - Treatment is similar to subspectacular abscess.
  - Conjunctivoralostomy can be attempted in large snakes by passing a curved 18G needle from the inferior conjunctival fornix into the roof of the mouth such that it emerges between the palatine and maxillary teeth. A 0.025-inch Silastic tubing, threaded through the needle and secured at each end with sutures, may work in some cases.
- Avulsion of the spectacle
  - Often the eye is so badly damaged that enucleation is required.
  - Otherwise treat as for repair of subspectacular abscess.
- Congenital defects
  - No treatment
  - Consider incubation parameters (temperature, humidity, etc.) as well as genetic factors when considering cause.

Endocrine disorders

Little studied in reptiles

Neoplasia

- Thyroid neoplasia (especially garter snakes, *Thamnophis* spp.)

Other noninfectious problems

- Hyperthyroidism (see "Dysecdysis" in *Skin Disorders*)

Findings on clinical examination

- Swollen cervical region (thyroid neoplasia—Fig. 11-11)
- Excessive repetitive skin shedding

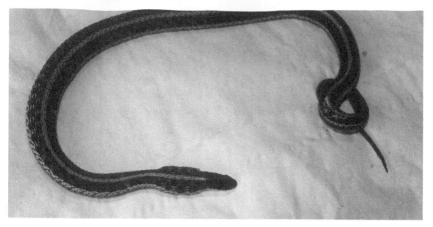

Fig 11-11. A garter snake with a cervical swelling; surgical resection revealed a thyroid carcinoma.

Investigations

1. Radiography
2. Routine hematology and biochemistry
    a. Blood T_4 levels (Table 11-7)
3. Culture and sensitivity
4. Endoscopy
5. Biopsy
6. Ultrasonography

Table 11-7 Blood T_4 levels		
Species	**T_4 concentration (nmol/L)**	
	Range	**Mean**
Corn snakes (Elaphe guttata)	0.45-6.06	2.75
Ball pythons (Python regius)	0.93-4.79	2.58
Milk snakes (Lampropeltis triangulum)	0.27-2.94	1.88
Boas (Boa constrictor constrictor)	0.24-3.98	2.50
Adapted from Greenacre et al (2001).		

Treatment/specific therapy

- Thyroid neoplasia
    - Surgical resection. Often metastasizes
- Hyperthyroidism (see *Skin Disorders*)

Renal disorders

Bacterial
• Bacterial kidney disease/abscessation

Fungal
• Mycetoma (e.g., *Aspergillus* spp.)

Parasitic
• Flukes (especially in king snakes, indigos, boas, tropical rat snakes, and bushmasters)
• Aberrant *Strongyloides* spp. infestation (Veazey et al 1994)

Neoplasia
• Renal adenocarcinoma (Gravendyck et al 1997)
• Renal cell carcinoma (may metastasize to lungs and liver)

Other noninfectious problems
• Gout
• Iatrogenic drug toxicity, especially nephrotoxic drugs, including the aminoglycosides

Findings on clinical examination

• Anorexia
• Lethargy
• Weight loss
• Polydipsia/polyuria
• Marked swelling of caudal third of coelom (renomegaly, renal neoplasia, extreme renal gout)
• Anuria
• Edema
• Pale mucous membranes
• Mortalities

Investigations

1. Radiography
   a. Renomegaly
2. Routine hematology and biochemistry
   a. No good single test. Snakes with renal disease may show hyperuricemia, hyperuremia, hyperphosphatemia, hyperkalemia, hyponatremia, and hyperproteinemia or hypoproteinemia.
3. Urinalysis
   a. Renal casts
   b. Inflammatory cells
4. Fecal examination (see *Gastrointestinal Tract Disorders*)
5. Culture and sensitivity
6. Endoscopy
   a. Abnormalities in shape, color, or size of kidneys
   b. Flukes in cloaca (and feces)

7. Biopsy/necropsy
   a. Flukes in kidneys (also on postmortem); can cause an interstitial nephritis and other renal abnormalities
   b. Ureteritis and nephritis caused by *Strongyloides* spp.
   c. Mycetoma
8. Ultrasonography
   a. Hyperechoic or hypoechoic, focal or multifocal changes; alteration of size

Treatment/specific therapy

- Flukes
  - Praziquantel at 5 mg/kg PO, SC, or IM. Repeat after 2 weeks.
  - Freeze food items (e.g., frogs, fish) for 3 days prior to feeding to eliminate intermediate stages.
- Aberrant *Strongyloides* infestation—see *Gastrointestinal Tract Disorders*
- Bacterial renal disease
  - Antibiotics (beware nephrotoxic medications)
  - Fluid therapy
- Mycetoma
  - Poor prognosis. Attempt antifungal therapy (see *Systemic Disorders*) as well as general renal supportive therapy.
- Gout
  - Fluid therapy
  - Allopurinol at 10 mg/kg PO s.i.d. *Note:* This will only prevent subsequent uric acid deposition.
  - Very guarded prognosis
  - May be linked with renal disease, chronic dehydration, or use of nephrotoxic drugs

Reproductive disorders

Snakes can be either oviparous (egg-laying) or viviparous (live-bearing). Typical oviparous snakes include the colubrids and pythons. Typical viviparous snakes include the boas and garter snakes (*Thamnophis* spp.).

Noninfectious problems
- Dystocia
- Preovulatory ovarian stasis (POOS)
- Egg stasis (postovulatory)
- Ectopic pregnancy (viviparous species)
- Prolapsed hemipene

Findings on clinical examination

- Eggs often palpable in the caudal third of the coelom
- Straining
- Poor condition
- Obesity
- Dehydration

- Presence of some eggs or young
- One or two large, swollen often spikey structures hanging from the cloaca (prolapsed hemipenes)

Investigations

1. Radiography
   a. Snake eggs are generally poorly calcified and so appear as rounded soft-tissue opacities in the caudal coelomic cavity.
   b. Fetal skeletons may be visible in advanced gestation in live-bearing snakes (e.g., boas)
   c. The hemipenes of some species are calcified and can be identified radiographically.
2. Routine hematology and biochemistry
3. Culture and sensitivity
4. Endoscopy
5. Biopsy
6. Ultrasonography
   a. Useful for POOS and identifying young in live-bearing snakes

Treatment/specific therapy

- Dystocia
  - Provision of correct environment, including appropriate temperature, humidity, and nesting chamber, may induce normal egg-laying or birth.
  - Medical induction
    - There is a small window of opportunity for the effective use of oxytocin; best used within 48 to 72 hours of obvious nesting or straining seen (Stahl 2000).
    - Use oxytocin at 5 to 20 IU/kg IM, starting at the lower dose; repeat 2 to 3 times at 6- to 12-hour intervals.
    - Vasopressin at 0.01 to 1.0 µg/kg IV, IM (more potent than oxytocin in reptiles)
    - Digital manipulation. In some cases eggs can be manipulated out of the cloaca. This should be done under GA as it is a very delicate procedure and there is a significant risk of trauma.
  - Percutaneous ovocentesis. Performed under anesthesia with sterile 20G needle. Beware of yolk leaking into coelomic cavity, aspiration of the viscera or their contents, both of which will trigger a serositis. Allow snake to pass collapsed eggs. If the eggs have been present for several days, then the yolk may be solid and resistant to aspiration.
  - Salpingotomy; easier than above; may require multiple incisions to remove all eggs
  - Ovariosalpingectomy. Make a paramedian incision along the junction between the ventral scales and the body wall to avoid incising into the ventral midline and the underlying ventral vena cava.
    - Consider ovariosalpingectomy for nonbreeding females to prevent future problems.
- Ectopic pregnancy
  - Surgery
- Prolapse of hemipene
  - Attempt replacement (with lubrication) and pursestring suture around the cloaca.
  - If severely swollen topical glycerin or concentrated sucrose solution may reduce the swelling enough to allow reduction.
  - Badly damaged, infected, or paralyzed hemipenes should be resected. Providing the snake still has one functional hemipene, it can still breed.

Noninfectious problems

- Prolapse of the umbilicus
- Congenital deformities
- Dead in shell (mid to late embryonic deaths)

Findings on clinical examination

- Bulging of tissue at the umbilicus of newborn or newly hatched snakes. Bulge may contain coelomic lining, yolk sac remnant, and coelomic fat.

Investigations

1. Radiography
2. Routine hematology and biochemistry
3. Culture and sensitivity
4. Endoscopy
5. Biopsy/necropsy
6. Ultrasonography

Treatment/specific therapy

- Prolapsed umbilicus
  - Clean and replace prolapse. Suture in place.
  - May require surgical resection of yolk sac remnant
  - This is particularly prevalent in hatchlings with incomplete yolk sac resorption, where the yolk sac membranes adhere to dry surfaces or to the inside of the shell (especially if the humidity is too low). Keep hatchlings with pronounced egg sacs in moist, clean surroundings until resorption takes place. Do not attempt to separate the hatchling from the egg, but increase humidity and/or remove the hatchling plus egg to a warm, humid environment to allow natural separation.
- Dead in shell. Can be due to a variety of conditions. Consider:
  - Nutritional status of parents, especially the female
  - Incubation parameters (temperature, humidity, hygiene, oxygen levels, CO_2 levels)
  - Bacterial and fungal infection
- Congenital abnormalities
  - Hereditary conditions
  - Incorrect incubation parameters

Tortoises and turtles

Chelonia, such as tortoises and their semi-aquatic relatives, terrapins (or turtles), are becoming very popular as pets, especially in Europe where there is a long history of keeping the Mediterranean *Testudo* species as house and garden pets. Although CITES II listed, this trade is being fueled by the increasing availability of captive-bred specimens, especially from Eastern Europe.

The internal anatomy of a tortoise is shown in Figure 12.1.

Table 12-1 Commonly encountered tortoises and turtles: Key facts

Species	Notes	Common disorders
The Mediterranean *Testudo* species, including the southern European Hermann's *(T. hermanni)*, members of the north African spur-thighed complex *(T. graeca)*, and the Russian tortoise *(T. horsfeldi)*	These are small to moderately large species; most can be safely hibernated, but see *Hibernation* for more details. Diet should primarily be leafy greens with added calcium supplementation. No animal protein should be given.	Metabolic bone disease, chelonian herpesvirus, ascarids
African spur-thighed tortoise *Centrochelys sulcata*	This species from sub-Saharan Africa is a potential monster that can weigh up to 50-80 kg. They require tropical heat with relatively low humidity. Diet as for *Testudo* spp.	Metabolic bone disease, chelonian herpesvirus
The leopard tortoise *(Geochelone pardalis)*	Another sub-Saharan African species. Requires tropical temperatures and a *Testudo*-like diet	Metabolic bone disease
Red-footed tortoises *(G. carbonaria)*	Tropical South America. They need tropical temperatures, high humidity (70%), and a diet with more fruit than *Testudo* spp. with a small amount of animal protein.	Metabolic bone disease
Red-eared slider *(Trachemys picta elegans)*	Less common in the European pet trade following several scares over *Salmonella* and concerns over alien releases. It is semi-aquatic and requires a dry, warm haul-out area on which to bask. They are carnivorous as hatchlings and feed on commercially available insect larvae (e.g., bloodworms); graduating up to sea-foods such as prawns, fish, mussels, and cockles plus calcium supplement. Commercial pelleted foods are available.	Metabolic bone disease, hypovitaminosis A
Box turtles *(Terrapene* spp.)	Omnivorous, requiring slugs, snails, earthworms, waxworms, mealworms, fruit, green loafed vegetables, and mushrooms	Metabolic bone disease, tympanic scale abscesses

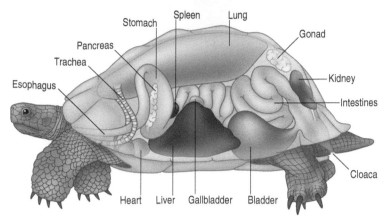

Fig 12-1. Internal anatomy of a tortoise (lateral).

Captive care

As with lizards, the long-term welfare of captive chelonia is intimately dependent on their environment. They must be provided with appropriate temperatures, full-spectrum diet, and correct nutrition, including a calcium supplement (see Chapter 10 for more detail). This especially applies to hatchlings of the *Testudo* spp., for whom a vivarium is mandatory despite the relative hardiness of the adults.

Importance of lighting

Light in the spectrum of 290 to 315 nm (ultraviolet-B, UVB) is required for endogenous vitamin D_3 production; ultraviolet-A (UVA) spectrum (320 to 400 nm) has been shown to have a beneficial influence on normal behavior.

Endogenous vitamin D_3 production in reptiles is a many-step process that involves not only exposure to UVB but also thermal isomerization and modification in the liver and kidneys. Therefore, correct environmental temperatures and healthy organs are required for normal vitamin D_3 synthesis.

Dietary supplementation with vitamin D_3 alone is not sufficient for chelonia. In addition, dietary calcium supplementation is essential for all captive chelonia. The commercially available leafy greens and vegetables usually offered to tortoises are inherently low in calcium but high in phosphates. Evidence suggests that in the wild tortoise select high-calcium foods. A Ca:P ratio of 3.5:1 is recommended.

Consultation and handling

Most terrestrial chelonia can be safely handled without fear of being bitten, but take care with larger terrapins or potentially dangerous species such as snapping turtles. These should be held at the rear of the carapace and, in the case of snappers, at the base of the tail.

Start the examination at the head, as this is likely to be withdrawn into the shell precluding further examination. Grasp the head behind the back of the skull and draw it out to its fullest extent. With most tortoises the mouth can now be opened and examined using the tip of a finger as a gag. With terrapins and similar a gag must be used. The rest of the body can then be examined systematically. Useful auscultation of the lung fields can sometimes be achieved by placing a damp towel over the carapace onto which the stethoscope is placed.

Weight: Length measurement as an indicator of health in Mediterranean tortoises

For Hermann's tortoise *(Testudo hermanii)* and the spur-thighed complex *(T. graeca)*, an indication of health can be gained by the following (Peter Heathcote, personal communication). This is achieved by the following actions:

1. Weigh the tortoise (in grams).
2. Measure the straight length of the carapace (cm). *Note:* This straight length of the carapace is a linear measurement from the most rostral point of the carapace to the most caudal. It is not a measurement over the dome of the carapace.
3. The weight of the tortoise (g) is then divided by the (straight length of the carapace (cm³)); i.e., tortoise weight (g)/straight length of the carapace (cm)³.
4. The resultant number is compared with the straight length of the carapace:
   a. Straight length of carapace >15 cm; normal ratio 0.21 to 0.23.
   b. Straight length of carapace <15 cm; normal ratio 0.23 to 0.25.
5. Tortoises with a ratio of 0.17 or less are considered critical.
6. Examples for tortoises with a high ratio are obesity (hepatic lipidosis), gravid (multiple eggs, averaging around 10 g each), or fluid retentive.

Sexing

As a general rule, males have longer tails, a slitlike opening to the cloaca, and a degree of concavity to the plastron, although this varies from species to species (Fig. 12-2). Chelonia have temperature-dependent sex determination and it is likely that variations in temperature at thermally sensitive stages of embryonic development may produce a range of such secondary sexual characteristics, meaning that in some cases sexing is not an exact science.

Male red-eared sliders have elongated claws on their front feet that are used to "tickle" the nose of the female during courtship.

Microchipping

- Subcutaneously in the left hind leg (intramuscularly in thin-skinned species) and subcutaneously in the tarsal area in giant species. *Note:* Hemorrhage is common with accidental intramuscular injection in smaller chelonia.
- Skin closure is achieved either by suture or with tissue glue.

Blood sampling

Optimum site for collection in most chelonia is the jugular vein or brachial vein. Collection from the dorsal coccygeal vein and the subcarapacial jugular anastomosis are readily contaminated with lymph.

Note: EDTA destroys chelonian red blood cells. Take a sample into heparin and make a smear immediately. EDTA is, however, good for WBC preservation.

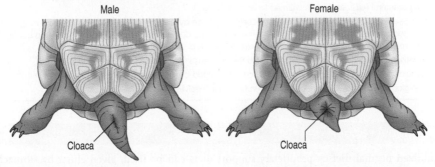

Male   Female

Cloaca   Cloaca

Fig 12-2. Sexing of chelonia.

Nursing care

Provide appropriate environment, including provision of:

1. Optimal temperature (basking lights, heat mats, etc., to allow thermoregulation). Use of max–min thermometers will assist in monitoring temperature ranges incumbent reptiles are exposed to.
2. Full-spectrum lighting (provision of UVA and UVB)
3. Humidity
4. Ventilation
5. Easily cleaned accommodation; use paper substrate and disposable/sterilizable hides and other vivarium furniture (see Fig. 10-3).
6. Keep individually to minimize intraspecies stress and competition for resources.

Large terrestrial chelonia often appear to have difficulty with transparent barriers and may spend a considerable amount of time attempting to walk through, over, or under glass vivarium sides and doors. Blanking off these sides with tape or paint may reduce this behavior.

With semi-aquatic chelonia such as terrapins, for general care they should be provided with a dry haul-out area that has an overhanging heat source to allow thorough drying of the carapace and sufficient water such that the terrapin can rest with its hind feet on the bottom and its nostrils above the surface. A weak terrapin is at risk of drowning. In some cases a terrapin may need to be "dry-docked" for a period of time. Where possible, this can entail only short periods in a deeper bath. This can be combined with feeding because healthy terrapins will often prefer to feed submerged. Alternatively, serious attention to and monitoring of its fluid status should be undertaken if access to water is felt inappropriate (see "Fluid Therapy" below).

Fluid therapy

See "Fluid Therapy" in Chapter 10.

The assessment of dehydration in chelonia can be difficult visually. An obvious sign in chelonia is sunken eyes, so it is better to monitor packed cell volume (PCV). This varies with species, but it should be around 26 to 32 L/L.

Fluid administration

1. Daily bathing in shallow, warm water is often beneficial; it encourages many chelonia to drink as well as defecate and urinate. Many chelonia can absorb fluids across the cloacal lining.
2. Stomach tubing is often feasible in small to medium-sized chelonia (Fig. 12-3). Large chelonia are often physically too strong to hold for stomach tubing (Fig. 12-4).
3. Esophagostomy tubes are often very useful for medium to long-term fluid and nutritional management.
4. All parenteral fluids should be warmed to around 26° C.
5. In chelonia, fluid can be given into the epicoelomic space by passing a 1- to 1.5-inch needle through the pectoral musculature such that the needle is inserted dorsal to and parallel with the plastron but is beneath the pectoral girdle. The needle is directed toward the contralateral hind leg.
6. Another site is by intraosseous catheter into the vertical plastrocarapacial bridge.
7. Whole-blood transfusions can be undertaken using blood obtained from the same or related species.
8. Oxyglobin at 10 mL/kg once only has been used successfully.

Nutritional support

Liquidized normal diet or proprietary support diets can be used, given either by stomach tube or by esophagostomy tube.

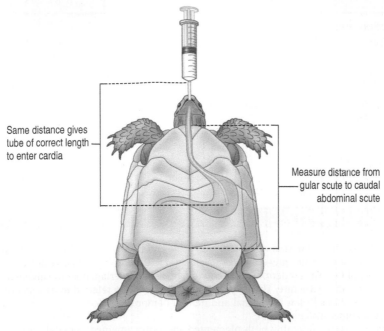

Same distance gives
tube of correct length
to enter cardia

Measure distance from
gular scute to caudal
abdominal scute

Fig 12-3. Measuring a stomach tube for tubing a tortoise.

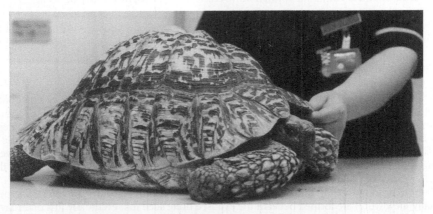

Fig 12-4. Large terrestrial chelonia such as this leopard tortoise are physically very strong.

Analgesia

- Morphine 1.5 mg/kg PO s.i.d. for 3 days
- Tramadol at 5.0 to 100 mg/kg PO s.i.d. (Baker et al 2011)
  Also see "Analgesia" in Chapter 10.

Anesthesia

For general notes, see "Anesthesia" in Chapter 10.

Induction and maintenance of anesthesia in *Chelonia*

1. Propofol at 12 to 15 mg/kg IV delivered into the jugular vein or the dorsal coccygeal vein. Adverse reactions have been noted occasionally when administered via the subcarapacial jugular anastomosis.
2. Alfaxalone at 2.0 to 5.0 mg/kg IV (Knotek 2014). Can be maintained either with further top-ups at 2.0 mg/kg or by gaseous anesthesia.
3. With prolonged intermittent positive-pressure ventilation the lungs may become permanently expanded, so regular deflation by flexion and compression of all four legs in toward the shell should be undertaken.
4. In chelonia, Doppler ultrasound can be used to monitor heartbeat by placing the ultrasound monitor into the clavicular fossa.
5. For large chelonia in whom IV access is impractical, ketamine at 5 to 10 mg/kg and dexmedetomidine 50 to 100 µg/kg IM. Reverse with same volume atipamazole.
6. Otherwise as for lizards (see Chapter 10)

Skin disorders

The structure of chelonian skin of the legs, tail, neck, and head is as in other reptiles. However, the chelonian shell is unique—in most species there are 54 epidermal scales covering 59 dermal bony plates. The epidermal and dermal seams rarely overlap, possibly giving increased strength to the shell structure. These epidermal scales are often referred to as *scutes* or *shields*. Even here, the skin still has epidermal and dermal components.

The scute epidermis consists of:

1. Horny material containing both pigmented and nonpigmented material. This layer contains a mixture of α- and β-type keratin.
2. Pseudostratified columnar epithelium. Occasional melanophores may be seen.
3. Dermis overlies the dermal bone.
4. In the seam between the scutes, the epidermal cell layers are 3 to 4 cells thick, and it is here that differentiation into keratin-producing cells occurs, and so new horny tissue is produced. Unlike in other reptiles, the keratin is usually retained, thereby producing the typical rings on the scutes.
5. Cellular proliferation and keratinization are continuous.

Chelonia generally shed their skin in a piecemeal and uncoordinated fashion. Semi-aquatic chelonia will often shed the older outer scutes.

In some species such as the spur-thighed tortoise *(Testudo graeca)*, there is a hinge between the abdominal and femoral scutes of the plastron, while in others (e.g., the Russian tortoise— *T. horsfieldii*), there is not. Box turtles (e.g., the Eastern box—*Terrapene carolina*) also have a hinged plastron that enables them to withdraw both the head and all four limbs within the shell, protecting them with the trapdoor-like plastron.

Following injury, exposed carapacial or plastral bone, if allowed to dry out, dies off superficially; new scutes are formed beneath the exposed bone such that eventually this outer layer is shed.

Differential diagnoses for skin disorders

Abnormal skin shedding (dysecdysis)

- In terrapins a form of dysecdysis is seen where there is a failure of the outer layers of the carapacial scutes to shed and air becomes trapped beneath these, producing silvery patches. This may occur if the terrapin is unable to haul out and bask properly to dry out the shell.

Pruritus

- Ectoparasites
- Dermatitis

Erosions, ulceration, and shell deficits

- Trauma
  - Often secondary to damage from another tortoise. Some males, especially the Turkish spur-thighed tortoise *(Testudo ibera)*, are very aggressive to conspecific and heterospecific males.
- Bacterial infection
- Keratinolytic bacteria from soil in the shell
- Other bacteria (e.g., *Aeromonas* spp. in damp conditions)
- *Benekea chitinovora* (terrapins)
- Septicemia (opportunistic species)
- Septicemic cutaneous ulcerative disease (SCUD), especially softshell turtles. Often due to *Citrobacter freundii* or *Pseudomonas* spp. Other gram-negative organisms may also cause this condition in aquatic chelonia.
- Mycobacteria (see *Systemic Disorders*)
- Fungal infections
- "Dry" lesions in terrestrial chelonia are often due to soil-derived keratinolytic mycotic infections, such as *Geotrichum candidum* and *Scolecobasidium humicola.*
- *Fusarium incarnatum* (gopher tortoises, *Gopherus berlandieri*—Rose et al 2001)
- *Microsporum* spp., *Mucor* spp. (ulcerative epidermitis in softshell *Trionyx* spp.)
- Chromomycosis (e.g., *Scolecobasidium humicola, Cladosporium herbarum, Phialophora* spp., *Hormodendrum* spp., *Curvularia* spp., *Fonsecaea* spp., *Rhinocladiella* spp., and *Drechslera* spp.)
- *Saprolegnia* can infect freshwater aquatic chelonia, often secondarily invading wounds and lesions. Appears as a cotton wool-like covering while submerged that collapses on removal from the water
- *Paecilomyces lilacinus* (Lafortune et al 2005)
- Iatrogenic hypervitaminosis A (a necrotic dermatitis leading to a full-thickness skin sloughing)
- Burns
- Spirochid flukes (terrapins)
- Renal failure (loss of scutes often accompanied by excess exudation and ascites)
- Shell fractures—see *Musculoskeletal Disorders*
- Dog or other predator attack
- Rat or rodent attack (gnawed lesions on the legs, especially the lateral surfaces of the front legs—Fig. 12-5)

Nodules and nonhealing wounds

- Abscess
- Granuloma (bacterial, including mycobacteria, fungal)
- *Cistudinomyia (Sarcophaga) cistudinis,* especially in the axillial and femoral fossae of box turtles (*Terrapene* spp.)
- Gas bubble disease in aquatic chelonia (rare)
- Spirochid flukes (terrapins)
- Subepidermal mites
- Dermal papillomatosis (sideneck turtles—*Platemys* spp.)
- Chelonian herpesvirus (CHV—see also *Respiratory Tract Disorders*)
- Poxlike virus in *T. hermanni*

Changes in pigmentation

- Erythema (septicemia)
- Burns

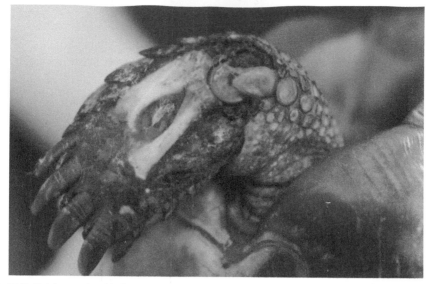

Fig 12-5. Rat damage in a Mediterranean spur-thighed tortoise. The elbow joint has been exposed.

- Liver disease (and other possible etiologies for coagulation abnormalities)
- Hemoprotozoans
- Renal failure (often accompanied by excess exudate and loss of scutes)
- Algal growths (aquatic chelonia)
- Scar tissue (depigmented)
- *Fusarium semitectum* is a cause of whitish skin blemishes in *Gopherus berlandieri.*
- Failure of the scutes to be able to dry out (semi-aquatic chelonia)

Ectoparasites

- Myiasis (fly strike; maggots)
- *Calliphora vicina*
- *Lucilia ampullacea, L. coeruleiviridis*
- *Cistudinomyia (Sarcophaga) cistudinis*
- Botfly larvae
- Ticks (e.g., *Amblyomma sparsum, A. marmoreum*)
- Subepidermal mites (African spurred tortoise *Centrochelys sulcata*—Nicasio et al 2002)
- Spirochid flukes (terrapins)
- Spirurids
- Leeches (wild-caught or feral freshwater chelonia)
- Barnacles (*Balanus* spp.) recorded on diamondback terrapins *(Malaclemys terrapin)* (Werner 2003)

Burns

Neoplasia

Shell deformities

- Excessive protein intake
- Metabolic bone disease (nutritional osteodystrophy)

- Old shell lesions (e.g., traumatic injuries)
- Dyskeratosis—cause unknown, but may be linked to systemic disease (Homer et al 2001)

Findings on clinical examination

- Reddened, thickened areas of skin suggest an underlying infection. These may be moist.
- Loss of dermal structures such as toenails
- Overgrowth of dermal structures such as the toenails, beak, and scutes
- Partial or complete loss of scutes
- Silvery patches on the scutes of semi-aquatic chelonia. Many of these, such as red-eared terrapins *(Chrysema scripta elegans)*, do routinely shed scutes. Failure to do so results in air trapped beneath loosened scutes.
- Exposure of underlying bone
- Flaking and fissuring of the keratin scutes
- Inflammation and exudate accompanied by separation of the scutes from the underlying bone can be indicative of severe septicemia or renal disease.
- Pruritus: The reptile may scratch against objects. The body plan of chelonia means that they are rarely able to scratch themselves in any meaningful manner, nor can they self-mutilate.
- Spirochid eggs cause vascular occlusion, causing focal and coalescing areas of ulcerative necrosis of the carapace and plastron.
- Obvious parasites
- Penetrating injuries through scutes into underlying bone; may reach into coelomic cavity or lungs (dog bites)
- Live maggots on or around open wounds; swellings under the skin (myiasis)
- Exfoliation of skin of head and neck associated with necrotic stomatitis (CHV)
- Papular lesions around the eyes *(T. hermanni)*—poxlike virus

Investigations

1. Radiography
2. Sterile swabs taken for bacterial or fungal culture
3. Impression smears or other samples taken for staining and cytology
4. Blood samples for general hematology and biochemistry
5. Biopsy of suspect lesions
   a. Dracunculid larvae may be present in the skin (spirurids). Adults lie in coelomic cavity.
6. Discuss environmental management with owner:
   a. Are calcium and vitamin D_3 supplements offered routinely?
   b. Is full-spectrum lighting provided?
   c. Are fluorescent tubes changed at the correct frequency (usually every 6 months)?
   d. Are high-protein foods being offered?
7. Endoscopy
8. Ultrasonography

Management

1. Any shell lesions should be investigated further by debridement around the lesion to remove fissures that could harbor persistent infections. This is potentially a very painful

procedure, and if large areas are to be debrided then general anesthesia (GA) should be considered.

2. Small to medium lesions can be managed with the application of topical iodine and/ or topical antimicrobials.

3. Larger lesions may require dressing:
   a. For terrestrial chelonia, application of a topical amorphous hydrogel dressing such as IntraSite Gel (Smith and Nephew Healthcare Ltd.) topically with a covering of a nonadhesive dressing promotes granulation and coverage of the underlying bone.
   b. For aquatic chelonia, applying Orabase (Squibb) or bone wax can be used to achieve a relatively watertight protective seal.

4. Consider fluid therapy if large areas of underlying bone are newly exposed and exuding.

5. Attempted covering of exposed bone with products such as methylmethacrylate or fiberglass should be delayed until all signs of infection have resolved.

6. Those chelonia on a high-protein diet may require burring back of excessively long toenails and upper and lower beak.

7. Long-term dry-docking of aquatic chelonia is contraindicated because dehydration and anorexia are common sequelae.

Treatment/specific therapy

- Ticks and maggots
  - These should be physically or surgically removed. Permethrin-based formulations are safe, although those products with synergists such as piperonyl butoxide should be avoided if possible. Fipronil may not affect a 10% kill of *Amblyomma* ticks (Burridge et al 2002). *Do not use ivermectin as this is toxic to chelonia.*
  - *Note:* Ticks are vectors for *Babesia/Hepatozoon* and *Ehrlichia*-like organisms.
  - *Note:* The tick *Amblyomma marmoreum* can transmit heartwater *(Cowdria ruminatium)* to domestic and native wildlife. This and other ectoparasites may act as vectors for other diseases.
- Bacterial and fungal infections
  - SCUD in freshwater terrapins is caused by *Citrobacter freundii* and other gram-negative bacteria. Often linked to high levels of environmental bacterial contamination so should be addressed
  - Antibiotics or antifungals as required
- Saprolegniosis: Salt solutions as low as 10 parts per thousand (ppt) (mg/100 mL) will inhibit infections.
- *Paecilomyces lilacinus* in the freshwater aquatic Fly River turtle *Carettochelys insculpta* was controlled (Lafortune 2005) with:
  - Permanent salt bath at 5 ppt (0.5%) for 14 days and then increased to 7 ppt
  - Malachite green and formalin dips (0.15 mg/L of 0.038% malachite green and 4.26% formaldehyde) for 15 minutes b.i.d. for 33 days
  - Itraconazole at 10 mg/kg PO every 48 hours for 20 days
- Spirochid flukes: Praziquantel at 10 mg/kg PO repeat after 4 weeks if necessary
- Address any dietary or environmental deficiencies.
- Dog attack
  - Covering antibiotics
  - Nonpenetrating injuries: Clean with topical iodine solution.
  - Dress any penetrating injuries with nonadhesive dressings. Only once any secondary infection is cleared should the lesion be sealed with synthetic polymers such as polymethylmethacrylate or fiberglass.

- Rat or rodent attack
  - Often during or shortly after hibernation when tortoises are sluggish
  - Commonly affects the lateral (outer) surfaces of the front legs, which are drawn across in front of the head for protection. Other limbs and the shell may be damaged as well.
  - The radius and ulna may be exposed, as may the elbow joint.
  - Clean and debride any devitalized tissue.
  - Application of topical amorphous hydrogel dressings such as IntraSite Gel (Smith and Nephew Healthcare Ltd.) will encourage secondary healing. A nonadhesive dressing should be applied.
  - Healing can take many months before reepithelialization occurs to a sufficient extent.
  - If the elbow joint is exposed:
    - Strap up the leg so that the tortoise cannot weight-bear on that leg.
    - Provide support by the attachment of a prop (e.g., half billiard ball; toy wheel) to the plastron of that quadrant.
    - In severe cases, one leg can be amputated at midhumeral or midfemoral level.
- Neoplasia
  - Rarely diagnosed or at least reported in the literature
  - Chemotherapy in reptiles is in its infancy, and most tumors are managed surgically. Accessible cutaneous tumors can be treated by injecting cisplatin directly into the tissue mass on a weekly basis as a debulking exercise. See Chapter 10

Respiratory tract disorders

Differential diagnoses for nasal tract disorders

Runny nose syndrome (RNS) is a poorly understood clinical syndrome. Linked with CHV, *Mycoplasma agassizii*, and various bacteria, but no single pathogenic agent has been established yet.

Viral

- CHV: A significant cause of RNS. Other commonly associated signs are stomatitis (with diphtheritic membranes on tongue, oropharynx, and nasopharynx), dysphagia, and hypersalivation. Less often there will be cervical edema, diarrhea, and CNS signs, including hind-limb paresis.
- Iridovirus: Can present similarly to CHV, especially with stomatitis and glossitis; may cause hepatitis
- Virus X: An as yet unidentified virus or group of viruses isolated from *Testudo* and *Geochelone* spp. that are linked to rhinitis, diphtheroid-necrotizing stomatitis/ pharyngitis, pneumonia, enteritis, and ascites (Marshang and Ruemenapf 2002).

Bacterial

- Often opportunistic bacterial infections—consider occult abscessation
- Mycobacteria (see *Systemic Disorders*)
- Mycoplasmosis
- *M. agassizii* identified as a cause of RNS in gopher tortoises

Fungal

- No definitive nasal fungal pathogens have been isolated, but a variety of fungi, regarded as commensals or secondary invaders, have been described in Sulawesi tortoises (*Indotestudo forstenii*—Innis et al 2003).

Protozoal

- Intranuclear coccidiosis: Undescribed protozoan found in the mucosal lining of the nares, conjunctiva, and eustachian tubes. May occur elsewhere (e.g., in renal and colonic mucosal epithelial cells). Linked, along with *Mycoplasma agassizii*, with severe necrotizing sinusitis (Innis et al 2003)

Nutritional

- Hypovitaminosis A (see *Nutritional Disorders*)

Neoplasia

Other noninfectious problems

- Poor husbandry (including nutrition) plus exposure to suboptimal temperatures

Findings on clinical examination

- Clear, serous to gelatinous or mucopurulent nasal discharge
- Necrosis of external nares, including the nasal septum, that may extend several millimeters caudally. The vomer and palatine bones may be severely damaged, and oronasal fistulae may develop.
- Occasionally accompanied by pharyngeal and tongue lesions
- Other, systemic clinical signs may be seen depending upon etiology.
- Aquatic and semi-aquatic chelonia may swim with one side held lower than the other (pneumonia—asymmetrical or unilateral pulmonary consolidation).

Investigations

1. Examination of discharge: Wet smear plus staining for cytology and Gram staining
2. Culture and sensitivity of discharge sample
   a. Submit mucus sample for mycoplasma PCR, isolation, or electron microscopy.
   b. Submit mucus sample for virus isolation
3. Radiography
4. Routine hematology and biochemistry
5. *Mycoplasma* serology
6. CHV serology
7. Endoscopy
8. Biopsy/necropsy
   a. Histopathology for intranuclear coccidiosis
9. Ultrasonography

Management

1. Covering systemic and/or topical antibiosis. Consider nebulization.
2. Topical iodine application to any areas of ulceration or exposed bone

3. Flushing of the nares: This should be attempted from both directions, with saline or an antibiotic ointment.
   a. With a syringe placed flush with the external nares such that any mucus or accumulated material is displaced caudally into the mouth, from where it can be removed
   b. Retrograde flushing can be achieved by placing antibiotic ointment onto the roof of the mouth at the nasopharynx, and displacing the antibiotic up and into the nasal cavity by compression with a cotton bud.
4. Surgical debridement may be required of any necrotic bone.
5. Supportive treatment—may require placement of an esophagostomy tube to bypass the buccal cavity.

Treatment/specific therapy

- CHV
  - Acyclovir at 80 mg/kg PO s.i.d. for cases of herpesvirus. Efficacy appears variable.
  - The author has found that lysine at 125 mg/kg PO b.i.d. PO may be useful to control CHV in some tortoises.
- Other viral infections: Supportive treatment only
- Nonspecific bacterial infections: Appropriate antibiotics
- Mycoplasmosis
  - Enrofloxacin at 5 to 10 mg/kg PO, SC s.i.d.
  - Doxycycline at 2.5 to 10 mg/kg PO s.i.d. or b.i.d. or 50 mg/kg IM (loading dose) followed by 25 mg/kg every 3 days
  - Tylosin at 5 mg/kg IM or PO s.i.d.
  - Clarithromycin at 15 mg/kg PO every 2 to 3 days
- Intranuclear coccidiosis
  - Potentiated sulfonamides (patient must be well hydrated)
  - Toltrazuril at 7.5 mg/kg PO s.i.d. for 2 days. Repeat after 12 days.

Lower respiratory tract disorders

Respiratory anatomy

The glottis is located at the base of the muscular, fleshy tongue relatively caudal in the oropharynx. The trachea has complete cartilaginous rings. It bifurcates into two bronchi a relatively short distance along the neck, and each of the two bronchi enters a lung dorsally. The lungs occupy the dorsal section of the shell and are adhered to the overlying dermal bones of the carapace. The lungs are paired and saclike with the gas exchanging alveoli situated at the periphery of these organs. The lack of a functional diaphragm allows inflammatory exudates to accumulate in the dependent portions of the lungs.

Common respiratory signs

Differential diagnoses of dyspnea:
1. Chelonia are unable to cough, so respiratory disease is likely to present as a dyspnea.
2. Pneumonia
3. Severe stomatitis/pharyngitis
4. Tracheal obstruction
5. Coelomic mass
6. Overheating

Differential diagnoses of respiratory noise:
1. RNS
2. Nasal foreign body
3. Tracheal obstruction/foreign body
4. Esophageal obstruction/foreign body
5. Pneumonia

Differential diagnoses for respiratory disorders

Viral

- CHV
- Iridovirus
- Virus X

Bacterial

- Various, especially environmental contaminants, including *Pseudomonas*
- Mycobacteria (see *Systemic Disorders*)

Fungal

- Mycotic pneumonia
- Often secondary to suboptimal temperatures or prolonged antibiotic use
- Many species described, including *Candida albicans* and *Paecilomyces*

Parasitic

- Migrant ascarids (often *Sulcascaris* or *Angusticaecum*), both in the trachea and the lungs
- Trematodes (aquatic chelonia—fish, amphibians, and crustaceans can act as intermediate hosts)

Nutritional

- Hypovitaminosis A predisposes to secondary lung infections.

Neoplasia

- Metastases

Other noninfectious problems

- Obstruction: Accumulations of mucus and inflammatory material from lower respiratory tract disease can act as obstructions.
- Drowning (typically terrestrial tortoises found in garden pond)
- Hyperthermia (overheating)—collapsed and may be salivating copiously

Findings on clinical examination

- Clearly audible respiratory sounds; may be quite moist in nature
- Dyspnea; exaggerated respiratory movements
- Discharge in mouth or at glottis
- Aquatic chelonia may consistently list to one side while swimming due to asymmetric consolidation in lungs.
- Aquatic chelonia may be reluctant to enter water.

Investigations

1. Radiography
   a. Lateral and craniocaudal views more useful than dorsoventral to detect areas of consolidation
   b. Compression of the lung fields may indicate an extrapulmonary lesion (e.g., obesity, hepatomegaly).
   c. Lung lesions can be accessed for swabbing, biopsy, etc., by carapacial osteotomy once position is ascertained by radiography.
2. Culture and sensitivity
3. Tracheal wash; staining of collected material and/or submission for culture and sensitivity
4. Endoscopy
5. Routine hematology and biochemistry
6. Endoscopy
7. Biopsy/necropsy
8. Ultrasonography

Management

- Systemic antibiosis plus any specific medication
- Nebulization may be effective if there is little build-up of inflammatory material.
- Direct application to lesions via carapacial osteotomy

Treatment/specific therapy

- Viral infections: Supportive treatment only
- CHV (see "Differential Diagnoses for Nasal Tract Disorders" in *Respiratory Tract Disorders*)
- Hypovitaminosis A
  - Vitamin A supplementation (see *Nutritional Disorders*)
- Bacterial pneumonia
  - As discussed under "Management" above
- Mycotic pneumonia
  - Difficult to treat. Use antimycotics within framework suggested under "Management" above.
  - Ketoconazole at 10 to 30 mg/kg PO s.i.d.
  - Itraconazole 5 mg/kg PO every other day
  - Griseofulvin 20 to 40 mg/kg PO every 3 days
- Ascarids
  - Fenbendazole at 50 to 100 mg/kg PO. Repeat every 2 weeks if necessary. *Note:* Fenbendazole is metabolized to oxfendazole by the liver. Note, however, that it may take up to 31 days to achieve maximum efficacy at 100 mg/kg (Giannetto et al 2007).
  - Oxfendazole at 68 mg/kg PO. Repeat every 2 weeks if necessary. Maximum efficacy after 12 days (Giannetto et al 2007)
  - Topical emodepside plus praziquantel preparations (Profender, Bayer) at 56 µL/100 g body weight (Mehlhorn et al 2005)
  - Prevention: Routine worming every 6 months (prehibernation and posthibernation for Mediterranean and other species where applicable), plus disposal of feces as soon as observed

- Trematodes
  - Praziquantel at 10 mg/kg PO or IM. Repeat after 2 weeks.
- Drowning
  - Vigorously pump water out of the lungs by holding the tortoise vertically with head downward and repetitively flexing the limbs into the inguinal and femoral fossae, thereby compressing the lungs.
  - Place in a high-oxygen atmosphere.
  - Furosemide at 5 mg/kg IM b.i.d. to encourage diuresis.
- Hyperthermia
  - Place in cool water.
  - Dexamethasone at 0.03-0.15 mg/kg IM, IV, or IO may be given.

Ear disorders

Differential diagnoses for tympanic scale (aural) abscess

Bacterial

- Ascending infection from the pharynx up the eustachian tube often reflects normal buccal flora, often gram-negative opportunistic bacteria, especially *Proteus vulgaris, Escherichia coli,* and *Aeromonas hydrophila* (Willer et al 2003)
- Mycoplasmosis

Fungal

- Yeasts

Parasitic

- Ascarid (*Angusticaecum* spp.) described in Mediterranean spur-thighed tortoise *Testudo graeca* (Cutler 2004)

Nutritional

- Possibly related to hypovitaminosis A

Neoplasia

Other noninfectious problems

- Poor husbandry and suboptimal temperatures
- Exposure to organochlorine pesticides

Findings on clinical examination

- More common in box turtles than other terrestrial chelonia
- Swollen tympanic scale—can be unilateral or bilateral (Fig. 12-6)
- A plug of purulent material may be visible in the pharynx at the site of the eustachian tube.

Investigations

1. Investigate oropharynx—if ascarid present, is likely to be visible
2. Routine culture and sensitivity of purulent material
3. Cytology
4. Radiography

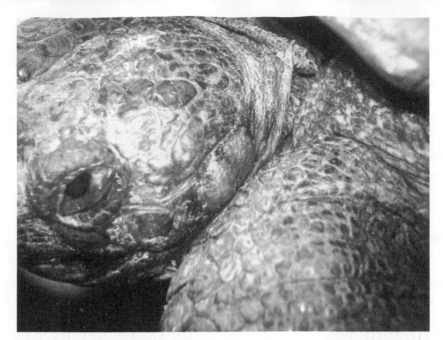

Fig 12-6. Tympanic abscess.

5. Endoscopy
6. Routine hematology and biochemistry
7. Endoscopy
8. Biopsy/necropsy
9. Ultrasonography

Management

1. Remove any ascarid present via the pharynx if possible.
2. Either under GA or local anesthetic, incise through tympanic scale.
3. Remove purulent material and flush. Check that the eustachian tube is patent by monitoring the pharyngeal ostium.
4. Tympanic scale can be sutured but is often left to heal by second intention, thereby allowing repeated flushing.

Treatment/specific therapy

- Bacterial infections: Appropriate antibiosis
- Yeasts
  - Nystatin at 100,000 units/kg PO daily for 10 days
- Ascarids
  - Fenbendazole at 50 to 100 mg/kg PO. Repeat every 2 weeks if necessary. *Note:* Fenbendazole is metabolized to oxfendazole by the liver.
  - Oxfendazole at 68 mg/kg PO. Repeat every 2 weeks if necessary.

- Topical emodepside plus praziquantel preparations (Profender, Bayer) at 56 μL/100 g body weight (Mehlhorn et al 2005)
  - Prevention: Routine worming every 6 months (prehibernation and posthibernation for Mediterranean and other species where applicable)
- Hypovitaminosis A: See *Nutritional Disorders.*

Gastrointestinal tract disorders

Disorders of the oral cavity

Viral

- CHV stomatitis (see also "Runny Nose Syndrome" in *Respiratory Tract Disorders*)
- Papillomavirus

Bacterial

- Stomatitis (see also "Runny Nose Syndrome" in *Respiratory Tract Disorders*)

Fungal

- Stomatitis

Parasitic

- Monogenetic trematodes (in semi-aquatic chelonia *Chrysemys, Trachemys,* and *Chelodina* spp.)

Nutritional

- Oak leaf toxicity (see *Urinary Disorders*)

Neoplasia
Other noninfectious problems

- Fractured jaw, especially at mandibular symphysis
- Overheating
- Overgrown beak

Findings on clinical examination

- Inflammation of the oral and pharyngeal membranes progressing to ulcerative lesions involving the palatine area and the trachea. A diphtheritic membrane may be present (CHV, bacterial and fungal stomatitis, oak leaf toxicity)
- Difficulty with prehension or processing of food
- Obvious lesion on lower jaw (fractured mandible); not always visible, however
- Loss of rostral lower jaw, including the intermandibular joint (sequel to bilateral mandibular fractures and/or osteomyelitis)
- Asymmetry of skull, swelling of one or both mandibles (metabolic bone disease—see *Musculoskeletal Disorders,* abscess/osteomyelitis, fracture, neoplasia)
- Icterus (see *Hepatic Disorders* and *Cardiovascular and Hematologic Disorders*). In some *Testudo* species (e.g., *T. cyrenacea*), the mucous membranes are naturally very yellow in appearance.
- Cyanosis
- Excessive ptyalism (overheating, stomatitis)

Investigations

1. Radiography
   a. Consider if risk of underlying osteomyelitis
   b. Likely to require GA to get head into suitable position for radiography
2. Routine hematology and biochemistry
3. Culture and sensitivity
4. Polymerase chain reaction (PCR) for CHV
5. Cytology
   a. Intranuclear inclusions (CHV), fungal hyphae
   b. Gram stain (bacteria, yeasts)
   c. Modified Ziehl-Neelsen (MZN) stain (mycobacteria)
6. Endoscopy
7. Biopsy
8. Ultrasonography

Treatment/specific therapy

- Fractured jaw
  - Can be due to traumatic handling (e.g., during stomach tubing) or may be pathological (e.g., infection, metabolic bone disease)
  - Placement of an esophagostomy tube will help with fluid and nutritional support during recovery.
  - Surgical repair is difficult in smaller chelonia; pins traversing the intermandibular space can interfere with tongue mobility.
  - Many terrestrial chelonia can manage surprisingly well following the loss of the intermandibular joint providing food is prepared in smaller pieces for them.
- Bacterial and fungal stomatitis
  - Topical antibiotics/antifungals plus topical povidone-iodine daily
  - Surgical debridement of necrotic tissue may be necessary, followed by systemic and topical treatment.
- Monogenetic trematodes
  - Usually seen in wild-caught piscivorous aquatic and semi-aquatic chelonia
  - Probably nonpathogenic
  - Praziquantel at 10 mg/kg PO or IM. Repeat after 2 weeks.
- Overgrown beak. Can be associated with:
  - Malocclusion following a jaw fracture (can be iatrogenic while stomach tubing)
  - Excessive protein intake, often accompanied by relative lack of dietary calcium (i.e., metabolic bone disease—see *Musculoskeletal Disorders*). In this case, there are often associated skull and shell deformities.
  - Burr back the beak into more appropriate shape.

Differential diagnoses for gastrointestinal disorders

Chelonia, like birds, will often produce both fecal and urinary components of their excretions at the same time, mixed to some extent inside the proctodeum of the cloaca. In herbivorous chelonia, the feces should be well formed. Loose feces suggest gastrointestinal disease, a low-fiber diet, excess fruit intake, or anxiety.

In all terrestrial chelonia the bladder is large and acts as a significant organ for water storage. Urination during handling as a sign of anxiety is not uncommon. The urine often consists of a combination of a mucilaginous portion stained white or yellow with urate crystals and a clear watery portion. The urate portion may not be present every time.

Viral

- Reovirus

Bacterial

- Salmonellosis (chelonia can act as asymptomatic reservoirs)
- *Campylobacter fetus*
- *Vibrio* spp.
- *Clostridium* spp.—can be linked to long-term antibiosis

Fungal

- Mycotic enteritis

Protozoal

- Cilates (e.g., *Balantidium* spp., *Nyctotherus* spp.)
- Flagellates (e.g., *Trichomonas*)
- *Entamoeba invadens* (usually asymptomatic in chelonia but can cause enterocolitis and myositis—Philbey 2006)
- *Cryptosporidium* spp.
- *Caryospora* spp.
- *Eimeria* spp.

Parasitic

- Nematodes
  - Ascarids: *Angusticaecum* and *Sulcascaris*
  - Oxyurids: *Tachygonetria* spp., *Alaeuris* spp., *Mehdiella* spp., *Thaparia* spp.
  - Acanthocephalans (especially aquatic and semi-aquatic chelonia)
  - Hookworms: *Camallanus* spp., *Spineoxys* spp. (freshwater chelonia)
- Cestodes
  - *Ophiotaenia* spp., *Glossocercus* spp., *Bancroftiella* spp. (freshwater chelonia)
  - Flukes

Nutritional

- Dysbiosis (lack of fiber, too much fruit in diet, long-term antibiosis)
- Poisoning
  - Oak leaf
  - Azaleas, rhododendrons, *Pieris* spp. (Pizzi et al 2005) and other members of the Ericaceae (see *Cardiovascular and Hematologic Disorders*)
  - Heavy metal (e.g., lead, zinc—see *Systemic Disorders*)

Neoplasia

Other noninfectious problems

- Green, well-formed feces—normal if fed mostly on pelleted foods
- Constipation
- Foreign body
- Gastric dilatation
- Cloacal prolapse
  - Cloacitis
  - Cloacoliths

- Intestinal foreign body
- Intussusception
- Extraintestinal mass (e.g., renal neoplasm, bladder stone)
- Dystocia
- Hypocalcemia/metabolic bone disease
- Parasitism

Findings on clinical examination

- Diarrhea: Voluminous, runny feces; may be foul smelling (flagellates, dysbiosis)
- Green, well-formed feces (pelleted food)
- Regurgitation (gastritis)
- Dehydration (sunken eyes)
- Lethargy
- Lack of feces (foreign body, bladder stone, renal neoplasia, intussusception)
- Ulceration of the oral mucous membranes
- Petechial hemorrhages (hookworms)
- Edematous swelling at cloaca (cloacal prolapse—differentiate from phallus in male)
- Death

Investigations

1. Microscopy (Fig. 12-7)
   a. Fresh fecal sample—"wet prep" (Table 12-2)
2. Radiography
   a. Contrast studies
   b. Barium sulfate suspension at 5 mL/kg by gavage in the leopard tortoise *(Geochelone pardalis)* (Table 12-3)
   c. Recommended timing for radiography following barium gavage is 0, 10 minutes, 2 hours, 6 hours, 12 hours, 24 hours, and 72 hours.
   d. Water-soluble iodine-based contrast media such as Gastrografin (at 1 mL per 130 g in Hermann's tortoise *Testudo hermanni* (Table 12-4)

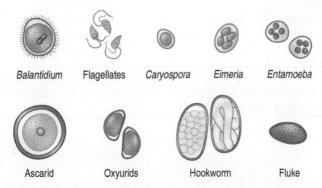

| Balantidium | Flagellates | Caryospora | Eimeria | Entamoeba |

| Ascarid | Oxyurids | Hookworm | Fluke |

Fig 12-7. Common gastrointestinal parasites of chelonia (not drawn to scale).

Table 12-2 Fecal parasites

Fecal parasite	Comments
Ascarid eggs (Angusticaecum, Sulcascaris)	Typical ascarid eggs
Hookworm eggs	Thin-walled, oval eggs
Strongyle eggs: Tachygonetria spp.	Thin-walled, often D-shaped eggs
Fluke eggs	Thin-shelled, often with single operculum. Orange or deep yellow color. Miracidium may be visible.
Flagellates	Numerous motile pear- to circular-shaped protozoa approximately 8 × 5 µm
Balantidium spp., Nyctotherus spp.	Large, motile ciliates
Cryptosporidium	Oocysts may be visible using phase contrast microscopy after flotation. Otherwise consider MZN staining.
Eimeria oocysts	Elongate
Caryospora	Circular, 1 sporocyst
Amebiasis (see also Hepatic Disorders). Common species of enteric amoeba below	Cysts are approx 11-20 µm. Trophozoites (ameboid form) have a single nucleus and average 16 µm when fixed. Distinguishing features of speciate cysts below
Entamoeba	Multinucleate cysts; nuclear endosomes measure up to nucleus diameter.
Acanthamoeba	Large cysts. Single nucleus containing endosome over one half diameter. Irregular outline
Hartmannella	As above but regular outline
Endolimax	Multinucleate; nuclear endosomes same diameter as nucleus, each of which has a dark-staining rim.

MZN, Modified Ziehl-Neelsen.

Table 12-3 Barium sulfate suspension at 5 mL/kg by gavage in the leopard tortoise (Geochelone pardalis)

Position of barium sulfate	Time following administration
Complete gastric emptying	5-9 hr
Entry to small intestine	0.2-1 hr
Entry to large intestine	5-8 hr
Exit from colon	144-166 hr
Still present in GI tract	8 days

Adapted from Taylor S K, Citino S B, Zdziarski J M et al 1996 Radiographic anatomy and barium sulphate transit time of the gastrointestinal tract of the leopard tortoise (Testudo pardalis). J Zoo Wildl Med 27(2):180–186.

Table 12-4 Water soluble iodine-based contrast media such as gastrografin (at 1 mL/130 g in Hermann's tortoise *Testudo hermanni*)

Body temperature (°C)	Average total gut transit time (hr)
15.2	8-24
21.5	3-8
30.6	1.5-4

Adapted from Meyer J 1998 Gastrografin as a gastrointestinal contrast agent in the Greek tortoise (Testudo hermanni). J Zoo Wildl Med 29(2):183–189.

    e. Hernandez-Divers and Hernandez-Divers (2001) suggest similar results with the nonionic iodine-based contrast medium iohexol at 7.5 to 10 mL/kg by gavage, with recommended timing for radiography following iohexol gavage given as 0, 20 minutes, 40 minutes, 60 minutes, 120 minutes, and 240 minutes at 30° C.

    f. Colonic contrast studies can be performed by retrograde introduction of the contrast media via a catheter into the colon via the cloaca.

    g. Foreign body: Small pieces of gravel or stone can be normal; large numbers suggest a gut stasis, obstruction, or pica.

    h. Ileus—common with dysbiosis

3. Routine hematology and biochemistry
4. Culture and sensitivity
5. Endoscopy
6. Biopsy
    a. Larvae encapsulated in gut wall (acanthocephalans) or other tissues, such as skin (spirurids—see *Skin Disorders*)
    b. Amebiasis
7. Ultrasonography

Management

- Fluid therapy (see *Nursing Care*)
- Covering antibiosis

Treatment/specific therapy

- Salmonellosis
  - Probably best considered as a normal constituent of chelonian cloacal/gut microflora
  - Rarely pathogenic to chelonia
  - Excretion likely to increase during times of stress (e.g., movement, illness)
  - Treatment usually not appropriate as unlikely to be effective long term and may encourage resistance
  - Recommendations for prevention of salmonellosis from captive reptiles issued by the Centers for Disease Control and Prevention in the United States include:
    - Pregnant women, children <5 years of age, and persons with impaired immune system function (e.g., AIDS) should not have contact with reptiles.

- All persons should wash hands with soap immediately after any contact with a reptile or reptile cage.
- Reptiles should be kept out of food preparation areas such as kitchens.
- Kitchen sinks should not be used to wash food or water bowls, cages or vivaria used for reptiles, or to bathe reptiles. Any sink used for these purposes should be disinfected after use.

- Mycotic enteritis
  - Nystatin at 100,000 units/kg PO daily for 10 days
  - Ketoconazole at 10 to 30 mg/kg PO s.i.d.
  - Itraconazole 5 mg/kg PO every other day
- Amebiasis
  - Metronidazole
    - 100 to 257 mg/kg PO body weight. Repeat after 2 weeks if necessary.
    - 20 mg/kg PO every other day until eradication
  - Chloroquine
    - 125 mg/kg PO every 48 hours for 3 treatments
    - 50 mg/kg IM every 7 days for 3 weeks
  - Iodoquinol/diiodohydroxyquin 50 mg/kg PO s.i.d. for 21 days. *Note:* Possibly toxic to black rat snakes
  - Paromomycin
    - 300 to 360 mg/kg PO every other day for 14 days
    - 25 to 100 mg/kg PO daily for 4 weeks
- *Caryospora*
  - Sulfadimethoxine at 50 mg/kg PO daily for 3 days; stop for 3 days, then repeat 3-day course.
- *Cryptosporidium*
  - Direct life cycle; infection by exposure to water containing infective oocysts
  - There is no recognized effective treatment.
  - Try metronidazole at 100 to 275 mg/kg PO once only.
  - Nitazoxanide at 5 mg/kg PO s.i.d.
  - Paromomycin at 300 to 800 mg/kg PO s.i.d. for 10 days
  - Oocysts *(C. parvum)* in water can be viable after 7 months at 15° C.
  - Disinfect by exposing to water above 64° C for >2 minutes.
  - *Cryptosporidium* oocysts are very resistant to chlorine or iodine.
- Ascarids, hookworms, and oxyurids
  - Fenbendazole at 50 to 100 mg/kg PO. Repeat every 2 weeks if necessary. *Note:* Fenbendazole is metabolized to oxfendazole by the liver.
  - Oxfendazole at 68 mg/kg PO. Repeat every 2 weeks if necessary.
  - Topical emodepside plus praziquantel preparations (Profender, Bayer) at 56 µL/100 g body weight (Mehlhorn et al 2005)
  - Prevention: Routine worming every 6 months (prehibernation and posthibernation for Mediterranean and other species where applicable), plus disposal of feces as soon as observed. *Note: Oxyuris* worms usually have a direct life cycle.
  - Hookworms have a direct life cycle; infective larvae can penetrate the skin or infect via contaminated food and water.
- Flukes and cestodes
  - Praziquantel at 10 mg/kg IM or PO once only. Repeat after 4 weeks.
- Ciliates
  - Usually part of normal gut fauna. Large numbers may indicate gut dysbiosis. Sensitive to metronidazole

- Flagellates
  - Metronidazole
    - 100 to 257 mg/kg PO body weight. Repeat after 2 weeks if necessary.
    - 20 mg/kg every other day until eradicated
  - Dysbiosis
    - High-fiber diets, reduced fruit intake, fluid and nutritional support
    - Antimicrobials often not necessary unless suspect bacterial or mycotic overgrowth.
- Gastric dilatation
  - Pass stomach tube to release gas.
    - Administer activated charcoal or simethicone through the tube.
    - Typically linked to an excess intake of fermentable carbohydrate; may be linked with abnormal gut motility or obstruction
- Cloacal prolapse
  - Prevent dessication and trauma by wrapping in nonadhesive protective film-wrap or equivalent.
  - Topical sugar may reduce edema by osmosis.
  - Place pursestring suture around cloaca for several weeks.
  - Limit feeding to reduce straining during defecation.
  - If repeated prolapses, consider cloacopexy.
  - Attend to underlying etiologies (e.g., uroliths).
- Oak leaf and other poisoning
  - If diagnosed antemortem, attempt removal of oak leaves from stomach either by endoscopy or via a coleotomy.
  - Supportive therapy, especially fluids, due to renal effects
  - Foreign body
  - If in stomach may be accessible with endoscopy
  - Use of lubricants such as liquid paraffin should be judicious as this may complicate subsequent therapy.
  - Surgical enterotomy
- Intussusception
  - Surgical enterectomy

Nutritional disorders

- Metabolic bone disease (see also *Musculoskeletal Disorders*)
- Hypovitaminosis A
  - Especially in young semi-aquatic chelonia (e.g., red-eared sliders, *Trachemys scripta elegans*)
  - A variety of ocular lesions, including swollen eyelids due to squamous metaplasia of the orbital glands and their ducts. A whitish cellular mass may develop behind the lower lid. Terrestrial chelonia may appear "bespectacled."
  - Squamous metaplasia also affects the renal tubules, causing kidney damage.
  - Affected chelonia are often anorexic, as they cannot see to locate food.
  - Treatment is with vitamin A given IM at 1000 to 5000 IU weekly for 4 weeks and the addition of dietary vitamin A supplements.
  - Ensure that diet contains natural sources of vitamin A precursors, especially with red, orange, and yellow vegetables, such as sweet peppers, plus leafy greens.
- Poisoning with azaleas, rhododendrons, and other members of the *Ericaceae* (see *Cardiovascular and Hematologic Disorders*)

- Hepatic lipidosis (see *Hepatic Disorders*)
- Dysbiosis
  - Excess fermentable carbohydrate intake, usually combined with insufficient fiber (too much fruit—see *Gastrointestinal Tract Disorders*)

Hepatic disorders

Viral

- CHV

Bacterial

- Abscessation
- *Salmonella typhimurium* (González Candela et al 2005)
- Mycobacteriosis (granulomas—may be multifocal)

Fungal

Protozoal

- Amebiasis

Nutritional

- Hepatic lipidosis
- Chronic debilitation
- Cholecystolithiasis (gallstones)

Neoplasia

Findings on clinical examination

- Malaise
- Listlessness
- Anorexia
- Weight loss
- Jaundice (icterus). *Note:* Some *Testudo* spp. (e.g., *T. cyrenacia*) naturally have yellowish oral mucous membranes.
- Greenish feces
- Diarrhea
- Death

Investigations

1. Microscopy
   a. Fecal examination: Cysts and trophozoites may be present (amebiasis).
2. Radiography
3. Routine hematology and biochemistry
4. Culture and sensitivity
5. Endoscopy
6. Biopsy/necropsy
   a. Granulomatous hepatitis (bacterial, fungal infection)
   b. Amebiasis
   c. Ziehl-Neelsen staining and PCR for mycobacteria
7. Ultrasonography

Management

- Milk thistle *(Silybum marianum)* is hepatoprotectant. Dose at 4 to 15 mg/kg PO b.i.d. or t.i.d.
- For ascites try furosemide at 2 to 5 mg/kg PO, SC s.i.d.
- Lactulose 0.05 mL/100 g PO s.i.d.

Treatment/specific therapy

- Mycobacteriosis—see *Systemic Disorders*
- Amebiasis
  - Metronidazole 20 mg/kg PO every other day until eradication
  - Chloroquine
    - 125 mg/kg PO every 48 hours for three treatments
    - 50 mg/kg IM every 7 days for 3 weeks
  - Iodoquinol/diiodohydroxyquin 50 mg/kg PO s.i.d. for 21 days. *Note:* Possibly toxic to black rat snakes
  - Paromomycin
    - 300 to 360 mg/kg PO every other day for 14 days
    - 25 to 100 mg/kg PO daily for 4 weeks
- Cholecystolithiasis and cholecystitis
  - Consider NSAIDs (e.g., meloxicam at 0.2 mg/kg IM, PO once daily or every other day) in the green iguana—see Hernandez-Divers (2006)—and covering antibiosis.
  - Surgery to remove gallstones may be feasible.
  - Linked to high dietary levels of processed dog and cat food (excessive protein, lipid, vitamin A and D_3 intake)
  - Feed a more appropriate herbivorous diet.

Pancreatic disorders

Diabetes mellitus (see *Endocrine Disorders*)

Cardiovascular and hematologic disorders

Cardiovascular anatomy

- Three-chambered heart consisting of two atria and one ventricle: A series of muscular ridges plus the timing of ventricular contraction tend to functionally divide the ventricle into two (the cavum venosum, the cavum pulmonale, and the cavum arteriosum), thereby separating systemic from pulmonary blood flow.
- The renal portal system (RPV): The RPV is a large vessel arising near the confluence of the epigastric and external iliac veins. It drains into the kidney. Blood returning from the tail, hind legs, and other closely situated structures may pass through these vessels or may bypass and enter the systemic circulation direct. This appears to depend on various factors, such as hydration status and core body temperature. May be more significant for drugs excreted by tubular secretion than by glomerular filtration.

Differential diagnosis for cardiovascular disorders

Viral

- Iridovirus (epicarditis but associated with other more typical iridovirus signs)

Bacterial

- Endocarditis

Fungal

Protozoal

- *Haemogregarina* spp.
- *Haemoproteus* spp.
- *Plasmodium* spp.
- *Pirhaemocyton* (may actually be iridoviral inclusions)

Parasitic

- Spirochid flukes, both adults and eggs

Nutritional

- Excessive calcium intake
- Excessive vitamin D$_3$ intake
- Ingestion of azaleas, rhododendrons, and other members of the *Ericaceae* (contain several toxins, including cardiac glycosides)

Neoplasia

Other noninfectious problems

- Metastatic mineralization
- Amyloidosis
- Renal disease
- Myocardial disease
- Hyperkalemia
- Pericardial effusion
- Visceral gout (uric acid in pericardial sac—see *Urinary Disorders*)

Findings on clinical examination

- Anorexia
- Edema
- Weakness
- Weight loss
- Areas of cutaneous mineralization (with metastatic mineralization)
- Spirochid fluke parasitism in freshwater turtles associated with subcutaneous edema, blood-tinged coelomic fluid, and hepatic, pancreatic, and splenic necrosis. Many organs can be affected due to microgranulomas triggered by the fluke eggs.

Investigations

1. Radiography
   a. May be useful to diagnose metastatic mineralization but unlikely to be useful for radiographic evaluation of the heart.
2. Routine hematology and biochemistry
3. Cytology (blood smear)
   a. *Haemogregarina* spp.
4. Blood culture and sensitivity
5. Endoscopy

Table 12-5 Normal ECG values in anesthetized red-eared slider *(Trachemys scripta elegans)* using a three-electrode, lead II trace, with comparative values from conscious terrapins

Variable	Normal ECG values*	Comparative values†
Body weight (kg)	0.45-1.81	
Heart rate (beats/min)	25 (16-37)	34
P, duration (s)	0.12 (0.04)	0.09
P, amplitude (mV)	0.030 (0.017)	
PR interval	0.51	0.41
QRS duration (s)	0.15 (0.02)	0.11
R, amplitude (mV)	0.254 (0.067)	
T, amplitude (mV)	0.068	
R–R interval (s)	2.38	
QT interval (s)	1.41 (0.38)	
ST interval (s)	1.05 (0.24)	0.81

*From Holz and Holz (1995).
†From Kaplan and Shwartz (1963), cited in Holz and Holz (1995).

6. Ultrasonography may be useful in large chelonia (Redrobe and Scudamore 2000).
7. Electrocardiography—potentially useful but few normal values established
   a. Normal ECG values in anesthetized red-eared slider *(Trachemys scripta elegans)* using a three-electrode, lead II trace, after Holz and Holz (1995). Some comparative values from conscious terrapins (from Kaplan and Shwartz [1963], cited in Holz and Holz [1995]) are given for comparison (Table 12-5).
   b. Note that the QRS complex was always in the form of a large R wave—no Q or S wave deflections were visible.
   c. Azalea toxicity: Paroxysmal tachycardia, atrial fibrillation, premature ventricular beats, extrasystoles, ectopic ventricular contractions (Frye and Williams 1995)
   d. Atrial fibrillation and first-degree heart block may be indicators of calcium deficiency.

Management

- The usual cardiac drugs are largely untried; therefore, treatment with these is speculative, although still worth attempting.
- Diuretics (e.g., furosemide at 5 mg/kg IM b.i.d. to encourage diuresis)

Treatment/specific therapy

- Hemoparasites
  - Loading dose of chloroquine phosphate (5 mg/kg PO) and primaquine phosphate (0.5 mg/kg PO)
  - Continue with chloroquine at 2.5 mg/kg PO once weekly and primaquine at 0.5 mg/kg once weekly for 12 to 16 weeks.
- Flukes: Praziquantel

- Azalea poisoning
  - Atropine sulfate at 0.04 mg/kg IV
  - After 2 minutes give calcium gluconate at 2 mg/kg by slow IV injection over the next 5 minutes
  - Once ECG normal, consider gastric lavage.
  - Supportive treatment
- Hypocalcemia: See *Musculoskeletal Disorders*.

Systemic disorders

Viral

- CHV
- Papilloma-like virus (see Drury et al 1998)

Bacterial

- Mycobacteria (see below)
- *Chlamydophila pneumoniae*
- Chlamydia-like organisms (possibly *Parachlamydia acanthamoeba, Simkania negevensis*—Soldati et al 2004)
- Spirochetes

Fungal

- *Exophiala* spp.

Protozoal

- Intranuclear coccidiosis

Nutritional

- Hypocalcemia (including metabolic bone disease)

Neoplasia
Other noninfectious problems

- Ivermectin toxicity
- Benzimidazole toxicity
- Anemia
- Gout (renal, visceral, and articular—see *Urinary Disorders*)
- Hypoglycemia (including posthibernational anorexia)
- Cardiac disease (see *Cardiovascular and Hematologic Disorders*)
- Heavy metal (e.g., lead, zinc)

Findings on clinical examination

- Weakness
- Emaciation and weight loss
- Anorexia
- Ocular and nasal discharge, stomatitis, with or without bouts of paralysis (CHV)
- Lethargy, anorexia, paralysis following ivermectin administration (ivermectin toxicity)
- Edema

Investigations

1. Radiography
   a. Heavy metal poisoning
2. Routine hematology and biochemistry
   a. Serum lead and zinc. Consider blood sampling other in-contact chelonia to establish normal ranges.
3. Serology and PCR for CHV
4. PCR for CHV
5. Ziehl-Neelsen staining and PCR for mycobacteria
6. Immunohistochemistry and PCR for *Chlamydophila* and *Chlamydia*-like organisms (Soldati et al 2004)
7. Culture and sensitivity
8. Endoscopy
9. Ultrasonography
10. Biopsy/necropsy
    a. Single or multiple granulomas (mycobacteria, fungi, *Chlamydophila pneumoniae*, *Chlamydia*-like organisms)
    b. Eosinophilic intranuclear protozoan-like organisms, typically in the renal epithelial cells, hepatocytes, pancreatic acinar cells, and intestinal epithelial cells (Jacobson et al 1994)

Management

- See *Nursing Care.*

Treatment/specific therapy

- CHV
  - No effective treatment, but consider acyclovir at 80 mg/kg PO s.i.d. Efficacy appears variable.
  - Supportive treatment only (but see *Respiratory Tract Disorders*)
- Bacterial infections
  - Appropriate antibiosis
  - General nursing care
- Mycobacteriosis
  - Potential zoonosis. Consider euthanasia.
  - No successful treatment for mycobacteriosis in reptiles reported
- Intranuclear coccidiosis
  - Potentiated sulfonamides at 30 mg/kg PO s.i.d.
- Ivermectin toxicity
  - IV fluids at 5 mL/kg per hour for up to 3 hours and then 5 to 10 ml/kg per day
  - Methylprednisolone 1 mg/kg IV s.i.d.
  - May require continued support for many weeks (see Divers et al 1999)
- Benzimidazole toxicity
  - Overdose with wormers (e.g., fenbendazole)
  - Lethargy, anorexia, secondary bacterial or fungal infections secondary to marked leukopenia

- Supportive treatment, including covering antimicrobials
- Care with compromised individuals as studies show (Neiffer et al 2005) an extended heteropenia with transient hypoglycemia, and hyperphosphatemia.
- Heavy metal poisoning
  - Remove metallic foreign bodies via endoscope if possible.
  - Sodium calcium edetate at 35 mg/kg by slow IV daily for 2 weeks

Musculoskeletal disorders

Bacterial

- Osteomyelitis
- *Corynebacterium aquaticum* (see Philbey et al 2006)

Fungal
Protozoal

- Amebiasis

Nutritional

- Metabolic bone disease—actually a complex of disorders including:
  - Dietary calcium deficiency
  - Dietary calcium/phosphorus imbalance
  - Protein excess
  - Hypovitaminosis D_3
    - Lack of exposure to ultraviolet light
    - Incorrect environmental temperatures
    - Lack of dietary vitamin D_3
  - Protein deficiency
  - Liver, kidney, and intestinal disease
  - Multiple factors may be involved.
  - Metastatic calcification of smooth muscle of various organs, including cardiovascular system, pulmonary system, gut, and urogenital system. Typically linked to excess dietary vitamin D_3 intake (e.g., oversupplementation, feeding with dog and cat food)

Neoplasia
Other noninfectious problems

- Metabolic bone disease (hepatic, renal, and intestinal disease—see also "Nutritional" above)
- Fractures of the shell or limbs (usually traumatic)
- Joint dislocations (traumatic)
- Degenerative joint disease due to:
  - Obesity
  - Articular gout (see *Urinary Disorders*)
  - Trauma
  - Septic arthritis
  - Osteochondritis
  - Coxofemoral arthritis (Philbey et al 2006)
  - Lawn mower trauma

Findings on clinical examination

- Soft shell (*Note:* In terrestrial chelonia, the shell should be hard by 12 months of age), flattened shell, doming of scutes (metabolic bone disease)
- Weakness—unable to support its own weight, hind legs articulated backward as if sliding rather than held beneath the body (metabolic bone disease)
- Beak abnormalities, including overgrowth
- Soft mandibles (metabolic bone disease)
- Claw abnormalities, including overgrowth (metabolic bone disease)
- Limb swellings (fractures, dislocations, osteomyelitis, myositis, septic or aseptic arthritis)
- Vague signs of ill health (anorexia, lack of movement, lethargy)

Investigations

1. Radiography
   a. Reduced bone density, cortical thinning, thickening of limb bones and shell (fibrous osteodystrophy)
   b. Fractures (shell, limbs)
   c. Lytic bone lesions (osteomyelitis)
   d. Areas of abnormal calcification (metastatic calcification)
2. Routine hematology and biochemistry
   a. Blood vitamin D_3 (25-hydroxycholecalciferol) levels; also total calcium, ionized calcium, phosphate
   b. Acierno et al 2006 measured 25-hydroxyvitamin D_3 in red-eared sliders (*Trachemys scripta elegans*) (Table 12-6)
3. Culture and sensitivity
4. Cytology (fine-needle aspiration)
5. Endoscopy
6. Biopsy/necropsy
   a. Amebiasis
7. Ultrasonography
8. ECG: Atrial fibrillation (see *Cardiovascular and Hematologic Disorders*)

Table 12-6 25-Hydroxyvitamin D_3 in red-eared sliders (*Trachemys scripta elegans*)

Red-eared slider turtles (*Trachemys scripta elegans*)	25-Hydroxyvitamin D_3 concentrations (nmol/L)	
	Mean	SD
Supplemental UV radiation	71.7	46.9
No provision of supplemental UV radiation	31.4	13.2

Adapted from Acierno M J, Mitchell M A, Roundtree M K et al 2006 Effects of ultraviolet radiation on 25-hydroxyvitamin D_3 synthesis in red-eared slider turtles (Trachemys scripta elegans). Am J Vet Res 67:2046–2049.

Management

- Close attention should be paid to environmental parameters, especially exposure to UV lighting, temperature, and dietary supplementation.

Treatment/specific therapy

- Amebiasis (see *Gastrointestinal Tract Disorders*)
- Metabolic bone disease
  - Usually due to secondary nutritional hyperparathyroidism linked with either failure to provide sufficient calcium supplementation or exposure to UVB
  - Parenteral calcium gluconate or lactate at 1.0 to 2.5 mg/kg daily
  - Oral vitamin D_3 at 1 to 4 IU/kg daily
  - Dietary calcium supplementation
  - Exposure to full-spectrum lighting as a UVB source
  - Calcitonin at 1.5 IU/kg SC s.i.d. if normocalcemic
- Metastatic calcification
  - No effective treatment
  - Reduce hypercalcemia by:
    - Calcitonin at 1.5 IU/kg SC s.i.d.
    - Fluid therapy: Hartmann's solution at 15 mL/kg intracoelomic until normocalcemic
  - Although often linked to excessive vitamin D_3 supplementation, many cases may be due to low levels of calcitrol, commonly secondary to renal disease. This leads to toxic levels of parathormone production with associated abnormal tissue mineralization and further renal damage.
- Osteochondritis
  - Arthrotomy and surgical removal of any loose bone fragments
  - NSAID therapy (e.g., meloxicam at 0.2 mg/kg once daily or every other day) in the green iguana—see Hernandez-Divers (2006)
- Joint dislocations
  - Reduce surgically if possible and immobilize as described for long bone fractures, below.
- Abscessation and osteomyelitis, myositis
  - Appropriate antibiosis
  - Consider amputation if damage is extensive.
- Fractures
  - Long bone fractures: Stabilization by confining the flexed limb into its fossa with strong adhesive tape may be sufficient to allow callus formation and healing; otherwise surgical reduction and internal/external fixation
  - Shell fractures may require closure. Some fractures may be reduced by placing clothing hooks attached by epoxy adhesives to the shell and connecting with surgical wire (Bogard and Innis 2008). Other cases may require surgical plating. Once all risk of infection has been ameliorated then shell deficits may require bridging with fiberglass or methylmethacrylate. Those fractures where the coelomic membrane has been breached carry a significantly poorer prognosis.
- Lawn mower trauma
  - Tortoises in long grass can be damaged during mowing, especially by "hover-mowers."
  - Injuries usually include injuries to the dorsal carapace, often with exposure of the lungs.
  - Because the lungs in tortoises are naturally rigid (attached to the inner surface of the carapace), respiration is usually not compromised.
  - Flush the lungs with sterile saline to remove any debris and treat as for *Respiratory Tract Disorders.*
  - As with other shell traumas (see *Skin Disorders*), do not place a permanent covering (e.g., methylmethacrylate) over the deficit until any infection has resolved.

Neurologic disorders

Viral
• CHV

Bacterial
• Septicemia
• Granuloma/meningitis
• Intracranial/extracranial abscess (vestibular syndrome)

Fungal
• Granuloma/meningitis

Protozoal
Parasitic
• Myiasis (aberrant—Sales et al 2003)

Nutritional
• Hypocalcemia (see "Metabolic Bone Disorder" in *Musculoskeletal Disorders*)

Neoplasia
• CNS neoplasia

Other noninfectious problems
• Ivermectin toxicity
• CNS gout (uric acid deposition—see *Urinary Disorders*)
• Heavy metal poisoning

Findings on clinical examination

• Weakness
• Hind-limb weakness; especially common in old female Hermann's tortoises. Often of unknown etiology but consider CHV or CNS gout.
• Lethargy, anorexia, paralysis following ivermectin administration (ivermectin toxicity)
• Vestibular syndrome (head tilt, circling to one side)
• Anorexia

Investigations

1. Radiography
   a. Skull
   b. Subtle spinal lesions unlikely to be seen on radiography
   c. Metallic objects in gut, especially nails, lead shot, etc.
2. Magnetic resonance imaging scan
3. Routine hematology and biochemistry
4. Blood lead or zinc levels
5. Culture and sensitivity
6. Endoscopy
7. Ultrasonography

Treatment/specific therapy

- Hypocalcemia (see "Metabolic Bone Disorder" in *Musculoskeletal Disorders*)
- Ivermectin toxicity (see *Systemic Disorders*)
- Aberrant myiasis
  - No safe systemic insecticidal preparation. Necrosis of dead larva may release toxins.
- Vestibular syndrome
  - Consider surgical removal or debridement if due to a contributing abscess, if feasible.
- Heavy metal toxicity
  - Remove metallic foreign body if possible.
  - NaCa-EDTA at 35 mg/kg IM s.i.d. until clinically normal (see Chitty 2003)

Ophthalmic disorders

Chelonia have both rods and cones but lack a fovea. Instead they have an area centralis or area temporalis: sections of retina sensitive to detail, edges, or movement. There is no conus papillaris. Chelonia have both lachrymal and harderian glands.

Examination of the posterior segment of the eye is difficult as the iris muscle fibers are striated and partly under voluntary control. Therefore, parasympatholytics (e.g., atropine) and sympathomimetics (e.g., phenylephrine) will not work. Consider examination by:
1. Using low light levels
2. General anesthesia
3. Nonparasympatholytic mydriatics such as vecuronium

Viral

- CHV
- Poxlike virus

Bacterial

- Secondary infection
- Eyelid granuloma (mycobacteriosis)
- *Pasteurella*

Fungal

- Keratitis (Fig. 12-8)
- *Exophiala* spp.

Parasitic

- Nematode larvae (red-eared slider, *Trachemys scripta elegans*)
- Microfilariae

Nutritional

- Hypovitaminosis A (especially semi-aquatic chelonia—Fig. 12-9)

Neoplasia

Other noninfectious problems

- Aging (cataracts)
- Subzero temperatures (cataracts, vitreal haze)
- Nutritional deficiencies (cataracts)
- Trauma
- Poor water quality (aquatic chelonia, especially snapping turtle—*Chelydra serpentina*)

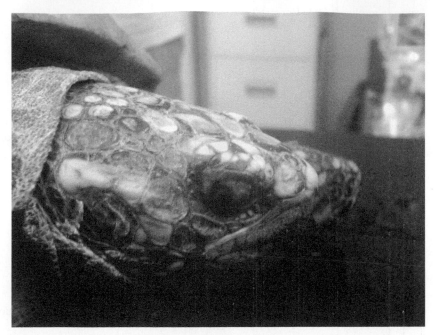

Fig 12-8. Fungal keratitis in a red-footed tortoise.

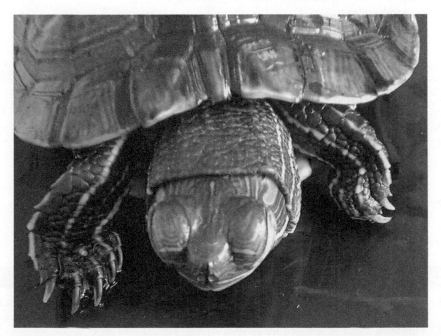

Fig 12-9. Hypovitaminosis A in a hatchling red-eared slider.

- Exposure to ultraviolet C (incorrect UV lighting)
- Congenital defects
- Cyclopia
- Microphthalmia
- Anophthalmia
- Arcus senilis
- Chronic hypertrophy of the nictitating membrane
- Coagulative keratopathy

Findings on clinical examination

- Conjunctivitis
- Blepharitis
- Ocular discharge
- Corneal ulceration
- Deep ulceration followed by perforation and iris collapse
- Hypopyon
- Uveitis
- Keratitis
- Cataracts
- Grossly swollen eyelids; unable to open one or both eyes (hypovitaminosis A, infection)
- In terrestrial chelonia, the eyelid lesions give a semblance of spectacles.
- A whitish cellular mass may develop behind the lower lid.
- Anorexia (cannot see to locate food). *Note:* Renal disease may be concurrent with hypovitaminosis A (see *Urinary Disorders*).
- Nematode larvae within the choroid (red-eared slider *Trachemys scripta elegans*)
- Obvious worm in the anterior chamber (microfilariae)
- Panophthalmitis
- Ocular signs possibly accompanied by stomatitis and rhinitis (CHV)
- Yellow papular lesions of the eyelids in *Testudo hermanni* (poxlike virus)

Investigations

1. Ophthalmic examination
2. Radiography
3. Routine hematology and biochemistry
4. Culture and sensitivity
5. Endoscopy
6. Biopsy/necropsy
   a. Ziehl-Neelsen staining and PCR for mycobacteria
7. Water quality testing for aquatic chelonia (especially pH, ammonia, nitrites, nitrates, temperature)
8. Ultrasonography
9. Reassess lighting (exposure to UVC).

Management

1. Many nonspecific ocular lesions respond well to vitamin A supplementation at 1000 to 5000 IU IM weekly for 4 weeks and the addition of dietary vitamin A supplements.
2. Enucleation may be required for severely damaged or infected eyes.

Treatment/specific therapy

- Hypovitaminosis A (see *Nutritional Disorders*)
- Eyelid granuloma
  - Topical treatment
  - Consider resection.
- Fungal keratitis
  - Topical antimycotics (e.g., clotrimazole)
  - Systemic antimycosis may be required.
- Congenital defects
  - No treatment
  - Consider incubation parameters (temperature, humidity, etc.) as well as genetic factors when considering cause.
- Cataracts
  - Phacoemulsification (see Kelly et al 2005)
  - Lens extraction
- Arcus senilis: Age related; no treatment
- Chronic hypertrophy of the nictitating membrane
  - Lavage of the conjunctival space
  - Topical application of ophthalmic corticosteroid preparation
- Coagulative keratopathy
  - Topical ophthalmic ointment containing proteolytic enzyme
  - May occur posthibernation
- Poor water quality
  - Identify abnormality and correct (see Chapter 15).
- Microfilariae and helminths
  - Fenbendazole at 50 to 100 mg/kg PO. Repeat every 2 weeks if necessary.
  - Do not use ivermectin (see *Systemic Disorders*).
- Exposure to UVC
  - Provision of incorrect lighting (e.g., UV-sterilization tubes, blacklights for tanning beds instead of the correct full-spectrum lighting)
  - Correct lighting; provision of a darkened area during the initial recovery period may be beneficial.
  - Supportive treatment as may be anorexic due to compromised vision

Urinary disorders

Bacterial
- Cystitis
- Pyelonephritis

Fungal
- Cystitis
- Pyelonephritis

Protozoal
- Hexamita
- *Myxidium* spp. (Myxozoa—crowned river turtle *Hardella thurjii*; see Garner et al 2003)

Parasitic

- Monogenetic trematodes (in semi-aquatic chelonia *Chrysemys, Trachemys,* and *Chelodina* spp.)

Nutritional

- Hypovitaminosis A (squamous metaplasia of the renal tubules)
- Oak leaf toxicity (see *Gastrointestinal Tract Disorders*)

Neoplasia

Other noninfectious problems

- Bladder calculi/stones
- Gout (renal)
- Iatrogenic (nephrotoxic drugs, such aminoglycosides)
- Pelvic obstruction (foreign body, coxofemoral arthritis—see *Musculoskeletal Disorders,* retained eggs)
- Interstitial nephropathy
- Tubulonephropathy
- Glomerulonephropathy

Findings on clinical examination

- Anorexia
- Lethargy
- Weight loss
- Polydipsia/polyuria
- Polyuria
- Urinary tenesmus
- Yellow urates (denotes prolonged retention)
- Anuria
- Edema
- Hind-limb weakness (see also *Neurologic Disorders*)
- Pale mucous membranes
- Ocular disease, especially in semi-aquatic chelonia (hypovitaminosis A)
- Mortalities

Investigations

1. Radiography
   a. Soft-tissue mineralization; increased soft-tissue or mineral density in renal region
   b. Uroliths. *Note:* The bladder is voluminous in chelonia, and bladder stones may appear farther cranial and more lateral than expected.
   c. Pneumocystography may help to differentiate eggs in the bladder from eggs in the reproductive tract (see *Reproductive Disorders*).

Pneumocystography in larger chelonia

1. Catheterize the urethra.
2. Flush out the bladder contents.
3. Infuse 10 to 20 mL/kg of air (stop if resistance encountered).
4. Administer 2 to 5 mL of iohexol to produce a double-contrast pneumocystogram.

(Hernandez-Divers S, Hernandez-Divers S 2001 Diagnostic imaging of reptiles. Practice 23:370–391.)

Intravenous urography

1. Fast chelonian for 2 to 3 days.
2. Maintain at 30°C.
3. Place IV catheter into right jugular vein.
4. Use suitable urography medium—inject 800 to 1200 mg iodine into the jugular vein.
5. Lateral and dorsoventral radiographs taken at 0, 1, 3, 5, 15, 30, and 60 minutes.
6. As an adjunct, inject medium into dorsal coccygeal tail vein. Radiographs taken after 30 seconds.

(Hernandez-Divers S, Hernandez-Divers S 2001 Diagnostic imaging of reptiles. Practice 23:370 391.)

---

2. Routine hematology and biochemistry
   a. Blood uric acid levels, urea, creatinine, calcium, and phosphorus
3. Urinalysis including cytology
   a. Renal casts
   b. Inflammatory cells
   c. Centrifuged urine (supernatant)
4. Detectable levels of alkaline phosphatase, aspartate transaminase (AST), alanine transaminase (ALT), urea, calcium, creatine kinase (CK), creatinine, glucose, lactate dehydrogenase (LDH), magnesium, ammonia, phosphorus, total bilirubin, total protein, and uric acid
5. Parameters raised with renal disease: AST, urea, calcium, CK, creatinine, glucose, LDH, ammonia, and phosphorus. Uric acid may be significantly raised or lowered than normal (Koelle and Hoffman 2002).
6. Culture and sensitivity
7. Endoscopy
8. Biopsy/necropsy
9. Ultrasonography

Management

- Fluid therapy (see *Nursing Care*)

Treatment/specific therapy

- Bacterial pyelonephritis and cystitis
  - Appropriate antibiosis
- Fungal pyelonephritis and cystitis
  - Appropriate mycosis (see *Respiratory Tract Disorders*)
- Myxozoans
  - No effective treatment
- Flukes
  - Probably nonpathogenic
  - Praziquantel at 10 mg/kg once. Repeat after 4 weeks if necessary.
- Hexamitiasis
  - Cause of renal tubular damage
  - Metronidazole
    - 100 to 257 mg/kg PO body weight. Repeat after 2 weeks if necessary.
    - 20 mg/kg PO every other day until eradicated
  - Dimetridazole at 40 mg/kg PO s.i.d. for 5 days

- Gout
  - Fluid therapy
  - Allopurinol at 10 mg/kg PO s.i.d. *Note:* This will only prevent subsequent uric acid deposition.
  - Very guarded prognosis
- Uroliths/bladder calculi
  - Adults: Surgical cystotomy; note that the chelonian bladder is very thin and difficulty can be experienced during closure. One method is by marsupialization of bladder to the body wall at the inguinal fossa.
  - Hatchling/small chelonia: Success can be achieved by long-term treatment with allopurinol at 10 mg/kg PO s.i.d. indefinitely; this helps prevent enlargement of the stone such that in time the growing chelonian may be able to pass the calculus.

Endocrine disorders

Thyroid activity in chelonia can be affected by temperature; low temperatures ($10°$ C for 15 days) inhibit thyroid activity, whereas high temperatures (32 to $34°$ C) stimulate thyroid activity in soft-shelled turtle *Lissemys punctata punctata* (Sengupta et al 2003).

Nutritional

- Thymic hyperplasia (goiter associated with iodine deficiency)

Neoplasia

- Multicentric lymphoblastic lymphoma (thyroid)

Other noninfectious problems

- Thymic hyperplasia (not diet related; possibly antigenic stimulation)
- Diabetes mellitus

Findings on clinical examination

- Marked swelling of ventral neck (goiter)
- Polydipsia, polyuria, inappetence (diabetes mellitus)

Investigations

1. Radiography
2. Routine hematology and biochemistry
   a. Hyperglycemia, normal renal parameters (diabetes mellitus); differentiate from stress hyperglycemia
   b. Serum insulin
   c. Serum glucagon (may be more important in glucose regulation than insulin)
   d. Serum thyroxine levels (consider sampling conspecifics to establish normal ranges)
   e. Normal $T_{3(total)}$ < 0.0154 nmol/L
   f. Normal $T_{4(total)}$ = 0.05 to 0.1 nmol/L
   g. However, Hulbert (2000) cites $T_{4(total)}$ values for growing red-eared sliders *(Trachemys scripta)* of 80 to 145.0 nM/L.
   h. *Note:* Thymic hyperplasia can occur with normal T_3 and T_4 levels (Fleming et al 2004).
3. Culture and sensitivity
4. Endoscopy

5. Biopsy/necropsy
6. Ultrasonography

Treatment/specific therapy

- Thymic hyperplasia (nutritional)
  - Supplement with iodine.
  - Sodium or potassium iodide solution at 0.25 to 0.5 mg/kg IV or PO every 7 days
  - Lugol's iodine solution at 0.5 to 2.0 mg/kg PO every 7 days
  - Other dietary supplements high in iodine include kelp tablets.
  - Usually associated with feeding high volumes of Brassicas (cabbage family), which contain goitrogens that antagonize thyroid function
  - Volcanic island herbivores (e.g., Galapagos tortoises) especially predisposed
- Thymic hyperplasia (nonnutritional)
  - Investigate other, nonnutritional, causes
- Diabetes mellitus
  - Rare but very guarded prognosis
  - Commercial insulin unlikely to work—reptilian insulin is different from mammalian.
  - Attempt feeding high-fiber, low-carbohydrate diet to allow natural modulation of glucose uptake.

Hibernation-associated disorders

Many species of chelonia undergo a seasonal period of dormancy. Typically this is a period of hibernation (brumation) to survive times of low temperatures and poor food resources, but occasionally it may be to survive times of high temperatures or drought (estivation).

Commonly kept species suitable for hibernation

1. Mediterranean species that are safe to hibernate include *Testudo ibera, T. whitei, T. marginata, T. hermanni*, and *T. horsfieldii*. Of the *T. graeca graeca* group, the Moroccan and Algerian races are safe to hibernate.
2. North American gopher tortoise *Gopherus agassizi*
3. Northern populations of the ornate box turtle *(Terrapene ornata)* and eastern box turtle *(T. carolina)*
4. Some populations of Bell's hinge-back tortoise *(Kinixys belliana)* will estivate during periods of drought.
5. Painted terrapins *(Chrysemys* spp.) and some sliders *(Trachemys* spp.—red-eared sliders, *T. scripta elegans)*

Commonly kept species that should not be hibernated

1. Mediterranean species: Egyptian tortoise *(Testudo kleinmanni)* and the Tunisian tortoise *(T. nabulensis)*. The Libyan race of *T. graeca graeca* should either not be hibernated or should only be allowed to do so for a relatively short time, such as 6 to 8 weeks.
2. Indian star tortoise *(Geochelone elegans)*, red-footed tortoise *(G. carbonaria)*, yellow-footed tortoise *(G. denticulata)*, leopard tortoise *(G. pardalis)*, and African spur-thighed tortoise *(G. sulcata)*
3. Serrated hinge-back tortoise *(Kinixys erosa)* and Homes' hinge-back tortoise *(K. homeana)*
4. Vietnamese leaf turtle *(Geoemyda spengleri)*
5. Keeled box turtle *(Pyxidea mouhoti)*

Hibernation triggered by environmental stimuli

1. Reducing ambient temperatures
2. Reducing photoperiod
3. Reducing light intensity

Testudo spp. during hibernation lose around 0.2 to 0.4 g/day, so expect a loss of around 1% of body weight per month. Water is lost via respiration, so PCV rises from 0.28 to 0.29 L/L to 0.34 to 0.38 L/L, while urea levels rise from <10 mmol/L to <103 mmol/L.

The ideal temperature for hibernation is around 5 to 6° C, while reemergence is initiated by temperatures rising consistently above 10° C. At this time, there is a major rise in blood glucose from liver glycogen stores to fuel initial foraging. *Testudo* spp. will eat when blood glucose is at least 3.2 mmol/L. As a general rule, a posthibernational tortoise:

1. Must drink or absorb water across the cloacal lining within 10 days to produce a reduction in blood urea levels and PCV
2. Must eat within 3 to 4 weeks

Posthibernational anorexia

Typically, this is due to inadequate preparation the previous summer and autumn, with poor/inappropriate nutrition, but it can also be due to unsuitable hibernation facilities or concurrent disease (e.g., stomatitis, CHV). Such tortoises will have utilized entire fat reserves, exhausted fat-soluble vitamin supplies, and are forced to break down muscle and other tissues as a protein source to provide an alternative energy and amino acid source.

Findings on clinical examination

- Cataracts and vitreal haze (see *Ophthalmic Disorders*)
- Frostbite
  - Covering antibiotics
  - Application of a topical amorphous hydrogel dressing, such as IntraSite Gel (Smith and Nephew Healthcare Ltd.) topically to lesions
  - Systemic NSAIDs (e.g., meloxicam)

Investigations

1. Radiography
2. Routine hematology and biochemistry
   a. As minimum, assess PCV, glucose, and urea. *Note:* LDH and CK levels are likely to be naturally higher in hibernating chelonia (see Birkedal and Gesser 2004).
3. Culture and sensitivity
4. Endoscopy
5. Ultrasonography
6. Assessment of hibernation environment

Treatment

- Fluid therapy (see *Nursing Care*)
- Vitamin supplementation
- Feeding by stomach tube or via pharyngostomy tube. Supplement with probiotics.
- Hospitalize in vivarium—summer temperatures (preferred body temperature for *Testudo* spp. is around 30° C) and 12 to 14 hours of full-spectrum lighting.
- Treat any concurrent disease.
- *Note:* Treatment can be prolonged.

Inappropriate hibernation-like behaviors

- Often seen in Horsfield's tortoise *(T. horsfieldii)*; some populations hibernate for up to 9 months of the year, and some individuals develop hibernation/brumation/estivation behaviors when exposed to inappropriate environmental stimuli, such as shortened photoperiods or excessively high or low temperatures.
- Individuals from species that do hibernate (see list above) that are exposed to inappropriate environmental stimuli immediately prior to hibernation (i.e., exposed to high temperatures or photoperiods at a time when they have been naturally preparing for hibernation)
- Differentiating such tortoises from those that are unwell can be difficult as both those that are ill and those showing inappropriate hibernation behaviors will cease feeding and reduce basking times, often hiding away.
- A detailed case history with recent husbandry management is vital (i.e., was the tortoise outside during the autumn, exposure to natural lighting such as a nearby window [and therefore responsive to day length changes], ambient temperatures).
- Tortoises that appear otherwise healthy can be monitored. If the tortoise is not excessively active, then the author finds that weight loss is limited to approximately 1% to 3% per month.
- Clinical investigations such as routine hematology and clinical pathology can be used to assess health status.

Treatment

- If underlying disease can be reasonably ruled out then:
  - Decide whether to allow a short hibernation of around 2 to 4 weeks or to attempt to keep active. If the latter, treat as for posthibernational anorexia.
  - If hibernating, should only lose around 1% body weight per month. Any concerns during hibernation are managed by bringing the tortoise out of hibernation and managing as a posthibernation anorexia plus dealing with any problems identified.

Reproductive disorders

Nutritional
- Poor plane of nutrition
- Hypocalcemia (see *Musculoskeletal Disorders*)

Neoplasia
- Obstructive dystocia

Other noninfectious problems
- Fractured egg
- Egg yolk serositis
- Preovulatory ovarian stasis (POOS)
- Egg stasis (postovulatory)
- Egg retention in the urinary bladder
- Prolapse of the phallus
- Hypersexuality in male tortoises

Findings on clinical examination

- Restlessness—may be extreme (egg retention). In males may be combined with mounting suitably sized or shaped objects (hypersexuality)
- Digging
- Abnormally low clutch of eggs
- Anorexia
- Depression
- Egg may be palpable on cloacal examination.
- Swollen reddish or grayish structure hanging from the vent (prolapsed phallus—differentiate from cloacal prolapse; Fig. 12-10)
- Phallic trauma—may be associated with hypersexuality

Investigations

1. Radiography
   a. Postovulatory eggs are heavily shelled and are readily demonstrable on radiography.
   b. Radiography of dystocic chelonia allows:
      i. Assessment of total number of eggs present
      ii. Any abnormal or fractured eggs
      iii. Any egg-pelvic disproportion
      iv. Presence of eggs in the bladder (occasionally following attempted oxytocin induction). These eggs typically have thick, uneven walls due to uric acid deposition.
      v. Some underlying causes (e.g., metabolic bone disorder, active or historical, bladder calculi or foreign bodies that may be causing an obstruction)
2. Cytology: Coelomic tap (yolk serositis)

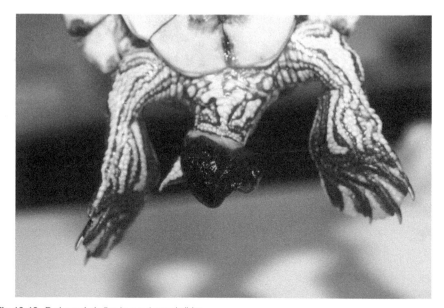

Fig 12-10. Prolapsed phallus in a red-eared slider.

3. Urine sample: High levels of spermatozoa in sexually active male tortoises
4. Routine hematology and biochemistry
5. Culture and sensitivity
6. Endoscopy
7. Biopsy/necropsy
8. Ultrasonography
   a. Place probe into inguinal fossa to pick up ova in POOS.
   b. Eggs in the bladder

Treatment/specific therapy

- POOS
  - Medical management with levothyroxine at 50 µg/kg PO s.i.d. This treatment can be prolonged over several months; monitor follicular regression with regular ultrasound scans.
  - Ovariectomy
- Egg stasis
  - Provision of correct environment, including appropriate temperature, humidity, and nesting chamber, may induce normal egg laying. Supplement with calcium (e.g., calcium gluconate at 1 mL/kg PO b.i.d.).
  - May be linked with stress
  - Medical induction
    - Calcium at 100 mg/kg IV, IM every 6 to 12 hours
    - 1 to 10 IU/kg oxytocin IM given 1 hour after last calcium. Unlike in snakes there appears to be a wide "window" of many weeks where oxytocin is effective for induction.
    - Repeat over 2 to 3 cycles if the reptile is otherwise healthy.
    - If some eggs still retained after 48 hours, consider surgery.
    - Vasopressin at 0.01 to 1.0 µg/kg IM, IV (more potent than oxytocin in reptiles)
      * Salpingotomy
    - Plastral coeliotomy
    - Prefemoral coeliotomy
      * Ovariosalpingectomy (as for "Salpingotomy")
- Egg retention in the urinary bladder
  - Cystotomy: Temporary marsupialization of the bladder via the inguinal fossa. Bladder closure can be problematic.
  - Ultrasound-guided snaring of eggs per cloaca
- Fractured egg
  - Risk of egg yolk serositis and trauma from sharp shell fragments
  - Consider either endoscopic or surgical retrieval.
- Egg yolk serositis
  - Coeliotomy followed by extensive lavage and removal of any egg fragments; surgical repair of oviduct or salpingectomy if necessary
- Hypersexuality
  - Delmadinone acetate at 1 to 2 mg/kg SC. Repeat after 4 to 6 weeks if needed.
  - Supplementary feeding (e.g., tube feeding) for tortoises with anorexia and weight loss
  - Environmental modification may be possible by shortening day length and dropping ambient temperatures by 2 to 3° C for a period of time for those tortoises kept inside.

- Prolapsed phallus
  - If fresh and relatively nontraumatized, replace and retain with a pursestring suture.
  - If badly damaged or if pursestring unsuccessful, consider resection. This will only interfere with reproduction, not with urination.

Pediatric and neonatal disorders

Bacterial

- Systemic infections

Fungal

Protozoal

Parasitic

- Nematodes (see *Gastrointestinal Tract Disorders*)

Nutritional

- Metabolic bone disease
- Uroliths (Fig. 12-11)

Other noninfectious problems

- Prolapse of the umbilicus
- Congenital abnormalities

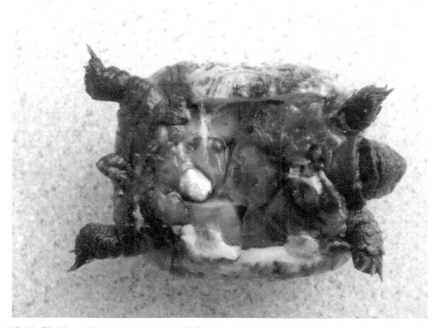

Fig 12-11. Bladder urolith in a hatchling spur-thighed tortoise (plastron removed).

Findings on clinical examination

- Lethargy
- Loss of appetite
- Cryptic behavior (hiding)
- Bulging of tissue at the umbilicus of newborn or newly hatched chelonia. Bulge may contain coelomic lining, yolk sac remnant, and coelomic fat.
- Edema

Investigations

1. Radiography
2. Routine hematology and biochemistry
   a. Serum calcium and ionized calcium
3. Culture and sensitivity
4. Endoscopy
5. Biopsy/necropsy
6. Ultrasonography

Treatment/specific therapy

- Systemic infections
  - Difficult to diagnose in hatchlings as small size precludes adequate sampling.
  - Covering antibiosis often gives a good clinical response.
- Metabolic bone disease—see *Musculoskeletal Disorders*
  - *Note:* Hatchling chelonia are naturally soft and somewhat flexible.
  - Often accompanied by hypovitaminosis A (especially semi-aquatic chelonia) and other signs of disease (e.g., anorexia, lethargy)
  - May be delayed if calcium status of female was good; signs only once calcium reserves utilized
  - If very early onset, may be due to poor calcification of egg, a reflection of poor calcium status of the mother
- Prolapsed umbilicus
  - Clean and replace prolapse. Suture in place.
  - May require surgical resection of yolk sac remnant
  - This is particularly prevalent in hatchlings with incomplete yolk sac resorption, where the yolk sac membranes adhere to dry surfaces or to the inside of the shell (especially if the humidity is too low). Keep hatchlings with pronounced egg sacs in moist, clean surroundings until resorption takes place. Do not attempt to separate the hatchling from the egg, but increase humidity and/or remove the hatchling plus egg to a warm, humid environment to allow natural separation.
- Edema
  - Occasionally seen in hatchling *Testudo* spp.
  - Swollen body
  - Soft shell
  - On postmortem the carcass is edematous; uroliths may be present.
  - Unknown etiology
- Uroliths
  - See *Urinary Disorders* for treatment.
  - Can occur individually or in groups

- May be linked to poor environmental conditions (e.g., marginal chronic dehydration)
- In some cases hatchlings may have inherited susceptibility (clutch mates under different husbandry regimens developed uroliths—personal observation).

Husbandry-related disorders

- Water quality
  - Poor water quality, especially high ammonia levels, can cause skin and ophthalmic disorders and mortalities in young semi-aquatic chelonia. (See Chapter 15 for details in "Management.")
- Metabolic bone disease (see *Musculoskeletal Disorders*)
- Posthibernational anorexia (see *Hibernation-Associated Disorders*)

Amphibians

Amphibians are a popular group of pets among herpetologists and some aquarists. Popular species include a number of *Anura* (frogs and toads) and some *Urodeles* (salamanders and newts).

Table 13-1 Popular species of amphibians: Key facts

Species	Notes	Common disorders
Horned frogs (*Ceratophrys* spp.)	From South America, these sit-and-wait predatory frogs grow large and have a strong bite.	*Aeromonas* infections, gout, corneal lipidosis
Poison-arrow frogs (*Dendrobates* spp.)	South American. Skin toxins are based on plant alkaloids ingested by native prey insects. Captive-bred and long-term captives usually safe to handle with appropriate precautions	Bacterial and fungal infections
White's tree frogs (*Littoria caerulea*)	A large Australian tree frog requiring high temperatures (26-32° C daytime; 20-24° C nighttime) and a comparatively low humidity (50%-60%)	Bacterial and fungal infections
African clawed toad (*Xenopus laevis*, in both wild and albino forms)	Totally aquatic. Extremely popular	Bacterial and fungal infections. Poor water quality
Axolotl (*Ambystoma mexicanum*)	A neotenous salamander originating from Mexico. Keep cool (15-20° C).	Poor water quality, ingestion of foreign bodies, bite injuries from other axolotls
Caecilians, such as *Typhlonectes compressicauda*	These aquatic and moist subterranean wormlike amphibians are occasionally available in aquarium outlets.	Fungal skin infections, poor water quality

Consultation and handling

Handle amphibians with damp hands and/or smooth latex gloves to protect the delicate skin and mucous covering. Amphibia can be very unpredictable and are excellent at leaping from the unsuspecting grasp of the veterinarian; therefore, beware of potentially traumatic falls to the floor. Wrapping them in very damp, thin paper towels enables some control; areas of interest are accessed by gently tearing through the paper.

Large frogs such as horned frogs (*Ceratophrys* spp.) and African giant frogs (*Pyxicephalus adspersus*) can inflict a painful bite and are likely to do so. Handle these by gently grasping them around the waist. Large marine toads (*Bufo marinus*) may eject toxins from their parotid glands if severely stressed. Wild-caught poison-arrow frogs can produce potentially very toxic skin secretions, which are manufactured from prey; captive-bred frogs usually do not produce such toxins, but caution is advised.

Most amphibia have very thin, moist skins, which allow significant absorption of topical medications. This should be borne in mind if using topical preparations designed for mammalian species, but these can be used advantageously, as therapeutic levels of active medications may be able to be achieved following topical application of injectable drugs (e.g., antibiotics). Drugs absorbed transcutaneously may be transported directly to the kidneys via the lymphatic fluid, so care must be taken with potentially nephrotoxic drugs.

Nursing care

Provide an appropriate environment, including provision of:
1. Optimal temperature (basking lights where appropriate, heat mats etc. to allow thermoregulation). Use of max–min thermometers will assist in monitoring temperature ranges to which incumbent amphibia are exposed.
2. Full-spectrum lighting appears to be relatively unimportant for the majority of amphibia; if in doubt, use a light with a minimal (2%) UV output.
3. Humidity is crucially important. A relative humidity of 80% or higher is generally recommended.
4. Ventilation: Important, but may need to be sacrificed somewhat to maintain high humidity levels
5. Easily cleaned accommodation; use damp paper substrate and disposable/sterilizable hides and other vivarium furniture.
6. Keep individually to minimize intraspecies stress and competition for resources.

Fluid therapy

Most amphibians can absorb fluids directly across the skin, with terrestrial anurans possessing a vascular ventral pelvic skin patch designed for transcutaneous water absorption. Dehydrated amphibians show increased tackiness of the skin mucous covering, tightening of the skin, sunken eyes, and weight loss. Dehydration can also affect cutaneous gaseous exchange, leading to hypercapnia and acidosis.

Oral fluids are of limited use in amphibians. Dehydrated terrestrial amphibians should be placed in a shallow bath of clean, dechlorinated, and well-oxygenated water.

Fluid therapy for amphibians
1. Intracoelomic fluids should be slightly hypotonic:
   a. 1:2 sodium chloride 0.9% : glucose 5%
   b. 1:2 Hartmann's solution : glucose 5%
   c. 9:1 saline : sterile water (Wright 1995)
2. Do not exceed 25 mL/kg as an initial dose.

Nutritional support

Offer commercially available live food if possible. If anorexic:
1. Place whole prey items into mouth.
2. Consider use of stomach tube; initially use commercially available "critical care" products for reptiles (usually containing amino acids, vitamins, and electrolytes) and graduate to available carnivore products or high-energy formulations available for domestic dogs and cats.

Analgesia

Morphine: Intracoelomic at 10 to 100 mg/kg in frogs. Given at 30 to 100 mg/kg IM, SC, or topically provides analgesia that peaks at 60 to 90 minutes in leopard frogs, *Lithobates pipiens* (Stevens 2011).

Meloxicam at 0.1 mg/kg IM s.i.d. in American bullfrogs, *Rana catesbiana* (Minter et al 2011)

Anesthesia

Terrestrial amphibians have several respiratory surfaces, which can complicate the control of anesthesia. These include the lungs, skin, and buccal lining. Aquatic amphibians respire largely through gills, although the skin is also an important respiratory organ, and many possess lungs too.

When inducing terrestrial amphibians in a water bath, always guard against the possibility of drowning. Once anesthetized, large amphibians can be intubated and maintained as for reptiles with isoflurane, but maintenance can be difficult due to alternative respiratory surfaces.

Transcutaneous anesthetic techniques in amphibians

1. Isoflurane at 4% to 5% bubbled into water and administered according to the amphibian's response, *or* place animal in damp towels in induction chamber.
2. Mix 3.0 mL of liquid isoflurane + 1.5 mL of water + 3.5 mL KY jelly:
   a. Apply this mixture to animal's dorsum at roughly 0.025 to 0.035 mL/g body weight depending on species. Use a lower dose for frogs and newts, higher for toads.
   b. Once the solution has been applied, place the animal in a small sealed container until induction has occurred (around 5 to 15 minutes). When righting and withdrawal reflexes are lost, wipe the dermis free of anesthetic. Should give 45 to 80 minutes of surgical time.
3. Fish anesthetics can be used, such as MS222 (see Chapter 14).

Parenteral anesthesia for amphibians

Propofol at 10 mg/kg IV in all large species; for salamanders use ventral tail vein; for frogs and toads use abdominal vein or heart or at 25 to 35 mg/kg intracoelomically (tiger salamander).

Skin disorders

The amphibian skin is thin and covered with a layer of mucus, which acts as an antibacterial and antifungal barrier. It is highly porous to medications and toxins; many treatments can be administered topically to achieve systemic effects. Normal flora are –gram-negative, such as *Aeromonas* spp., *Pseudomonas* spp., *Proteus* spp., and *Escherichia coli*. However, these can also be pathogenic, and so results may require a degree of interpretation.

Hypovitaminosis A may contribute to secondary skin infections (e.g., chytridiomycosis), possibly by reducing cutaneous mucus production (see also "Hypovitaminosis A" in *Gastrointestinal Disorders*).

Pruritus

- Trombiculid mites (terrestrial forms)
- Poor water quality, especially high ammonia levels, can cause skin irritation in both adults and tadpoles.
- Environmental tobacco smoke

Erosions and ulceration

- Traumatic wounds (e.g., bites)
- Bacterial (see also "Changes in Pigmentation," below)

- Iridovirus (ranavirus, including frog virus 3—see *Systemic Disorders*)
- Mycobacteriosis
- Cutaneous capillariasis: *Pseudocapillaroides xenopi* (African clawed toads)
- Fungal infections include *Batrachochytrium dendrobatidis* (chytridiomycosis) and *Basidiobolus ranarum*
- Microsporidia
- Trombiculids in terrestrial amphibians (erythematous vesicles)

Nodules and nonhealing wounds

- *Ichthyophonus hoferi*
- Trematodes *(Clinostomum attenuatum)*

Changes in pigmentation

- Erythema and ulceration ("red leg")
- Environmental pathogens (*Aeromonas* spp., *Pseudomonas* spp.)
- Environmental irritants
- Iridovirus (ranavirus)
- *Chlamydophila* in *Xenopus laevis*
- Chromomycosis
- Chytridiomycosis
- *Saprolegnia* (aquatic amphibians): Cotton wool-like growth on the skin
- Trombiculids in terrestrial amphibians (erythematous vesicles)
- Whitish patches on caecilians (fungal infection, water too hard, poor water quality)
- Environmental toxins (see also *Systemic Disorders*)
  - Chlorhexidine
  - Povidone-iodine
  - Chlorine
  - Quaternary ammonium compounds
  - Ammonium

Ectoparasites

- Aquatic adult and larval amphibians
- *Oodinium pillularis*
- Ciliated protozoa
- Crustaceans
- Argulus (large, disc-shaped crustacean)
- Copepods
- Leeches
- Terrestrial amphibians
- Trombiculids
- *Bufolucilia* spp. (toadfly—see *Respiratory Disorders*)

Neoplasia

- Hemangioma

Findings on clinical examination

- Inflammation and ulceration (see "Erosions and Ulceration" and "Changes in Pigmentation," above). Septicemic infections may be accompanied by systemic signs such as inappetence, lethargy, convulsions, swelling of the body (either with fluid or gas), and obvious eye abnormalities.

- Wasting (often despite an apparently good appetite), ulceration, swellings either at the skin or deeper (mycobacteriosis)
- Graying of the skin (excess mucus production) and gills, respiratory impairment, debilitation, and death (ectoparasites, including *Oodinium pillularis*)
- Dark, raised nodules in the skin, debilitation and weight loss (chromomycosis—see also *Systemic Disorders*)
- Skin sloughing, splayed leg (chytridiomycosis)
- Inactivity
- Anorexia
- Damage and deformity to the head, especially the nares, in toads *(Bufolucilia)*
- Raised mass (granuloma, neoplasia)

Investigations

1. Skin scrapings
   a. *Oodinium:* Can be quite large, up to 1.0-mm diameter, oval-shaped with a very dark appearance because of chloroplasts, not usually mobile
   b. *Pseudocapillaroides xenopi:* Eggs and worms visible
   c. Copepods
   d. Trombiculid mites
2. PCR for chytridiomycosis
3. Radiography
4. Routine hematology and biochemistry
5. Culture and sensitivity
6. Endoscopy
7. Biopsy/necropsy
8. Ultrasonography
9. Water quality testing

Management

1. Fluid therapy—see *Nursing Care*
2. Wound management
   a. Debride and clean by flushing with sterile saline solution.
   b. Iodine compounds, chlorhexidine, isopropyl alcohol, and quaternary ammonium compounds are potentially toxic and should be used with care.
   c. Wounds (and hemostasis achieved) should be sealed either by suturing or with cyanoacrylate.

Treatment/specific therapy

- Trauma—see "Management" above
- *Aeromonas* and *Pseudomonas*
  - Appropriate antibiosis
  - Often secondary to immunocompromise from poor environmental conditions (e.g., inappropriate temperature, poor nutrition)
- *Chlamydophila*
  - Appropriate antibiosis (e.g., doxycycline at 10 to 50 mg/kg PO s.i.d.)

- Mycobacteriosis
  - Treatment is rarely effective and so euthanasia should be considered.
- *Saprolegnia*
  - Removing visible hyphae by swabbing the affected area with a 10% povidone-iodine solution s.i.d.
  - Salt-water baths (10 to 25 mg sea salt per liter) s.i.d. for 10 to 30 minutes
  - Often secondary to poor water quality and high biologic contamination of water
- *Basidiobolus ranarum*
  - Benzalkonium chloride dips, at 0.25-2 mg/L water for 30 minutes every 48 hours for 3 treatments
- Chromomycosis
  - No effective treatment. Consider euthanasia.
- Chytridiomycosis
  - Larval stages lack keratinized skin so are less susceptible to infection, so heavy mortalities may follow metamorphosis (postmetamorphic death syndrome, PMDS). Can be carried on mouthparts of larvae
  - Very virulent; consider euthanasia.
  - Some cases respond to itraconazole baths. Create 0.01% itraconazole solution (dilute a 10 mg/mL itraconazole suspension in 0.6% saline solution), and give 5-minute baths in this solution daily for 11 days. *Note:* Chlorhexidine is potentially toxic to amphibians.
  - *B. dendrobatidis* is susceptible to temperatures above 23° C, but beware that amphibians with chytridiomycosis will have reduced heat tolerance, so use hyperthermia with caution.
- *Oodinium* and ciliated protozoa
  - Try a proprietary *Oodinium* (velvet) treatment formulated for aquarium fish.
  - Metronidazole at 10 to 14 mg/L for up to 24 hours daily for 10 days
  - Quinine hydrochloride at 10 to 20 mg/L indefinitely. Some amphibians may be sensitive to this.
  - The encysted stage is relatively resistant to chemical attack.
  - Antibiotic cover should be considered, as secondary infections are common at the areas where the skin is damaged.
  - Eliminate the parasite from a show aquarium by removing all amphibians (and fish), reducing or cutting out the light levels, and raising the temperature to 30 to 32° C for 3 weeks.
- *Microsporidia*
  - Chloramphenicol sodium succinate (5 to 10 mg/kg intracoelomic) plus topical oxytetracycline and polymyxin B s.i.d.
- *Pseudocapillaroides xenopi*
  - Fenbendazole at 50 to 100 mg/kg PO repeat after 2 weeks
  - Thiabendazole at 50 to 100 mg/kg PO once only. Repeat after 2 weeks.
  - Levamisole (100 to 300 mg/L) bath for up to 24 hours once weekly for up to 12 weeks
- Leeches
  - Individual removal
- Copepods
  - Hypertonic bath (10 to 25 g NaCl—not table salt) for 5 to 30 minutes
  - Treat with lufenuron at 0.088 mg/L as a single dose.
- *Argulus* (fish louse)
  - Individual removal of parasites
  - Treat with lufenuron at 0.088 mg/L as a single dose.

- A potassium permanganate bath at 10 ppm (mg/L) for 5 to 60 minutes can be used to rid both individual amphibians and plants of this parasite.
- Trombiculids
  - Physical removal of mites with damp cotton bud
  - Topical ivermectin: Dilute 1:50 in Hartmann's solution and apply topically to dorsal surface.
  - Selamectin topically at 6 mg/kg (D'Agostino et al 2007)
- *Bufolucilia* (toadfly)
  - Physical removal of parasites if possible
  - Flush the nares and oropharynx with ivermectin or levamisole.
  - Covering antibiosis

Respiratory tract disorders

Amphibians respire through a variety of organs—namely, the lungs, buccopharyngeal lining, skin, and gills (larval amphibia). In terrestrial amphibians dehydration may affect gaseous exchange at the skin, leading to hypercapnia and acidosis.

Bacterial
- Pneumonia

Fungal
- Pneumonia

Protozoal
- *Oodinium* and other aquatic protozoa (larval amphibian; see *Respiratory Disorders* in Chapter 15)

Parasitic
- *Rhabdias* spp.
- Trematodes (wide variety—see *Systemic Disorders*)

Neoplasia
Other noninfectious problems
- Acute pulmonary emphysema
- Poor water quality, especially larval amphibians. High ammonia and nitrite levels may predispose to gill damage and secondary bacterial and fungal infections.

Findings on clinical examination

- Increased respiratory rate (especially larval amphibians)
- Open-mouthed breathing
- "Wet" or unusual respiratory noises
- Discharge around the glottis or inside the proximal trachea
- Occluded nostrils
- Sudden death

Investigations

1. Microscopy
2. Fecal examination

3. Embryonated eggs or rhabditiform larvae (*Rhabdias* spp.)
4. Transillumination of very small or transparent amphibian
   a. May see large adult worms in lungs
5. Radiography
6. Routine hematology and biochemistry
7. Culture and sensitivity
8. Endoscopy
9. Biopsy
10. Ultrasonography
11. Water quality testing

Management

1. For aquatic amphibians, transfer to a shallow container and increase aeration to maximally oxygenate water.
2. For terrestrial amphibians, transfer to a high-oxygen environment. *Note:* High air flow rates may increase the risk of dehydration from moisture loss across the skin.

Treatment/specific therapy

- Pneumonia
- Appropriate antimicrobials
- *Oodinium*
  - Proprietary fish treatments
  - Metronidazole at 50 mg/L for up to 24 hours daily for 10 days
  - Quinine hydrochloride at 10 to 20 mg/L indefinitely. Some amphibians may be sensitive.
  - The encysted stage is relatively resistant to chemical attack.
  - Can colonize the intestines of fish and possibly larval amphibians, where again it can be protected from medications
  - Antibiotic cover should be considered, because secondary infections are common at the areas where the skin is damaged.
  - Eliminate the parasite from a show vivaria/aquaria by removing all amphibians, reducing or cutting out the light levels and raising the temperature to 30 to 32° C for 3 weeks.
- *Rhabdias*
  - Ivermectin
    - Dilute 1:50 in Hartmann's solution and apply topically to dorsal surface.
    - 10 g/L bath for 1 hour weekly for up to 12 weeks
  - Selamectin topically at 6 mg/kg once only (D'Agostino et al 2007)
  - Levamisole (100 to 300 mg/L) bath for up to 24 hrs once weekly for up to 12 weeks
  - Fenbendazole at 50 to 100 mg/kg PO. Repeat after 2 weeks
- Acute pulmonary emphysema
  - Repetitive aspiration of coelomic air until pulmonary lesion seals
  - Covering antibiosis

Gastrointestinal tract disorders

Bacterial
- Enteritis (rarely encountered)

Fungal
- Enteritis (rarely encountered)

Protozoal
- *Entamoeba ranarum*
- Ciliates

Parasitic
- *Strongyloides* spp.
- A variety of nematode species may be detected.
- Acanthocephalans
- Cestodes (wide variety—see *Systemic Disorders*)
- Trematodes (wide variety—see *Systemic Disorders*)

Nutritional
- Short-tongue syndrome of frogs (suspected hypovitaminosis A)

Neoplasia
- Myxoma (especially tree frogs)

Other noninfectious problems
- Gastric impaction (especially large frogs, such as horned frogs, *Ceratophrys* spp.): May be the result of gastric overload (i.e., offered too large food item)
- Gastric prolapse
- Intestinal foreign body
- Cloacal prolapse (especially tree frogs)

Findings on clinical examination

- Diarrhea, blood in feces, wasting, loss of appetite *(Entamoeba)*
- Firm swelling from lining of oral cavity; if large, can affect frog's ability to feed (myxoma)
- Inability to catch prey
- Weight loss
- Swollen, often gassy coelom (gastric impaction)
- Anorexia
- Inactivity
- Cloacal prolapse (intestinal parasitism, enteritis, toxins)

Investigations

1. Fecal examination
   a. *Entamoeba:* Multinucleate cysts; nuclear endosomes measure up to nucleus diameter
   b. Ciliated protozoa
2. Radiography
3. Routine hematology and biochemistry
4. Culture and sensitivity
5. Endoscopy
6. Biopsy/necropsy
   a. Squamous metaplasia of the mucus-secreting glands of the tongue (short-tongue syndrome)
   b. Hepatic retinol levels in suspected hypovitaminosis A (Table 13-2)

Table 13-2 Hepatic retinol levels in suspected hypovitaminosis A

Species	Short-tongue syndrome affected Wyoming toad (*Bufo baxteri*) (*n* = 6)	Healthy Wyoming toad (*Bufo baxteri*) (*n* = 3)	Healthy southern toad (*Bufo terrestris*) (*n* = 4)	Healthy American toad (*Bufo americanus*) (*n* = 2)
Hepatic retinol (µg/g)	0.004-7.3	81-138	96-243	418-569

Adapted from Pessier et al (2002).

7. Ultrasonography
8. Water quality testing

Management

- See *Nursing Care*.

Treatment/specific therapy

- *Entamoeba ranarum*
  - Metronidazole at 10 to 14 mg/L bath for 1 hour unless showing signs of distress.
- Ciliated protozoa
  - These are usually considered normal gut commensals.
  - If high numbers and amphibians showing consistent clinical signs, treat as for *Entamoeba*
- *Strongyloides* spp.
  - Ivermectin
    - Dilute 1:50 in Hartmann's solution and apply topically to dorsal surface.
    - 10 g/L bath for 1 hour weekly for up to 12 weeks
  - Selamectin topically at 6 mg/kg once only. (D'Agostino et al 2007)
  - Levamisole (100 to 300 mg/L) bath for 1 hour once weekly for up to 12 weeks
- Nematodes and acanthocephalans
  - As for *Strongyloides* spp. above
  - Fenbendazole 50 to 100 mg/kg PO. Repeat after 2 weeks as necessary.
- Acanthocephalans require intermediate arthropod host so can be self-limiting.
- Myxoma
  - Surgical resection
  - Radiosurgery
  - Likely to recur but grow very slowly
- Short-tongue syndrome
  - Supplement with vitamin A. *Note:* Commercial injectable vitamin A preparations are too concentrated for amphibians.
  - 2 IU/g IM every 72 hours or 1 IU/g PO or topically s.i.d.
  - May require hand-feeding as prey-capturing adhesive qualities of the tongue are significantly reduced.

- Gastric impaction
  - Removal of impaction contents by gastric lavage, endoscopic retrieval, or gastroenterotomy
  - Broad-spectrum covering antibiotics
- Gastric prolapse
  - Appears as a fleshy structure above the tongue
  - Can be a normal activity in some frogs
  - Can be pathologic—often linked to starvation or increased intracoelomic pressure
  - Gently replace stomach and fill with liquid food to maintain position.
  - Often fatal
- Intestinal foreign body
  - Laxatives often beneficial due to short GI tract.
  - May require enterotomy
- Cloacal prolapse
  - Investigate possible underlying etiologies (e.g., endoparasites).
  - Surgical replacement often poorly tolerated
  - Prognosis is guarded.

Nutritional disorders

- Hypocalcemia (metabolic bone disease—see *Musculoskeletal Disorders*)
- Hypervitaminosis D_3 accompanied by hypercalcemia (see *Systemic Disorders*)
- Hypovitaminosis A (see also *Gastrointestinal Disorders* and *Ophthalmic Disorders*)
- Obesity (especially horned frogs *Ceratophrys* spp.)
  - Manage by switching to a low-energy diet (e.g., substituting more invertebrate prey for mammalian) plus supplement with vitamin E especially.
- Lipid keratopathy (see *Ophthalmic Disorders*)

Hepatic disorders

Bacterial
- *Aeromonas* spp., *Pseudomonas* spp.
- Mycobacteria

Fungal
Protozoal
- Amebiasis

Parasitic
Neoplasia
- Cholangiocellular carcinoma

Findings on clinical examination

- Ascites (see *Systemic Disorders*)
- Anasarca

485

Investigations

1. Radiography
2. Routine hematology and biochemistry
3. Culture and sensitivity
4. Endoscopy
   a. Multifocal abscessation (mycobacteriosis)
5. Biopsy/necropsy
6. Ultrasonography
7. Water quality testing

Management

- Milk thistle *(Silybum marianum)* is hepatoprotectant. Dose at 4 to 15 mg/kg PO b.i.d. or t.i.d.
- Aspirate excess fluid from the coelom if ascitic.
- Furosemide at 2.5 mg/kg IM b.i.d.
- For aquatic and semi-aquatic amphibia attempt to correct osmotic imbalance by keeping in either salt solution (0.55 to 1.0%) or magnesium sulfate solution.

Treatment/specific therapy

- Bacterial hepatitis
  - Appropriate antibiosis
- Mycobacteriosis
  - Potential zoonosis
  - Considering euthanasia as treatment is often unrewarding (but see *Systemic Disorders* in Chapter 15).
- Hepatic amebiasis
  - Metronidazole at 100 mg/kg PO every 14 days (Wright 1995)

Cardiovascular and hematologic disorders

Amphibians have a well-developed lymphatic system with a significant exchange rate with the vascular system (up to 10 mL/hr in the frog). Lymph is circulated with a varying number of lymph hearts. Cardiac and/or lymph heart disease and insufficiency is likely to lead to fluid accumulation in the coelom and lymphatics, presenting as an ascites or anasarca-like condition.

Bacterial

- Endocarditis

Fungal

Protozoal

- Trypanosomes
- *Haemogregarina* spp.
- *Hepatozoon* spp.

Parasitic

- Microfilaria (see *Systemic Disorders*)

Dietary

Neoplasia

Other noninfectious problems

- Cardiomyopathy
- Lymph heart insufficiency

Findings on clinical examination

- Edema, ascites (may be gross and present with swollen coelom or confined to one or more limbs)
- Anorexia
- Mortalities

Investigations

1. Radiography
2. Routine hematology and biochemistry
3. Culture and sensitivity
4. Endoscopy
5. Biopsy
6. Ultrasonography
7. Electrocardiogram
8. Water quality testing

Management

1. Fluid accumulation causes a reduction in circulating fluid volume, tissue hypoxia, and lung compression.
2. Aspirate excess fluid from the coelom.
3. Furosemide at 2.5 mg/kg IM b.i.d.
4. For aquatic and semi-aquatic amphibians, attempt to correct osmotic imbalance by keeping in either salt solution (0.55% to 1.0%) or magnesium sulfate solution.
5. Treat any underlying specific causes.

Treatment/specific therapy

- Bacterial and fungal disorders
  - Appropriate antimicrobials
- Trypanosomes
  - Bathe in quinine sulfate (30 mg/L) for 1 hour daily.
- *Haemogregarina* spp. and *Hepatozoon* spp.
  - Potentiated sulfonamides may relieve symptoms; chloroquine and primaquine regimens as outlined for treating hemoparasites in snakes (see Chapter 11) may be modified.
  - May be self-limiting as an invertebrate vector such as mosquito or leech is usually required

Systemic disorders

Viral

- Frog virus 3 (iridovirus; tadpole edema disease—see also *Renal and Urinary Disorders*)
- Bohle iridovirus (in Australian amphibians)

Bacterial

- *Aeromonas* spp., *Pseudomonas* spp.
- *Flavobacterium* spp.
- Mycobacteriosis, especially *M. marinum, M. chelonae, M. ranae, M. xenopi, M. fortuitum,* and rarely *M. avium* complex (*M. intracellulare* and *M. avium avium*)

Fungal

- Chromomycosis (see also *Skin Disorders*), such as *Veronaea botryosa* (Mayer et al 2000)
- *Batrachochytrium dendrobatidis* (chytridiomycosis)
- *Mucor amphibiorum*

Protozoal

- Microsporidia (e.g., *Pleistophora, Microsporidium*)

Parasitic

- Microfilaria
- Cestodes (wide variety—see *Systemic Disorders*)
- Trematodes (wide variety—see *Systemic Disorders*)

Nutritional

- Hypervitaminosis D_3/hypercalcemia (see *Nutritional Disorders*)
- Hypocalcemia (see *Musculoskeletal Disorders*)

Neoplasia

- Fibrosarcoma
- Thymoma (Jacobson et al 2004)
- Gonadal neoplasia

Other noninfectious problems

- Acute pulmonary emphysema (see *Respiratory Disorders*)
- Renal disease
- Cardiovascular disease
- Failure of lymph hearts
- Intestinal disease (gaseous bloating—see *Gastrointestinal Disorders*)
- Keeping in very soft water (inducing osmotic imbalance)
- Thermal shock (Green et al 2003)
- Environmental toxins
  - Chlorhexidine
  - Povidone-iodine
  - Chlorine toxicity (tadpoles, aquatic amphibians)
  - Quaternary ammonium compounds
  - Ammonium
  - Heavy metal, especially zinc, lead, or copper (see also *Neurologic Disorders*)

Findings on clinical examination

- Weight loss
- Anorexia (consider brumation)
- Unwilling/unable to move
- Splayed legs, skin sloughing (chytridiomycosis); high mortality following metamorphosis (PMDS)
- Swollen coelom (ascites, anasarca, lymphedema, septicemia, renal disease, acute pulmonary emphysema, hypervitaminosis D_3)
- Septicemic infections may be indicated by signs typical of "red leg" (see *Skin Disorders*), such as inflammation, ulceration, inappetence, lethargy, convulsions, coelomic swelling, and obvious eye abnormalities.
- Dark, raised nodules in the skin, debilitation, and weight loss (chromomycosis)
- Increased mucus production, erythema, agitation, lethargy, dyspnea, convulsions, paralysis, diarrhea, and death following exposure to chlorhexidine (chlorhexidine toxicity)
- Mortalities

Investigations

1. Radiography
2. Routine hematology and biochemistry
   a. Cold-adapted amphibians show an increased RBC count, hemoglobin concentration, heterophilia, lymphopenia, and eosinopenia
3. Culture and sensitivity
4. Endoscopy
   a. Microfilaria free in coelomic cavity
5. Biopsy/necropsy
   a. Microfilaria in vasculature or encysted in a variety of tissues and organs
   b. A wide variety of trematodes and cestodes at different developmental stages may be encountered in a variety of tissues.
6. Ultrasonography
7. Water quality testing

Management

1. Ascites and anasarca
   a. Fluid accumulation causes a reduction in circulating fluid volume, tissue hypoxia, and lung compression.
   b. Aspirate excess fluid from the coelom.
   c. Furosemide at 2.5 mg/kg IM b.i.d.
   d. For aquatic and semi-aquatic amphibians, attempt to correct osmotic imbalance by keeping in either salt solution (0.55% to 1.0%) or magnesium sulfate solution.
   e. Treat any underlying specific causes.

Treatment/specific therapy

- Bacterial infections *(Aeromonas, Pseudomonas, Flavobacterium)*
  - Appropriate antibiosis

- Mycobacteriosis
  - Potential zoonosis, so consider euthanasia
- Hypervitaminosis D_3/hypercalcemia
  - Metastatic calcification in many organs (e.g., heart, liver, kidneys) leads to marked ascites.
  - Treat symptomatically.
  - Investigate possible causes of dietary imbalance.
- Chromomycosis
  - Treatment often ineffective
  - Some apparent success with fluconazole (Mayer et al 2000)
  - Consider euthanasia.
- Chytridiomycosis
  - Larval stages lack keratinized skin so are less susceptible to infection, so heavy mortalities may follow metamorphosis (PMDS). Can be carried on mouthparts of larvae
  - Very virulent; consider euthanasia.
- Microsporidia
  - No effective treatment. Consider:
    - Toltrazuril at 30 mg/L bath for 60 minutes repeated every other day for 3 treatments
    - Feeding a diet of 0.1% fumagillin
- Microfilaria
  - Ivermectin
    - Dilute 1:50 in Hartmann's solution and apply topically to dorsal surface.
    - 10 g/L bath for 1 hour weekly for up to 12 weeks
  - Mortality may occur following treatment.
- Trematodes and cestodes
  - Praziquantel at 10 mg/L bath for 3 hours as a single dose or 8 to 24 mg/kg PO or SC daily for 14 days
- Thermal shock
  - Usually diagnosed postmortem
  - History of sudden temperature change—either to a markedly low or high temperature
  - If identified soon enough, return to clean, well-oxygenated water close to previous temperature.
  - Supportive treatment
- Environmental toxins
  - Bathe amphibian in clean water.
  - Supportive therapy (e.g., parenteral fluids)
- Ammonia toxicity
  - If due to poor water quality, undertake partial water changes to dilute the ammonia levels.
  - Adding zeolite will absorb large quantities of ammonia.
  - Longer-term control may include addition of commercially available *Nitrosomonas* bacterial cultures or equivalent.
- Chlorine toxicity
  - Place in aged water.
  - Avoid either by use of aged water or commercial dechlorinators as used for aquarium fish.

- Brumation
  - A period of inactivity characterized by anorexia, withdrawal from the environment, and immobility and reduced responsiveness.
  - Typically can be associated with periods of adverse environmental conditions in the wild (e.g., low temperatures or arid conditions).
  - Most likely seen in Chacoan horned frogs (Ceratophrys cranwelli), but other species may present.
  - If unsure whether brumating or not, monitor weight: Weight loss is negligible, of the order of 1% to 2% body weight per month, in brumation, whereas it can be very pronounced in the presence of disease.
  - Assess exposure to possible brumation triggers such as low temperatures, shortened day lengths, reduced light intensity, and reduced humidity.

Musculoskeletal disorders

Bacterial
- Bacterial osteomyelitis
- Mycobacteriosis

Fungal
- Mycotic osteomyelitis
- Chromomycosis

Protozoal
- Pleistophora (Microsporidia)

Parasitic
- Ribeiroia ondatrae (trematode)

Nutritional
- Metabolic bone disease (especially at time of metamorphosis)
- Fluorosis (Shaw et al 2012)

Neoplasia
Other noninfectious problems
- Gout (articular and periarticular), especially in horned frogs (Ceratophrys spp.)
- Trauma (fractures)

Findings on clinical examination

- Swellings (abscess, gout, fracture)
- Any limb or spinal swelling, fracture, or paralysis should be considered as a possible sign of a pathologic fracture.
- Soft mandibles, foreshortening of the maxillae, swollen midshaft of long bones, kyphosis/scoliosis, weakness, inability to support own body weight (metabolic bone disease)
- Signs consistent with metabolic bone disease but increased cortical density and bone volume; water fluoride levels >0.2 mg/L (fluorosis/osteofluorosis)
- Muscle weakness, inability to support body or hunt/locate food
- Muscle fasciculations and other neurologic signs

- Kyphosis (microsporidial myositis)
- Supernumerary limbs, limb abnormalities (*Ribeiroia ondatrae,* trematode)

Investigations

1. Radiography
2. Cytology
   a. Fine-needle aspirate
   b. Gout tophi
3. Routine hematology and biochemistry
4. Culture and sensitivity
5. Endoscopy
6. Biopsy
7. Ultrasonography

Treatment/specific therapy

- Gout
  - In large amphibians (e.g., horned frogs), may be linked to excessive mammalian prey intake; these are often fed on small mice, whereas their natural diet would be mostly insectivorous.
  - Allopurinol at 10 mg/kg PO s.i.d.
- Metabolic bone disease
  - Classically a nutritional secondary hyperparathyroidism due to relative lack of calcium
  - May be especially pronounced at time of metamorphosis
  - Postmetamorphic amphibians may exhibit signs of metabolic bone disease even on a good diet, as a result of a larval calcium deficit. *Note:* In many adult Urodeles and larval anurans, prolactin is an important hypercalcemic hormone as well as parathormone and 1,25-hydroxy vitamin D_3.
  - Daily baths in a high calcium and vitamin D_3 solution (2 to 3 IU/mL)
  - Oral or injectable calcium and vitamin D_3 supplementation (may be absorbed transcutaneously, so try applying to skin of back of terrestrial amphibians).
  - Supplement with dietary calcium.
  - Provide appropriate levels of UVB lighting.
  - Some species endemic to hard water areas may have a higher calcium requirement.
- Fluorosis/osteofluorosis
  - Exacerbated by hypocalcemia
  - Use water filter through chemical media to remove fluorine.
  - Increase calcium intake in diet (see "Metabolic Bone Disease" above).
  - Provide UVB.
- Abscessation and osteomyelitis, myositis
  - Appropriate antibiosis
  - Consider amputation if damage is extensive.
- Fracture
  - Differentiate between pathological fracture (chromomycosis, neoplasia) and traumatic fracture with radiography.
  - For compound fractures, deal with skin lesions, as described under *Skin Disorders*.
  - Extensive trauma to limbs is often best dealt with by amputation. Many Urodeles are able to regenerate lost limbs and tails.

Neurologic disorders

Bacterial
- Septicemia
- CNS granuloma

Fungal
- CNS granuloma

Neoplasia
Other noninfectious problems
- Hypoglycemia (weakness)
- Environmental toxins (see also *Systemic Disorders*)
  - Chlorhexidine
  - Povidone-iodine
  - Chlorine toxicity (tadpoles, aquatic amphibians)
  - Quaternary ammonium compounds
  - Ammonium
  - Poor water quality
  - Cleaning agents
  - Heavy metal, especially zinc, lead, or copper (see also *Systemic Disorders*)

Findings on clinical examination

- Abnormal behavioral signs, especially in larval amphibia (poor water quality)
- Flaccid paralysis
- Disorientation
- Seizures
- Loss of righting reflex
- Mortality

Investigations

1. Radiography
2. Routine hematology and biochemistry
   a. Blood glucose levels: In the North American bullfrog *(Rana catesbeiana)* normal resting glucose levels around 0.4 mmol/L; 1.3 mmol/L when stressed (Crawshaw 1998)
3. Culture and sensitivity
4. Endoscopy
5. Biopsy
6. Ultrasonography
7. Water quality testing

Management

See *Nursing Care.*

Treatment/specific therapy

- Bacterial and fungal diseases
  - Appropriate antimicrobials
  - Supportive care
- Hypoglycemia
  - Oral glucose, but see "Cataracts" under *Ophthalmic Disorders*
- Environmental toxins (see *Systemic Disorders*)
- Heavy metal poisoning
  - Remove suspected source.
  - Remove to unaffected water.
  - Oxygenate or aerate water well.

Ophthalmic disorders

The amphibian eye changes during metamorphosis. At hatching, each larva has a duplex cornea with an inner cornea and a second, outer, cornea. At metamorphosis, these fuse into a single, mammalian-like cornea. Pupillary dilation is best achieved under general anesthesia with tricaine methanesulfonate (MS222). Otherwise, intracameral muscle relaxants such as vecuronium, succinylcholine, or D-tubocurarine are required.

Bacterial

- Subspectacular abscess (larval amphibians)
- Keratitis and ulceration
- Uveitis

Fungal

- Keratitis and ulceration
- Uveitis

Protozoal

Parasitic

Nutritional

- Calcium lesions in the cornea
- Cholesterol lesions (lipid keratopathy)
- Hypovitaminosis A

Neoplasia

Other noninfectious problems

- Corneal trauma
- Crickets and other prey insects
- Collision with environmental objects, including transparent barriers

Findings on clinical examination

- Keratitis
- Calcium and cholesterol lesions in the cornea
- Bilateral conjunctival swellings (hypovitaminosis A)
- Fluorescein-positive corneal lesions (corneal ulceration)

- Buphthalmos
- Cataracts

Investigations

1. Ophthalmic examination
2. Radiography
3. Routine hematology and biochemistry
4. Culture and sensitivity
5. Endoscopy
6. Biopsy
7. Ultrasonography
8. Water quality testing, especially for aquatic amphibians

Treatment/specific therapy

- Hypovitaminosis A (see *Gastrointestinal Disorders*)
- Lipid and calcium keratopathies
  - If only small part of cornea affected, then monitor
  - Partial keratectomy if cornea largely affected plus topical antibiosis
  - Lipid keratopathy may be linked with:
    - Fat mobilization during oogenesis in females
    - Failure to achieve (high) preferred body temperatures
    - Diets high in mammalian fat (e.g., rodents)
- Corneal ulcers and secondarily infected corneal traumas
  - Under anesthesia, swab for culture and sensitivity, clean, and debride lesion.
  - Apply appropriate antibiosis and allow time for absorption.
  - Seal with cyanoacrylate (Bicknese & Cranfield 1995).
- Uveitis
  - Topical and systemic antibiosis
  - Enucleation. *Note:* Many frogs and toads use the eyes during swallowing, so enucleation may affect feeding ability.
  - In cases of buphthalmus, if enucleation is decided against, consider tarsorrhaphy to protect cornea from desiccation.
- Cataracts
  - Various etiologies, including nutritional, toxic, and infectious, should be considered.
  - Temporary cataracts in poison-arrow frogs linked with provision of 5% dextrose as part of supportive therapy (Williams & Whitaker 1994)

Endocrine disorders

Despite extensive studies into the amphibian endocrine system, especially with regard to metamorphosis, pathology of the endocrine system is little documented. Supplementation with thyroxine is known to trigger metamorphosis in the axolotl; prolonged larval stages may reflect a hypothalamic-pituitary-thyroidal dysfunction.

Neoplasia

- Thymoma (see *Systemic Disorders* and *Renal and Urinary Disorders*)

Renal and urinary disorders

Viral

- Frog virus 3 (iridovirus; tadpole edema disease—see also *Systemic Disorders*)
- Lucké tumor herpesvirus (induces renal adenocarcinoma in leopard frogs, *Lithobates pipiens*)

Bacterial

- Nephritis

Fungal

- Nephritis

Protozoal

- *Entamoeba ranarum* (renal amebiasis)
- Myxosporea

Parasitic

- Trematodes (wide variety—see *Systemic Disorders*)

Neoplasia

- Renal adenocarcinoma (in the leopard frog *Lithobates pipiens*, likely to be induced by a herpesvirus)
- Thymoma (see also *Systemic Disorders*)

Other noninfectious problems

- Prolapse of the urinary bladder (differentiate from cloacal or oviductal prolapse)
- Cystic calculi (tree frogs)

Findings on clinical examination

- Ascites (see also *Systemic Disorders*)
- Ascites in tadpoles (frog virus 3, but see also *Systemic Disorders*)
- Loss of appetite, anorexia
- Weight loss
- Inactivity

Investigations

1. Urinalysis of terrestrial amphibian
   a. Renal casts
   b. Inflammatory cells
   c. Bacteria
2. Radiography
3. Routine hematology and biochemistry
   a. Inverse calcium: phosphorus ratio, hypoproteinemia, and hypoalbuminemia suggest renal disease (or hepatic disease).
   b. Nephrotic syndrome (may be linked with thymoma—Jacobson et al 2004)
4. Culture and sensitivity
5. Endoscopy

6. Biopsy/necropsy
   a. Hemorrhage into Bowman's capsule, necrosis of glomerular endothelial cells, and tubular necrosis (frog virus 3)
7. Ultrasonography
8. Water quality testing

Management

- See *Nursing Care.*

Treatment/specific therapy

- Ranavirus (frog virus 3)
  - No effective treatment. Potentially very infectious, so consider euthanasia.
- Bacterial and fungal nephritis
  - Appropriate antimicrobials
- Myxosporea
  - No effective treatment available. Try fumagillin as for fish at 1 g/kg food for 10 to 14 days for prevention.
- Renal amebiasis
  - Metronidazole at 100 mg/kg PO every 14 days
- Renal neoplasia
  - Partial or unilateral nephrectomy
- Lucké tumor herpesvirus
  - Lethal in tadpoles, but adults relatively resistant
  - Virus production associated with low temperatures (e.g., during hibernation)
- Urinary bladder prolapse
  - Clean and aspirate out any urine.
  - Gently replace.
  - Consider cystopexy following a coeliotomy.
  - Percutaneous cystopexy: Achieved by inserting a small probe into the bladder per cloaca as a guide to identify the position of the bladder. Hold the probe against the coelomic wall while transcutaneous sutures are positioned.

Reproductive disorders
• •

Neoplasia

Other noninfectious problems

- Oviductal prolapse
- Ovarian prolapse

Findings on clinical examination

- Ovary or oviduct partially protruding from cloaca, usually following egg-laying

Investigations

1. Radiography
2. Routine hematology and biochemistry

3. Culture and sensitivity
4. Endoscopy
5. Biopsy
6. Ultrasonography
7. Water quality testing

Management

See *Nursing Care.*

Treatment/specific therapy

- Oviductal and ovarian prolapse
  - Attempt surgical resection.
  - Very guarded prognosis
- Gonadal neoplasia
  - Surgical resection

Goldfish and koi

This chapter covers those disorders likely to be seen in goldfish and koi, which constitute the most popular section of fish-keeping. Tolerance of wide temperature ranges means that these species can be kept outside, as well as inside, in most temperate countries such as those of Europe and North America. However, they are also happy at more tropical temperatures and in those countries such as Singapore, Malaysia, and southern China, where they are kept alongside "tropical species." Hence, this disorders chapter should be read in conjunction with Chapter 15.

Fish-keeping is a huge worldwide hobby and industry. Unfortunately, veterinarians are often last to be consulted over a fish-related problem, or else they are approached purely as a source of antibiotics and other regulated medications. This is because:
1. There are a great many proprietary products available for the treatment of ornamental fish, which aquarists are able to access from their aquarium retailer without recourse to the veterinarian. Most of these products are poorly regulated, and, therefore, their efficacy is often very poor in contrast to the claims made for them, a problem compounded by inadequate diagnostics by both aquarists and helpful retailers. Ectoparasitic preparations are usually sufficiently efficacious to justify their use when their safety and ease of use is also brought into consideration.
2. This ready availability of proprietary medications devalues professional input.
3. There is a low economic cost for many widely kept fish.
4. There is a historical perception that veterinarians know little about fish and fish diseases.

Consultation and handling

The key to successful fish-keeping, and a major stumbling point, is water quality. Recommended water quality parameters for koi and goldfish are listed in Table 14-1.

Hobbyist test kits are available to measure these parameters, and they give reasonable results; accurate testing requires professional equipment.

If possible, fish should be examined in their home aquarium or pond. However, if the pond is large it may pay to ask for the fish to be caught and separated before arrival, as much time can be wasted attempting to catch the fish. Ponds are rarely built with recapture in mind. Once caught, place the fish on a damp towel for examination. If necessary sedate with tricaine methonesulfonate (MS222) or benzocaine (see "Anesthesia" below).

Always examine the ventral surface, as lesions here may not be obvious when viewed from above. Skin scrapes should be taken from the operculae, the flank, and around the base of the fins. Examine the gills and oral cavity.

Blood sampling

This is best done under anesthesia. Blood can be drawn using a well-heparinized syringe from the ventral tail vein, which runs midline just below the caudal vertebrae. In small fish this can be accessed via the ventral midline; in larger fish, a lateral approach is often better. This same approach can be used for intravenous injections.

For the internal anatomy of a goldfish, see Figure 14-1.

Table 14-1 Recommended water quality parameters for koi and goldfish

Parameter	Value
Temperature (°C)	10-30 (preferred range = 22-28 for koi)
pH	6.0-8.4 (preferred 7.0-8.0)
Hardness (CaCO₃) (mg/L)	100-250
Conductivity (mS/cm)	180-480
Ammonia (total) (mg/L)	<0.02
Nitrite (mg/L)	<0.2
Nitrate (above ambient tapwater levels) (mg/L)	<40
Oxygen (mg/L)	5.0-8.0
Chlorine (mg/L)	0.002
Adapted from Jepson (2001).	

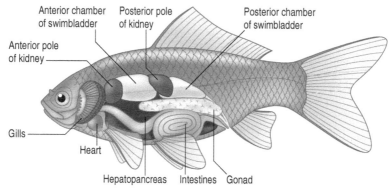

Fig 14-1. Internal anatomy of goldfish. *Note:* Goldfish and koi do not possess a true stomach. Adhesions between the internal organs are normal and not the result of coelomitis.

Nursing care

Provision of optimal water quality is essential to maximize recovery. A separate hospital aquarium or vat can be used, but the water quality in this facility should be as good as in a main display (Fig. 14-2). The water should be filtered, but because of the use of medications such as antibiotics, biological filtration cannot be used. After each patient, the aquarium or vat should be dismantled and cleaned out with an iodine-based disinfectant.

Reliance is placed on physical and chemical methods of water purification. Zeolite will absorb ammonia excreted by the fish, while activated charcoal will adsorb many harmful chemicals from the water. If salt is used, a small protein skimmer would be of great benefit. Ozonizers and ultraviolet sterilization are also useful adjuncts. Keep decorations to a minimum, giving just sufficient for nervous fish to hide behind. All materials used should be readily cleanable, such as plastic—and avoid live plants and bogwood where possible, as these can act as disease reservoirs. Temperature can be maintained at the optimum using commercial aquarium heaters. For koi and goldfish, a temperature of 18 to 25°C should be considered. Keeping fish in a permanent 5-g/L solution of salt (use aquarium or sea salt, not table or rock salt) will reduce the osmotic load on a sick koi or goldfish. Salt concentrations of over 10 g/L have been shown to be toxic to goldfish (Burghdorf-Moisuk et al 2011).

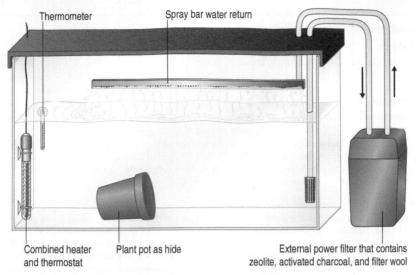

Fig 14-2. Clinical aquarium setup.

Antibiotics can be administered either by:
1. Injection. Optimum site is either immediately in front or behind the dorsal fin in the midline.
2. In feed (but note that many sick fish are inappetant)
3. Bath (may damage biological filtration)
4. Gavage.

Analgesia

Butorphanol at 0.05 to 0.5 mg/kg IM

Anesthesia

There are a number of anesthetic preparations and protocols described, but the author has found MS222 and benzocaine to be the most useful.

Suitable anesthetic agents

1. MS222
   a. This is a benzocaine derivative with a sulfonate radical, giving it water solubility (and increased acidity). It is absorbed and primarily excreted across the gill epithelium. Hypoxia can be a problem.
   b. MS222 can be added directly to water in incremental doses, but fish may show mild signs of distress due to a rapid fall in pH. As a rough guide, sedation is achieved at 20 to 50 mg/L and anesthesia at 50 to 100 mg/L.
   c. To avoid this, dissolve in saturated solution of $NaHCO_3$ to form a buffered stock solution of 10 g/L (10,000 ppm). *Note:* This is unstable in light.
   d. Recovery from short procedures is rapid (<10 minutes), but after lengthy operations it can be prolonged (<6 hours), especially in large fish.
2. Benzocaine
   a. Must be dissolved in ethanol or acetone (stock solution of 100 g/L). Unstable in light. The author finds it less reliable than MS222, possibly due to the effects of solute.

Anesthetic protocol for fish anesthesia

Induction

1. During anesthesia, the water quality should be optimal for that species.
2. There is a risk of hypoxia due to respiratory depression; therefore, aerate/oxygenate the water well.
3. Fish are ectotherms; therefore, higher temperatures speed up induction and recovery, but water at higher temperatures holds less oxygen.
4. Withhold food for one feeding cycle—regurgitation can clog gill rakers and foul water.
5. Handle fish carefully with wet hands to avoid damage to mucous layers.
6. Before induction prepare two supplies of well-oxygenated water of the same suitable water quality—one with anesthetic solution and one without.
7. Induction is either by addition of the anesthetic to the bath with the fish already in situ, or fish is placed into a bath containing the anesthetic solution.

Maintenance

1. Fish can be maintained out of water for prolonged periods of time for surgery providing the gills are constantly bathed in oxygenated water. The simplest method is for an assistant to constantly and gently syringe water into the mouth such that it flows over the gills and out beneath the operculae. Water is selected from either the anesthetic-containing or anesthetic-free container as required.
2. For more advanced anesthetic techniques, the fish can be placed over a water reservoir, with water continuously pumped from this reservoir and introduced into the oral cavity via a tube. The water exiting the operculae flows back into the reservoir below.
3. Anesthesia is usually maintained at a concentration of MS222 of 50 to 100 mg/L.
4. If performing multiple anesthetics, beware build-up of ammonia and proteinaceous material from sloughed mucus.
5. During recovery, water flow over gills should be in physiologically normal direction as reversal short-circuits the normal counter-current gaseous exchange mechanism.

Skin disorders

Skin structure

The skin is a large and complex organ that is constantly in contact with the immediate environment of the fish. Its functions include an osmotic barrier, disease barrier, protection, intraspecies signaling, and camouflage. Histologically it consists of:
1. Cuticle—a thin mucopolysaccharide layer containing mucus, sloughed cells, and antibodies
2. Epidermis—stratified squamous epithelium plus mucus-secreting cells
3. Dermis
   a. Stratum spongiosum—this contains chromatophores
   b. Scales (flat plates of bone) are also present in this layer.
   c. Stratum compactum—this is a dense, collagenous tissue
4. Hypodermis—loosely arranged, often vascular, and may contain adipose tissue; attaches integument to underlying muscle

   Note: The scales of fish are dermal structures (not epidermal thickenings, as seen in reptiles); therefore, the loss of scale involves damage to the overlying epidermis and a potential breach in the fish's immune and osmotic barrier.

Differential diagnoses for skin disorders

Pruritus

- Scratching against surfaces, sometimes termed "flashing" or "flicking"
- Ectoparasites
- Poor water quality

Erosions and ulceration, including fin rot

- Bacterial disease, typically *Aeromonas* spp., *Cytophaga*-like bacteria, *Flavobacterium* spp.; also mycobacteriosis (see *Musculoskeletal Disorders*). With *Cytophaga psychrophila*, infection is often on the dorsal fin spreading toward the base, where a large ulcer forms—this is sometimes referred to as *saddleback disease* (Figs. 14-3 and 14-4).

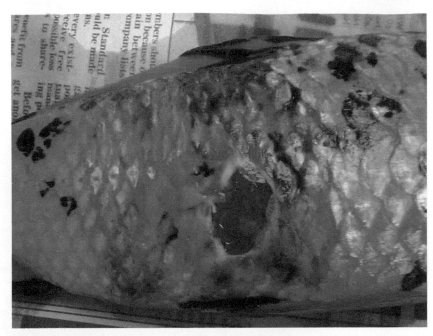

Fig 14-3. Bacterial ulceration in a koi.

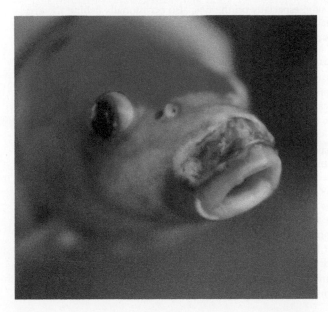

Fig 14-4. Mouth ulceration due to *Flavobacteria*.

- Fungal disease, such as *Fusarium* spp. (see also *Ophthalmic Disorders*)
- Protozoa *(Trichodina, Epistylis)*, *Thelohanellus hovorkai* (Yokohama et al 1999)
- Large ectoparasites (e.g., *Argulus, Learnea*)
- Trauma with secondary bacterial infections—often damage to skin and/or loss of eyes and fins; may occur due to predator attack (e.g., heron, raccoon, cat) or during handling or spawning
- Sunburn will affect only the white or unpigmented areas of the dorsal surface.

Nodules and nonhealing wounds

- Nuptial tubercles (normal in sexually mature goldfish and other cyprinids; usually confined to the operculae and leading rays of the pectoral fins. In some fancy goldfish, those on the fins can be very large and nodular, resembling neoplasia.)
- White spot disease—obvious discrete pinhead white spots *(Ichthyophthirius multifiliis)*; also often breathing difficulties, irritation; fins clamped
- Carp pox (cyprinid herpesvirus 1, CHV-1)—candle-wax masses on skin and fins on cyprinids, especially carp/koi; retarded growth in young koi. *Note:* May cause mass mortalities in young (2-week-old) carp (Sano et al 1991—see *Systemic Disorders*)
- *Dermocystidium koi* (see also *Musculoskeletal Disorders*)
- Lymphocystis (iridovirus)—large, cauliflower-like masses on fins and skin; does not usually infect cyprinids, but may be seen in other pond or coldwater fish, such as sunfish (*Lepomis* spp.)
- Epitheliocystis—looks like lymphocystis, but can infect cyprinids, including carp
- Myxosporidae—obvious nodules; often fish displays dark or accentuating coloring, weight loss, whirling, and fin rot
- *Henneguya koi*—small, smooth rounded cystlike nodules in the skin; can also affect the gills and internal organs
- *Ichthyophonus hoferi*—wasting, darkening of skin color, and obvious boil-like swellings in the skin; in extreme cases it may have a sandpaper effect, due to the large number of granulomas present. Also exophthalmia, abnormal behavior, and abnormal swimming patterns (if the central nervous system is invaded). See also *Neurologic and Swimming Disorders, Ophthalmic Disorders,* and *Systemic Disorders.*
- Gas-filled bubbles in the skin, especially on the fins; also occasionally behind the eye (gas bubble disease—usually secondary to oxygen supersaturation)
- Hypersensitivity reactions at attachment sites of parasites such as *Argulus* and *Lernea*

Changes in pigmentation or color

- Reddened fin and skin. Bacterial infection (see "Erosions and Ulceration" above), golden shiner virus (*Notemigonus crysoleucas* only), spring viremia of carp (SVC; see *Systemic Disorders*), grass carp rheovirus (*Ctenopharygodon idella* only)
- Graying skin secondary to excessive mucus production (ectoparasites, especially *Chilodonella, Trichodina*—Fig. 14-5)
- White tufts on surface, may look like cotton wool (*Epistylis, Saprolegnia, Cytophaga*-like bacteria). In pond fish, fungal infections that have been present for some time may be green or brown due to secondary colonization by algae. *Note:* Mucous strands hanging from the skin can strongly resemble *Saprolegnia.*
- Staff's disease—*Saprolegnia* fungal growths present only in the nostrils; seen in common carp in Poland during the winter months in 1- to 2-year-old carp
- Obvious discrete white spots *(Ichthyophthirius)*. In koi, there is often a "salt and pepper" dusting appearance rather than distinct white spots.
- Dark or accentuating coloring *(Myxosporidae)*
- Dusty effect over body surface (*Oodinium*, velvet disease)
- Gray spots on gills and fins (*Glocchidia*, larval freshwater mussels)

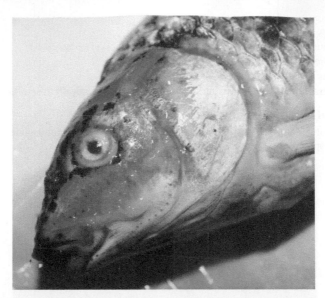

Fig 14-5. Excess mucus on a koi with a *Chilodonella* infestation.

- Whitish mucous tufts on hood (or wen) of fancy goldfish (see also *Ophthalmic Disorders*)
- Color fading—in goldfish and koi it is likely to be a nutritional lack of appropriate carotenoids. Some goldfish on good diets do spontaneously turn white—this is likely to be genetic.
- Occasionally areas of dark pigment develop on the red areas of koi, particularly seen in kohakus. Known to koi keepers as *shimmies,* these are merely changes in pigmentation and do not warrant removal except for aesthetic purposes.

Ectoparasites
- Protozoa
  - *Chilodonella* (see also *Respiratory Tract Disorders*)
  - *Trichodina, Trichodonella,* and *Triparciella* (see also *Respiratory Tract Disorders*)
  - *Ichthyodo necator* (*Costia necatrix*—see also *Respiratory Tract Disorders*)
  - *Epistylis* (*Heteropolaria*)
  - *Ichthyophthirius multifiliis* (white spot—see also *Respiratory Tract Disorders*)
  - *Oodinium* (velvet disease)
  - *Myxosporidea*
    - *Henneguya koi*
    - *Thelohanellus nikolskii*
    - *Thelohanellus hovorkai* (myxosporean—Yokohama et al 1999)
- Helminths
  - *Gyrodactylus* (skin flukes)
  - *Dactylogyrus* (gill flukes—see also *Respiratory Tract Disorders*)
  - Leeches (e.g., *Piscicola geometra*)
- Molluscs
  - *Glocchidia* (larval freshwater mussels—see also *Respiratory Tract Disorders*)
- Crustaceans
  - *Argulus* spp. (fish louse)—large, mobile disc-shaped parasite
  - *Learnea* spp. (anchor worm)—obvious Y-shaped parasites

- Neoplasia
  - Carp pox (CHV-1, see above)
  - Squamous cell carcinoma (possibly triggered by CHV-1—Fig. 14-6)
  - *Erythrophoroma* (especially koi)
  - Fibromas (especially goldfish—Fig. 14-7)
  - Papillomas. *Note:* The lesions induced by CHV-1 histologically resemble papillomas.

Disorders of the fins

- Disorders of the fins largely follow those of the skin and are usually symptomatic of a more widespread dermal problem.

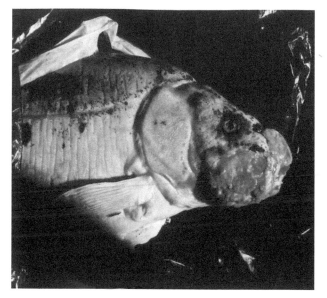

Fig 14-6. Squamous cell carcinoma in a carp.

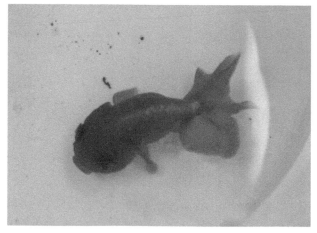

Fig 14-7. Fibroma on a lionhead goldfish.

- Occasionally fins suffer traumatic injury and will split between the rays or even fracture the rays. Often these heal uneventfully. Occasionally suturing may be undertaken to improve the aesthetic result.
- Damaged or diseased distal sections of the fins can be resected, and usually the fin will regenerate over time.

Other findings on clinical examination

- Clamped fins, depression, sudden death (*Chilodonella*, golden shiner virus)
- Skin ulceration, respiratory breathing problems
- Fish usually appear depressed, fins clamped shut, may "wobble" as they swim or even "shimmy," skin appears dull and grayish; ulceration may be seen, respiratory signs (*Ichthyobodo*)
- Breathing difficulties, irritation; fins clamped (*Ichthyophthirius, Oodinium*)
- Dark or accentuating coloring, weight loss, whirling and fin rot (*Myxosporidea*)
- Open skin sores, wasting and protruding eyes, possible spinal curvature (*Mycobacteriosis*)
- Exophthalmia, hemorrhages in grass carp (grass carp rheovirus)
- Gas bubbles behind eye (gas bubble disease)
- Darkened body color, ascites, skin hemorrhages, anal prolapse (SVC)

Investigations

1. Skin scrape and microscopy (Fig. 14-8)
   a. Protozoa
      i. *Trichodina, Trichodonella,* and *Triparciella:* Circular, rotating parasites around 40 μm
      ii. *Ichthyophthirius:* Large ciliate, horseshoe-shaped nucleus
      iii. *Chilodonella:* Large protozoan (30 to 70 μm) that has an almost oval, flattened appearance. Obvious cilia; moves with gliding, slow circular movement
      iv. *Oodinium:* Can be quite large, up to 1.0-mm diameter, oval-shaped with a very dark appearance because of chloroplasts. Not usually mobile

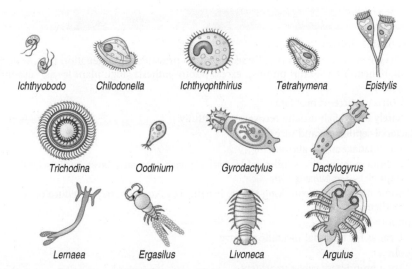

Fig 14-8. Common fish ectoparasites (freshwater—not drawn to scale).

b. Flukes
   i. *Gyrodactylus*: Live-bearing; can usually see large H-shaped hooks of both adult and unborn young
   ii. *Dactylogyrus*: Egg layer. Usually four black spots at caudal end. Can be quite large flukes
2. Radiography
3. Routine hematology and biochemistry
4. Culture and sensitivity
5. Endoscopy
6. Biopsy
   a. Intranuclear inclusions present with CHV-1 infections
   b. Polymerase chain reaction (PCR) for SVC
7. Ultrasonography
8. Postmortem examination
9. Viral isolation for SVC
10. Water quality parameters: Check temperature, ammonia, nitrite, nitrate, and pH values.

Management

1. See under *Nursing Care.*
2. Skin lesions and ulcers
   a. Maintain good water quality.
   b. Clean once with topical iodine.
   c. If large/deep, then cover with barrier substance such as Orabase (Squibb) to reduce further secondary contamination and form a partial osmotic barrier.
3. Antibiotic cover:
   a. Enrofloxacin at 5 mg/kg IM every other day or as a bath at 2.5 mg/L for 5 hours s.i.d.
   b. Marbofloxacin at 5 mg/kg IM every 3 days
4. Alter management to reduce risk of recurrence.

Treatment/specific therapy

- Gas bubble disease
  - Oxygen supersaturation usually secondary to pressurized oxygenation (e.g., waterfalls, malfunctioning Venturi pumps), excess photosynthesis (high plant levels, suspended algae)
  - Correct source of problem.
  - Rarely fatal—fish usually recover uneventfully.
- Bacterial septicemia and ulceration
  - See "Management" above.
  - Debridement of ulcers followed by packing with protective layer, such as Orabase (Squibb)—see *Nursing Care*
  - Some may benefit from long-term salt bath (see *Nursing Care*) to reduce osmotic gradient.
- Sunburn
  - Treat as for bacterial ulceration above.
- *Oodinium*
  - Try a proprietary velvet treatment.
  - Metronidazole bath at 50 mg/L bath for up to 24 hours daily for 10 days

- Quinine hydrochloride added to water at 10 to 20 mg/L tank water indefinitely. Some fish are sensitive to this.
- The encysted stage is relatively resistant to chemical attack.
- Can colonize the intestines of fish, where again it can be protected from medications
- Antibiotic cover should be considered as secondary infections are common at the areas where the skin is damaged.
- Eliminate the parasite from a show aquarium by removing all fish, reducing or cutting out the light levels, and raising the temperature to 30 to 32° C for 3 weeks.
- *Ichthyophthirius multifiliis*—white spot
  - Proprietary white spot remedy
  - Raising water temperature 1 or 2° C speeds up life cycle, promoting the exposure of the chemical-sensitive motile theront stage.
- *Epistylis (Heteropolaria)*
  - Commercial ectoparasitic preparations
- *Chilodonella*
  - Proprietary ectoparasitic medications
  - Glacial acetic acid dips at 8 mL/gallon for 30 to 45 seconds; may kill weak fish
  - *Chilodonella* prefers temperatures of 18 to 22° C, but for *Chilodonella cyprini*, temperatures of 5 to 10° C seem to be close to its optimum.
- *Trichodina, Trichodonella,* and *Triparciella*
  - Proprietary ectoparasitic medication
- *Ichthyobodo*
  - Standard proprietary antiprotozoan treatments
  - Remove all of the fish from the infected aquarium or pond for 24 to 48 hours as the parasite can only survive without a host for a few hours.
  - *Ichthyobodo* is able to survive temperatures down to 2° C and can cause mortality in overwintering carp.
- *Henneguya koi* and *Thelohanellus* spp.
  - No effective treatment
  - Common carp are more susceptible to *Thelohanellus nikolsii* than koi or goldfish (Molnar 2002).
  - *T. hovorkai* requires an intermediate oligochaete host.
  - Feeding a diet of 0.1% fumagillin prevented mortality in *Thelohanellus*-infected koi (Yokohama et al 1999).
- Flukes (skin, gill)
  - Proprietary ectoparasitic preparations
  - Praziquantel at 10 mg/kg body weight PO; as a 1- to 2-hour bath at 15 to 20 mg/L. With larger fish, in-feed medication at a rate of 400 mg/100 g food daily for 7 days
  - Dactylogyrids are egg layers; the egg stage is resistant to treatment and so infestations require multiple treatments up to 4 weeks apart depending on water temperature.
- *Glocchidia* (larval freshwater mussels): Usually self-limiting. Larvae only transiently parasitic
  - Whitish tufts on hood. This is normal and may be linked to normal hood growth. No treatment needed
- Grass carp rheovirus
  - No treatment. Symptomatic treatment only
- Golden shiner virus
  - No treatment. Symptomatic treatment only
- SVC
  - No treatment. Symptomatic treatment only

- Leeches
  - Remove individual parasites.
  - Treat with organophosphates (where legal to do so).
- *Learnea* (anchor worm)
  - Remove individual parasites.
  - Treat with lufenuron (Program, Novartis) at 0.088 mg/L as a once-only treatment.
  - Treat with organophosphates (where legal to do so).
- *Argulus* (fish louse)
  - Remove individual parasites.
  - Treat with lufenuron (Program, Novartis) at 0.088 mg/L as a once-only treatment.
  - Treat with organophosphates (where legal to do so).
  - A potassium permanganate bath at 10 ppm (mg/L) for 5 to 60 minutes can be used to rid both individual fish and plants of this parasite.
- *Dermocystidium koi*
  - Surgical removal
  - Consider itraconazole at 1.0 to 5.0 mg/kg PO every 1 to 7 days, either in feed or gavage.
- *Saprolegnia* (fungal disease)
  - Proprietary medications containing malachite green
  - Remove visible hyphae and swab the affected area with a 10% povidone-iodine solution once daily.
  - Maintain the fish in a salt solution as this will not only help to control the fungal infection but will also help with the osmotic imbalance resulting from the infection. Even salt solutions as low as 10 parts per thousand (mg/100 mL) will inhibit *Saprolegnia* infections. Ideally aim for 1 to 3 g/L as a permanent solution until the problem has resolved.
- Carp pox (CHV-1)
  - No treatment. Will usually clear up in warmer water, but recrudescence common
- Lymphocystis
  - No direct cure. Usually self-limiting
  - Ozone or ultraviolet sterilization may reduce spread.
  - Attempted surgical removal is usually followed by recurrence.
- Epitheliocystis
  - *Chlamydophila*-like organism
  - Some antibiotics (e.g., chloramphenicol) recorded as effective
- SVC—see *Systemic Disorders*
- Neoplasia
  - Chemotherapy in fish is in its infancy.
  - Surgical removal followed by treatment of surgical wound as described under "Management" above
  - Surgical debulking followed by injection of cisplatin directly into the tissue mass on a weekly basis

Respiratory tract disorders

Viral

- Koi herpesvirus (KHV; cyprinid herpesvirus 3, CHV-3)
- Gill necrosis virus

Bacterial
- Bacterial (environmental) gill disease

Fungal
- Branchiomycosis

Protozoal
- White spot *(Ichthyophthirius)*
- *Chilodonella* (see also *Skin Disorders*)
- *Ichthyobodo (Costia) necatrix*
- Oodinium (velvet disease) (see also *Skin Disorders*)
- *Trichodina, Trichodonella,* and *Triparciella* (see also *Skin Disorders*)
- *Henneguya koi* (see also *Skin Disorders*)
- *Myxosoma dujardini*

Parasitic
- *Dactylogyrus* spp. (gill flukes)
- *Glocchidia* (larval freshwater mussels)
- *Ergasilus* (gill maggot—large crustacean parasite)

Neoplasia
- Gill neoplasia

Other noninfectious problems
- Hypoxia (high stocking levels, high temperatures, low atmospheric pressure)
- Poor water quality; can cause gill damage that predisposes to bacterial gill disease
- Ammonia toxicity (see also *Neurologic and Swimming Disorders*)
- Nitrite toxicity
- Malachite green toxicity
- Stress

Findings on clinical examination

- Moderate to extreme respiratory effort
- Rapid gill ventilation
- Apparent gasping at water surface
- Hemorrhage from the gills in koi following handling (stress)
- Gray spots on gills and fins (*Glocchidia*, larval freshwater mussels)
- Mottled colored gills, necrotic gills, or patches on gills; weak, lethargic (branchiomycosis; severe bacterial gill disease; in carp, koi—KHV, gill necrosis virus; Fig. 14-9)
- Mass deaths in koi only; goldfish, rudd, orfe, etc., unaffected (KHV)
- Extensive gill damage and hemorrhage (*Sanguinicola inermis*)
- Damaged gills, obvious large parasites (*Ergasilus*)
- Excess mucus production, clamped fins, depression, sudden death (*Chilodonella, Ichthyobodo*)
- Clamped fins; scratching and flashing; inactivity (gill flukes)
- Thickened gills, mucus trailing from gills (bacterial gill disease)
- Dusty effect over body surface (*Oodinium*—velvet disease)
- Cystic nodules on the gills (*Myxosoma dujardini, Henneguya koi*)

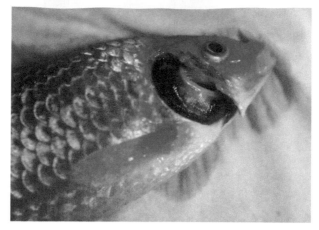

Fig 14-9. Gill lesions of koi herpesvirus.

- Permissive temperature range for KHV (18 to 25° C)
- Brown discoloration of gills (nitrite toxicity—methemoglobin formation)

Investigations

1. Water quality tests, especially ammonia, nitrite, nitrate, pH, temperature
2. Check dissolved oxygen levels.
3. Gill scrape ("wet" prep under light microscope)
4. Radiography
5. Routine hematology and biochemistry
6. Culture and sensitivity
7. PCR for KHV
8. Endoscopy
9. Biopsy
   a. Gill and other organs: Typical intranuclear inclusions for KHV. *Note:* Also seen with carp pox (CHV-1)
10. Ultrasonography
11. Water quality parameters: Check temperature, ammonia, nitrite, nitrate, and pH values.

Management

1. See *Nursing Care.*
2. Improve water quality.
3. Vigorous aeration

Treatment/specific therapy

- Ammonia toxicity
  - Partial water changes to dilute the ammonia levels
  - Adding zeolite will absorb large quantities of ammonia.
  - Longer-term control may include addition of commercially available *Nitrosomonas* bacterial cultures or equivalent.

- Nitrite toxicity
  - Adding salt to the water to a concentration of 0.3%, the equivalent of 3.0 kg/1000 L, can be beneficial (chloride ions compete with the absorption of nitrite ions).
  - Partial water changes
  - Addition of extra-bacterial (Nitrobacter) cultures in the form of commercially available freeze-dried or suspended cultures may be of some benefit.
  - Dietary vitamin C may have a protective function, although its effect is less than that of salt.
- Malachite green toxicity
  - Improved management only
  - Malachite green binds irreversibly to respiratory enzymes, so increased aeration may not be beneficial.
- Hypoxia
  - Increase water turnover by use of pumps and airstones to maximize gaseous exchange at the surface.
  - Reduce stocking density.
  - Pump liquid oxygen into water.
- Gill necrosis virus: No treatment
- KHV
  - No treatment
  - Reducing temperatures to below the permissive range may halt mortalities.
  - Koi can be "vaccinated" by exposing them to the virus at 23° C for 3 to 5 days and then transferring these fish to water held at the nonpermissive temperature of 30° C. Such koi usually have high levels of KHV-specific antibodies.
  - KHV is notifiable in the UK and reportable in USA, Canada and Australia.
- Bacterial gill disease
  - Correct any underlying environmental problem.
  - Chloramine-T at 10 mg/L in pond/aquarium—use less in soft water, down to 2 mg/L
  - Appropriate antibiosis
- Branchiomycosis
  - No known effective antifungals
  - Consider itraconazole at 1.0 to 5.0 mg/kg PO every 1 to 7 days, either in feed or gavage.
- Chilodonella
  - Proprietary ectoparasitic medications
  - Glacial acetic acid dips at 8 mL per gallon for 30 to 45 seconds; may kill weak fish
  - Chilodonella prefers temperatures of 18 to 22° C, but for Chilodonella cyprini, temperatures of 5 to 10° C seem to be close to optimum.
- Ichthyobodo necator (Costia necatrix)
  - Usual ectoparasitic treatments
  - Remove all of the fish from the infected aquarium for 24 to 48 hours, as the parasite can only survive outside the host for a few hours.
  - Ichthyobodo is able to survive temperatures down to 2° C and can cause mortalities in overwintering carp.
- Oodinium (velvet disease)
  - Proprietary velvet treatment
  - Metronidazole bath at 50 mg/L bath for up to 24 hours daily for 10 days
  - Quinine hydrochloride added to water at 10 to 20 mg/L pond/aquarium indefinitely; some fish are sensitive to this
  - The encysted stage is relatively resistant to chemical attack.
  - Can colonize the intestines of fish, where again it can be protected from medications

- Antibiotic cover should be considered as secondary infections are common at the areas where the skin is damaged.
- Eliminate the parasite from a show aquarium by removing all fish, reducing or cutting out the light levels. and raising the temperature to 30 to 32° C for 3 weeks.
- *Ichthyophthirius multifiliis*—white spot
  - Proprietary white spot remedy
  - Raising water temperature 1 or 2° C speeds up life cycle, promoting the exposure of the chemical-sensitive motile theront stage.
- *Trichodina, Trichodonella,* and *Triparciella*
  - Proprietary ectoparasitic medication
- *Myxosoma dujardini* and *Henneguya koi*
  - No effective treatment
- *Glocchidia* (larval freshwater mussels)—usually self-limiting. Larvae only transiently parasitic
- Flukes (skin, gill)
  - Proprietary ectoparasitic preparations
  - Praziquantel at 10 mg/kg PO or at 10 mg/L for a 3-hour bath
  - *Dactylogyrus* spp. are egg layers; the egg stage is resistant to treatment, so praziquantel should be repeated every 2 to 4 weeks depending on temperature, for at least 3 doses.
- *Sanguinicola*
  - Praziquantel at 10 mg/kg PO in food
  - Control of snail intermediate hosts where possible
- *Ergasilus*
  - Individual removal of parasites
  - Organophosphates (where legal to do so)
  - Ivermectin at 0.1 to 0.2 mg/kg IM. May be toxic to goldfish; may be persistent in environment
  - Treat with lufenuron (Program, Novartis) at 0.088 mg/L as a once-only treatment.

Gastrointestinal tract disorders

Protozoal

- *Eimeria* spp., esp. *E. carpelli* and *E. subepithelialis* (young carp and koi)

Parasitic

- Nematodes
  - *Camallanus* spp.
  - *Raphidascaris acus* (Dezfuli et al 2000)
- Helminths
  - *Bothriocephalus* spp.
  - *Khawia* spp.

Nutritional

- Constipation/diarrhea (especially fancy goldfish—see also *Nutritional Disorders*)

Neoplasia

- Buccopharyngeal neoplasia
- Gill neoplasia
- Intestinal adenocarcinoma

Other noninfectious disorders

- Foreign body (e.g., piece of gravel), especially goldfish

- Emaciation, sunken eyes
- Diarrhea
- Anorexia
- Long trails of feces; may contain gas bubbles. Loss of balance (constipation/diarrhea)
- Weight loss; big head in carp. Swollen abdomen. May cause mass mortalities in young koi (tapeworms)
- Obvious red worms protruding from anus, especially with live-bearers. Ulceration around anus may be apparent. Weight loss *(Camallanus)*
- Dysphagia (buccopharyngeal neoplasia, pharyngeal foreign body)
- Swimming with mouth permanently open (pharyngeal foreign body)

1. Light microscopy
2. Fecal sample
   a. Flotation
3. Radiography
4. Routine hematology and biochemistry
5. Culture and sensitivity
6. Endoscopy
7. Biopsy/necropsy
   a. Larvae of *Raphidascaris acus* (European minnow *Phoxinus phoxinus*)
8. Ultrasonography
9. Water quality parameters: Check temperature, ammonia, nitrite, nitrate, and pH values.

- *Eimeria* spp.
  - May respond to anticoccidial drugs such as amprolium as a continuous bath at 10 mg/L for 7 to 10 days or to sulfonamide antibiotics
- Constipation/diarrhea
  - Feed higher fiber foods, such as shelled peas, live or frozen invertebrates (e.g., *Daphnia* or bloodworm, *Chironomus* larvae).
- Nematodes
  - Levamisole bath at 2 mg/L for up to 24 hours
  - Fenbendazole at 20 mg/kg body weight given 7 days apart
  - Mebendazole at 20 mg/kg for 3 treatments given at weekly intervals
  - *Camallanus* has both a direct and indirect life cycle (small crustaceans such as *Cyclops* act as intermediate hosts).
- Tapeworms
  - Praziquantel at 10 mg/kg mixed in food once only
  - Control of intermediates
    - *Bothriocephalus:* Intermediate stages in copepods
    - *Khawia:* Intermediate stages in tubulicid worms

- Neoplasia
  - Usually inoperable by the time it is identified
  - Accessible tumors may be managed by injecting cisplatin directly into the tissue mass on a weekly basis as a debulking exercise.

Nutritional disorders

- Hypovitaminosis E (sekoke disease—carp/koi)
  - Wasting when fed on vitamin E–deficient diet—classically a diet of silkworm larvae only
  - Supplement with vitamin E or feed a commercially complete diet.
- Hypovitaminosis C
  - Poor immune function; spinal deformities, possibly secondary to effects of collagen and cartilage integrity
- Hepatic lipidosis
  - Too high a protein and carbohydrate diet; often fed to achieve maximum growth rates in koi
  - Switch to lower energy foods and supplement with vitamin E.
- Constipation/diarrhea
  - Difficult in practice to distinguish between the two
  - Typically a problem with fancy goldfish characterized by long trails of feces
  - Gas bubbles may be present in the feces; in the gut these may cause a loss of balance, mimicking swimbladder disease.
  - Feed higher fiber foods, such as shelled peas, live or frozen invertebrates (e.g., *Daphnia* or bloodworm—*Chironomus* larvae).

Hepatic disorders

Protozoal

- *Chloromyxum cyprini* and *C. koi*

Nutritional

- Hepatic lipidosis (see *Nutritional Disorders*)

Neoplasia

- Hepatocellular tumors

Findings on clinical examination

- Vague signs of ill health
- Unexpected mortalities in "healthy" fish
- Large females particularly susceptible (hepatic lipidosis)
- Incidental finding of protozoa in gallbladder (*Chloromyxum* spp.)

Investigations

1. Radiography
2. Routine hematology and biochemistry
3. Culture and sensitivity

4. Endoscopy
5. Biopsy
6. Ultrasonography
7. Water quality parameters: Check temperature, ammonia, nitrite, nitrate, and pH values.

Treatment/specific therapy

- Hepatic neoplasia
  - Usually no viable treatment; often sizable by the time of diagnosis
- *Chloromyxum* spp.
  - Usually incidental finding. No effective treatment

Pancreatic disorders

Parasitic
- Nematodes

Neoplasia

Findings on clinical examination

- Vague signs of ill health
- May be incidental finding

Investigations

1. Radiography
2. Routine hematology and biochemistry
3. Culture and sensitivity
4. Endoscopy
5. Biopsy
6. Ultrasonography
7. Water quality parameters: Check temperature, ammonia, nitrite, nitrate, and pH values.

Treatment/specific therapy

- Nematodes (see *Gastrointestinal Tract Disorders*)

Cardiovascular and hematologic disorders

Bacterial
- Endocarditis

Protozoal
- Hemoparasites (see *Systemic Disorders*)
- *Trypanoplasma borreli* (see also *Urinary Disorders*)
- *Trypanosoma carassii*
- *Trypanosoma danilewskyi*

Parasitic

- *Sanguinicola inermis* (see *Respiratory Tract Disorders*)

Neoplasia

Other noninfectious problems

- Cardiomyopathy

Findings on clinical examination

- Apparent respiratory disease secondary to anemia (see also *Respiratory Tract Disorders*)
- Ascites, bloated abdomen
- Exophthalmos (see also *Ophthalmic Disorders*)

Investigations

1. Radiography
2. Routine hematology and biochemistry
   a. Cytology: Stained blood smears for hemoparasites
3. Culture and sensitivity
4. Endoscopy
5. Biopsy/necropsy
6. Ultrasonography
7. Water quality parameters: Check temperature, ammonia, nitrite, nitrate, and pH values.

Management

- See *Nursing Care.*
- Keeping fish in a permanent 5-g/L solution of salt (not table or rock salt) will reduce the osmotic load on a sick koi or goldfish.

Treatment/specific therapy

- Vegetative endocarditis
  - Antibiotics
  - Guarded prognosis
- Hemoparasites
  - Methylene blue at 60 mg/kg leave as is per day PO for 4 days
  - Metronidazole at 50 mg/kg PO per day
  - *Note:* The leech *Piscicola geometra* acts as a vector for *Trypanosoma danilewskyi.*

Systemic disorders

Viral

- SVC (rhabdovirus)
- Lymphocystis *(iridovirus)*—usually forms masses on skin but rarely occurs in coelom (see *Skin Disorders*)
- CHV-1 (in carp fry <8 weeks old—see also *Skin Disorders*)
- Cyprinid herpesvirus 2 (CHV-2), also known as infectious hematopoetic necrosis (IHN) virus or goldfish herpesvirus (GHV)

Bacterial

- Mycobacteriosis (see *Musculoskeletal Disorders*)
- Septicemia
- Typically *Aeromonas* spp., *Pseudomonas* spp., *Flavibacterium* spp.; rarely *Vibrio cholerae*

Fungal

- *Ichthyophonus hoferi* (see also *Neurologic and Swimming Disorders, Ophthalmic Disorders, and Skin Disorders*)

Protozoal

- Hemoparasites
- *Trypanosoma* spp.
- *Trypanoplasma borreli* (Bunnajirakul et al 2000)
- *Hoferellus carassii* (goldfish only—see *Urinary Disorders*)

Nutritional

- Vitamin E deficiency (sekoke disease)

Neoplasia

- Gonadal neoplasia (see *Reproductive Disorders*)
- Liver neoplasia
- Renal neoplasia, polycystic kidney disease (see *Urinary Disorders*)
- Oral/pharyngeal neoplasia (fish unable to feed)

Other noninfectious problems

- Polycystic renal disease (goldfish—see *Urinary Disorders*)
- Metabolic acidosis/delayed capture mortality

Findings on clinical examination

- Lethargy
- Wasting (mycobacteriosis, hemoparasites, neoplasia—especially oral, hypovitaminosis E); see also *Gastrointestinal Tract Disorders*
- Wasting, darkening of skin color, and obvious boil-like swellings in the skin; also exophthalmia, abnormal behavior, and abnormal swimming patterns *(Ichthyophonus hoferi)*
- Swollen abdomen
  - Hemorrhages, mucoid fecal casts from rectum, lethargy. Seen in carp, koi, goldfish, grass carp, tench, and occasionally pike *(Esox)* and Wels catfish *(Siluris glanis)*. Differentiate from non-SVC ascites (SVC).
  - Scales protruding, hemorrhages (ascites, known to aquarists as *dropsy*). Usually secondary to multiorgan failure, especially heart, gill, and kidney disease
  - Goldfish only—scales not protruding (*Hoferellus carassii*, polycystic renal disease)
  - Nonsymmetrical swelling, ulceration, loss of balance (internal neoplasia)
  - Exophthalmos, swimming disorders ("sleeping sickness") in carp *(T. borreli)*
- Mass mortalities in young (<8 weeks old) carp fry. Typically show swimming abnormalities, hemorrhages, swollen abdomen (CHV-1—Sano et al 1991)
- Listlessness in goldfish, anemia (pale gills), some gill necrosis, loss of skin mucus, mass mortalities in goldfish (CHV-2)

- Following a difficult capture, fish may exhibit incoordination, weakness, poor vision, and mortalities (often several days later—metabolic acidosis; see Jepson 2001)
- Tumors

Investigations

1. Radiography
2. Routine hematology and biochemistry
   a. Cytology/blood smears (hemoparasites)
   b. Anemia (hemoparasites, CHV-2)
3. Culture and sensitivity
4. PCR test for SVC (notifiable in UK, reportable in United States, Canada, and Australia)
5. Virus isolation for SVC
6. Endoscopy
7. Biopsy
8. Ultrasonography
9. Water quality parameters: Check temperature, ammonia, nitrite, nitrate, and pH values.

Treatment/specific therapy

- Bacterial disease
  - Appropriate antibiosis
- Hemoparasites
  - Methylene blue at 60 mg/kg per day PO for 4 days
  - Metronidazole at 50 mg/kg PO per day
- SVC: No effective treatment
- Neoplasia
  - Surgery or euthanasia
- Ascites
  - Poor prognosis
  - Often involves multiorgan failure
  - Attempt to correct osmotic imbalance by keeping in either salt solution (0.55%) or magnesium sulfate solution.
  - Often bacterial in origin, so consider antibiotics
- Lymphocystis
  - No treatment—usually self-limiting but may cause significant problems internally
- *Ichthyophonus hoferi*
  - No efficacious treatment available
- CHV-1
  - No efficacious treatment available
- CHV-2
  - Triggered by stress and more common in temperatures in low 20s° C. In United States more common in spring and fall when temperatures are suitable
  - No treatment, but losses can be reduced by transferring out of permissive temperature range (e.g., 26 to 30° C)
- Metabolic acidosis
  - Difficult to treat; best avoided by patient, low-stress capture techniques involving two nets (use one net to guide the fish toward the other)

Musculoskeletal disorders

Bacterial

- Mycobacteriosis (fish tuberculosis), primarily *Mycobacterium marinum, M. fortuitum, M. cheloni,* occasionally other *Mycobacterium* spp. implicated

Fungal

- *Dermocystidium koi*

Nutritional

- Hypovitaminosis C (see *Nutritional Disorders*)
- Tryptophan deficiency
- Sekoke disease (see *Nutritional Disorders*)

Neoplasia

Other noninfectious problems

- Electrocution (see *Neurologic and Swimming Disorders*)
- Organophosphate exposure
- Trauma

Findings on clinical examination

- Spinal curvature/scoliosis (mycobacteriosis, electrocution, trauma, hypovitaminosis C, tryptophan deficiency, organophosphates)
- Open skin sores, wasting, and protruding eyes with or without spinal curvature (mycobacteriosis)
- Cysts in skin and muscles *(Dermocystidium)*

Investigations

1. Radiography
2. Routine hematology and biochemistry
3. Culture and sensitivity
4. Endoscopy
5. Biopsy
6. Ultrasonography
7. Water quality parameters: Check temperature, ammonia, nitrite, nitrate, and pH values.

Treatment/specific therapy

- Mycobacteriosis
  - Antibiotic treatment often not very effective
  - Kanamycin bath at 50 mg/L every 48 hours for four treatments was successful in guppies (Conroy and Conroy 1999)
  - Consider euthanasia, especially because of zoonotic risk.
- *Dermocystidium koi*
  - See *Skin Disorders*.
- Spinal curvature/scoliosis
  - Treatment difficult. Surgical internal fixation to stabilize condition has been attempted (Govett et al 2004).

- Tryptophan deficiency
  - Supplement with tryptophan.

Neurologic and swimming disorders

Viral

- SVC (swimbladder inflammation—see *Systemic Disorders*)

Bacterial

- CNS infection/granuloma

Fungal

- *Ichthyophonus hoferi*
- CNS infection/granuloma

Protozoal

- Myxosporidea (see also *Skin Disorders*)
- *Myxosoma encephalina*
- *Sphaerospora renicola*

Neoplasia

- Internal neoplasia compressing swimbladder

Other noninfectious problems

- Electrocution/lightning strike—sudden-onset spinal deformities, sudden death, especially in pond fish (Pasnik et al 2003)
- Whirling and erratic swimming, dark or accentuating coloring, weight loss, and fin rot; there may be obvious nodules *(Myxosporidea)*
- Poor water quality, especially high ammonia and/or nitrite levels—new tank/pond syndrome
- Sudden-onset poisoning, such as from zinc (galvanized buckets, etc.), pesticides
- Swimbladder dysfunction, a particular problem with fancy goldfish. Often due to anatomical malformation of swimbladder in fancy breeds of goldfish but can be due to infection (bacterial, fungal) or compression from surrounding organs (e.g., gonadal neoplasia)
- Abnormal swimbladder functioning secondary to compression from internal space-occupying lesions (e.g., neoplasia)
- Swimbladder torsion
- Hypothermia (koi)

Findings on clinical examination

- Sudden darting movements, loss of balance, rapid respiration (water quality, poisoning)
- Loss of balance—unable to swim down from surface or up from bottom (swimbladder dysfunction, enteritis, SVC)
- Fish, especially koi, may need to permanently swim in order to maintain position in water column; may regularly gulp at surface as attempts to inflate swimbladder via pneumatic duct (swimbladder disease/compression)
- Koi lying on side at bottom, sluggish movements, water temperature close to freezing (hypothermia)
- Swimbladder signs but in carp fry *(Sphaerospora)*

- Wasting, darkening of skin color, and obvious boil-like swellings in the skin; also exophthalmia, abnormal behavior, and abnormal swimming patterns *(Ichthyophonus)*
- Abnormal swimming posture, whirling *(Myxosporidea, Myxosoma encephalina)*

Investigations

1. Water quality tests
2. Radiography for swimbladder disease (Figs. 14 10 to 14-12)
3. Routine hematology and biochemistry
4. Culture and sensitivity
5. PCR test for SVC (notifiable in UK, reportable in United States, Canada, and Australia)
6. Virus isolation for SVC
7. Endoscopy
8. Biopsy
9. Ultrasonography
10. Water quality parameters: Check temperature, ammonia, nitrite, nitrate, and pH values.

Management

- Maintain optimum water conditions.

Treatment/specific therapy

- Poor water quality
  - Address which parameter(s) are abnormal. Multiple partial water changes often beneficial in short term. Many need to review stocking, filtration system, or husbandry management.

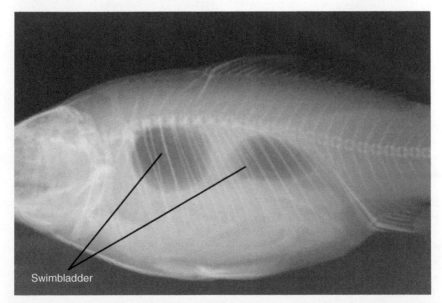

Swimbladder

Fig 14-10. Comparative radiograph of a normal goldfish showing relative size and position of the cranial and caudal sections of the swimbladder (labeled).

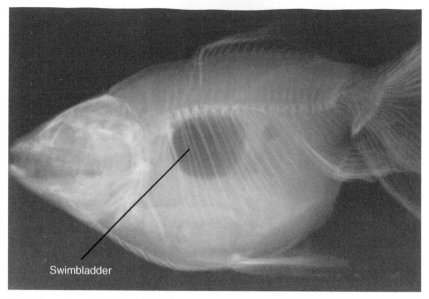

Swimbladder

Fig 14-11. Same view of a fantail goldfish showing poor inflation of the caudal portion of the swimbladder.

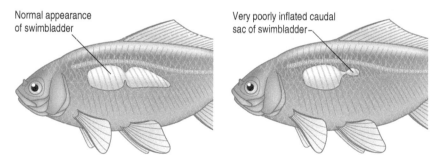

Normal appearance of swimbladder

Very poorly inflated caudal sac of swimbladder

Fig 14-12. Diagrammatic explanation of Figures 14-10 and 14-11.

- Ammonia toxicity
  - Partial water changes to dilute the ammonia levels
  - Adding zeolite will absorb large quantities of ammonia.
  - Longer term control may include addition of commercially available *Nitrosomonas* bacterial cultures or equivalent.
- Swimbladder disease
  - Usually no effective treatment for fancy goldfish. May develop ulceration on areas persistently floating above water level
  - Pneumocystocentesis can provide temporary relief, but the problem is likely to recur.
  - Try antibiotics if suspect bacterial infection
  - If goldfish is floating can implant small sterile counterweight into ventral coelomic cavity, but is difficult to judge correct weight
  - Pneumocystoplasty has been attempted (Britt et al 2002) and with refinement could prove useful.

- Enteritis may trigger gas formation in the gut, mimicking swimbladder dysfunction. Offer high-fiber feeds such as live or frozen bloodworm or *Daphnia.*
  - Surgical removal of internal neoplasia
- SVC (see *Systemic Disorders*)
- Swimbladder torsion
  - Surgical correction
- Hypothermia
  - Usually seen in larger koi kept in ponds that are too shallow and where the temperature falls close to freezing. Typically these koi were introduced as small specimens but have since grown. For large koi the pond should be at least 120 cm deep.
  - Where possible, remove koi to warmer water or more suitable accommodation.
  - Will usually self-correct as conditions improve but may predispose to further swimbladder complications
- *Sphaeropsora renicola*
  - Fumigillin at 1 g/kg food for 10 to 14 days for prevention
- Myxosporidea/*Myxosoma encephalina*
  - No effective treatment. Try fumigilin as above.
- *Ichthyophonus hoferi*
  - No efficacious treatment available
- CNS infection/granuloma
  - Attempt antibiotic or antimycotic treatment. Poor prognosis
- Electric shock
  - Supportive treatment

Ophthalmic disorders

Viral

- Grass carp rheovirus (grass carp *Ctenopharyngodon idella*—see *Skin Disorders*)

Bacterial

- Mycobacteriosis (see also *Musculoskeletal Disorders* and *Skin Disorders*)
- Retrobulbar granuloma
- Bacterial keratitis (often *Cytophaga*-like bacteria).

Fungal

- *Fusarium* spp. (see also *Skin Disorders*)
- *Ichthyophonus hoferi* (see also *Neurologic and Swimming Disorders*, *Skin Disorders*, and *Systemic Disorders*)
- Retrobulbar granuloma

Protozoal

- *Ichthyophthirius*

Parasitic

- *Diplostomum* (intermediate stage of avian tapeworm)

Nutritional

- Riboflavin deficiency
- Ascorbic acid deficiency
- Hypovitaminosis A

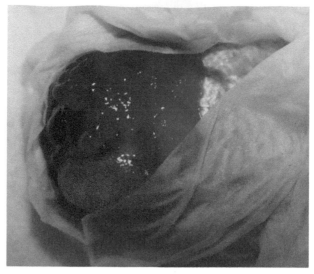

Fig 14-13. Overgrowth of the eye by the hood of an oranda goldfish.

Neoplasia
- Retrobulbar neoplasm

Other noninfectious problems
- Overgrowth of the eye by the hood in certain breeds of fancy goldfish, such as lionheads and orandas (Fig. 14-13)
- Gas bubble disease (see *Skin Disorders*)
- Cataracts
- *Erythrophoroma*
- Cardiomyopathy

Findings on clinical examination

- Exophthalmia (grass carp rheovirus, SVC, retrobulbar mass, cardiomyopathy)
- Opacity of the cornea—keratitis
- Opacity of lens in eye
- Corneal ulceration
- Blindness. Fish may be able to compensate to some extent by use of lateral line.
- Exophthalmia accompanied by wasting, darkening of skin color, and obvious boil-like swellings in the skin, abnormal behavior, and abnormal swimming patterns (*Ichthyophonus hoferi*)
- Gas bubbles around and behind eye (gas bubble disease)
- Glaucoma (usually secondary to intraocular disease)
- Overgrowth of both eyes by exuberant growth of the hood in fancy goldfish

Investigations

1. Ophthalmic examination
2. Radiography

3. Routine hematology and biochemistry
4. Culture and sensitivity
5. PCR test for SVC (notifiable in UK, reportable in United States, Canada, and Australia)
6. Virus isolation for SVC
7. Endoscopy
8. Biopsy
9. Ocular ultrasonography
10. Water quality parameters: Check temperature, ammonia, nitrite, nitrate, and pH values.

Treatment/specific therapy

- *Ichthyophonus hoferi*
  - No efficacious treatment available.
- *Diplostomum*
  - No effective treatment
  - Consider praziquantel at 10 mg/kg body weight PO; as a 1- to 2-hour bath at 15 to 20 mg/L. With larger fish, in-feed medication at a rate of 400 mg/100 g food daily for 7 days. This should eliminate the cestode, but there is unlikely to be any resolution of ocular damage.
  - Attempt to break life cycle by:
    - Control of aquatic snails as source of disease
    - Preventing predation by birds (primary hosts)
- Glaucoma
  - Enucleation
- Cataracts
  - Aging change; occasionally can be due to nutritional deficiencies (e.g., riboflavin deficiency or parasitism), but these are rare.
  - In globe-eyed goldfish is very common
- Corneal ulceration
  - Systemic antibiosis
  - Scarification and application of tissue glue can protect the cornea and aid reepithelialization.
- *Erythrophoroma*
  - If partially or completely covering the cornea, then a superficial keratectomy may be necessary. Treat subsequently as for corneal ulceration.
- Overgrowth of hood
  - Resect part of hood covering eye under general anesthesia.

Urinary disorders

Bacterial

- Nephritis

Protozoal

- *Hoferellus carassii* (goldfish)
- *Hoferellus cyprini* (carp)
- *Trypanoplasma borreli*—see *Cardiovascular and Hematologic Disorders* (Meyer et al 2002)

Neoplasia

Other noninfectious problems

- Polycystic renal disease (goldfish)

Findings on clinical examination

- Lethargy
- Ascites
- Swollen abdomen in goldfish, loss of balance, scales not protruding (*Hoferellus carassii*, polycystic renal disease); differentiate from ascites—see *Systemic Disorders*
- Carp cease feeding, are "off color," deaths after 7 to 14 days *(H. cyprini)*
- Abdominal distension, exophthalmus, swimming disorders ("sleeping sickness"— *T. borreli*)

Investigations

1. Radiography
2. Routine hematology and biochemistry
3. Culture and sensitivity
4. Endoscopy
5. Biopsy/necropsy
   a. Progressive nephritis *(T. borreli)*
   b. Dilated renal tubules and collecting ducts; trophozoites or spores visible *(H. carassii)*
   c. Trophozoites or spores visible *(H. cyprini)*
6. Ultrasonography
7. Water quality parameters: Check temperature, ammonia, nitrite, nitrate, and pH values.

Treatment/specific therapy

- Polycystic renal disease
  - Genetic disorder—autosomal recessive. No treatment
- *Hoferellus* spp.
  - No reliable treatment
  - Try toltrazuril at 30 mg/L as a 60-minute bath every other day for 3 treatments.
  - Intermediate stages found in tubulicid worms.
- *Trypanoplasma*—see *Cardiovascular and Hematologic Disorder.*

Reproductive disorders

Neoplasia

- Ovarian neoplasia
- Testicular neoplasia

Other noninfectious problems

- Egg retention

Findings on clinical examination

- Pronounced swelling of the coelomic cavity; may be asymmetrical (gonadal neoplasia) or symmetrical (egg retention)
- Other differentials for a symmetrical swollen coelom
  - Scales not prominent (in goldfish consider also *Hoferellus*, polycystic kidney disease—see *Urinary Disorders*)
  - Scales prominent—ascites (see *Systemic Disorders*)

Investigations

1. Radiography
2. Routine hematology and biochemistry
3. Culture and sensitivity
4. Endoscopy
5. Biopsy
6. Ultrasonography
7. Water quality parameters: Check temperature, ammonia, nitrite, nitrate, and pH values.

Treatment/specific therapy

- Gonadal neoplasia
  - Surgical resection
- Egg retention

Treatment of egg retention

Goldfish

1. Buserelin at a 1:10 dilution applied to the gills or 10 μg/kg IM
2. hCG at 700 to 1000 IU/kg IM
3. In both cases, followed by manual stripping 6 to 12 hours later

Koi

1. In general koi will only respond to injections of carp pituitary extract.
2. Maintain temperature around 25°C.
3. Priming dose of 0.3 mg/kg of reconstituted carp pituitary extract
4. Second dose of 3.0 mg/kg 12 to 18 hours later
5. Attempt manual stripping 6 to 12 hours later.
6. Cool temperatures (<20°C) and/or lack of sufficient or large enough sexually active males contribute to the etiology of this condition.
7. Koi may, however, respond to GnRH analogues in combination with dopamine antagonists (e.g., domperidone or metoclopramide—Patino 1997).

CHAPTER

15

Tropical freshwater fish

Around 80% to 90% of tropical freshwater fish are captive bred, with typical hot spots of production being Singapore (e.g., Fig. 15-1), Malaysia, Israel, Florida, and the Czech and Slovak Republics. Some important fish to the industry, such as the cardinal tetra *(Parachei-rodon axelrodi)* from the Amazon basin, are still wild-caught, however.

For general information on fish consultations, examination, nursing care, and anesthesia, see Chapter 14.

Recommended water quality parameters for different aquariums are listed in Table 15-1. Water hardness is measured in a variety of different ways, with mg $CaCO_3$ as the international standard. Conversion factors from other units are given in Table 15-2. Common species of tropical freshwater fish presented to the veterinarian are listed in Table 15-3.

Skin disorders

Structure and function of skin (see Chapter 14)

Differential diagnoses for skin disorders

Pruritus

- Ectoparasites
- Poor water quality

Erosions and ulceration including fin rot

- Bacterial disease, typically *Aeromonas* spp., *Cytophaga*-like bacteria, and *Flavobacterium* spp.; also mycobacteriosis (see *Musculoskeletal Disorders*)
- Ulceration, hemorrhage, darkening of color, and exophthalmos in cichlids (streptococcal infections)
- Often secondary to trauma or ectoparasites (especially *Tetrahymena, Ichthyobodo*)
- *Flexibacter columnaris*—whitish erosive areas, especially along back of fish, mouth fungus and shimmying (mollies), and tail rot (guppies). Sometimes known as false neon tetra disease when it occurs on small tetras.
- In snakehead, striped snakehead skin ulcerative disease (rhabdovirus)
- *Fusarium* mycosis—may also cause blindness
- *Aphanomyces invadens* mycosis (epizootic ulcerative syndrome, EUS). Susceptible species include striped snakehead *(Channa striata)*, giant gourami *(Osphronemus goramy)*, and silver barb *(Barbodes gonionotus)*; see Miles et al 2001
- Channel catfish virus disease is a herpesvirus that affects fry and fingerling catfish. Infected fish swim erratically, are pale with multiple skin hemorrhages, severe exophthalmia, and swollen abdomens.
- Lymphosarcoma (see "Neoplasia")

Nodules and nonhealing wounds

- Large, cauliflower-like masses on fins and skin (*Lymphocystis*—an iridovirus; Fig. 15-2)
- Uneven skin surface in angelfish, *Pterophyllum* spp. (*Pleistophora*)
- Lip fibroma in angelfish, *Pterophyllum* spp. (suspected retrovirus; Francis-Floyd et al 1993)

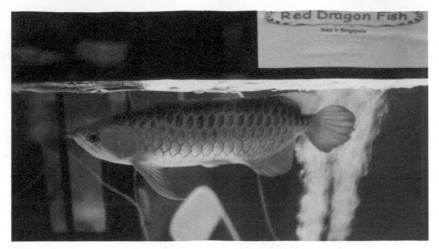

Fig 15-1. The Asian dragonfish *(Scleropages formosus)*.

Table 15-1 Recommended parameters for typical community aquarium, rift lake aquarium, and discus aquarium

Parameter	Typical community aquarium	Rift Lake aquarium (Lake Malawi/ Tanganyika)	Discus aquarium
Temperature (°C)	22-26	22-26	26-30 (higher for spawning)
pH	6.8-7.5	8.0-8.3	5.0-7.5 (lower range for wild-caught discus)
General hardness (GH) (mg CaCO₃)	60-200	200 +	50-100
Carbonate hardness (KH) (mg CaCO₃)	50-100	>80	20-80
Conductivity (μs/cm)	500-800	800 +	180-480
Ammonia (total) (mg/L)	<0.02	<0.02, but the high pH requires that ammonia should be 0.0 mg/L	<0.02
Nitrite (mg/L)	<0.02	<0.02	<0.02
Nitrate (mg/L)	<40 mg above ambient tapwater levels	<40 mg above ambient tapwater levels	<40 mg above ambient tapwater levels
Oxygen (mg/L)	5.0-8.0	5.0-8.0	5.0-8.0
Chlorine (mg/L)	<0.002	<0.002	<0.002

- Obvious skin nodules (*Myxosporidea*, see below)
- Hole in the head disease (head and lateral line disease—*Spironucleus*), especially in discus, angelfish, oscars, and other cichlids; ulceration on the head and along lateral line (see also *Gastrointestinal Tract Disorders*)
- Wasting, darkening of skin color, and obvious boil-like swellings in the skin; in extreme cases it may have a sandpaper effect, due to the large number of granulomas present. Also exophthalmia, abnormal behavior, and abnormal swimming patterns (if the CNS

Table 15-2 Water hardness conversion factors

Unit	Conversion factor to (mg CaCO₃)
dH	17.85
Clark	0.07
f (French)	0.1
Hardness	1
Milliequivalent (mEq)	0.02

Table 15-3 Common species of tropical freshwater fish: Key facts

Species	Temperature (°C)	pH	Hardness	Common disorders
Discus (*Symphysodon* spp.)	26-30	5.0-7.5	Soft	*Capillaria*, *Hexamita*, and *Spironucleus* are common diseases encountered with discus. "Discus plague" may be another up and coming disease.
Angelfish (*Pterophyllum* spp.)	23-28	6.5-7.6	Soft to medium hard (aquarium stocks)	*Capillaria*, gill flukes, *Hexamita*, and *Spironucleus* can be troublesome. Also *Pleistophora* and bacterial infections occasionally. Deep angelfish herpesvirus should be considered for unexplained deaths in this species.
Oscar (*Astronotus occellatus*)	23-30	6.5-7.8	Moderately soft to moderately hard	Veil-tail varieties have their fins easily damaged and should be kept individually or in mated pairs. Very good at begging; this can lead to overfeeding and degeneration of water quality. *Hexamita* and *Spironucleus* can be a problem. Trauma from damage, with a consequent risk of bacterial or fungal infection. Many oscars die from poor water quality due to overfeeding and inadequate filtration.
Rift Lake cichlids (originating from Lakes Malawi, Tanganyika, and Victoria)	22-26	8.0-8.3	Hard to very hard	Many species such as the Mbuna group require a higher vegetable intake than cichlids from other continents, and failure to provide this may predispose to gut-related problems. Also overfeeding leads to some individuals attaining a larger size than they would in the wild. Such "giants" can dominate an aquarium, leading to stress and trauma-related damage. Best kept in crowded communities where no one individual can dominate and where aggression is dissipated among a group. Bacterial diseases are common, as are external parasites such as white spot. *Cryptobia* is considered by many to be the main cause of Malawi bloat. Outbreaks of this may be related to an improper diet.

Table 15-3 Common species of tropical freshwater fish: Key facts—cont'd

Species	Temperature (°C)	pH	Hardness	Common disorders
Arowanas; dragonfish (*Osteoglossum* and *Scleropages* spp.) (see Fig. 15-1)	24-30	6.5-7.5	Moderately soft to moderately hard	Many arowanas die either from poor water quality (high ammonia levels) or injuries sustained from leaping—either hitting the lid or lighting apparatus, or from periods spent drying outside of water. Common parasites include fish lice, anchor worm, and white spot. Two common but poorly understood conditions in captive arowanas are overturned gill covers and "drop eye."
Freshwater stingrays (*Potamotrygon* spp.)	24-27	6.0-7.0	Soft to medium hard	The sting is often damaged during transit and can become infected—it may need removal under sedation. Stingrays will bite each other, especially during courtship, and such bites can become secondarily infected. Fungal infections are common—usually *Saprolegnia*. Bacterial infections, especially of the fins around the disc, are also regularly seen. Protozoan parasites appear to be a rare problem, although fish lice such as *Argulus* and *Livoneca* may be seen on recently caught specimens. Very sick stingrays will often show obvious upward curling of the disc. Heater burns may be seen. These are live-bearers so dystocia is occasionally encountered.

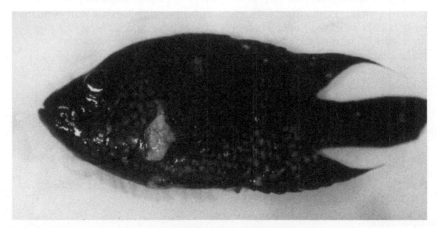

Fig 15-2. Lymphocystis on a Texas cichlid (*Herichthys cyanoguttatus*).

is invaded; *Ichthyophonus hoferi*—see also *Neurologic and Swimming Disorders, Ophthalmic Disorders* and *Systemic Disorders*)
- Pentastomids
- Gas-filled bubbles in the skin, especially on the fins; also occasionally behind the eye (gas bubble disease—usually secondary to oxygen supersaturation)
- Yellowish cystic lesions up to 5 mm diameter (*Clinostomum* spp., a digenetic trematode; Wildgoose 1998)

Changes in pigmentation and color

- Lethargy and reddened areas of skin; fish stop feeding (bacterial septicemia, *Edwardsiella ictaruli* in catfish)
- Obvious discrete white spots visible on skin and fins (*Ichthyophthirius multifiliis*, white spot disease)
- Whitened areas of muscle, often accompanied by loss of color, especially with neon tetras, other small tetras, and killifish. Also may see emaciation and spinal curvature (*Pleistophora*—neon tetra disease). In white angelfish may cause localized accumulations of melanophores producing "black holes"
- Dark or accentuating coloring, obvious nodules, weight loss, whirling, and fin rot (*Myxosporidea*)
- Darkened colors, emaciation, abnormal swimming behavior, and mortalities in tilapia (*Piscirickettsia*-like organisms, PLO); some respiratory signs (gill hyperplasia)
- Enhanced coloration, especially Malawi cichlids (hemoparasites); may see wasting
- White tufts on surface that may resemble cotton wool (*Epistylis, Saprolegnia, Flexibacter columnaris*). *Note:* Mucous strands hanging from the skin can strongly resemble *Saprolegnia.*
- "Mouth fungus" (along with fin rot) is often described as a fungal infection, especially in live-bearers such as mollies and guppies. This is usually due to *Cytophaga*-like bacteria such as *Flexibacter columnaris.*
- Graying skin (due to excessive mucus production—ectoparasites, typically *Trichodina, Chilonodella, Ichthyobodo, Gyrodactylus, Dactylogyrus*)
- Multiple small black spots in the skin and deeper in the muscles (so-called black spot disease; Digenetic trematodes, e.g., *Neascus*). The blackened cysts appear particularly obvious in light-colored fish such as silver dollars (*Metynnus argentius*).
- Darkening of body coloration, lethargy, loss of appetite, abdominal distension, and mortalities in varieties of the three spot gourami (*Trichogaster trichopterus*); also mortalities in the dwarf gourami (*Colisia lalia*)—an unspecified iridovirus
- Black spots—melanin concentrations—described in *Mycobacterium marinum* skin granulomas in *Oreochromis mossambassicus* (Noga et al 1990)
- Darkened color, weight loss, excessive mucus production, rapid respiration, lethargy (discus plague—discus, occasionally angelfish, *Pterophyllum* spp.; see *Systemic Disorders*)
- Algal dermatitis in farmed *Metriaclima zebra* has been described associated with deep invasion and persistent skin infections with *Chlorochytrium* and *Scenedesmus* spp. of algae.
- Color fading—likely to be nutritional lack of appropriate carotenoids
- Planaria (flatworms) visible in aquaria—rarely cause problems; usually due to overfeeding. Consider praziquantel (toxic to *Corydoras* catfish).

Ectoparasites

- Protozoa
  - *Ichthyophthirius multifiliis* (white spot disease)
  - *Oodinium* (velvet disease)—dusty effect over body surface

- *Tetrahymena*—whitish areas or "spots" often with ulceration; more common on live-bearers, cichlids (particularly dwarf cichlids), and tetras; often associated with bacterial infections and white spot
- *Ichthyobodo necator (Costia necatrix)*—common on catfish, killifish, anabantids, swordtails (*Xiphophorus* spp.) and cichlids; see also *Respiratory Tract Disorders*
- *Epistylis (Heteropolaria)*
- *Chilodonella*
- *Spironucleus*
- *Trichodina, Trichodonella*, and *Triparciella*
- Myxosporidea, including *Henneguya, Myxidium*, and *Mitaspora*
- Helminths
  - *Gyrodactylus, Enterogyrus*, and *Cichlidogyrus* spp. (skin flukes)
  - Digenetic trematodes (black spot disease)
  - *Clinostomum* spp.
  - Leeches
  - *Batracobdella tricarinata* (Negm-Eldin and Davies 1999; see also *Cardiovascular and Hematologic Disorders*)
  - Flatworms on glass and substrate *(Planaria)*—not parasitic, but may indicate overfeeding
- Molluscs
  - *Anodonites trapesialis* (Silva-Souza and Eiras 2002)
- Crustaceans
  - *Argulus* (fish louse)
  - *Livoneca* (usually on wild-caught South American fish); see also *Respiratory Tract Disorders*
- Pentastomes

Neoplasia

- Lymphosarcoma—start as nodules in the skin; eventually the overlying skin becomes devitalized and sloughs, leaving an ulcer. Internal lesions may also occur. Lymphosarcoma has been identified in pike (*Esox* spp.) and Malawi cichlids (*Metriaclima* spp.)
- *Xiphophorus* (swordtails and platies) hybrids are very prone to developing melanomas and neuroblastomas. *Note:* At least three viruses, a papovavirus and two retroviruses, have been implicated as predisposing factors.
- Papillomas
- Odontomas appear as swellings around the mouth on freshwater angelfish (*Pterophyllum* spp.).
- Lip fibroma in angelfish (*Pterophyllum* spp.)—suspected retrovirus (Francis-Floyd et al 1993)

Other findings on clinical examination

- Loss of fins and/or eyes
- Irritation, ulceration (ectoparasites)
- Breathing difficulties, irritation, fins clamped (*Ichthyophthirius, Oodinium, Trichodina*—see also *Respiratory Tract Disorders*)
- Clamped fins, depression, sudden death *(Chilodonella)*
- Slimey droppings, weight loss, no appetite, secondary infections *(Spironucleus)*

Investigations

1. Skin scrape under light microscopy (see Fig. 14-8)
   a. Protozoa
      i. *Chilodonella* is a large protozoan (30 to 70 μm) that has an almost oval, flattened appearance. Obvious cilia; moves with gliding, slow circular movement
      ii. *Ichthyobodo:* Even on high power, a small comma-shaped, very mobile parasite seen gyrating through the water
      iii. *Oodinium:* Can be quite large, up to 1-mm diameter, oval-shaped with a very dark appearance because of chloroplasts; not usually mobile
      iv. *Trichodina, Trichodonella,* and *Tripartiella:* Circular, rotating parasites around 40 μm
      v. *Ichthyophthirius:* Large ciliate, horseshoe-shaped nucleus
      vi. *Epistylis:* Stalked, cup-shaped ciliates in colonies
   b. Flukes
      i. *Gyrodactylus:* Live-bearing; can usually see large H-shaped hooks of both adult and unborn young
      ii. *Dactylogyrids:* Egg layer; usually four black spots at caudal end; can be quite large
   c. Fungi
      i. *Saprolegnia:* A meshwork of mycelium and fruiting bodies should be easily identifiable.
      ii. *Ichthyophonus:* Squash preparation of nodule. The spores can be readily seen as spherical bodies, varying from 10 to 100 μm in diameter. There is much variation in the appearance of these multinucleated spores.
2. Radiography
3. Routine hematology and biochemistry
4. Culture and sensitivity
5. Endoscopy
6. Biopsy
7. Ultrasonography
8. Water quality parameters: Check temperature, ammonia, nitrite, nitrate, and pH values.

Management

- See *Nursing Care.*

Treatment/specific therapy

- Gas bubble disease
  - Oxygen supersaturation usually secondary to pressurized oxygenation (waterfalls, malfunctioning Venturi pumps, etc.), excess photosynthesis (high plant levels, suspended algae)
  - Correct source of problem.
  - Rarely fatal—fish usually recover uneventfully.
- Algal dermatitis
  - No treatment; usually of no consequence to the fish
- *Lymphocystis*
  - No direct cure. Usually self-limiting
  - Ozone or ultraviolet sterilization may reduce spread.
  - Attempted surgical removal is usually followed by recurrence.

- Striped snakehead skin ulcerative disease (viral infection)
  - No treatment
- Channel catfish virus disease
  - No treatment
  - Covering antibiotics as it may be secondary infections that cause mortalities
- Bacterial infections
  - Antibiotics
  - Debridement of ulcers followed by packing with protective layer, such as Orabase (Squibb)
  - Change management system (e.g., separation of aggressive individuals, removal of damaging aquarium furniture, improved water quality).
- *Flexibacter columnaris*
  - Antibiotics
  - Copper-based medications can work.
  - Surfactants such as benzalkonium chloride are useful as a bath. *Note:* Toxicity of benzalkonium chloride is increased in soft water, so doses should be reduced if used in soft water (or if hardness not known) and the fish monitored closely for signs of distress.
  - Recommended dose rate for benzalkonium chloride (Table 15-4)
  - Improved management
- PLO
  - Antibiotics
- Mycobacteriosis
  - Difficult to treat; potential zoonosis
  - Kanamycin bath at 50 mg/L every 48 hours for 4 treatments was successful in guppies (Conroy and Conroy 1999).
- *Ichthyophonus hoferi*
  - No efficacious treatment available.
- *Ichthyophthirius multifiliis* white spot
  - Proprietary white spot remedy
  - Raising water temperature 1 or 2° C speeds up life cycle, promoting the exposure of the chemical-sensitive motile theront stage.
- *Oodinium*
  - Proprietary velvet treatment
  - Metronidazole bath at 50 mg/L for up to 24 hours daily for 10 days
  - Quinine hydrochloride at 10 to 20 mg/L indefinitely. *Some fish are sensitive.*
  - The encysted stage is relatively resistant to chemical attack.
  - Can colonize the intestines of fish, where again it can be protected from medications

Table 15-4 Recommended dose rate for benzalkonium chloride

Benzalkonium chloride concentration (mg/L)	Duration of bath (min)
10	5-10
5	30
2	60
1	Several hours

- Antibiotic cover should be considered, as secondary infections are common at the areas where the skin is damaged.
- Eliminate the parasite from a show aquarium by removing all fish, reducing or cutting out the light levels, and raising the temperature to 30 to 32° C for 3 weeks.
- *Tetrahymena*
  - Predisposes to secondary infections
  - Often found associated with *Ichthyophthirius*
  - Poor environmental conditions (high ammonia, high organic load, low water temperatures) predispose (Pimenta Leibowitz et al 2005).
  - Try proprietary ectoparasitic medication. Can spread internally through the body musculature, so treatment may not work.
  - Chloramine-T at an average dose rate of 10 mg/L—use less in soft water, down to 2 mg/L.
  - Recommended chloramine-T concentrations for different pH and water hardness combinations (Table 15-5)
- *Epistylis (Heteropolaria)*
  - Commercial ectoparasitic preparations
- *Chilodonella*
  - Proprietary ectoparasitic medications
  - Glacial acetic acid dips at 8 mL/gallon for 30 to 45 seconds; may kill weak fish
- *Trichodina*
  - Proprietary ectoparasitic medication
  - Flukes (skin, gill)
  - Proprietary ectoparasitic preparations
  - Praziquantel at 10 mg/kg body weight by mouth; as a 1- to 2-hour bath at 15 to 20 mg/L. With larger fish, in-feed medication at a rate of 400 mg/100 g food daily for 7 days. *Toxic to* Corydoras *catfish*
- *Dactylogyrids* are egg layers; the egg stage is resistant to treatment and so infestations require multiple treatments up to 4 weeks apart depending on water temperature.
- Digenetic trematodes
  - Complex life cycle involving a primary host such as a piscivorous bird, reptile or fish, and secondary snail hosts, so they rarely become a problem in aquaria.
  - Treat with praziquantel as described above for skin flukes.
  - Alternatively treat in a bath for 1 hour with a combination of salt, acriflavine, and formalin or in the aquarium with acriflavine and salt only for 36 hours. *Care with* Corydoras *catfish*

Table 15-5 Recommended chloramine-T concentrations for different pH and water hardness combinations

pH	Concentration in soft water (mg/L)	Concentration in hard water (mg/L)
6.0	2.5	7.0
6.5	5.0	10.0
7.0	10.0	15.0
7.5	18.0	18.0
8.0	20.0	20.0

- Hemoparasites (e.g., *Trypanosoma* spp.)
  - Methylene blue at 60 mg/kg per day PO for 4 days, or metronidazole at 50 mg/kg PO per day
- Myxosporidea. No treatment available. Try fumagillin at 1 g/kg food for 10 to 14 days for prevention.
- Neon tetra disease *(Pleistophora)*
  - No good treatment. Options would include:
    - Feeding a diet of 0.1% fumagillin
    - Toltrazuril at 30 mg/L as a 60-minute bath every other day for 3 treatments
  - Transmitted via consumption of infected cadavers or food crustaceans (cyclops)
- *Spironucleus*
  - Treat with metronidazole.
  - Dimetridazole appears to be linked with sterility in fish.
- *Fusarium* mycosis
  - No effective treatment
- *Aphanomyces invadens* (EUS)
  - No effective treatment
  - Temperature-dependent pathology; EUS not seen at 32° C but does occur at lower temperatures (20° C)
- *Saprolegnia* (fungal disease)
  - Proprietary medications containing malachite green
  - Remove visible hyphae and swab the affected area with a 10% povidone-iodine solution once daily.
  - Maintain the fish in a salt solution, as this will not only help to control the fungal infection but will also help with the osmotic imbalance resulting from the infection. Salt solutions as low as 10 parts per thousand (ppt) (mg/100 mL) will inhibit *Saprolegnia* infections. Ideally aim for 1 to 3 g/L as a permanent solution until the problem has resolved. *Care with* Corydoras *catfish*
  - Usually secondary invader, so may need to treat underlying ulceration and secondary bacterial infections
- *Anodontites trapesialis*
  - Larval stages described as parasitizing the epidermis of the cichlid *Tilapia rendalli* and the suckermouth catfish *Hypostomus regani* (Silva-Souza & Eiras 2002)
  - Little inflammatory response, but multiple microscopic skin lesions may predispose to secondary skin infections.
  - Usually self-limiting. Larvae only transiently parasitic
- Fish louse *(Argulus)* or *Livoneca*
  - Individual removal of parasites
  - Treat with lufenuron (Program, Novartis) at 0.088 mg/L as a once-only treatment.
  - Treat with organophosphates where legal.
  - Placing fish in a potassium permanganate bath at 10 ppm (mg/L) for 5 to 60 minutes can be used to rid both individual fish and plants of this parasite. Care with sensitive species
- Pentastomids
  - No treatment
  - Prevent by removal of other hosts from life cycle, especially reptile predators (e.g., turtles, snakes).
- Discus plague
  - Unknown cause. No effective treatment. May be linked to, or initiated by, stress

- Lip fibromas, odontomes, neoplasia
  - Debulking/surgical removal
  - Surgical debulking followed by injection of cisplatin directly into the tissue mass on a weekly basis

Respiratory tract disorders

Note that many freshwater fish can utilize atmospheric air. Lungfish (*Protopterus* spp.), anabantids—including the popular gouramis (*Trichogaster* spp.), fighting fish (*Betta* spp.), and paradise fish (*Macropodus* spp.)—and some South American catfish, such as *Hypostomus punctatus* and *Corydoras*, are common examples. Gulping for air in these species may not necessarily indicate a respiratory problem.

Bacterial

- Bacterial gill disease
- PLO in tilapia—see also *Skin Disorders*

Fungal

- Fungal gill diseases

Protozoal

- *Oodinium* (velvet disease—see *Skin Disorders*)
- *Trichodina* (see *Skin Disorders*)
- *Ichthyophthirius* (white spot), especially catfish (see *Skin Disorders*)
- *Ichthyobodo necator* (*Costia necatrix*—see also *Skin Disorders*)
- *Cryptobia iubilans* (indirect—respiratory signs secondary to anemia—see *Systemic Disorders*)
- Myxosporidea, including *Henneguya* (especially *Corydoras* catfish), *Myxidium*, and *Myxobolus*

Parasitic

- Helminths—*Dactylogyrus* (gill flukes)
- Crustaceans—*Livoneca*

Neoplasia

- Gill tumors are common in *Poecilia* hybrids (molly-guppy).

Other noninfectious problems

- Hypoxia
- Ammonia toxicity (see also *Neurologic and Swimming Disorders*)
- Nitrite toxicity
- Malachite green toxicity
- Overturned operculae in dragonfish (*Sclerophages* spp.) and arowanas (*Osteoglossum* spp.)
- Complete or partial absence of operculae (unilateral or bilateral)

Findings on clinical examination

- Moderate to extreme respiratory effort
- Rapid gill ventilation

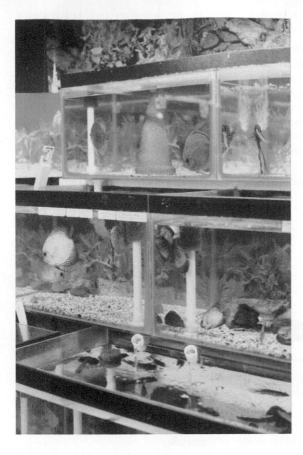

Fig 15-3. A group of discus with high respiratory rates aggregate at the surface in one corner. Contrast this with the behavior of fish in the other aquaria.

- Apparent gasping at water surface or at areas of high turbulence, such as water inlets (Fig. 15-3)
- Anemia (chronic disease, *Cryptobia*)
- Breathing difficulties, dusty effect over body surface *(Oodinium)*
- White spots on skin/fins *(Ichthyophthirius)*; white spots not always obvious
- Visible gill flukes
- Respiratory distress, clamped fins, flashing; one-sided breathing in discus *(Dactylogyrus)*
- Fish usually appear depressed, fins clamped shut, may "wobble" as they swim or even "shimmy"; skin appears dull and grayish; ulceration may be seen; respiratory signs *(Ichthyobodo)*
- Brown color to gills (nitrite toxicity)
- Respiratory signs, darkened colors, emaciation, abnormal swimming behavior, and mortalities in tilapia (PLO)
- Large woodlouse-resembling parasite *(Livoneca)*—up to 2.5 cm long; the adult parasites burrow into the gills and mouth cavity, but they may also attach and burrow into the flank. *Livoneca* are protoandrous hermaphrodites. The larger female is often found in the mouth, while the smaller male is attached to the gills.
- The soft edging to the operculum gradually curls outward and can become permanently deformed (overturned operculae).

Investigations

1. Gill scrape under light microscopy
   a. Thickening of the secondary lamellae (gill hyperplasia)
   b. Large ciliate, horseshoe-shaped nucleus *(Ichthyophthirius)*
   c. *Chilodonella:* A large protozoan (30 to 70 μm) that has an almost oval, flattened appearance; obvious cilia; moves with gliding, slow circular movement
   d. *Oodinium:* Can be quite large, up to 1-mm diameter, oval-shaped with a very dark appearance because of chloroplasts; not usually mobile
   e. Circular, rotating parasites around 40 μm *(Trichodina, Trichodonella,* and *Triparciella)*
2. Radiography
3. Routine hematology and biochemistry
4. Culture and sensitivity
5. Endoscopy
6. Biopsy
7. Ultrasonography
8. Water quality parameters
   a. Check temperature, ammonia, nitrite, nitrate, and pH values.
   b. Recommended levels of oxygen are above 6 mg/L at 25° C for tropical freshwater fish.

Management

- Improve circulation and/or aeration.

Treatment/specific therapy

- Ammonia toxicity
  - Partial water changes to dilute the ammonia levels
  - Adding zeolite will absorb large quantities of ammonia.
  - Longer-term control may include addition of commercially available *Nitrosomonas* bacterial cultures or equivalent.
- Nitrite toxicity
  - Partial water changes
  - Salt (chloride ions compete with nitrite binding sites at the gills). Ideally aim for 1 to 3 g/L as a permanent solution until the problem has resolved. *Care with* Corydoras *catfish*
  - Commercially available *Nitrobacter* cultures (long term)
- Malachite green toxicity
  - Improved management only
  - Malachite green binds irreversibly to respiratory enzymes, so increased aeration may not be beneficial.
- Bacterial gill disease
  - Correct any underlying environmental problem.
  - Consider surfactants such as:
    - Chloramine-T (see "*Tetrahymena*" in *Skin Disorders*)
    - Benzalkonium chloride (see "*Flexibacter*" in *Skin Disorders*)
- Fungal gill disease
  - As for bacterial gill disease
  - Salt at 1 to 3 g/L as a permanent solution until the problem has resolved if *Saprolegnia* involved. Caution: Corydoras catfish may be sensitive to salt.

- PLO
  - Antibiotics
- *Oodinium* (velvet disease—see *Skin Disorders*)
- *Chilodonella*
  - Proprietary ectoparasitic medications
  - Glacial acetic acid dips at 8 mL/gallon for 30 to 45 seconds; may kill weak fish
  - *Chilodonella* prefers temperatures of 18 to 22° C.
- *Ichthyobodo*
  - Standard proprietary antiprotozoan treatments
  - With species of fish able to cope with high temperatures (like discus and fighting fish, *Betta* spp.), raise the temperature to over 30° C.
  - Remove all of the fish from the infected aquarium for 24 to 48 hours as the parasite can only survive away from the host for a few hours.
- *Dactylogyrus* spp.
  - Proprietary ectoparasitic preparations
  - Praziquantel at 10 mg/kg PO once only or at 10 mg/L for a 3-hour bath. *Toxic to* Corydoras *catfish*
  - *Dactylogyrus* spp. are egg layers; the egg stage is resistant to treatment, so praziquantel should be repeated every 2 to 4 weeks depending on temperature, for at least 3 doses. *Toxic to* Corydoras *catfish*
- *Livoneca*
  - See *Skin Disorders*.
- Overturned gill covers
  - Linked to poor water quality, especially high ammonia and nitrite levels
  - If caught in the early stages, transferring the arowana to highly oxygenated, good-quality water may reverse the condition.
  - For advanced cases, surgical removal of the affected part is undertaken.
  - This operation is regularly described for the highly prized Asian dragonfish (see Fig. 15-1), but it may be more for aesthetic reasons than of benefit to the fish.
- Partial or complete absence of operculum
  - Congenital problem. No treatment

Gastrointestinal tract disorders

Bacterial
- Enteritis

Protozoal
- *Protopalina* (very large ciliate), especially discus, kissing gouramis
- *Spironucleus*—especially in discus, angelfish, oscars, and other cichlids (see *Skin Disorders*)
- *Hexamita*—especially in cichlids and anabantids
- *Cryptosporidium*—especially angelfish (*Pterophyllum* spp.)
- *Coccidia*
- *Piscicryptosporidium cichlidaris*—uncertain pathogenicity; encysts deep in the lining of the stomach, so has the potential to cause much damage
- *Crytobia iubilans*

Parasitic

- Nematodes
  - *Camallanus* spp.
  - *Spirocamallanus rebecae* (Vidal-Martinez and Kennedy 2000)
  - *Raillietnema kritscheri* (Vidal-Martinez and Kennedy 2000)
  - *Capillaria* spp. (esp. discus)
  - *Atractis vidali* (in wild *Vieja intermedia* and *Cichlasoma pearsei*) (Gonzalez-Solis and Moravec 2002)
  - *Contracaecum* spp. (in *Oreochromis leucostictus*)
- Cestodes
  - Tapeworms
    - *Crassicutis cichlasomae* (Vidal-Martinez and Kennedy 2000)
    - *Amirthalingamia* spp. (Aloo 2002)
    - *Cyclustera* spp. *(Aloo 2002)*
    - *Enterogyrus cichlidarum* (tilapine cichlids)
- Thorny-headed worms
  - *Acanthocephalus* spp. (especially wild-caught Malawi cichlids)
  - *Neoechinorhynchus golvani* (Vidal-Martinez and Kennedy 2000)
  - *Polyacanthorhynchus kenyensis* (Aloo 2002)

Nutritional

- Lack of dietary fiber, especially Lake Malawi cichlids: In highly adapted vegetarian cichlids, such as many of the Rift Lake species, a diet low in dietary fiber appears to predispose to *Cryptobia iubilans*.
- Lack of bogwood: Some loricarid catfish (South American sucking catfish)—particularly some of the panaques—have specialist dietary requirements including bogwood on which to feed. Failure to provide this causes a progressive fading and loss of condition.
- Hypovitaminosis C: Classic sign is spinal curvature, typically in live-bearers. Supplement with vitamin C and increase greens/algae in diet. See *Musculoskeletal Disorders*.
- Vitamin E deficiency: Muscle wastage, especially large, fast-growing predatory fish fed on dead fish. Supplement with vitamin E, and alter diet appropriately.
- Hepatic lipidosis: Seen often in rapidly growing large fish, such as red-tailed catfish *(Phractocephalus)*, which are fed excessively to maximize growth rate. Reduce feeding and supplement with vitamin E.

Neoplasia

- Buccopharyngeal neoplasia
- Gill neoplasia

Other noninfectious problems

- Incisor teeth overgrowth in pufferfish
- Foreign body

Findings on clinical examination

- Weight loss
- Stunting/poor growth (intestinal parasites)
- Listlessness and weight loss, especially in wild-caught Malawi cichlids *(Acanthocephalus)*
- Emaciation (coccidiosis)
- Stringy, white feces *(Protopalina, Spironucleus, Capillaria, Cryptobia)*

- Diarrhea, darkened coloration in discus *(Capillaria)*
- Anorexia, regurgitation of food, diarrhea, death in angelfish *(Pterophyllum spp.—Cryptosporidium)*
- Weight loss, poor growth (tapeworms, *Enterogyrus cichlidarum*)
- Slimy droppings, head and lateral line lesions, weight loss, no appetite, secondary infections *(Spironucleus)*
- Anorexia, lethargy, and weight loss; some fish may develop ascites *(Hexamita)*
  - In Siamese fighting fish *(Betta splendens)*, *Hexamita* can cause dropsy-like signs due to multiorgan damage. The liver and kidneys are especially affected.
  - In kissing gouramis *(Helostoma temmincki)*, it has been linked to swimming abnormalities, emaciation, white stringy feces, and secondary bacterial infections of the skin.
  - Severely affected angelfish will show a distended abdomen and may lie flat at the water surface.
  - Less severely affected adult cichlids may have reduced fertility, egg hatchability, and increased loss of fry.
- Obvious red worms protruding from anus, especially with live-bearers; ulceration around anus may be apparent; weight loss *(Camallanus)*
- Weight loss in spite of good appetite in pufferfish (incisor teeth overgrowth)
- Dysphagia (buccopharyngeal or gill neoplasia, overgrown incisors)

Investigations

1. Anesthetize and examine teeth/oral cavity (especially pufferfish).
2. Light microscopy of feces
   a. Large, capsule-shaped ciliated protozoan *(Protopalina)*
   b. Typical capillarid eggs *(Capillaria)*
3. Radiography
4. Routine hematology and biochemistry
5. Culture and sensitivity
6. Endoscopy
7. Biopsy/necropsy with histopathology
   a. Granulomatous gastritis; other organs affected *(Cryptobia,* mycobacteriosis). Use modified Ziehl-Neelsen (MZN) stain to differentiate (positive for mycobacteriosis).
8. Ultrasonography
9. Water quality parameters: Check temperature, ammonia, nitrite, nitrate, and pH values.

Management

- Routine removal of dead fish to prevent scavenging (and hence cross-infection) by other aquarium inhabitants

Treatment/specific therapy

- *Protopalina* (protozoal parasite)
  - Proprietary ectoparasitic medication
- *Hexamita*
  - Metronidazole at 50 mg/L as a bath for up to 24 hours daily for 10 days or as a bath at 5 mg/L every other day for a total of 3 treatments

- *Coccidia*
  - May respond to amprolium as a continuous bath at 10 mg/L for 7 to 10 days
  - Potentiated sulfonamide antibiotics:
    - 30 mg/kg IM s.i.d. for 7 to 10 days
    - 30 mg/kg body weight in feed every 24 hours for 10 to 14 days
  - Toltrazuril at 30 mg/L as a 60-minute bath every other day for 3 treatments
- *Cryptosporidium*
  - Treatment is difficult. Consider sulfonamide antibiotics, but success is unlikely.
- *Cryptobia iubilans*—see *Systemic Disorders*
- Tapeworms (including *Enterogyrus cichlidarum*)
  - Worming with praziquantel at 10 mg/kg body weight PO; as a 1- to 2-hour bath at 15 to 20 mg/L. With larger fish, in-feed medication at a rate of 400 mg/100 g food daily for 7 days. *Toxic to* Corydoras *catfish*
  - Avoid feeding live foods to complete life cycle.
- *Enterogyrus cichlidarum* may escape from the stomach and anterior intestine to invade other organs, such as liver, coelomic cavity, swimbladder, and braincase—see *Systemic Disorders* (Noga and Flowers 1995).
- *Camallanus, Capillaria*, and *Acanthocephalus*
  - Levamisole at 2 mg/L for up to 24 hours
  - Fenbendazole at 20 mg/kg body weight given 7 days apart
  - Mebendazole at 20 mg/kg PO for 3 treatments given at weekly intervals
  - *Camallanus* has both a direct and indirect life cycle (small crustaceans, such as cyclops act as intermediate hosts).
- Incisor teeth overgrowth
  - Burr back under anesthetic.
  - Offer foods that increase normal wear (e.g., cockles still in shell).
- Foreign body
  - Retrieval from stomach, possibly with aid of endoscopy
  - Coeliotomy and surgical retrieval

Hepatic disorders

Bacterial

- Hepatitis
- Mycobacteriosis (see *Systemic Disorders*)

Nutritional

- Hepatic lipidosis (see *Nutritional Disorders*)

Neoplasia

Other noninfectious problems

- Hypoxia/anoxia (e.g., gill disease—areas of liver necrosis)
- Heavy metal toxicity

Findings on clinical examination

- Nonspecific signs of ill health
- Anorexia
- Loss of balance (displacement of swimbladder)

- Swollen coelom
- Ascites (see *Systemic Disorders*)

Investigations

1. Radiography
   a. Abnormal position of swimbladder secondary to hepatomegaly
2. Routine hematology and biochemistry
   a. Raised liver enzymes
3. Culture and sensitivity
4. Endoscopy
5. Biopsy
6. Ultrasonography
7. Water quality parameters: Check temperature, ammonia, nitrite, nitrate, and pH values.

Management

- Try milk thistle mixed in feed or via gavage.

Treatment/specific therapy

- Neoplasia
  - No treatment
- Heavy metal poisoning
  - Remove suspected source.
  - Remove to unaffected water.
  - Oxygenate or aerate water well.

Cardiovascular and hematologic disorders

Bacterial
- Endocarditis

Protozoal
- *Cryptobia iubilans* (see *Systemic Disorders*)
- *Trypanosoma mukasai* (Negm-Eldin and Davies 1999)
- *Babesiosoma mariae* (Negm-Eldin and Davies 1999)
- *Cyrilia nili* (Negm-Eldin and Davies 1999)

Neoplasia
Other noninfectious problems
- Cardiomyopathy

Findings on clinical examination

- High respiratory rate, anemia (hemoparasites)
- Death occurring within 24 hours of respiratory disease *(Cryptobia)*
- Ascites (see *Systemic Disorders*)

Investigations

1. Radiography
2. Routine hematology and biochemistry
3. Cytology (hemoparasites)
4. Culture and sensitivity
5. Endoscopy
6. Biopsy
7. Ultrasonography
8. Water quality parameters: Check temperature, ammonia, nitrite, nitrate, and pH values.

Treatment/specific therapy

- Bacterial endocarditis
  - Antibiosis
- *Cryptobia*—see *Systemic Disorders*
- Hemoparasites (*Trypanosoma, Babesiosoma,* and *Cyrilia*)
  - Methylene blue at 60 mg/kg per day PO for 4 days
  - Metronidazole at 50 mg/kg per day PO
- Cardiomyopathy
  - No treatments described, possibly due to difficulty in diagnosis. May be worth adapting reptile protocols

Systemic disorders

Viral

- Lymphocystis (iridovirus—see *Skin Disorders*). Lymphocystis-induced masses can occur internally, acting as space-occupying lesions.
- Rio Grande perch rhabdovirus: Texas cichlid *(Herichthys cyanoguttatus)*, convict cichlid *(Archocentrus nigrofasciatum),* and *Tilapia zilli*
- Ramirez dwarf cichlid virus: Ramirez dwarf cichlid *(Microgeophagus ramirezi)*
- Channel catfish virus disease (herpesvirus)
- PLO: Blue-eyed panaque *(Panaque suttonorum)*

Bacterial

- Multiorgan systemic infections
- Mycobacteriosis
- *Lactococcus garvieae*
- *Clostridium difficile*—possible link with Malawi bloat

Fungal

- *Ichthyophonus hoferi*—see also *Neurologic and Swimming Disorders, Ophthalmic Disorders, Reproductive Disorders,* and *Skin Disorders.*

Protozoal

- *Hexamita*—see *Gastrointestinal Tract Disorders*
- *Cryptobia*—see *Musculoskeletal Disorders*
- *Cryptosporidiosis:* Angelfish, *Pterophyllum* spp.—see *Gastrointestinal Tract Disorders*

Parasitic

- *Enterogyrus cichlidarum*—visceral invasion from gut; see *Gastrointestinal Tract Disorders*

Infectious conditions of unknown etiology

- Discus plague

Nutritional

- See *Nutritional Disorders.*

Neoplasia

Other noninfectious problems

- Nitrite toxicity

Findings on clinical examination

- Fish may separate themselves from the main group.
- Weight loss, obvious loss of muscle mass of epaxial muscles
- Ascites: Known to aquarists as *dropsy,* this is often considered a disease in its own right. Typical signs include a swollen abdomen, raised scales, and protruding eyes. Commonly due to multiorgan failure from systemic bacterial infection
- In Siamese fighting fish *(Betta splendens)*, *Hexamita* can cause dropsy-like signs due to multiorgan damage, in particular the liver and kidneys.
- Hemorrhages and mortalities: Systemic bacterial infections, *Lactococcus garvieae*
- Spinal curvature, open skin sores, protruding eyes—especially anabantids (mycobacteriosis)
- Erratic swimming, pallor, multiple skin hemorrhages, severe exophthalmia, and swollen abdomens in fry and fingerling channel catfish *(Ictarulus punctatus*—channel catfish virus disease)
- Progressive loss of appetite and wasting *(Cryptobia)*—can affect all cichlid species, but it is a particular cause of mortalities in the Rift Lake cichlids. Some of these fish will develop ascites known as *Malawi bloat. Note: C. difficile* has also been implicated in Malawi bloat.
- Weight loss, darkened color, excessive mucus production, rapid respiration, lethargy (discus plague)—seen in discus *(Symphysodon* spp.), occasionally angelfish *(Pterophyllum* spp.); see *Skin Disorders*
- Lethargy and mortalities in Texas cichlid, convict cichlid, and *Tilapia zilli* (Rio Grande perch rhabdovirus)
- Lethargy, loss of appetite, incoordination, emaciation, and death in Ramirez dwarf cichlids (Ramirez dwarf cichlid virus)
- Head standing (tiger barbs); respiratory signs (nitrite toxicity)
- Wasting, darkening of skin color, and obvious boil-like swellings in the skin; also exophthalmia, abnormal behavior, and abnormal swimming patterns (if the CNS is invaded); sex reversal in guppies (female to male): *Ichthyophonus*
- Mortalities in blue-eyed panaque *(Panaque suttonorum)*: PLO

Investigations

1. Radiography
2. Routine hematology and biochemistry
3. Culture and sensitivity
4. Endoscopy

5. Biopsy
6. Postmortem
   a. Multiple granulomas in internal organs (mycobacteriosis, *Cryptobia*); differentiate with MZN (positive for mycobacteria)
7. Ultrasonography
8. Water quality parameters: Check temperature, ammonia, nitrite, nitrate, and pH values.

Management

- See *Nursing Care.*

Treatment/specific therapy

- Rio Grande perch rhabdovirus: No treatment
- Ramirez dwarf cichlid virus: No treatment
- Channel catfish virus: No effective treatment
  - Antibiotics, as secondary infection is often cause of mortalities
- Ascites (dropsy)
  - Without definite diagnosis, prognosis is poor. Attempt use of antibiotic.
- Bacterial infections (including *Lactococcus garvieae*)
  - Antibiotics
- Mycobacteriosis
  - Difficult. Potential zoonosis, so euthanasia. See *Musculoskeletal Disorders.*
- PLO
  - Can be treated with a variety of antibiotics
- *Cryptobia*
  - Metronidazole helps but does not appear to eradicate the organism. See *"Hexamita"* in *Gastrointestinal Tract Disorders* for suggested dose rates. Yanong et al (2004) found metronidazole ineffective in discus *(Symphysodon aequifasciatus)*, but dimetridazole (80 mg/L for 24 hours repeated daily for 3 days) or 2-amino-5-nitrothiazole (10 mg/L for 24 hours repeated daily for 3 days) reduced infection.
  - In some collections, virtually all the cichlids can be infected and the disease will show itself as a low-grade loss of fish over a period of time.
- *Ichthyophonus hoferi*
  - No efficacious treatment available
- Discus plague
  - Unquantified disease; may actually be outbreaks of other undiagnosed diseases such as *Hexamita* or *Capillaria*. However, there is some suggestion that an as-yet unidentified infectious agent may be responsible.
  - Concentrate on maintaining optimum water quality and minimize stress (e.g., provide hiding places).
  - Quarantine all new stock.

Musculoskeletal disorders

Viral

- Chromide iridovirus (chromide cichlids *Etroplus maculates*, *E. canariensis*, and *E. suratensis*)

Bacterial

- Mycobacteriosis—typically *M. marinum*, *M. cheloni*, and *M. fortuitum*

Fungal

Protozoal

- *Pleistophora* (neon tetra disease)
- *Cryptobia iubilans*—see *Systemic Disorders*

Nutritional

- Hypovitaminosis C (especially live-bearers—see *Nutritional Disorders*)
- Starvation; inappetence, through failure to provide correct environment or diet.

Neoplasia

Other noninfectious problems

- Electroshock (Pasnik et al 2003).

Findings on clinical examination

- Weight loss, muscle wastage (see also *Systemic Disorders* and *Gastrointestinal Tract Disorders*)
- In freshwater stingrays (*Potamotrygon* spp.), weight loss over the pelvic bones can be prominent
- Spinal curvature (hypovitaminosis C, mycobacteriosis, *Pleistophora*)
- White patches, loss of color, and emaciation (*Pleistophora*—see *Skin Disorders*)
- Open skin sores, wasting, and protruding eyes (mycobacteriosis)
- Poor growth (hypovitaminosis C)
- Weight loss and weakness in chromide cichlids *Etroplus* spp. (chromide iridovirus)

Investigations

1. Radiography
2. Routine hematology and biochemistry
3. Culture and sensitivity
4. Endoscopy
5. Biopsy
6. Postmortem—Multiple granulomas in internal organs (mycobacteriosis, *Cryptobia*, *Flavobacteria*); differentiate with MZN (positive for mycobacteria)
7. Ultrasonography
8. Water quality parameters: Check temperature, ammonia, nitrite, nitrate, and pH values.

Treatment/specific therapy

- Chromide iridovirus: No treatment
- *Pleistophora*—see *Skin Disorders*
- Mycobacteriosis
  - Potential zoonosis, so consider euthanasia.
  - Treatment problematic; kanamycin bath at 50 mg/L every 48 hours for 4 treatments was successful in guppies (Conroy and Conroy 1999).
- Hypovitaminosis C—see *Nutritional Disorders*

Neurologic and swimming disorders

Viral

- Ramirez dwarf cichlid virus in Ramirez dwarf cichlid *(Microgeophagus ramirezi)*
- Deep angelfish disease (herpesvirus): Altum (deep) angelfish *(Pterophyllum altum)* only. Other *Pterophyllum* species unaffected

Bacterial

- *Flavobacterium* spp. (especially live-bearers)
- Streptococcal infections, especially *S. iniae*
- Bacterial meningitis
- CNS infection/granuloma

Fungal

- *Ichthyophonus hoferi*—see also *Systemic Disorders, Ophthalmic Disorders, Reproductive Disorders,* and *Skin Disorders*
- CNS infection/granuloma

Protozoal

- *Myxosporidea*—see *Skin Disorders*
- *Hexamita*—see *Gastrointestinal Tract Disorders*

Neoplasia

Other noninfectious problems

- Ammonia toxicity—see also *Respiratory Tract Disorders*
- Abnormal swimbladder functioning secondary to compression from internal space-occupying lesions (e.g., neoplasia)
- Swimbladder disease
- Swimbladder torsion
- Nicotine toxicity

Findings on clinical examination

- Whirling swimming pattern, dark or accentuating coloring, sudden death (meningitis, *Myxosporidea*—especially if obvious nodules visible); there may be weight loss and fin rot.
- Swimming abnormalities, emaciation, white stringy feces, and secondary bacterial infections of the skin in kissing gouramis *(Helostoma temmincki); Hexamita*—see *Gastrointestinal Tract Disorders*
- Incoordination, muscle spasms, lethargy, loss of appetite, emaciation, and death in Ramirez dwarf cichlids
- Aimless swimming (shimmying), loss of balance, death *(Flavobacterium)*
- Loss of balance, spinning, pale gills, ulcers, death in altum angelfish (deep angelfish disease)
- Abnormal behavior and abnormal swimming patterns accompanied by wasting, darkening of skin color, and obvious boil-like swellings in the skin; in extreme cases it may have a sandpaper effect, due to the large number of granulomas present; exophthalmia; sex reversal in guppies (female to male): *Ichthyophonus*
- All or most fish affected: Consider environmental disease (e.g., water quality).
- Upward curling of the disc in freshwater stingrays *(Potamotrygon* spp.) is often a sign of ill health and is usually either poor water quality or bacterial infection.
- Stiffened pectoral fins, muscular spasms (nicotine toxicity)

Investigations

1. Radiography
2. Routine hematology and biochemistry
3. Culture and sensitivity
4. Endoscopy
5. Biopsy or postmortem
   a. Multiple granulomas (*Flavobacterium*, mycobacteriosis—see *Systemic Disorders*)
6. Ultrasonography
7. Water quality parameters: Check temperature, ammonia, nitrite, nitrate, and pH values.
8. Assessment of environment (nicotine toxicity).

Treatment/specific therapy

- Ammonia toxicity
  - Partial water changes to dilute the ammonia levels
  - Adding zeolite will absorb large quantities of ammonia.
  - Longer term control may include addition of commercially available *Nitrosomonas* bacterial cultures or equivalent.
- Deep angelfish disease
  - No treatment—supportive only
- *Flavobacterium* and bacterial meningitis
  - Antibiotics
- *Ichthyophonus hoferi*
  - No efficacious treatment available
- Swimbladder disease
  - Usually no effective treatment. May develop ulceration on areas persistently floating above water level
  - Pneumocystocentesis can provide temporary relief, but the problem is likely to recur.
  - Try antibiotics if suspect bacterial infection.
  - If the fish is floating, may implant small sterile counterweight into ventral coelomic cavity, but is difficult to judge correct weight
  - Pneumocystoplasty (Britt et al 2002) and pneumocystectomy (Lewbart et al 1995) have been attempted and with refinement could prove useful.
- Swimbladder torsion
  - Surgical correction
- CNS infection/granuloma
  - Attempt antibiotic or antimycotic treatment. Poor prognosis
- Nicotine toxicity
  - 10 ppm can kill guppies within 5 minutes.
  - Lower doses can cause low-grade mortalities, infertility, and other reproductive problems.
  - No direct treatment. Situate air pumps away from smoky atmospheres.

Ophthalmic disorders

Viral

- Channel catfish virus (herpesvirus)—see also *Skin Disorders* and *Systemic Disorders*

Bacterial

- Systemic bacterial infection/multiorgan failure
- Retrobulbar granuloma
- Streptococcal infections, especially *S. iniae*
- *Edwardsiella ictaruli* (catfish)—see also *Skin Disorders*

Fungal

- *Fusarium* mycosis
- *Ichthyophonus hoferi*—see also *Systemic Disorders, Neurologic and Swimming Disorders, Reproductive Disorders,* and *Skin Disorders*
- Retrobulbar granuloma

Protozoal

- *Ichthyophthirius*
- *Tetrahymena*

Nutritional

- Riboflavin deficiency
- Ascorbic acid deficiency
- Hypovitaminosis A

Neoplasia

- Retrobulbar neoplasia

Other noninfectious problems

- Traumatic damage or loss of eye; often due to interspecific or conspecific aggression, especially cichlids
- Gas bubble disease—see *Skin Disorders*
- Cardiomyopathy
- "Drop eye" in dragonfish (*Sclerophages* spp.) and arowanas (*Osteoglossum* spp.); (Fig. 15-4).

Findings on clinical examination

- Blindness (*Fusarium*)
- Exophthalmos, often accompanied by ascites

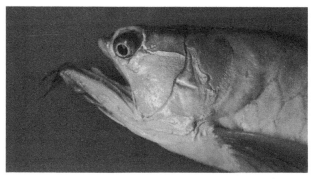

Fig 15-4. "Drop-eye" in a large silver arowana *(Osteoglossum birchirrosum)*.

- Exophthalmos, lethargy, pale skin, sex reversal in guppies (female to male): *Ichthyophonus*
- Exophthalmos, panophthalmitis, darkening of color, hemorrhage, ulceration in cichlids (streptococcal infections)
- Exophthalmos in channel catfish fry and fingerlings, accompanied by skin hemorrhages, severe abnormal swimming, and swollen abdomen (channel catfish virus)
- Glaucoma—usually secondary to intraocular disease
- One or both eyes is turned permanently downward in arowanas (drop eye).

Investigations

1. Ophthalmic examination
2. Radiography
3. Routine hematology and biochemistry
4. Culture and sensitivity
5. Endoscopy
6. Biopsy
7. Ultrasonography
8. Water quality parameters: Check temperature, ammonia, nitrite, nitrate, and pH values.

Management

- Maintain optimum water quality.
- See *Nursing Care.*

Treatment/specific therapy

- Traumatic damage/loss of eye
  - Consider antibiotic therapy.
  - Remove aggressive individuals, sharp aquarium furniture, etc.
- Bacterial infections
  - Antibiotics
- *Fusarium* mycosis: No effective treatment
- *Ichthyophonus*
  - No effective treatment
  - Enucleation
- Glaucoma
  - Enucleation
- "Drop eye"
  - Etiology unknown
  - Likely to be a neurologic problem leading to loss of function of the muscles that control the eye, possibly as a result of head trauma while jumping
- Neoplasia
  - Enucleation
  - Euthanasia
- Cardiomyopathy—see *Cardiovascular and Hematologic Disorders*
- Nutritional disorders
  - Feed analysis
  - Correction with dietary supplements

Anorexia

Episodes of anorexia can occur, especially in large predatory fish. These may be associated with poor environmental conditions (incorrect water parameters, inadequate space, incorrect social or species mix), pathology including pharyngeal masses, foreign body or other physical obstructions, and physiologic factors such as reproductive status. Condition loss may be minimal to begin with.

1. Review and correct environmental conditions.
2. Review diet, including presentation—live foods may be required for reluctant predators to stimulate feeding behavior. For many predators, mimicking prey movement by impaling food items on a clear stick may work.
3. Gavage under heavy sedation or anesthesia (see "Anesthesia" in Chapter 14). Cat urinary catheters make suitable gavage tubes for smaller fish; larger fish will tolerate silicone tubing or similar. The esophagus of predatory fish is often short and distensible and is very amenable to tubing. Aim the tube toward the back of the pharynx—if deflected it will exit through one or other opercular opening. Give 2% to 4% body weight at intervals that are felt a suitable compromise between the stress of handling and anesthesia against the benefit of feeding. Regurgitation upon recovery can be a problem. In some cases gavage feeding may be needed for several weeks or even months.
4. Note that some cyprinids such as carp and goldfish do not have a distinct stomach, and care should be taken when gavaging to account for this.

Endocrine disorders

• Goiter in freshwater stingrays—see *Endocrine Disorders* in Chapter 16

Renal disorders

In many fish, the kidney is divided into two sections. The caudal pole excretes urine and, along with the gills, is important in osmoregulation. The other section is involved with hematopoiesis and immune function, including white blood cell production and antibody formation. The osmoregulatory function means that freshwater fish excrete prodigious amounts of dilute urine to eliminate the excess water entering across the skin and gills. Severe renal disease may result in severe osmoregulatory upset, with extreme cases developing into ascites.

Bacterial

• Nephritis

Fungal

Protozoal

• Myxozoans

Neoplasia

• Renal cyst adenomas (possibly genetic in red oscars, *Astronotus occellatus*)

Other noninfectious problems

• Prolonged exposure to free CO_2 levels >10 to 20 mg/L has been associated with nephrocalcinosis, mineral deposits forming in the renal tubules, collecting ducts, and ureters.

Findings on clinical examination

- Wasting and general malaise
- Anemia
- Ascites due to osmoregulatory disruption
- Mortalities
- Swollen abdomen

Investigations

1. Radiography
   a. Swimbladder displacement (renal and other coelomic neoplasia)
2. Routine hematology and biochemistry
3. Culture and sensitivity
4. Endoscopy
5. Biopsy
6. Ultrasonography
7. Postmortem examination
8. Water quality parameters
   a. Check temperature, ammonia, nitrite, nitrate, and pH values.
   b. High CO_2 levels may be linked with low pH levels, high stocking densities, poor water circulation, and excess CO_2 infusion in planted aquaria.

Treatment/specific therapy

- CO_2 excess
  - Assess possible underlying causes and correct (see Investigations 8b above).
- Neoplasia
  - Surgical resection
  - Euthanasia

Reproductive disorders

Fungal
- *Ichthyophonus hoferi*—see also *Skin Disorders, Neurologic and Swimming Disorders, Ophthalmic Disorders,* and *Systemic Disorders*

Protozoal
- *Hexamita*

Other noninfectious problems
- Functional sterility is seen in fancy strains of live-bearers (guppies, swordtails) where there is increased length or branching of the gonopodium—the modified anal fin used for sperm transfer in these fish. In these strains it is usually only young males without full gonopodial development that are used for breeding. In the guppy this is an autosomal dominant mutation, in which increased branching of the fins produces a veil-tail appearance.
- Lethal gene in certain strains of black Siamese fighting fish *(Betta splendens)*; such strains must be outcrossed to be propagated.

- Nicotine toxicity—see also *Neurologic and Swimming Disorders*
- Egg retention—see *Reproductive Disorders* in Chapter 14
- Dystocia in live-bearing species (e.g., freshwater stingrays)

Findings on clinical examination

- Poor reproductive performance in cichlids *(Hexamita)*
- Sex reversal in guppies (female to male); also lethargy, pale skin, protruding eyes *(Ichthyophonus)*
- Swollen body cavity (dystocia in stingrays)

Investigations

1. Radiography
2. Routine hematology and biochemistry
3. Culture and sensitivity
4. Endoscopy
5. Biopsy
6. Ultrasonography
   a. Check for fetal heartbeats in dystocic stingrays.
7. Water-quality parameters: Check temperature, ammonia, nitrite, nitrate, and pH values.

Treatment/specific therapy

- *Ichthyophonus:* No treatment. Consider euthanasia.
- *Hexamita*
  - See *Gastrointestinal Tract Disorders.*
- Nicotine toxicity—see also *Neurologic and Swimming Disorders*
- Dystocia
  - If possible, calculate if over due date (in stingrays gestation is around 2.5 to 3 months; young females will have 1 to 2 young; older, full-sized females can have 8 or more).
  - Under general anesthesia, assess if young are alive either by observation/palpation of young or ultrasonography.
  - Young may be delivered per cloaca or via surgical salpingotomy.

Tropical marine fish

Over 90% of tropical marine fish are wild-caught. This means that, although they are robust as individuals (they are the Darwinian survivors of the rigors of planktonic survival), the stress of capture and transportation plus the mingling of species from different continents and biotopes at the wholesaler and retailer mean that disease outbreaks are not uncommon. Some captive breeding does occur, principally with those species with either short or no planktonic larval stage, such as clownfish (*Amphiprion* spp.), seahorses (*Hippocampus* spp.), and Banggai cardinalfish *(Pterapogon kauderni)*.

Most marine fish are net-caught, but in some countries there is still an unacceptable willingness to use cyanide to catch fish hidden in coral crevices, an action that causes both immediate and later mortalities when the fish have entered the ornamental fish trade.

Recommended water-quality parameters are listed in Table 16-1.

Table 16-1 Recommended water quality parameters: Fish-only community aquarium and reef aquarium

Parameter	Fish-only community aquarium	Reef aquarium (with photosynthetic invertebrates)
Temperature (° C)	22-26	24-28
pH	8.0-8.3	8.0-8.4
Salinity (measured as specific gravity)	1.020-1.027	1.022-1.027
Carbonate hardness (KH) (mg $CaCO_3$)	116	116-267
Ammonia (total) (mg/L)	<0.02	<0.02, but the high pH requires ammonia should be 0.0 mg/L
Nitrite (mg/L)	<0.02	<0.02
Nitrate (mg/L)	<40 mg above ambient tapwater levels	<5-10
Calcium (mg/L)	300-500	300-500
Oxygen (mg/L)	5.0-8.0	5.0-8.0
Phosphate (mg/L)	<0.2	<0.036
Water volume turnover	Dependent on fish housed in aquarium	15-20 times per hour
Lighting	Dependent on fish housed in aquarium	10-14 hours daylight; 0.6-5.5 watts/L

Consultation and handling

See Chapter 14.

Nursing care

The same principles apply as for goldfish and koi but differ significantly in some areas. Salt water holds less oxygen than fresh water at an equivalent temperature, so stocking densities are more critical. The high pH of marine aquaria means that excreted ammonia is more toxic. Lowering the salinity to a specific gravity of 1.020 is often beneficial—it reduces osmotic stress on the fish and is less well tolerated by many ectoparasites. Protein skimming is an important method of removing proteinaceous and other dissolved and suspended materials from salt water. However, zeolite is ineffective in salt water.

Proprietary products containing copper are commonly available medications for marine fish. Copper is toxic to certain groups of fish, including the elasmobranchs (sharks and rays) and many invertebrate species. It may also interfere with the normal gut flora of herbivorous fish such as tangs and surgeonfish. Signs of toxicity include stress coloration, loss of appetite, excessive mucus production, and respiratory distress. Copper levels, therefore, require daily monitoring with a copper test kit (Table 16-2). Never use copper-based treatments in aquaria containing invertebrates, and ideally always use a separate dedicated treatment aquarium.

Table 16-2 Therapeutic use of copper

Free copper ion concentration	Result
0.2 ppm	Therapeutic
<0.15 ppm	Nontherapeutic
>0.25 ppm	Toxic

Analgesia and anaesthesia

See Chapter 14.

Species commonly presented to the veterinarian include those listed in Table 16-3.

Table 16-3 Species of tropical marine fish commonly encountered: Key facts

Species	Notes	Common disorders
Clownfish (*Amphiprion* spp.)	Most species available are captive bred. Host anemone not often required in captivity	Ectoparasites, especially *Cryptocaryon, Brooklynella, Uronema,* and *Amyloodinium*
Angelfish (*Pomacanthus, Holacanthus,* and *Centropyge* spp.)	Natural diet high in algae and sponges	*Cryptocaryon*, skin flukes, head and lateral line disease. Variably susceptible to poor water quality
Lionfish (*Pterois* spp. and *Dendrochirus* spp.)	Venomous dorsal spines	Hepatic lipidosis
Seahorse (*Hippocampus* spp.)	Live-bearers; commercially bred for both the ornamental fish trade and traditional Chinese medicine	Ectoparasites, brood pouch emphysema

Skin disorders

Structure and function of skin (see Chapter 14).

Pruritus

- *Note:* For wrasses, apparent scratching against the substrate can be normal behavior thought to be linked to foraging for hidden invertebrates.
- Scratching and irritation (flukes, protozoa)
- Sudden darting movements, loss of balance, rapid respiration (sudden-onset water poisoning; new tank syndrome—see *Systemic Disorders* and *Neurologic and Swimming Disorders*)
- Seahorses with *Glugea* (see below) appear pruritic and induce serious excoriation by rubbing affected areas.

Erosions and ulceration including fin rot

- Respiratory distress, irritation, ulceration (*Brooklynella, Uronema marinum* and *Miamiensis avidus,* especially in seahorses—see *Respiratory Tract Disorders*)
- Damage to skin and/or loss of eyes and fins (bacterial infections—typically *Vibrio* spp.; [for *Vibrio parahaemolyticus,* see also *Gastrointestinal Tract Disorders*], but *Pasteurella, Myxobacteria,* and streptococci are also recorded; also mycobacteriosis, *Nocardia kampachi,* trauma)
- Weight loss, thickened areas of inflammation, ulceration, fin rot *(Nocardia)*
- Ulcers on snout and mouth of puffer fish (*Tetraodon* spp.), increased aggression (tiger puffer virus)
- Erosions at cephalic sensory pits and along lateral line, often involving surrounding muscles, in marine angelfish, surgeonfish, and tangs; slimy feces (head and lateral line disease, HLLD)
  - Linked to an aquareovirus in marine angelfish (*Pomacanthus* spp.) (Varner and Lewis 1991)
  - Possible hypovitaminosis A
  - Suggested protozoal etiology (see Skin Disorders, Chapter 15), but unconfirmed in marine fish
- Foreign body reaction to fiberglass in moray eels
- Neoplasia
- Excessively low pH

Nodules and nonhealing wounds

- Wasting, darkening of skin color, and obvious boil-like swellings in the skin; in extreme cases it may have a sandpaper effect, due to the large number of granulomas present. Also exophthalmia, abnormal behavior, and abnormal swimming patterns (if the CNS is invaded—*Ichthyophonus hoferi*). See also *Neurologic and Swimming Disorders, Ophthalmic Disorders,* and *Systemic Disorders.*
- Nonulcerative skin masses in seahorses (*Hippocampus* sp.), lethargy, and disorientation (exophthaliosis)
- Whitish skin nodules in seahorses, especially *H. erectus (Glugea heraldi)* (Vincent and Clifton-Hadley 1989)
- Nodules, darkened coloring, emaciation, abnormal swimming *(Myxosporidea)*
- Cauliflower-like growths on fins and skin (*Lymphocystis*—Fig. 16-1)
- Epitheliocystis—looks like lymphocystis (*Chlamydophila*-like organism)
- Goiter in marine elasmobranchs—see *Endocrine Disorders*
- Gas-filled bubbles in the skin, especially on the fins, also occasionally behind the eye (gas bubble disease—usually secondary to oxygen supersaturation; see also "Seahorse Gas Bubble Disease" in *Systemic Disorders*)
- Neoplasia

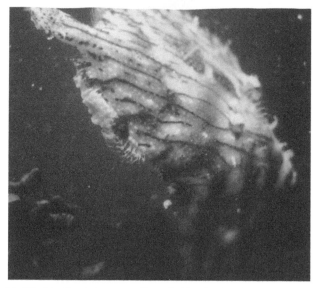

Fig 16-1. A tesselated file fish *(Chaetoderma pencilligerus)* with yellow lymphocystic lesions on the ventral fin.

Changes in pigmentation

- Large discrete white spots, labored breathing, flashing (*Cryptocaryon irritans*, marine white spot)
- Fine white "dusting" on skin, labored breathing, flashing (*Amyloodinium*—coral fish disease, *Crepidoodinium*)
- Gray skin due to excessive mucus production, reddened skin, ulceration (skin flukes, ectoparasites)
- Hemorrhages, ulceration, abnormal swimming, shimmying (bacterial disease)
- Small black spots over body, cloudy skin, respiratory distress, especially in laterally compressed fish such as yellow tangs (*Zebrasoma flavescens, Turbellaria*)
- Fingerprint-like marks on skin of tangs and surgeonfish (tang fingerprint disease virus)
- Color fading—likely to be nutritional lack of appropriate carotenoids
- Light gray patches that are multifocal, well defined, and ovoid in blacktip sharks (*Carcharinus limbatus)—Dermopthirus*; see Bullard et al 2000

Ectoparasites

- Protozoa
  - *Cryptocaryon irritans*—see also *Respiratory Tract Disorders*
  - *Amyloodinium* and *Crepidoodinium*—see also *Respiratory Tract Disorders*
  - *Brooklynella hostilis*—see also *Respiratory Tract Disorders*
  - *Uronema marinum*—see also *Respiratory Tract Disorders*
  - *Miamiensis marinum*, especially seahorses
  - *Turbellaria*—see also *Respiratory Tract Disorders*
  - Microsporidians (e.g., *Glugea, Pleistophora, Sprauga* spp.)
- Helminths
  - Skin flukes (*Gyrodactylus*)
  - Gill flukes (dactylogyrids—see also *Respiratory Tract Disorders*)
  - *Dermopthirius penneri*

- Crustacea
  - *Livoneca*
  - *Lerneascus* spp.

Neoplasia

- Nonsymmetrical swelling, ulceration, loss of balance
- Epithelioma
- Papillomas

1. Skin scrape and light microscopy
   a. Protozoa
      i. *Brooklynella:* Large (55 to 85 µm) and mobile ciliates, with the basket-shaped "mouth" and cilia very apparent
      ii. *Cryptocaryon:* Large (48 × 27 to 450 × 350 µm) oval-shaped ciliated protozoa with a characteristic four-lobed nucleus
      iii. *Amyloodinium:* Can be quite large, up to 1.0-mm diameter, oval-shaped with a very dark appearance because of chloroplasts; not usually mobile
      iv. *Uronema:* Motile, oval-shaped protozoan parasites
   b. Flukes
      i. *Gyrodactylus:* Live-bearing; can usually see large H-shaped hooks of both adult and unborn young
      ii. *Dactylogyrids:* Egg-layer; usually four black spots at caudal end. Can be quite large
   c. Fungi
      i. *Ichthyophonus:* Squash preparation of nodule. The spores can be readily seen as spherical bodies, varying from 10 to 100 µm in diameter. There is much variation in the appearance of these multinucleated spores.
2. Radiography
3. Routine hematology and biochemistry
4. Culture and sensitivity
5. Endoscopy
6. Biopsy
7. Ultrasonography
8. Water-quality parameters: Check as a minimum: temperature, ammonia, nitrite, nitrate, and pH values.

- Gas bubble disease—see also "Seahorse Gas Bubble Disease" in *Systemic Disorders*
  - Oxygen supersaturation usually secondary to pressurized oxygenation (e.g., malfunctioning Venturi pumps), excess photosynthesis (high algae levels)
  - Correct source of problem
  - Rarely fatal—fish usually recover uneventfully
- HLLD
  - No treatment for aquareovirus
  - Vitamin A supplementation, either in commercial supplement or as "greens" (e.g., suchi seaweed wraps)
  - Metronidazole at 50 mg/kg PO per day if suspect protozoal involvement

- Tiger puffer virus
  - No treatment available. Supportive care only
- Tang fingerprint disease virus
  - No treatment available. Supportive care only
- Lymphocystis
  - No direct cure; usually self-limiting
  - Ozone or ultraviolet sterilization may reduce spread.
  - Attempted surgical removal is usually followed by recurrence.
- Epitheliocystis
  - Some antibiotics (e.g., chloramphenicol) recorded as effective
- Bacterial infections
  - Antibiotics
  - Debridement of ulcers followed by packing with protective layer, such as Orabase (Squibb)
- *Nocardia* and mycobacteriosis
  - Antibiotic treatment not very effective
  - Consider euthanasia, especially because of zoonotic risk.
- *Exophthaliosis*
  - Ketoconazole at 5.0 mg/kg PO s.i.d.
  - Itraconazole at 1 to 10 mg/kg PO. (in feed) s.i.d. for 1 to 7 days
- *Ichthyophonus hoferi*
  - No efficacious treatment available. Try treatment as for *Exophthaliosis,* above.
- *Glugea*
  - No effective treatment. Consider:
    - Toltrazuril at 30 mg/L bath for 60 minutes repeated every other day for 3 treatments
    - Feeding a diet of 0.1% fumagillin
- Myxosporidea
  - No effective treatment—try as for *Glugea* above
- *Cryptocaryon irritans*—marine white spot
  - Sensitive to copper-based ectoparasitic treatments (see *Nursing Care,* above)
  - Formalin baths
  - Freshwater dips
  - *Cryptocaryon tomonts* cannot survive at salinities with a specific gravity below around 1.015 (a salinity of around 16 ppt). Maintaining *Cryptocaryon*-infested fish at 1.015 or below for a minimum of 6 days can effect a cure at standard tropical temperatures. Examples of fish groups able to adapt to such low levels of salt include the blennies *(Blennidae)*, groupers *(Serranidae)*, target fish *(Theraponidae)*, jacks *(Carangidae)*, snappers *(Lutja)*, rabbitfishes *(Siganidae)*, damselfish and clownfish *(Pomacentridae)*, left-eye flounders *(Bothidae)*, and even some marine angelfish *(Pomacanthids)*. Estuarine and rock pool fish will also have little difficulty osmoregulating at such low salinities. Some invertebrates such as cleaner shrimps *(Lysmata* spp.) may well not survive such treatment.
- *Amyloodinium* and *Crepidoodinium*
  - Sensitive to copper-based ectoparasitic treatments
  - The encysted stage is relatively resistant to chemical attack.
  - Can colonize the intestines of fish, where again it can be protected from medications
  - In such cases, treat with metronidazole at 50 mg/L daily for 10 days, changing the water daily.
  - Antibiotic cover should be considered, as secondary infections are common at the areas where the skin is damaged.
  - Eliminate the parasite from a show aquarium by removing all fish, reducing or cutting out the light levels, and raising the temperature to 30 to 32° C for 3 weeks.

- *Brooklynella, Uronema,* and *Miamiensis*
  - Sensitive to proprietary formalin/malachite green and/or copper-based ectoparasitic treatments
  - Freshwater baths for larger/tougher fish
  - Covering antibiosis
- Skin flukes
  - Proprietary ectoparasitic preparations
  - Praziquantel at 10 mg/L for a 3-hour bath, or in feed at a rate of 400 mg/100 g food daily for 7 days (but see *Neurologic and Swimming Disorders*)
  - Freshwater dips 5 minutes once daily for 5 days
- *Dermophthirius penneri*
  - Consider praziquantel as above.
- *Turbellaria*
  - Formalin bath at 2 mL/L for up to 1 hour
  - 5-minute freshwater bath daily for 5 days
- Crustacean ectoparasites
  - Individual removal of parasites
  - Treat with lufenuron (Program, Novartis) at 0.088-0.13 mg/L as a once-only treatment.
  - Treat with organophosphates if legal to do so.
- Neoplasia
  - Surgery or euthanasia
  - Surgical debulking followed by injection of cisplatin directly into the tissue mass on a weekly basis.

Respiratory tract disorders

Bacterial

- Bacterial gill disease, especially Flavobacteria (sygnathids)
- *Epitheliocystis* (sygnathids)

Fungal

- Fungal gill disease

Protozoal

- *Cryptocaryon irritans*—see also *Skin Disorders*
- *Amyloodinium* and *Crepidoodinium*—see also *Skin Disorders*
- *Brooklynella hostilis*—see also *Skin Disorders*
- *Uronema marinum*—see also *Skin Disorders*
- *Miamiensis marinum,* especially seahorses
- *Turbellaria*—see also *Skin Disorders*
- *Coccomyxa hoffmani* (Myxosporidean)

Parasitic

- Gill flukes (*Dactylogyrus, Microcotyle, Haliotrema, Ancyrocephalus, Pseudoancyrocephalus, Cleithrarticus, Neohaliotrema,* and *Pseudempleurosoma*)

Neoplasia

Other noninfectious problems

- Hypoxia
- Ammonia toxicity—see also *Neurologic and Swimming Disorders*
- Copper toxicity

Findings on clinical examination

- Moderate to extreme respiratory effort
- Rapid gill ventilation
- Apparent gasping at water surface
- Abnormal color of gills, necrosis, exposure of underlying cartilage
- Respiratory distress, irritation, ulceration *(Brooklynella, Uronema)*
- Respiratory distress, small black spots over body with cloudy skin *(Turbellaria)*
- Respiratory distress, clamped fins, scratching and flashing, inactivity (gill flukes)
- Gill or intraoral mass

Investigations

1. Gill scrape and light microscopy
   a. Protozoa
      i. *Brooklynella:* Large (55 to 85 µm) and mobile ciliates, with the basket-shaped "mouth" and cilia very apparent
      ii. *Cryptocaryon:* Large (48 × 27 to 450 × 350 µm) oval-shaped ciliated protozoa with a characteristic four-lobed nucleus
      iii. *Amyloodinium:* Can be quite large, up to 1.0-mm diameter, oval-shaped with a very dark appearance because of chloroplasts; not usually mobile
      iv. *Uronema* and *Miamiensis:* Motile, oval-shaped protozoan parasites
      v. *Coccomyxa hoffmani:* Cartilage of the gill filaments of coral catfish *(Plotosus anguillaris)*
   b. Flukes
      i. *Gyrodactylus:* Live-bearing; can usually see large H-shaped hooks of both adult and unborn young
      ii. *Dactylogyrus:* Egg-layer; usually four black spots at caudal end. Can be quite large
2. Radiography
3. Routine hematology and biochemistry
4. Culture and sensitivity
5. Endoscopy
6. Biopsy
7. Ultrasonography
8. Water quality parameters: Check as a minimum: temperature, ammonia, nitrite, nitrate, and pH values.

Management

- Good oxygenation of water; recommended level of oxygen is above 5.5 mg/L at 25° C for tropical marine fish.

Treatment/specific therapy

- Ammonia toxicity
  - Partial water changes to dilute the ammonia levels
  - Longer-term control may include addition of commercially available *Nitrosomonas* bacterial cultures or equivalent.

- Bacterial gill disease
  - Correct any underlying environmental problem.
  - Chloramine-T at 5 to 10 mg/L
  - Appropriate antibiosis
- *Epitheliocystis*
  - *Chlamydophila*-like organism
  - Considered nonpathogenic in sygnathids
  - Some antibiotics (e.g., chloramphenicol) recorded as effective.
- Fungal gill disease
  - Consider itraconazole at 1.0 to 5.0 mg/kg PO every 1 to 7 days, either in feed or gavage.
- *Brooklynella, Uronema,* and *Miamiensis*
  - Sensitive to proprietary formalin/malachite green and/or copper-based ectoparasitic treatments
  - Freshwater baths for larger/tougher fish
  - Covering antibiosis
- *Cryptocaryon irritans* (marine white spot)
  - Sensitive to copper-based ectoparasitic treatments (see *Nursing Care* above)
  - Formalin baths
  - Freshwater dips
- *Amyloodinium* and *Crepidoodinium*
  - Sensitive to copper-based ectoparasitic treatments (see *Nursing Care* above)
  - The encysted stage is relatively resistant to chemical attack.
  - Can colonize the intestines of fish, where again it can be protected from medications
  - In such cases, treat with metronidazole added to water at 50 mg/L daily for 10 days, changing the water daily.
  - Antibiotic cover should be considered, as secondary infections are common at the areas where the skin is damaged.
  - Eliminate the parasite from a show aquarium by removing all fish, reducing or cutting out the light levels, and raising the temperature to 30 to 32° C for 3 weeks.
- *Turbellaria*
  - Formalin bath at 2 mL/L for up to 1 hour
  - 5-minute freshwater bath daily for 5 days
- Gill flukes
  - Proprietary ectoparasitic preparations
  - Praziquantel at 10 mg/L for a 3-hour bath or in feed at a rate of 400 mg/100 g food daily for 7 days (but see *Neurologic and Swimming Disorders*)
  - Freshwater dips 5 minutes daily for 5 days
  - *Dactylogyrus* spp. are egg-layers; the egg stage is resistant to treatment, so treatment should be repeated every 2 to 4 weeks depending on temperature, for at least 3 doses.
- *Coccomyxa hoffmani*
  - No treatment
- Copper toxicity
  - Multiple partial water changes
  - See also *Nursing Care* above.
- Neoplasia
  - Surgical debulking followed by injection of cisplatin directly into the tissue mass on a weekly basis
  - Euthanasia if inoperable

Gastrointestinal tract disorders

Bacterial

- *Vibrio parahaemolyticus* (Oestmann 1985)

Protozoal

- *Cryptosporidium* (tangs, sygnathids)
- *Eimeria sygnathi* and *E. phillopterycis* (sygnathids)

Parasitic

- Tapeworms
  - *Tetraphyllidea*
  - *Spathebothriidea*
  - *Trypanorhyncha*
  - *Pseudophyllidea*
- Nematodes
  - *Spirocamallanus*
  - *Cucullanus*
  - *Camallanus*

Nutritional

- Inappropriate feeding

Neoplasia

- Intestinal carcinoma in sygnathids (LePage et al 2014)

Other noninfectious problems

- Overgrowth of incisor teeth in pufferfish, parrotfish, and trigger fish
- Foreign body
- Air ingestion by neonatal seahorses

Findings on clinical examination

- Weight loss, poor growth, swollen abdomen (tapeworms)
- A cluster of worms protruding from the anus of an infested fish often accompanied by extensive damage and erosion around this area *(Spirocamallanus)*; also weight loss, failure to thrive, stringy or slimy feces, and a susceptibility to secondary infections, including tail and fin rot
- Weight loss, regurgitation, undigested food in feces, and anorexia in tangs *(Cryptosporidium)*
- Chronic weight loss in pufferfish, triggerfish, or parrotfish; appetite still good, difficulty feeding (incisor overgrowth)
- Hemorrhagic feces, reddening around cloaca; also erythematous skin lesions and boil-like lesions following septicemia *(Vibrio parahaemolyticus)*
- Swollen coelom, lethargy (foreign body, inappropriate nutrition, neoplasia, egg retention—see *Reproductive Disorders*)
- Neonatal seahorses with gas bubbles visible in their guts; trapped floating at surface

Investigations

1. Fecal examination
2. Anesthetize and examine teeth/buccal cavity

3. Radiography
4. Routine hematology and biochemistry
5. Culture and sensitivity
6. Endoscopy
7. Biopsy
8. Ultrasonography
9. Water quality parameters: Check as a minimum: temperature, ammonia, nitrite, nitrate, and pH values.

Treatment/specific therapy

- *Vibrio parahaemolyticus*
  - Antibiotics
  - Quarantining/removal of infected fish
- *Cryptosporidium nasoris*—no effective treatment
- Tapeworms
  - Praziquantel at 10 mg/L for a 3-hour bath (but see *Neurologic and Swimming Disorders*)
- *Cucullanus, Camallanus,* and *Spirocamallanus*
  - Levamisole at 10 mg/L as a single dose added to the water. This is particularly good for killing larval worms. Suspend carbon filtration.
  - Piperazine at 2.5 mg/g of feed, added to the food. This may only kill adult worms.
  - Fenbendazole at 50 mg/kg body weight added to feed, or by stomach tube if the fish is large enough. Fish are quick to refuse medicated food, so it is best to starve for 24 to 48 hours prior to offering such feed.
  - *Camallanus* has both a direct and indirect life cycle (small crustaceans, such as cyclops act as intermediate hosts).
- Incisor teeth overgrowth
  - Burr back under anesthetic.
  - Offer foods that increase normal wear (e.g., cockles still in shell).
- Inappropriate nutrition
  - Some marine fish fed on foods designed for other fish (e.g., koi foods) can develop a gastric or intestinal bloat and ileus as a result of excessive carbohydrate intake.
  - Starve for 24 to 48 hours.
  - Gavage activated charcoal.
  - Covering antibiosis
- Neoplasia
  - Surgical resection
- Air ingestion in neonatal seahorses
  - Neonatal seahorses are often fed on *Artemia nauplii* (brine shrimp); these larvae are positively phototactic and accumulate at the surface where the light intensity is strongest. Neonatal seahorses accidentally ingest air at the surface while feeding.
  - Cover the surface so as to darken it and light from below and to the side to attract the *Artemia* (and so the neonates) away from the surface.
- Foreign body
  - Retrieval from stomach, possibly with aid of endoscopy
  - Coeliotomy and surgical retrieval

Nutritional disorders

- Hypovitaminosis A
  - Suggested as a cause of HLLD in marine angelfish and tangs (see *Skin Disorders*)
  - Provide either with a commercial vitamin A supplement or offer more vegetable foods (e.g., suchi mori seaweed wraps or lightly boiled greens)
- Highly unsaturated fatty acid (HUFA) deficiency
  - Commonly seen in captive-bred marine fry (e.g., clownfish, *Amphiprion* spp.) fed wholly or largely on unsupplemented brine shrimp *Artemia nauplii*. Jerky spasmic swimming and mass deaths are often triggered by external stimuli such as a loud noise or water change.
  - Supplement with commercially available HUFA products.
- Hepatic lipidosis
  - Frequently seen in large predatory species such as groupers *(Serranidae)* and lionfish (*Pterois* spp.) that are overfed; often exacerbated by the feeding of freshwater fish such as goldfish that are deficient in HUFA
  - Failure to provide appropriate foods

Note: Many marine fish are specialist feeders. Those that prey primarily on coral polyps such as the exquisite butterflyfish *(Chaetodon austriacus)* or sponges (such as the rock beauty *Holocanthus tricolor*) may receive inadequate diets and fail to thrive.

- Underfeeding
  - Some aquarists may deliberately underfeed to reduce the levels of metabolites in reef systems.
- Overfeeding
  - In addition to hepatic lipidosis and other obesity-related problems, overfeeding can cause rapid and dangerous changes in the water quality, particularly triggering falls in the pH and KH.

Findings on clinical examination

- Weight loss
- Inappetence
- Lethargy
- Mass mortality of larvae or fry (HUFA insufficiency)
- Ulcerative lesions on the head and lateral line of marine angelfish, surgeonfish, and tangs

Investigations

1. Review species identification and husbandry.
2. Radiography
3. Routine hematology and biochemistry
4. Culture and sensitivity
5. Endoscopy
6. Biopsy
7. Ultrasonography
8. Water quality parameters: Check as a minimum: temperature, ammonia, nitrite, nitrate, and pH values.
9. Postmortem
   a. Lack of food in stomach/intestines
   b. Loss of body fat

570

Treatment/specific therapy

- Address obvious deficiencies.
- Otherwise as described above

Hepatic disorders

Bacterial
- Hepatitis

Fungal
- Hepatitis

Protozoal
- Myxosporideans (e.g., *Ceratomyxa*, *Myxidium*, *Leptotheca*, and *Sphaeromyxa* spp.)

Nutritional
- Hepatic lipidosis (see *Nutritional Disorders*)

Neoplasia
- Liver neoplasia

Findings on clinical examination

- Weight loss
- Inappetence
- Lethargy

Investigations

1. Radiography
2. Routine hematology and biochemistry
3. Culture and sensitivity
4. Endoscopy
5. Biopsy
   a. Histopathology
      i. Myxosporideans in the gallbladder. Large numbers may affect function of gallbladder
      ii. *Sphaeromyxa* spores in the gallbladder of seahorses (*Hippocampus* spp.—Vincent and Clifton-Hadley 1989)
6. Ultrasonography
7. Water quality parameters: Check as a minimum: temperature, ammonia, nitrite, nitrate, and pH values.

Treatment/specific therapy

- Myxosporideans
  - No treatment. Usually an incidental finding
- Bacterial and fungal hepatitis
  - Treat as for similar infections in *Systemic Disorders*.

Pancreatic disorders

Viral

- Infectious pancreatic necrosis virus—see *Systemic Disorders*

Neoplasia

- Exocrine pancreatic carcinoma in sygnathids (LePage et al 2014)

Cardiovascular and hematologic disorders

Bacterial

- Endocarditis

Protozoal

- Hemoparasites (e.g., *Trypanosoma, Trypanoplasma, Haemogrergarina* spp.—see *Systemic Disorders*

Neoplasia

- Mesothelioma (Shields and Popp 1979)
- Cardiac rhabdomyosarcoma in sygnathids (LePage et al 2014)

Other noninfectious problems

- Cardiomyopathy

Findings on clinical examination

- Anemia, abnormal swellings (*Trypanoplasma* spp.)
- Lethargy
- Anorexia
- Nonspecific signs of ill health

Investigations

1. Radiography
2. Routine hematology and biochemistry
3. Culture and sensitivity
4. Endoscopy
5. Biopsy
6. Ultrasonography
7. Water quality parameters: Check as a minimum: temperature, ammonia, nitrite, nitrate, and pH values.

Treatment/specific therapy

- Hemoparasites
  - Try methylene blue at 60 mg/kg per day PO for 4 days.
  - Metronidazole at 50 mg/kg PO per day
- Bacterial endocarditis
  - Likely to be diagnosed on postmortem
  - Appropriate antibiosis

- Cardiomyopathy
  - Likely to be diagnosed on postmortem

Systemic disorders

Viral

- Infectious pancreatic necrosis virus
- Angelfish encephalitis virus (*Pomacanthus, Holocanthus,* and *Centropyge* spp.—see also *Neurologic and Swimming Disorders*)
- Banggai cardinal iridovirus (BCIV; megalocytivirus) in Banggai cardinalfish (*Pterapogon kauderni*)

Bacterial

- Abnormal swimming, shimmying; may also see hemorrhages, ulceration (bacteremia, septicemia)
- *Mycobacteria,* especially *M. marinum, M. fortuitum,* and *M. cheloni* (fish tuberculosis), especially seahorses (*Hippocampus* spp.—see also *Skin Disorders* and *Musculoskeletal Disorders*)
- *Nocardia asteroides*
- *Renibacterium (Corynebacterium)* spp.

Fungal

- *Ichthyophonus hoferi*—see also *Skin Disorders, Neurologic and Swimming Disorders,* and *Ophthalmic Disorders*

Protozoal

- Hemoparasites—see *Cardiovascular and Hematologic Disorders*

Neoplasia

Other noninfectious problems

- Sudden-onset water quality toxicity; new tank syndrome
- Pouch and systemic emphysema of male seahorses (seahorse gas bubble disease)
- Cyanide toxicity (in recently caught wild marine fish)

Findings on clinical examination

- Sudden darting movements, loss of balance, rapid respiration (poor water quality)
- Anorexia, lethargy, abdominal fluid accumulation, sudden death (infectious pancreatic necrosis virus)
- Weight loss, thickened areas of inflammation, ulceration, fin rot (*Nocardiosis, mycobacteriosis*)
- Loss of balance in male seahorses (*Hippocampus* spp.) accompanied by obviously swollen brood pouch. May float at surface. Emboli may also be found subcutaneously, especially at the tail (Fig. 16-2) (seahorse gas bubble disease)
- Weakness, wasting, and anemia (hemoparasites)
- Lethargy, weight loss, excessive mucus production, loss of balance, and death in marine angelfish (angelfish encephalitis virus)
- Wasting, darkening of skin color, and obvious boil-like swellings in the skin; exophthalmia, abnormal behavior, and abnormal swimming patterns (*Ichthyophonus hoferi*)
- Swollen abdomen, ascites (*Renibacterium* spp.)

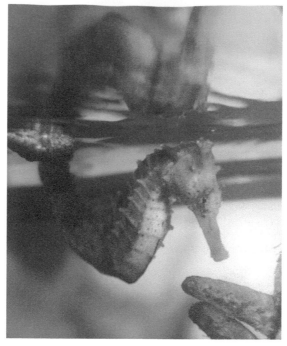

Fig 16-2. Seahorse with systemic emphysema affecting the tail. Note how the tail floats at the surface.

- Anorexia, excessive bright colors, deaths in recently caught fish (cyanide toxicity)
- Banggai cardinalfish: lethargy, darkening of body pigmentation, inappetence, listlessness, increased respiratory rate, white fecal casts, mortalities within 2 days; often mass mortalities (BCIV)

Investigations

1. Radiography
2. Routine hematology and biochemistry
3. Culture and sensitivity
4. Endoscopy
5. Biopsy
6. Ultrasonography
7. Histopathology (BCIV)
8. Assay for cyanide on postmortem
9. Water quality parameters: Check as a minimum: temperature, ammonia, nitrite, nitrate, and pH values.

Treatment/specific therapy

- Water quality problem
  - Identify and address problem.
- Infectious pancreatic necrosis virus: No treatment. Supportive only

- BCIV: No treatment. Isolate and euthanize to confirm diagnosis and prevent transfer to other Banggai cardinalfish.
- Angelfish encephalitis virus: No treatment. Supportive only
- Bacterial disease (bacteremia, septicemia)
  - Antibiotics
- *Nocardiosis*—see *Skin Disorders*
- *Mycobacteriosis*—see *Musculoskeletal Disorders*
- *Ichthyophonus hoferi:* No efficacious treatment available
- Hemoparasites
  - Methylene blue at 60 mg/kg per day PO for 4 days
  - Metronidazole at 50 mg/kg PO per day
- Seahorse gas bubble disease (pouch and systemic emphysema of male seahorses)
  - Unknown etiology—often linked to subclinical mycobacteriosis, metabolic disturbances, and occasionally brood pouch infections
  - Gently release trapped air from brood pouch. For systemic emphysema aspirate gas from obvious gas pockets.
  - Acetazolamide. Three treatment options:
    - 2 to 3 mg/kg IM every 5 to 7 days for up to 3 treatments
    - Flush the brood pouch with an acetazolamide solution daily for 3 days.
    - 2 to 4 mg/L as a 24-hour treatment over 3 consecutive days. Perform a 100% water change between treatments. *Note:* Acetazolamide may temporarily affect both vision (Fairbanks et al 1974) and balance (Beier et al 2002), potentially giving rise to apparent inappetence.
  - High-pressure treatment (exposing affected seahorses to great depth) has been successful in curing this condition.
  - Antibiotics if appropriate
  - In *H. erectus*, incidence of seahorse gas bubble disease was lowest at 26° C rather than 23° C, which may support a metabolic etiology (Lin et al 2010). Therefore, reassess environmental parameters, including preferred temperature range.
- Cyanide toxicity
  - No effective treatment—supportive therapy only

Musculoskeletal disorders

Bacterial

- *Mycobacteria*, especially *M. marinum, M. fortuitum,* and *M. cheloni* (fish tuberculosis—see also *Skin Disorders* and *Systemic Disorders*)

Parasitic

- Tapeworms—see *Gastrointestinal Tract Disorders*

Neoplasia
Other noninfectious problems

- Electrocution (Pasnik et al 2003)
- Idiopathic myopathy of seahorses *(H. kuda)*—LePage et al 2014)

Findings on clinical examination

- Spinal curvature, ulceration, weight loss (mycobacteriosis, electrocution)
- Chronic weight loss, skin ulceration (mycobacteriosis)

- Weight loss (mycobacteriosis, tapeworms)
- Sudden multiple mortalities (electrocution)

Investigations

1. Check electrical equipment for faults.
2. Radiography
   a. Vertebral fractures (electric shock)
3. Routine hematology and biochemistry
4. Culture and sensitivity
5. Endoscopy
6. Biopsy
7. Ultrasonography
8. Water quality parameters: Check as a minimum: temperature, ammonia, nitrite, nitrate, and pH values.

Treatment/specific therapy

- Mycobacteriosis
  - Antibiotic treatment not very effective
  - Kanamycin at 50 mg/L every 48 hours for four treatments was successful in guppies (Conroy and Conroy 1999).
  - Consider euthanasia, especially because of zoonotic risk.
- Electrocution
  - No specific treatment

Neurologic and swimming disorders

Viral

- Angelfish encephalitis rhabdovirus (*Pomacanthus, Holocanthus,* and *Centropyge* spp.—see also *Systemic Disorders*)

Bacterial

- CNS infection/granuloma
- *Eubacterium tarantellus*

Fungal

- *Ichthyophonus hoferi*—see also *Skin Disorders, Ophthalmic Disorders,* and *Systemic Disorders*
- Central nervous system infection/granuloma

Protozoal

- *Septemcapsula plotosi (Myxosporidea)* in coral catfish *(Plotosus anguillaris)*

Nutritional

- HUFA deficiency—see *Nutritional Disorders*

Neoplasia

Other noninfectious problems

- Sudden-onset water quality problem; new tank syndrome
  - Ammonia toxicity—see also *Respiratory Tract Disorders*

- Abnormal swimbladder functioning secondary to compression from internal space-occupying lesions (e.g., neoplasia)
- Swimbladder torsion
- Praziquantel toxicity
- Nicotine toxicity
- Heavy metal poisoning

Findings on clinical examination

- Sudden darting movements, loss of balance, rapid respiration (water quality problem)
- Lethargy, weight loss, excessive mucus production, loss of balance, and death in marine angelfish (angelfish encephalitis virus)
- Abnormal behavior and swimming patterns *(Ichthyophonus)*; also wasting, darkening of skin color, and obvious boil-like swellings in the skin (exophthalmia)
- Spasmic, jerky swimming movements accompanied by sudden mass deaths in captive-bred marine fish (e.g., clownfish) fed wholly or largely on brine shrimp *Artemia nauplii* (Ω-3-fatty acid deficiency)
- Whirling behavior, death in coral catfish *(Septemcapsula)*
- Stiffened pectoral fins, muscular spasms (nicotine toxicity)

Investigations

1. Radiography
2. Routine hematology and biochemistry
3. Culture and sensitivity
4. Endoscopy
5. Biopsy
6. Ultrasonography
7. Water quality parameters: Check as a minimum: temperature, ammonia, nitrite, nitrate, and pH values.

Treatment/specific therapy

- Water quality problem
  - Identify and address problem.
  - Ammonia toxicity
    - Partial water changes to dilute the ammonia levels
    - Longer term control may include addition of commercially available *Nitrosomonas* bacterial cultures or equivalent
- Angelfish encephalitis rhabdovirus: No treatment. Supportive only
- *Ichthyophonus hoferi:* No efficacious treatment available
- Swimbladder torsion
  - Surgical correction
- CNS infection/granuloma
  - Attempt antibiotic or antimycotic treatment. Poor prognosis
- *Eubacterium tarantellus*
  - Antibiotic therapy
- *Septemcapsula plotosi*
  - No effective treatment

- Praziquantel toxicity
  - Terminate treatment.
- Nicotine toxicity
  - No direct treatment. Situate air pumps away from smoky atmospheres.
- Heavy metal poisoning
  - Partial water changes
  - Remove possible sources (e.g., piping, equipment not designed for marine aquaria, such as central heating pumps).

Ophthalmic disorders

Bacterial
- Bacterial granuloma
- Uveitis

Fungal
- Fungal granuloma
- *Ichthyophonus hoferi*—see also *Skin Disorders, Neurologic and Swimming Disorders,* and *Systemic Disorders*
- Uveitis

Protozoal
- *Cryptocaryon*
- *Henneguya*

Nutritional
- Lipid keratopathy (in green moray eels; see Greenwell and Vainisi 1994)
- Riboflavin deficiency
- Ascorbic acid deficiency
- Hypovitaminosis A

Neoplasia
- Thyroid neoplasia
- Lymphoma

Other noninfectious problems
- Blindness secondary to exposure to excessive bright light in nocturnal species, especially lionfish (*Pterois* and *Dendrochirus* spp.)
- Gas bubble disease—see also *Skin Disorders, Reproductive Disorders,* and *Systemic Disorders*
- Trauma (Carrillo et al 1999)
- Cardiomyopathy

Findings on clinical examination

- Blindness (may present as inability to locate food in predatory species)
- Cataracts
- Exophthalmos
- Exophthalmia accompanied by wasting, darkening of skin color, and obvious boil-like swellings in the skin; abnormal behavior and abnormal swimming patterns if the CNS is invaded (*Ichthyophonus*)

- Glaucoma, usually secondary to intraocular disease
- Gas bubbles around and behind eye (gas bubble disease)

Investigations

1. Ophthalmic examination (under sedation/general anesthesia)
2. Radiography
3. Routine hematology and biochemistry
4. Culture and sensitivity
5. Endoscopy
6. Biopsy
7. Ultrasonography
8. Water quality parameters: Check as a minimum: temperature, ammonia, nitrite, nitrate, and pH values.

Treatment/specific therapy

- Bacterial or fungal uveitis
  - Appropriate antibiosis
  - Enucleation
- Gas bubble disease
  - If only eyes affected (frequently in seahorses), consider acetazolamide:
    - 2 to 3 mg/kg IM every 5 to 7 days for up to 3 treatments
    - 2 to 4 mg/L as a 24-hour treatment over 3 consecutive days. Perform a 100% water change between treatments. *Note:* Acetazolamide may temporarily affect vision, giving rise to apparent inappetence.
  - Species other than seahorses: Likely to be connected to supersaturation of water—see *Skin Disorders*
- Blindness secondary to excessive exposure to bright light
  - Reduce lighting levels.
  - Supplement with vitamin A.
- *Ichthyophonus hoferi*
  - No efficacious treatment available
- Glaucoma
  - Enucleation
- Lipid keratopathy
  - Keratoplasty; see Greenwell and Vainisi 1994

Anorexia
• •

See "Anorexia" in Chapter 15.

Endocrine disorders
• •

Neoplasia
- Thyroid adenoma
- Thyroid adenocarcinoma (Blasiola et al 1981)

Other noninfectious problems

- Goiter (hypothyroidism) in marine elasmobranchs

Findings on clinical examination

- Swelling in the thyroid region (especially visible in sharks and rays)

Investigations

1. Radiography
2. Routine hematology and biochemistry
   a. Blood thyroid levels (Table 16-4)

Table 16-4	Blood thyroid levels
Species	**Total T_4 (µg/dL)**
Dusky shark (Carcharinus obscurus)	4.5
Scalloped hammerhead shark (Sphyrna lewini)	2.9
Sharpnose shark (Scoliodon terraenovae)	2.9
Adapted from Stoskopf (1993).	

3. Culture and sensitivity
4. Endoscopy
5. Biopsy
6. Ultrasonography
7. Water quality parameters
   a. Check as a minimum: Temperature, ammonia, nitrite, nitrate, and pH values.
   b. High nitrate levels antagonize iodine uptake.

Treatment/specific therapy

- Goiter
  - Supplement with dietary iodine at 20 µg/kg PO or IM every 48 hours.
  - Reduce nitrate levels to below 40 mg/L, preferably below 10 mg/L.
- Thyroid adenoma
  - May require surgery but likely to be technically very difficult.

Urinary disorders

Bacterial

- Renibacterium spp. (Corynebacterium)

Fungal

Protozoal

- Myxosporidea

Neoplasia

- Renal adenoma, renal adenocarcinoma, renal round cell tumor in sygnathids (LePage et al 2014)

Other noninfectious problems

Findings on clinical examination

- Swollen body, ascites (*Renibacterium* spp.)
- Nonspecific signs of ill health, including anorexia and lethargy

Investigations

1. Radiography
2. Routine hematology and biochemistry
3. Culture and sensitivity
4. Endoscopy
5. Biopsy
6. Ultrasonography
7. Water quality parameters: Check as a minimum: temperature, ammonia, nitrite, nitrate, and pH values.

Treatment/specific therapy

- *Renibacterium*
  - Appropriate antibiosis
  - Reduce salinity to 1.020 to reduce osmotic stress.
- *Myxosporidea*
  - No effective treatment, but see *Skin Disorders*

Reproductive disorders

See *Reproductive Disorders* in Chapters 14 and 15.

Noninfectious problems

- Pouch emphysema of seahorses—see *Systemic Disorders*
- Egg retention—see *Reproductive Disorders* in Chapters 14 and 15.

Bibliography

Chapter 1

Batchelder M A, Bell J A, Erdman S E et al 1999 Pregnancy toxaemia in the European ferret *(Mustela putorius furo)*. Lab Anim Sci 49(4):372–379

Beck W 2007 Ectoparasites, endoparasites, and heartworm control in small animals. Comp Cont Edu Vet 29(5 A):3–8

Bell J A 1997 Periparturient and neonatal diseases. In: Hillyer E V, Quesenberry K E (eds) Ferrets, rabbits, and rodents, 1st ed. Saunders, Philadelphia, p 60

Brown S A 1997 Neoplasia. In: Hillyer E V, Quesenberry K E (eds) Ferrets, rabbits, and rodents, 1st ed. Saunders, Philadelphia, p 108

Bublot I B, Randolph R W, Chalvet-Monfrey K et al 2006 The surface electrogram in domestic ferrets. J Vet Card 8:87–93

Erdman S E, Kanki P J, Moore F M et al 1996 Clusters of lymphoma in ferrets. Cancer Invest 14(3):225–230

Erdman S E, Reimann K A, Moore F M et al 1995 Transmission of a chronic lymphoproliferative syndrome in ferrets. Lab Invest 72(5):539–546

Govorkova E A, Rehg J E, Krauss S et al 2005 Lethality to ferrets of H5N1 influenza viruses isolated from humans and poultry in 2004. J Virol 79(4):2191–2198

Hanley C S, Wilson G H, Frank P et al 2004 T cell lymphoma in the lumbar spine of a domestic ferret *(Mustela putorius furo)*. Vet Rec 155(11):329–332

Helm J R, Morgan E R, Jackson M W et al 2010 Canine angiostrongylosis: an emerging disease in Europe. J Vet Emerg Crit Care (San Antonio) 20(1):98–109

Hillyer E V 1997 Urogenital diseases. In: Hillyer E V, Quesenberry K E (eds) Ferrets, rabbits, and rodents, 1st ed. Saunders, Philadelphia, p 47

Johnson-Delaney C A, Nelson W B 1992 A rapid procedure for filling fractured canine teeth of ferrets. J Small Exot Anim Med 1(3):100–102

Keeble E 2001 Endocrine diseases in small mammals. In Pract 23(10):570–585

Larsen K S, Siggurdsson H, Mencke N 2005 Efficacy of imidacloprid, imidacloprid/permethrin and phoxim for flea control in the Mustelidae (ferrets, mink). Parasitol Res 97:S107–S112

Lu D, Lamb C R, Patterson-Kane J C et al 2004 Treatment of a prolapsed lumbar intervertebral disc in a ferret. JSAP 45(10):501–503

Lunn J A, Martin P, Zaki S et al 2005 Pneumonia due to *Mycobacterium abscessus* in two domestic ferrets *(Mustela putorius furo)*. Aust Vet J 83(9):542–546

Malik R, Alderton B, Finlaison D et al 2002 Cryptococcus in ferrets: a diverse spectrum of clinical disease. Aust Vet J 80(12):749–755

Manning D D, Bell J A 1990 Lack of detectable blood groups in domestic ferrets: implications for transfusions. J Am Vet Med Assoc 197:84–86

Martorell J, Espada Y, Ramis A 2005 Bilateral adrenalectomy in a ferret *(Mustela putorius furo)* with hyperadrenocortism. Clin Vet Peq Anim 25(3):173–177

Miller D S, Eagle R P, Zabel S et al 2006 Efficacy and safety of selamectin in the treatment of *Otodectes cynotis* infestation in domestic ferrets. Vet Rec 159:748

Montiani-Ferreira F et al 2006 Reference values for ophthalmic diagnostic tests in ferrets. Vet Ophthalmol 9(4):209–213

Moore G E, Glickman N W, Ward M P et al 2005 Incidence of and risk factors for adverse events associated with distemper and rabies vaccine administration in ferrets. J Am Vet Med Assoc 226(6):909–912

Mullen H 1997 Soft tissue surgery. In: Hillyer E V, Quesenberry K E (eds) Ferrets, rabbits, and rodents, 1st ed. Saunders, Philadelphia, p 143

Munday J S, Brown C A, Richey L J 2004 Suspected metastatic coccygeal chordoma in a ferret *(Mustela putorius furo)*. J Vet Diagn Invest 16(5):454–458

NOAH Suprelorin datasheet http://www.noahcompendium.co.uk/Virbac_Limited/Suprelorin_9_4_mg_Implant_for_Dogs_and_Ferrets/-56993.html. Accessed 12/01/2015

Nolte D M, Carberry C A, Gannon K M et al 2002 Temporary tube cystotomy as a treatment for urinary obstruction secondary to adrenal disease in four ferrets. J Am Anim Hosp Assoc 38:527–532

Orcutt C J 1998 Emergency and critical care of ferrets. In Critical Care. Vet Clin North Am Exot Anim Pract 1(1):99–126

Patterson M M, Rogers A B, Schrenzel M D et al 2003 Alopecia attributed to neoplastic ovarian tissue in two ferrets. Comp Med 53(2):213–217

Sasai H, Kato K, Sasaki T et al 2000 Echocardiographic diagnosis of dirofilariasis in a ferret. JSAP 41: 172–174

Schoemaker N J, Mol J A, Lumeij J T et al 2003 Effects of anaesthesia and manual restraint on the plasma concentrations of pituitary and adrenocortical hormones in ferrets. Vet Rec 152:591–595

Schoemaker N J, van der Hage M H, Flik G et al 2004 Morphology of the pituitary gland in ferrets *(Mustela putorius furo)* with hyperadrenocortism. J Comp Path 130:255–265

Schoemaker N J, Teerds K J, Mol J A et al 2002 The role of luteinizing hormone in the pathogenesis of hyperadrenocortism in neutered ferrets. Mol Cell Endocrinol 197:117–125

Stamoulis M E, Miller M S, Hillyer E V 1997 Cardiovascular diseases. In: Hillyer E V, Quesenberry K E (eds) Ferrets, rabbits, and rodents, 1st ed. Saunders, Philadelphia, p 66

Stepien R L, Benson K G, Forrest L J 1999 Radiographic measurement of cardiac size in normal ferrets. Vet Radiol Ultrasound 40(6):606–610

Une Y, Wakimoto Y, Nakano Y et al 2000 Spontaneous Aleutian disease in a ferret. J Vet Med Sci 62(5):553–555

Wagner R A, Piche C A, Jochle W et al 2005 Clinical and endocrine responses to treatment with deslorelin acetate implants in ferrets with adrenocortical disease. Am J Vet Res 66(5):910–914

Chapter 2

Beck W 2007 Ectoparasites, endoparasites, and heartworm control in small mammals. Comp Cont Edu Vet 29(5A):3–8

Biricik H S, Oguz H, Sindak N et al 2005 Evaluation of the Schirmer and phenol red thread tests for measuring tear secretion in rabbits. Vet Rec 156:485–487

Bonvehi C, Ardiaca M, Barrera S et al 2014 Prevalence and types of hyponatraemia, its relationship with hyperglycaemia and mortality in ill pet rabbits. Veterinary Record doi: 10.1136/vr.102054

Boucher S, Gracia E, Villa A et al 2001 Pathogens in the reproductive tract of farm rabbits. Vet Rec 149:677–678

Brown S A 1997 Neoplasia. In: Hillyer E V, Quesenberry K E (eds) Ferrets, rabbits, and rodents, 1st ed. Saunders, Philadelphia, p 108

Coletti M, Passamonti F, Del Rossi E 2001 *Klebsiella pneumoniae* infection in Italian rabbits. Vet Rec 149:626–627

Fontes-Sousa A P N, Brás-Silva C, Moura C et al 2006 M-mode and Doppler echocardiographic reference values for male New Zealand white rabbits. Am J Vet Res 67(10):1725–1729

Gómez L, Gázquez A, Roncero V et al 2002 Lymphoma in a rabbit: histopathological and immunohistochemical findings. J Small Anim Pract 43:224–226

González-Gil A, Silván G, García-Partida P et al 2006 Serum glucocorticoid concentrations after halothane and isoflurane anaesthesia in New Zealand white rabbits. Vet Rec 159:51–52

Greig A, Stevenson K, Perez V et al 1997 Paratuberculosis in wild rabbits *(Oryctolagus cuniculus)*. Vet Rec 140:141–143

Hack R J, Walstrom D J, Hair J A 2002 Efficacy and safety of two different dose rates of selamectin against natural infestations of *Psoroptes cuniculi* in rabbits. Clinical Research Abstracts presented at BSAVA Congress 2001. J Small Anim Pract 43:ix

Harcourt-Brown F M, Harcourt-Brown S F 2012 Clinical value of blood glucose measurement in pet rabbits. Veterinary Record doi: 10.1136/vr.100321

Hulbert A J 2000 Thyroid hormones and their effects: a new perspective. Biol Rev 75:519–631

Jass A, Matiasek K, Henke J et al 2008 Analysis of cerebrospinal fluid in healthy rabbits and rabbits with clinically suspected encephalitozoonosis. Vet Rec 162(19):618–622

Lennox A M, Chitty J 2006 Adrenal neoplasia and hyperplasia as a cause of hypertestosteronism in two rabbits. J Exot Pet Med 15(1):56–58

Mancinelli E, Keeble E, Richardson J et al 2014 Husbandry risk factors associated with hock pododermatitis in UK pet rabbits *(Oryctolagus cuniculus)*. Veterinary Record doi: 10.1136/vr.101830

Marini R P, Li X, Harpster N K et al 1999 Cardiovascular pathology possibly associated with ketamine/xylazine anaesthesia in Dutch belted rabbits. Lab Anim Sci 49:153–160

Miwa Y, Mochiduki M, Nakayama H et al 2006 Apocrine adenocarcinoma of possible sweat gland origin in a male rabbit. J Small Anim Pract 47:541–544

Pinter L 1999 *Leporacarus gibbus* and *Spilopsyllus cuniculi* infestation in a pet rabbit. J Small Anim Pract 40:220–221

Pizzi R, Hagan R U, Meredith A L 2007 Intermittent colic and intussusception due to a caecal polyp in a rabbit. J Exot Pet Med 16(2):113–117

Reusch B 2005 Investigation and management of cardiovascular disease in rabbits. In Pract 27:418–435

Reusch B, Boswood A 2003 Electrocardiography of the normal domestic pet rabbit (Abstract). J Small Anim Pract 44:514

Richardson V 2001 Rabbits. The digestive system. UK Vet 6(4):72–76

Sanchez-Migallon D G, Mayer J, Gould J et al 2006 Radiation therapy for the treatment of thymoma in rabbits (Oryctolagus cuniculus). J Exot Pet Med 15(2):138–144

Vangeel I, Pasmans F, Vanrobaeys M et al 2000 Prevalence of dermatophytes in asymptomatic guinea pigs and rabbits. Vet Rec 146:440–441

Weisbroth S H, Flatt R E, Krauss A L (eds) 1974 The Biology of the Laboratory Rabbit. Academic Press, New York

Whitbread T J, Genovese L, Hargreaves J et al 2002 Sebaceous adenitis in the rabbit, a presentation of three cases and comparison with sebaceous adenitis in the dog and the cat. Clinical Research Abstracts presented at BSAVA Congress 2001. J Small Anim Pract 43:ix

White R N 2001 Management of calcium ureterolithiasis in a French Lop rabbit. J Small Anim Pract 42:595–598

Chapter 3

Azuma Y, Maehara K, Tokunaga T et al 1999 Systemic effects of the occlusal destruction in guinea pigs. In Vivo 13(6):519–524

Beck W 2007 Ectoparasites, endoparasites, and heartworm control in small mammals. Comp Cont Edu Vet 29(5A):3–8

Castro M I, Alex S, Young R A et al 1986 Total and free serum thyroid hormone concentrations in fetal and adult pregnant and non-pregnant guinea pigs. Endocrinology 118:533–537

Crossley D A 2001 Dental disease in chinchillas in the UK. J Small Anim Pract 42(1):12–19

Fehr M 2014 Dental diseases in small mammals. British Veterinary Zoological Society Proceedings of the Spring Meeting 2014. 15-17

Fujieda K, Goff A K, Pugeat M et al 1982 Regulation of the pituitary-adrenal axis and corticosteroid-binding globulin–cortisol interaction in the guinea pig. Endocrinology 111:1944–1950

Hammer M, Klopfleisch R, Teifke J P et al 2005 Cavernous or capillary haemangioma in two unrelated guinea pigs. Vet Rec 157:352–353

Huerkamp M J, Murray K A, Orosz S E 1996 Guinea pigs. In: Laber-Laird K, Swindle M, Flecknell P (eds) Handbook of rodent and rabbit medicine. Pergamon, Oxford

Keeble E 2001 Endocrine diseases in small mammals. In Pract 23(10):570–585

Kenagy G J, Veloso C, Bozinovic F 1999 Daily rhythms of food intake and feces reingestion in the degu, an herbivorous Chilean rodent: optimizing digestion through coprophagy. Physiol Biochem Zool 72(1):78–86

Kimoto A 1993 Change in trigeminal mesencephalic neurons after teeth extraction in guinea pig [Abstract, in Japanese]. Kokubyo Gakkai Zasshi 60(1):199–212

Linde A, Summerfield N J, Johnston M et al 2004 Echocardiography in the chinchilla. J Vet Intern Med 18:772–774

Linek M, Bourdeau P 2005 Alopecia in two guinea pigs due to hypopodes of Acarus farris (Acaridae: Astigmata). Vet Rec 157:58–60

Meingassner J G, Burtscher H 1977 Double infection of the brain with Frenkelia species and Toxoplasma gondii in Chinchilla laniger. Vet Pathol 14(2):146–153

Najecki D, Tate B 1999 Husbandry and management of the degu. Lab Anim 28(3):54–62

Nielsen T D, Holt S, Ruelokke M L et al 2003 Ovarian cysts in guinea pigs: influence of age and reproductive status on prevalence and size. J Small Anim Pract 44:257–260

Richardson V C G 2003 Diseases of small domestic rodents, 2nd ed. Blackwell, Oxford

Singh B R, Alam J, Hansda D 2005 Alopecia induced salmonellosis in guinea pigs. Vet Rec 156:516–518

Strake J G, Davis L A, LaRegina M et al 1996 Chinchillas. In: Laber-Laird K, Swindle M, Flecknell P (eds) Handbook of rodent and rabbit medicine. Pergamon, Oxford, p 172

Van Gestel J F E, Engelen M A C M 2004 Comparative efficacy of lufenuron and itraconazole in a guinea pig model of cutaneous Microsporum canis. Free Comm Abst. Session 1: Fungal and Bacterial diseases. Vet Dermatol 15(Suppl 1):20–40

Wasson K, Criley J M, Clabaugh M B et al 2000 Therapeutic efficacy of oral lactobacillus preparation for antibiotic-associated enteritis in guinea pigs. Contemp Top Lab Anim Sci 39(1):32–38

Zeugswetter F, Fenske M, Hassan J et al 2007 Cushing's syndrome in a guinea pig. Vet Rec 160:878–880

Chapter 4

Beck W, Pfister K 2004 Mites as newly emerging disease pathogens in rodents and human beings. Free Comm Abst Vet Dermatol 15(Suppl 1):20–40

Beco L, Petite A, Olivry T 2001 Comparison of subcutaneous ivermectin and oral moxidectin for the treatment of notoedric acariasis in hamsters. Vet Rec 149:324–327

Bowman M R, Pare J A, Pinckney R D 2004 Trichosomoides crassicauda infection in a pet hooded rat. Vet Rec 154:374–375

Fallon M T 1996 Rats and mice. In: Laber-Laird K, Swindle M, Flecknell P (eds) Handbook of rodent and rabbit medicine. Oxford, Pergamon, p 28

Fox M T, Baker A S, Farquhar R et al 2004 First record of *Ornithonyssus bacoti* from a domestic pet in the United Kingdom. Vet Rec 154:437–438

Hulbert A J 2000 Thyroid hormones and their effects: a new perspective. Biol Rev Camb Philos Soc 75:519–631

Jepson L 2004 Management of small rodent emergencies. BSAVA Congress. Scientific Proceedings 39:373–376

Keeble E 2001 Endocrine diseases in small mammals. Practice 23:570–585

Kubiak M, Denk D 2014 Chemotherapy use in a case of dermal lymphoma in a pet rat. Proceedings of the Autumn Meeting 2014, p 25

Laber-Laird K 1996 Gerbils. In: Laber-Laird K, Swindle M, Flecknell P (eds) Handbook of rodent and rabbit medicine. Oxford, Pergamon, p 48

Mehlhorn H, Schmahl G, Frese M et al 2005a Effects of a combination of emodepside and praziquantel on parasites of reptiles and rodents. Parasitol Res 97:S64–S69

Mehlhorn H, Schmahl G, Mevissen I 2005b Efficacy of a combination of imidacloprid and moxidectin against parasites of reptiles and rodents: case reports. Parasitol Res 97:S97–S101

Richardson V C G 2003 Diseases of small domestic rodents, 2nd ed Blackwell, Oxford

Schmidt R E, Reavill D R 2007 Cardiovascular disease in hamsters: review and retrospective study. J Exot Pet Med 16(1):49–51

Chapter 5

Adams A P, Aronson J F, Tardif S D et al 2008 Common marmosets *(Callithrix jacchus)* as a nonhuman primate model to assess the virulence of eastern equine encephalitis virus strains. J Virol 82(18):9035–9042

Brack M, Rothe H 1981 Chronic tubulointerstitial nephritis and wasting disease in marmosets (Callithrixjacchus). Vet Pathol 18:45–54

Chamanza R, Parry N M A, Rogerson P et al 2006 Spontaneous lesions of the cardiovascular system in purpose-bred laboratory nonhuman primates. Toxicol Pathol 34:357–363

Davies J A 1969 Some aspects of the physiology of the anaesthetized marmoset. Lab Anim 3:151–156

Favoretto S R, de Mattos C C, Morais N B et al 2001 Rabies in marmosets *(Callithrix jacchus)*, Ceara, Brazil. Emerg Infect Dis 7(6):1062–1065

Fox J G 2002 Nonhuman primates. In: Fox J G, Anderson L C, Loew F M, et al (eds) Laboratory animal medicine, 2nd ed. Academic Press, New York, p 675–791.

Furr P M, Hetherington C M, Taylor-Robinson D 1979 Ureaplasmas in the marmoset *(Callithrix jacchus)*: Transmission and elimination. J Med Primatol 8(5):321–326

Giannico A T, Somma A T, Lange R R et al 2013 Electrocardiographic values in marmosets *(Callithrix penicillata)*. Pesq Vet Bras 33(7). http://dx.doi.org/10.1590/S0100-736X2013000700016. Accessed 29/03/2015

Gore M A, Brandes F, Kaup F J et al 2001 Callitrichid nutrition and food sensitivity. J Med Primatol 30(3):179–184

Hahn N E, Capuano S V 2010 Successful treatment of cryptosporidiosis in 2 common marmosets *(Callithrix jacchus)* by using paromomycin. J Am Assoc Lab Anim Sci 49(6):873–875

Jarcho M R, Power M L, Layne-Colon D G et al 2013 Digestive efficiency mediated by serum calcium predicts bone mineral density in the common marmoset *(Callithrix jacchus)*. Am J Primatol 75(2):153–160

Johnson-Delaney C A 2008 Nonhuman primate dental care. J Exotic Pet Med 17(2):138–143

Juan-Sallés C, Prats N, Resendes A et al 2003 Anemia, myopathy, and pansteatitis in vitamin E-deficient captive marmosets (Callithrix spp). Vet Pathol 40:540–547

Juan-Sallés C, Marco A, Ramos-Vara J A et al 2002 Islet hyperplasia in callitrichids. Primates 43(3):179–190

Kramer J A, Hachey A M, Wachtman L M et al 2009 Treatment of giardiasis in common marmosets *(Callithrix jacchus)* with tinidazole. Comp Med 59(2):174–179

Kramer J A, Grindley J, Crowell A M et al 2015 The common marmoset as a model for the study of nonalcoholic fatty liver disease and nonalcoholic steatohepatitis. Vet Pathol 52(2):404–413

Kuehnel F, Grohmann J, Buchwald U et al 2012 Parameters of haematology, clinical chemistry and lipid metabolism in the common marmoset and alterations under stress conditions. J Med Primatol 41(4):241–250

Kuehnel F, Mietsch M, Buettner T et al 2013 The influence of gluten on clinical and immunological status of common marmosets *(Callithrix jacchus)*. J Med Primatol 42(6):300–309

Lange R R, Lima L, Montiani-Ferreira F 2012 Measurement of tear production in black-tufted marmosets *(Callithrix penicillata)* using three different methods: modified Schirmer's I, phenol red thread and standardized endodontic absorbent paper points. Vet Ophthalmol 15(6):376–382

Lazaro-Perea C, Snowdon C T, Arruda M F 1999 Scent-marking behavior groups of common marmosets *(Callithrix jacchus)*. Behav Ecol Sociobiol 46:313–324

Ludlage E, Mansfield K 2003 Clinical care and diseases of the common marmoset *(Callithrix jacchus)*. Comp Med 53(4):369–382

Mano M T, Potter B J, Belling G B et al 1985 Low-iodine diet for the production of severe I deficiency in marmosets *(Callithrix jacchus jacchus)*. Br J Nutr 4(2):367–372

Miller G F, Barnard D E, Woodward R A et al 1997 Hepatic hemosiderosis in common marmosets, *Callithrix jacchus*: Effect of diet on incidence and severity. Lab Anim Sci 47(2):138–142

Morin M L 1980 Progress report #8 on "Wasting Marmoset Syndrome." HEW, PHS, NIH, Bethesda, Md.

National Research Council (NRC) 1978 Nutrient requirements of nonhuman primates. National Academy of Sciences, Washington, D.C.

Otovic P, Smith S, Hutchinson E 2015 The use of glucocorticoids in marmoset wasting syndrome. J Med Primatol 44(2015):53–59

Power M L, Tardif S D, Layne D G et al 1999 Ingestion of calcium solutions by common marmosets *(Callithrix jacchus)*. Am J Primatol 47:255–261

Smith K M, Calle P, Raphael B L et al 2006 Cholelithiasis in four callitrichid species *(Leontopithecus, Callithrix)*. J Zoo Wildl Med 37(1):44–48

Tardif S D, Power M L, Ross C N et al 2009 Characterization of obese phenotypes in a small nonhuman primate, the common marmoset *(Callithrix jacchus)*. Obesity (Silver Spring) 17(8):1499–1505

Tardif S D, Mansfield K G, Ratnam R et al 2011 The marmoset as a model of aging and age-related diseases. ILAR J 52(1):54–65

Tochitani T, Matsumoto I, Hoshino K et al 2013 Spontaneous rhabdomyosarcoma in a common marmoset *(Callithrix jacchus)*. J Toxicol Pathol 26(2):187–191

Turton J A, Ford D J, Bleby J et al 1978 Composition of the milk of the common marmoset *(Callithrix jacchus)* and milk substitutes used in hand-rearing programmes, with special reference to fatty acids. Folia Primatol 29:64–79

Vanselow B A, Pines M K, Bruhl J J et al 2011 Oxalate nephropathy in a laboratory colony of common marmoset monkeys *(Callithrix jacchus)* following the ingestion of *Eucalyptus viminalis*. Vet Rec 169(4):100

Wachtman L M, Pistorio A L, Eliades S et al 2006 Calcinosis circumscripta in a common marmoset *(Callithrix jacchus jacchus)*. J Am Assoc Lab Anim Sci 45(3):54–57

Weber M, Junge R 2000 Identification and treatment of *Moniliformis clarki (Acanthocephala)* in cotton-topped tamarins *(Saguinus oedipus)*. J Zoo Wildl Med 31(4):503 507

Yamada N, Sato J, Kanno T et al 2013 Morphological study of progressive glomerulonephropathy in common marmosets *(Callithrix jacchus)*. Toxicol Pathol 41:1106–1115

Yamaguchi I, Myojo K, Sanada H et al 2013 Spontaneous malignant T cell lymphoma in a young male common marmoset *(Callithrix jacchus)*. J Toxicol Pathol 26(3):301–307

Yokouchi Y, Imaoka M, Sayama A et al 2013 Inflammatory fibroid polyp in the duodenum of a common marmoset *(Callithrix jacchus)*. Toxicol Pathol 41(1):80–85

Ziegler T E, Colman R J, Tardif S D et al 2013 Development of metabolic function biomarkers in the common marmoset, callithrix jacchus. Am J Primatol 75(5):500–508

Ziegler T E, Sosa M E, Peterson L J et al 2013b Using snacks high in fat and protein to improve glucoregulatory function in adolescent male marmosets *(Callithrix jacchus)*. J Am Assoc Lab Anim Sci 52(6):756–762

Zöller M, Mätz-Rensing K, Fahrion A et al 2008 Malignant nephroblastoma in a common marmoset *(Callithrix jacchus)*. Vet Pathol 45(1):80–84

Chapter 6

Augee M L, Raison J K, Hulbert A J 1979 Seasonal changes in membrane lipid transitions and thyroid function in the hedgehog. Am J Physiol 236(6):E589–E593

Benoit-Biancamano M O, D'Anjou M A, Girard C et al 2006 Rib osteoblastic osteosarcoma in an African hedgehog *(Atelerix albiventris)*. J Vet Diagn Invest 18(4):415–418

Black P A, Marshall C, Seyfried A W et al 2011 Cardiac assessment of African hedgehogs *(Atelerix albiventris)*. J Zoo Wildl Med 42(1):49–53

Burballa A, Martinez J, Martorell J 2012 Splenic lymphoma with cerebellar involvement in an African hedgehog *(Atelerix albiventris)*. J Exot Pet Med 21:255–259

Chung T H, Kim H J, Choi U S 2014 Multicentric epitheliotropic T-cell lymphoma in an African hedgehog *(Atelerix albiventris)*. Vet Clin Pathol 43(4):601–604

Delk K W, Eshar D, Garcia E et al 2013 Diagnosis and treatment of congestive heart failure secondary to dilated cardiomyopathy in a hedgehog. J Small Anim Pract 55:174–177

Finkelstein A, Hoover J P, Caudell D et al 2008 Cutaneous epithelioid variant hemangiosarcoma in a captive African hedgehog *(Atelerix albiventris)*. J Exot Pet Med 17(1):49–53

Fukuzawa R, Fukuzawa K, Abe H et al 2004 Acinic cell carcinoma in an African pygmy hedgehog *(Atelerix albiventris)*. Vet Clin Pathol 33(1):39–42

Ghaffari M S, Hajikhani R, Sahebjam F et al 2012 Intraocular pressure and Schirmer tear test results in clinically normal long-eared hedgehogs *(Hemiechinus auritus)*: Reference values. Vet Ophthalmol 15(3):206–209

Graczyk T K, Cranfield M R, Dunning C et al 1998 Fatal cryptosporidiosis in a juvenile captive African hedgehog *(Ateletrix albiventris)*. J Parasitol 84(1):178–180

Hallam S L, Mzilikazi N 2011 Heterothermy in the southern African hedgehog, *Atelerix frontalis*. J Comp Physiol [B] 181:437–445

Han J-I, Lee S-J, Jang H-J et al 2011 Isolation of *Staphylococcus simulans* from dermatitis in a captive African pygmy hedgehog. J Zoo Wildl Med 42(2):277–280

Hedley J, Benato L, Fraga G et al 2013 Congestive heart failure due to endocardiosis of the mitral valves in a African pygmy hedgehog. J Exot Pet Med 22:212–217

Helmer P J 2000 Abnormal hematologic findings in an African hedgehog *(Atelerix albiventris)* with gastrointestinal lymphosarcoma. Can Vet J 41(6):489–490

Juan-Sallés C, Raymond J T, Garner M M et al 2006 Adrenocortical carcinoma in three captive African hedgehogs *(Atelerix albiventris)*. J Exot Pet Med 15(4):278–280

Kim K R, Ahn K S, Oh D S et al 2012 Efficacy of a combination of 10% imidacloprid and 1% moxidectin against *Caparinia tripilis* in African pygmy hedgehog *(Atelerix albiventris)*. Parasit Vectors 7(5):p158

Kim H J, Kim Y B, Park J W et al 2010 Recurrent sebaceous carcinoma in an African hedgehog *(Atelerix albiventris)*. J Vet Med Sci 72(7):947–949

Kváč M, Hofmannová L, Hlásková L et al 2014a *Cryptosporidium erinacei* n. sp. (Apicomplexa: Cryptosporidiidae) in hedgehogs. Vet Parasitol 201(12):9–17

Kváč M, Sakovác K, Květoňováa D et al 2014b Gastroenteritis caused by the *Cryptosporidium* hedgehog genotype in an immunocompetent man. J Clin Microbiol 52(1):347–349

Lee S-Y, Park H-M 2012 Gastroeosphageal intussusception with megaesophagus in a hedgehog *(Atelerix albiventris)*. J Exot Pet Med 21:168–171

Madarame H, Ogihara K, Kimura M et al 2014 Detection of a pneumonia virus of mice (PVM) in an African hedgehog *(Atelerix arbiventris)* with suspected wobbly hedgehog syndrome (WHS). Vet Microbiol 173(1–2):136–140

Martínez L S, Juan-Sallés C, Cucchi-Stefanoni K et al 2005 *Actinomyces naeslundii* infection in an African hedgehog *(Atelerix albiventris)* with mandibular osteomyelitis and cellulitis. Vet Rec 157(15):450–451

Miller D L, Styer E L, Stobaeus J K et al 2002 Thyroid-C-cell carcinoma in an African Pygmy hedgehog *(Atelerix albiventrix)*. J Zoo Wildl Med 33(4):392–396

Moreira A, Troyo A, Calderón-Arguedas O 2013 First report of acariasis by *Caparinia tripilis* in African hedgehogs, *(Atelerix albiventris)*, in Costa Rica. Rev Bras Parasitol Vet 22(1):155–158

Pantchev N, Hofmann T 2006 Notoedric mange caused by *Notoedres cati* in a pet African pygmy hedgehog *(Atelerix albiventris)*. Vet Rec 158:59–60

Pei-Chi H, Yu J-F, Wang L-C 2015 A retrospective study of the medical status on 63 African hedgehogs *(Atelerix albiventris)* at the Taipei Zoo from 2003 to 2011. J Exot Pet Med 24(1):105–111

Phair K, Carpenter J W, Marrow J et al 2011 Management of an extraskeletal osteosarcoma in an African hedgehog *(Atelerix albiventris)*. J Exot Pet Med 20(2):151–155

Raymond J T, Aguilar R, Dunker F et al 2009 Intervertebral disc disease in African hedgehogs *(Atelerix albiventris)*: Four cases. J Exot Pet Med 18(3):220–223

Raymond J T, Garner M M 2000 Cardiomyopathy in captive African hedgehogs *(Atelerix albiventris)*. J Vet Diagn Invest 12(5):468–472

Rhody J L, Schiller C A 2006 Spinal osteosarcoma in a hedgehog with pedal self-mutilation. Vet Clin North Am Exot Anim Pract 9(3):625–631

Roh Y-S, Kim E J, Cho A et al 2014 Chylous ascites in a hedgehog *(Atalerix albiventris)*. J Zoo Wildl Med 45(4):951–954

Snider T A, Joyner P H, Clinkenbeard K D 2008 Disseminated histoplasmosis in an African pygmy hedgehog. J Am Vet Med Assoc 232(1):74–76

Spugnini E P, Pagotto A, Zazzera F et al 2008 Cutaneous T-cell lymphoma in an African hedgehog *(Atelerix albiventris)*. In Vivo 22(1):43–45

Webster W M 1957 Susceptibility of the hedgehog *(Erinaceus europaeus)* to infection with *Leptospira pomona*. Nature 80(4598):1372

Wheler C L, Grahn B H, Pocknell A M 2001 Unilateral proptosis and orbital cellulitis in eight African hedgehogs *(Atelerix albiventris)*. J Zoo Wildl Med 32(2):236–241

Wolff C F, Corradini P R, Cortés G 2005 Congenital erythropoietic porphyria in an African hedgehog *(Atelerix albiventris)*. J Zoo Wildl Med 36(2):323–325

Chapter 7

Bradley A J, Stoddart D M 1990 Metabolic effects of cortisol, ACTH, adrenalin and insulin in the marsupial sugar glider, *Petaurus breviceps*. J Endocrinol 127:203–212

Brust D M 2009 Sugar gliders. Exotic DVM 11(3):32–41

Brust D M 2013 Gastrointestinal diseases of marsupials. J Exotic Pet Med 22:132–140

Carboni D, Tully T N 2009 Marsupials. In: Mitchell M, Tully T (eds) Manual of Exotic Pet Practice. Saunders Elsevier, St. Louis, p 299–325.

Clauss M, Paglia D E 2012 Iron storage disorders in captive wild mammals: The comparative evidence. J Zoo Wildl Med 43(3):S6–S18

Corriveau L A 2015 Sugar Gliders. Purdue University Veterinary Teaching Hospital. https://www.vet.purdue .edu/vth/files/documents/Sugar%20Gliders.pdf. Accessed 16 March 2015

Dierenfeld E S, Thomas D, Ives R 2006 Comparison of commonly used diets on intake, digestion, growth, and health in captive sugar gliders *(Petaurus breviceps)*. J Exotic Pet Med 15(3):218–224

Endo H, Yokokawa K, Kurohmaru M et al 1998 Functional anatomy of gliding membrane muscles in the sugar glider *(Petaurus breviceps)*. Ann Anat 180(1):93–96

Gallego Agúndez M, Villaluenga Rodríguez J E, Juan-Sallés C et al 2014 First report of parasitism by *Ophidascaris robertsi* (Nematoda) in a sugar glider *(Petaurus breviceps,* Marsupialia). J Zoo Wildl Med 45(4): 984–986

Holloway J C, Geiser F 2000 Development of thermoregulation in the sugar glider *Petaurus breviceps* (Marsupialia: Petauridae). J Zool Lond (2000) 252:389–397

Holloway J C, Geiser F 2001 Seasonal changes in the thermoenergetics of the marsupial sugar glider *(Petaurus breviceps)*. J Comp Physiol B 171:643–650

Hough I, Miller R, Mitchell G et al 1992 Cutaneous lymphosarcoma in a sugar glider. Aust Vet J 69(4):93–94

Jones I H, Stoddart D M, Mallick J 1995 Towards a sociobiological model of depression: A marsupial model *(Petaurus breviceps)*. Br J Psychiatry (1995) 166:47–49

Keller K K, Nevarez J G, Rodriguez D et al 2014 Diagnosis and treatment of anaplastic mammary carcinoma in a sugar glider *(Petaurus breviceps)*. J Exotic Pet Med 23:277–282

Körtner G, Geiser F 2000 Torpor and activity patterns in free-ranging sugar gliders *Petaurus breviceps* (Marsupialia). Oecologia (2000) 123:350–357

Marrow J C, Carpenter J W, Lloyd A et al 2010 AEMV forum: A transitional cell carcinoma with squamous differentiation in a pericloacal mass in a sugar glider *(Petaurus breviceps)*. J Exotic Pet Med 19(1):92–95

Nolan T J, Zhu X, Ketschek A et al 2007 The sugar glider *(Petaurus breviceps)*: A laboratory host for the nematode *Parastrongyloides trichosuri*. J Parasitol 93(5):1084–1089

Parks and Wildlife Commission of the Northern Territory Guidelines for caring for injured and orphaned Gliders. http://parksandwildlife.nt.gov.au/__data/assets/pdf_file/0009/348498/Draft_Guidelines-for-caring -for-Gliders.pdf. Accessed 21 March 2015

Punzo F, Laird A, Pedrosa E 2003 Prenatal protein malnutrition and visual discrimination learning in the sugar glider, *Petaurus breviceps*. J Mammal 84(4):1437–1442, 2003

Rivas A E, Pye G W, Papendick R 2014 Dermal hemangiosarcoma in a sugar glider *(Petaurus breviceps)*. J Exotic Pet Med 23(4):384–388

Spratt D M 2003 *Rilleyella petauri* gen. nov., sp. nov. (Pentastomida : Cephalobaenida) from the lungs and nasal sinus of *Petaurus breviceps* (Marsupialia : Petauridae) in Australia. Parasite (2003) 10:235–241

Stoddart D M, Bradley A J 1991 The frontal and gular dermal scent organs of the marsupial sugar glider *(Petaurus breviceps)*. J Zool Lond 225:1–12

Chapter 8

Barton C E, Phalen D N, Snowden K F 2003 Prevalence of microsporidian spores shed by asymptomatic lovebirds: evidence for a potential emerging zoonosis. J Avian Med Surg 17(4):197–202

Bavelaar F J, Beynen A C 2003 Plasma cholesterol concentrations in African grey parrots fed diets containing psyllium. J Appl Res Vet Med 1:97–104

Bavelaar F J, van der Kuilen J, Hovenier R et al 2005 Plasma lipids and fatty acid composition in parrots in relation to the intake of α-linolenic acid from two feed mixtures. J Anim Physiol Anim Nutr 89:359–366

Berrocal A 2004 Cryptococcal granulomatous dermatitis in an African parrot. ESVD and ACVD Vet Dermatol 15(Suppl 1):68

Casares M, Enders F, Montoya J A 2000 Comparative electrocardiography in four species of macaws (Genera Anodorhynchus and Ara). J Vet Med 47(5):277–281

de Carvalho F M, Gaunt S D, Kearney M T et al 2009 Reference intervals of plasma calcium, phosphorus and magnesium for African grey parrots *(Psittacus erithicus)* and Hispaniolan parrots *(Amazona ventralis)*. J Zoo Wildl Med 40(4):675–679

De Voe R S, Trogdon M, Flammer K 2004 Preliminary assessment of the effect of diet and L-carnitine supplementation on lipoma size and body weight in budgerigars *(Melopsittacus undultatus)*. J Avian Med Surg 18(1):12–18

Diaz-Figueroa O, Garner M M, Tulley T N 2004 What is your diagnosis? J Avian Med Surg 18(1):51–53

Diaz-Figueroa O, Garner M M, Tulley T N 2005 What is your diagnosis? J Avian Med Surg 19(4):313–315

Doneley R J T, Miller R I, Fanning T E 2007 Proventricular dilatation disease: an emerging exotic disease of parrots in Australia. Aust Vet J 85:119–123

Doolan M 1994 Adriamycin chemotherapy in a blue-front Amazon with osteosarcoma. Proc Annu Conf Assoc Avian Vet 88–91

Ferrer L, Ramis A, Fernández J et al 1997 Granulomatous dermatitis caused by *Mycobacterium genavense* in two psittacine birds. Vet Dermatol 8:213–219

Flammer K, Nettifee Osborne J A, Webb D J et al 2008 Pharmacokinetics of voriconazole after oral administration of single and multiple doses in African grey parrots *(Psittacus erithacus timneh)*. Am J Vet Res 69(1):114–121

Flammer K, Trogdon M T, Papich M 2003 Assessment of plasma concentrations of doxycycline in budgerigars fed medicated seed or water. J Am Vet Med Assoc 223:993–998

France M 1993 Chemotherapy treatment of lymphosarcoma in a Moluccan cockatoo. Proc Annu Conf Assoc Avian Vet 15–19

Gancz A Y, Malka S, Sandmeyer L et al 2005 Horner's syndrome in a red-bellied parrot *(Poicephalus rufiventris)*. J Avian Med Surg 19(1):3–34

Garner J P, Meehan C L, Famula T R et al 2005 Genetic, environmental, and neighbor effects on the severity of stereotypies and feather picking in orange-winged Amazon parrots *(Amazona amazonica)*: An epidemiological study. Appl Anim Behav Sci 96(1–2):153–168

Girling S 2003 Diagnosis and management of viral diseases in psittacine birds. In Pract 25:396–407

Girling S 2004 Diseases of the digestive tract of psittacine birds. In Pract 26:146–153

Graham J E, Tell L A, Lamm M G et al 2004 Megacloaca in a moluccan cockatoo *(Cacatua moluccensis)*. J Avian Med Surg 18(1):41–49

Greenacre C B, Young D W, Behrend E N et al 2001 Validation of a novel high-sensitivity radioimmunoassay procedure for measurement of total thyroxine concentration in psittacine birds and snakes. Am J Vet Res 62(11):1750–1754

Gregory C R, Latimer K S, Campagnoli R P et al 1996 Histologic evaluation of the crop for diagnosis of proventricular dilatation syndrome in psittacine bird. J Vet Diagn Invest 8:70–80

Hanley C S, Wilson G H, Latimer K S et al 2005 Interclavicular haemangiosarcoma in a double yellow-headed Amazon parrot *(Amazona ochrocephala oratrix)*. J Avian Med Surg 19(2):130–137

Harcourt-Brown N H 1986 Diseases of birds in quarantine, with special reference to the treatment of *Salmonella typhimurium* by vaccination: A novel technique. Proc Vet Zoo Soc London

Harcourt-Brown N 2004 Development of the skeleton and feathers of dusky parrots *(Pionus fuscus)* in relation to their behaviour. Vet Rec 154:42–48

Hermans K, Devriese L A, De Herdt P et al 2000 *Staphylococcus aureus* infections in psittacine birds. Avian Pathol 29:411–415

Hoppes S, Heatley J J, Guo J et al 2013 Meloxicam treatment in cockatiels *(Nymhicus hollandicus)* infected with avian bornavirus. J Exot Pet Med 22:275–279

Jayson S L, Williams D L, Wood J L N 2014 Prevalence and risk factors of feather plucking in African grey parrots (*Psittacus erithacus erithacus* and *Psittacus erithacus timneh*) and cockatoos (*Cacatua* spp.). J Exot Pet Med 23:250–257

Klaphake E, Beazley-Keane S L, Jones M et al 2006 Multisite integumentary squamous cell carcinoma in an African grey parrot *(Psittacus erithacus erithacus)*. Vet Rec 158:593–596

Krautwald-Junghanns M, Braun S, Pees M et al 2004 Research on the anatomy and pathology of the psittacine heart. J Avian Med Surg 18(1):2–11

Lanteri G, Sfacteria A, Macrì D et al 2011 Penicillinosis in an African grey parrot *(Psittacus erithacus)*. J Zoo Wildl Med 42(2):309–312

Leber A C, Bürge T 1999 A dermoid of the eye in a blue-fronted Amazon parrot *(Amazona aestiva)*. Vet Ophthalmol 2:133–135

Lloyd C 2003 Control of nematode infections in captive birds 2003. In Pract 25:198–206

Malley D 1996 Handling and clinical examination of psittacine birds. In Pract 18:302–311

Mans C 2014 Sedation of pet birds. J Exot Pet Med 23:152–157

Manucy T K, Bennet R A, Greenacre C B et al 1998 Squamous cell carcinoma of the beak in a Buffon's macaw *(Ara ambigua)*. J Avian Med Surg 12:158–166

Meehan C L, Millam J R, Mench J A 2003a Foraging opportunity and increased physical complexity both prevent and reduce psychogenic feather picking by young Amazon parrots. Appl Anim Behav Sci 80:71–85

Meehan C L, Garner J P, Mench J A 2003b Isosexual pair housing improves the welfare of young Amazon parrots. Appl Anim Behav Sci 81:73–88

Meehan C L, Garner J P, Mench J A 2004 Environmental enrichment and development of cage stereotypy in orange-winged Amazon parrots *(Amazona amazonica)*. Dev Psychobiol 44:209–218

Monks D J, Carlisle M S, Carrigan M et al 2005 Angiostrongylus cantonensis. As a cause of cerebrospinal disease in a yellow-tailed black cockatoo *(Calyptorhynchus funereus)* and two tawny Frogmouths *(Podargus strigoides)*. J Avian Med Surg 29(4):289–293

Musulin S E, Adin D B 2006 Vet med today: ECG of the month. J Am Vet Med Assoc 229(4):505–507

Oglesbee B L, Lehmkuhl L 2001 Congestive heart failure associated with myxomatous degeneration of the left atrioventricular valve in a parakeet. J Am Vet Med Assoc 218(3):376–380, 360

Pees M, Schmidt V, Coles B et al 2006 Diagnosis and long-term therapy of a right-sided heart failure in a yellow-crowned Amazon (Amazona ochrocephala). Vet Rec 158:445–447

Phalen D N, Logan K S, Snowden K F 2006 Encephalitozoon hellem infection as the cause of a unilateral chronic keratoconjunctivitis in an umbrella cockatoo (Cacatua alba). Vet Ophthalmol 9:59–63

Philbey A W, Andrew P L, Gestier A W et al 2002 Spironucleosis in Australian king parrots (Alisterus scapularis). Aust Vet J 80(3):154–160

Pizarro M, Höfle U, Rodríguez-Bertos A et al 2005 Ulcerative enteritis (quail disease) in lories. Avian Dis 49:606–608

Polo F J, Peinado V I, Viscor G et al 1998 Hematologic and plasma chemistry values in captive psittacine birds. Avian Dis 42:523–535

Preziosi D E, Morris D O, Johnston M S et al 2006 Distribution of Malassezia organisms on the skin of unaffected psittacine birds and psittacine birds with feather-destructive behavior. J Am Vet Med Assoc 228:216–221

Rees Davies R 2001 Polyuria/polydipsia in parrots. UK VET 6(5):75–80

Rubbenstroth D, Brosinskib K, Rinderb M et al 2014 No contact transmission of avian bornavirus in experimentally infected cockatiels (Nymphicus hollandicus) and domestic canaries (Serinus canaria forma domestica). Vet Microbiol 172(1–2):146–156

Rupiper D J, Carpenter J W, Mashima T Y 2000 Formulary. In: Olsen G H, Orosz S E (eds) Manual of avian medicine. Mosby, Philadelphia, p 560.

Schmidt R E 1997 Immune system. In: Altman R B, Clubb S L, Dorrenstein G M (eds) Avian medicine and surgery. Saunders, Philadelphia, p 645–652.

Shaw S N 2013 Hypocalcaemia. Clinical veterinary advisor: birds and exotic pets. Saunders, p 197–198

Staeheli P, Rinder M, Kaspers B 2010 Avian bornavirus associated with fatal disease in psittacine birds. J Virol 84(13):6269–6275

Stanford M, 2003 Use of interferon to treat circovirus infection in grey parrots. Proceedings of the Autumn Meeting, British/Veterinary Zoological Society 35-36

Stockdale B, 2004 Detecting avian malnutrition-part 2. Veterinary Times 2nd August

Straub J, Pees M, Krautwald Junghanns M 2002 Measurement of the cardiac silhouette in psittacines. J Am Vet Med Assoc 221(1):76–79

Torregrossa A, Puschner B, Tell L et al 2005 Circulating concentrations of vitamins A and E in captive psittacine birds. J Avian Med Surg 19(3):225–229

Van Hoek C S, King C E 1997 Causation and influence of environmental enrichment on feather picking of the crimson bellied conure (Pyrrhura perlata perlata). Zoo Biol 16:161–172

Verstappen F A L M, Dorrestein G M 2005 Aspergillosis in Amazon parrots after corticosteroid therapy for smoke-inhalation injury. J Avian Med Surg 19(2):138–141

Wade L, 2004 Herbal therapy for liver disease: milk thistle (Silybum marianum). AAV Newsletter and Clinical forum: March-May

Werquin G J D L, De Cock K J S, Ghysels P G C 2005 Comparison of the nutrient analysis and calorific density of 30 commercial seed mixtures (in toto and dehulled) with 27 commercial diets for parrots. J Anim Physiol Anim Nutr 89:215–221

Wolf P, Rabehl N, Kamphues J 2003 Investigations on feathering, feather growth and potential influences of nutrient supply on feather's regrowth in small pet birds (canaries, budgerigars and lovebirds). J Anim Physiol Anim Nutr 87:134–141

Zandvliet M M J M, Dorrstein G M, van der Hage M 2001 Chronic pulmonary interstitial fibrosis in Amazon parrots. Avian Pathol 30:517–524

Zenoble R D, Kemppainen R J, Young D W et al 1985 Endocrine responses of healthy parrots to ACTH and thyroid stimulating hormone. J Am Vet Med Assoc 187(11):1116–1118

Chapter 9

Cornelissen H, Ducatelle R, Roels S 1995 Successful treatment of a channel-billed toucan (Rhamphastos vitellinus) with iron storage disease by chelation therapy: sequential monitoring of the iron content of the liver during the treatment period by quantitative chemical and image analyses. J Avian Med Surg 9:131–137

Dorrestein G M 2000 Passerines and exotic softbills. In: Tully T N, Lawton M P C, Dorrestein G M (eds) Avian medicine, 7th ed. Butterworth-Heinemann, Oxford, p 165

Dorrestein G M, Van der Hage M H, Grinwis G 1993 A tumour-like pox lesion in masked bullfinches (Pyrrhula erythaca). Proc 2nd Eur AAV, Utrecht, p 232–240

Gibbens J C, Abraham E J, MacKenzie G 1997 Toxoplasmosis in canaries in Great Britain. Vet Rec 140:370–371

Panigrahy B, Senne D A 1991 Diseases of mynahs. J Am Vet Med Assoc 199(3):378–381

Rodríguez F, Herráez H, Lorenzo H et al 2006 Intracutaneous keratinising epithelioma in a mynah bird (Gracula religiosa). Vet Rec 158:57–58

Rupiper D J, Carpenter J W, Mashima T Y 2000 Formulary. In: Olsen G H, Orosz S E (eds) Manual of avian medicine. Mosby, Philadelphia, p 560

Wade L 2004 Herbal therapy for liver disease: Milk thistle (Silybum marianum) AAV Newsletter and Clinical forum, March-May

Worell A B 1997 Toucans and mynahs. In: Altman R B, Clubb S L, Dorrestein G M (eds) Avian medicine and surgery. Saunders, Philadelphia, p 910–917

Chapter 10

Boyer T H 2002 Autoimmune haemolytic anemia in a Parson's chameleon, Calumma parsonii parsonii. Proc Assoc Reptil Amphib Vet 81–85

Drury S E N, Gough R E, Welschman D de B 2002 Isolation and identification of a reovirus from a lizard, Uromastyx hardwickii, in the United Kingdom. Vet Rec 151:637–638

Girling S J, Fraser M A 2004 Listeria monocytogenes septicaemia in an inland bearded dragon Pogona vitticeps. J Herpet Med Surg 14(3):6–9

Hall A J, Lewbart G A 2006 Treatment of dystocia in a leopard gecko (Eublepharus macularius) by percutaneous ovocentesis. Vet Rec 158:737–739

Hernandez-Divers S J 2006a Advances in reptile renal diagnostics: Identifying changes in renal function, not renal failure. Br Vet Zoo Soc Proc May:70–71

Hernandez-Divers S J 2006b Single-dose oral and intravenous pharmacokinetics of meloxicam in the green iguana (Iguana iguana). Br Vet Zoo Soc Proc May:54–55

Hulbert A J 2000 Thyroid hormones and their effects: A new perspective. Biol Rev 75:519–631

Kenny M J, Shaw S E, Hillyard P D et al 2004 Ectoparasite and haemoparasite risks associated with imported exotic reptiles. Vet Rec 154:434–435

Martin J C, Moore A S, Ruslander D et al 2003 Successful radiation treatment of leukaemia in a sungazer lizard (Cordylus giganteus). Proc Assoc Reptil Amphib Vet 8.

Martinez-Silvestre A, Mateo J A, Pether J 2003 Electrocardiographic parameters in a Gomeran giant lizard (Gallotia bravoana). J Herpet Med Surg 13(3):22–25

Martorell J, Ramis A, Espada Y 2002 Use of ultrasonography in the diagnosis of hepatic spindle-cell sarcoma in a Savannah monitor (Varanus exanthematicus). Vet Rec 150:282–284

McBride M, Koch T F, Hernandez-Divers S et al 2004 Preliminary evaluation of resting and post-prandial bile acid levels and a novel biliverdin assay in the green iguana (Iguana iguana). Proc Assoc Reptil Amphib Vet 105:81–85

Mehlhorn H, Schmahl G, Mevissen I 2005a Efficacy of a combination of imidacloprid and moxidectin against parasites of reptiles and rodents: Case reports. Parasitol Res 97:S97–S101

Mehlhorn H, Schmahl G, Frese M et al 2005b Effects of a combination of emodepside and praziquantel on parasites of reptiles and rodents. Parasitol Res 97:S64–S69

Orós J, Ruiz A, Castro P et al 2002 Immunohistochemical detection of microfilariae of Foleyella species in an Oustalet's chameleon (Furcifer oustaleti). Vet Rec 150:20–22

Patterson-Kane J C, Redrobe S P 2005 Colonic adenocarcinoma in a leopard gecko (Eublepharis macularis). Vet Rec 157:294–295

Scott S, Warwick C 2002 Behavioural problems in a monitor lizard. UK Vet 7(3):73–75

Smith D, Dobson H, Spence E 2001 Gastrointestinal studies in the green iguana: Technique and reference values. Vet Radiol Ultrasound 42(6):515–520

Soldati G, Lu Z H, Vaughan L et al 2004 Detection of mycobacteria and chlamydiae in granulomatous inflammation of reptiles: A retrospective study. Vet Pathol 41:388–397

Stahl S, 2000 Diseases of bearded dragons (Pogona vitticeps). Exotic Animal Medicine and Surgery BSAVA Continuing Education Course 3 November–5th November

Taylor M A, Geach M R, Cooley W A 1999 Clinical and pathological observations on natural infections of cryptosporidiosis and flagellate protozoa in leopard geckos (Eublepharis macularis). Vet Rec 145:695–699

Walter D E, Shaw M 2002 First record of the mite Hirstiella diolii Baker (Prostigmata pterygosomatidae) from Australia, with a revue of mites found on Australian lizards. Aust J Entomol 41(1):30–34

Wellehan J F X, Jarchow J L, Regiardo C et al 2003a A novel herpesvirus associated with hepatic necrosis in a San Esteban chuckwalla, Sauromalus varius. J Herpet Med Surg 13(3):15–19

Wellehan J F X, Johnson A J, Jacobson E R et al 2003b Nested PCR amplification and sequencing of reptile adenoviruses including a novel gecko adenovirus associated with enteritis. Proc Assoc Reptil Amphib Vet 14.

Wellehan J F X, Johnson A J, Jacobson E R et al 2003c Novel herpesviruses associated with stomatitis in lizards. Proc Assoc of Reptil Amphib Vet 57.

Wilson G H, Fontenot D K, Brown C A et al 2004 Pseudocarcinomatous biliary hyperplasia in two green iguanas, *Iguana iguana*. J Herpet Med Surg 14(4):12–18

Chapter 11

Abou-Madi N, Jacobson E R, Buergelt C D et al 1994 Disseminated undifferentiated sarcoma in an Indian rock python *(Python morulus morulus)*. J Zoo Wildl Med 25(1):143–149

Gravendyck M, Marschang R E, Schröder-Gravendyck A S et al 1997 Renal adenocarcinoma in a reticulated python *(Python reticulatis)*. Vet Rec 140:374–375

Greenacre C B, Young D W, Behrend E N et al 2001 Validation of a novel high-sensitivity radioimmunoassay procedure for measurement of total thyroxine concentration in psittacine birds and snakes. Am J Vet Res 62(11):1750–1754

Hernandez-Divers S, Hernandez-Divers S 2001 Diagnostic imaging of reptiles. In Pract 23:370–391

Jacobson E, Origgi F, Heard D et al 2002 An outbreak of chlamydiosis in emerald tree boas *Corallus caninus*. Proc Assoc Reptil Amphib Vet 47–48

Kenny M J, Shaw S E, Hillyard P D et al 2004 Ectoparasite and haemoparasite risks associated with imported exotic reptiles. Vet Rec 154:434–435

Mehlhorn H, Schmahl G, Frese M et al 2005a Effects of a combination of emodepside and praziquantel on parasites of reptiles and rodents. Parasitol Res 97:S64–S69

Mehlhorn H, Schmahl G, Mevissen I 2005b Efficacy of a combination of imidacloprid and moxidectin against parasites of reptiles and rodents: Case reports. Parasitol Res 97:S97–S101

Pees M C, Kiefer I, Ludewig E W et al 2007 Computed tomography of the lungs of Indian pythons *(Python molurus)*. Am J Vet Res 68:428–434

Raiti R, Garner M M, Wojcieszyn J 2002 Lymphocytic leukemia and multicentric T-cell lymphoma in a diamond python, *Morelia spilota spilota*. J Herp Med and Surg 12(1):26–29

Reavil D R, Helmer P, Scmidt R E 2003 Reovirus outbreak in Arizona mountain king snakes *(Lampropeltis pyromelana pyromelana)*. Proc Assoc Reptil Amphib Vet 58–59

Rosenthal K 1994 Chemotherapeutic treatment of a sarcoma in a corn snake. Proc Assoc Reptil Amphib Vet 46

Soldati G, Lu Z H, Vaughan L et al 2004 Detection of mycobacteria and chlamydiae in granulomatous inflammation of reptiles: A retrospective study. Vet Pathol 41:388–397

Stahl S 2000 Reptile obstetrics. *Exotic Animal Medicine and Surgery* BSAVA Continuing Education Course, 3 November–5 November

Stenglein M D, Jacobson E R, Wozniak E J et al 2014 Ball python nidovirus: A candidate etiologic agent for severe respiratory disease in *Python regius*. mBio 5(5):e01484–14

Stenglein M D, Sanders C, Kistler A L et al 2012 Identification, characterization, and in vitro culture of highly divergent arenaviruses from boa constrictors and annulated tree boas: Candidate etiological agents for snake inclusion body disease. mBio 3(4):e00180–12

Valentinuzzi M E, Hoff H E, Geddes L A 1969a Electrocardiogram of the snake: Observations on the electrical activity of the snake heart. J Electrocardiol 2(1):39–50

Valentinuzzi M E, Hoff H E, Geddes L A 1969b Electrocardiogram of the snake: Effect of the location of the electrodes and cardiac vectors. J Electrocardiol 2(3):245–252

Valentinuzzi M E, Hoff H E, Geddes L A 1969c Electrocardiogram of the snake: Intervals and durations. J Electrocardiol 2(4):343–352

Veazey R S, Stewart T B, Snider T G 1994 Ureteritis and nephritis in a Burmese python *(Python morulus bivittatus)* due to *Strongyloides* sp infection. J Zoo Wildl Med 25(1):119–122

Chapter 12

Acierno M J, Mitchell M A, Roundtree M K et al 2006 Effects of ultraviolet radiation on 25-hydroxyvitamin D$_3$ synthesis in red-eared slider turtles *(Trachemys scripta elegans)*. Am J Vet Res 67:2046–2049

Baker B B, Sladky K K, Johnson S M 2011 Evaluation of the analgesic effects of oral and subcutaneous tramadol administration in red-eared slider turtles. J Am Vet Med Assoc 238:220–227

Birkedal R, Gesser H 2004 Effects of hibernation on mitochondrial regulation and metabolic capacities in myocardium of painted turtle *(Chrysemys picta)*. Comp Biochem Physiol 139(Pt A):285–291

Bogard C, Innis C 2008 A simple and inexpensive method of shell repair in *Chelonia*. JHMS 18(1):12–13

Burridge M J, Peter T F, Allan S A et al 2002 Evaluation of safety and efficacy of acaricides for control of the African tortoise tick *(Amblyomma marmoreum)* on leopard tortoises *(Geochelone pardalis)*. J Zoo Wildl Med 33:52–57

Chitty J R 2003 Lead toxicosis in a Greek tortoise *(Testudo graeca)*. Proc Assoc Reptil Amphib Vet 101:16

Cutler S L 2004 Nematode-associated aural abscess in a Mediterranean tortoise, *Testudo graeca*. J Herp Med Surg 14(3):4–5

Divers S J, Lawton M P C, Stoakes L C 1999 Anthelminthic treatment of chelonians. Vet Rec Nov 20:620

Drury S E N, Gough R E, McArthur S et al 1998 Detection of herpesvirus-like and papilloma-like particles associated with diseases of tortoises. Vet Rec 143:639

Fleming G J, Heard D J, Uhl E W et al 2004 Thymic hyperplasia in subadult Galapagos tortoises, *Geochelone nigra*. J Rept Med Surg 14(1):24–27

Frye F L, Williams D L 1995 Self-assessment colour review of reptiles and amphibians. Manson, London, p 30

Garner M M, Raiti P, Bartholomew J L et al 2003 Renal myxozoanosis in two crowned river turtles *(Hardella thurjii, Emydidae)*. Proc Assoc Reptil Amphib Vet 93–95

Giannetto S, Brianti E, Poglayen G et al 2007 Efficacy of oxfendazole and fenbendazole against tortoise *(Testudo hermanni)* oxyurids. Parasitol Res 100(5):1069–1073. [Epub 2006 Nov 21]

González Candela M, Martín Atance P, Seva J et al 2005 Granulomatous hepatitis caused by *Salmonella typhimurium* in a spur-thighed tortoise *(Testudo graeca)*. Vet Rec 157:236–237

Hernandez-Divers S J 2006 Single-dose oral and intravenous pharmacokinetics of meloxicam in the green iguana *(Iguana iguana)*. Br Vet Zoo Soc Proc 106–107

Hernandez-Divers S, Hernandez-Divers S 2001 Diagnostic imaging of reptiles. Practice 23:370–391

Holz R M, Holz P 1995 Electrocardiography in anaesthetised red-eared sliders *(Trachemys scripta elegans)*. Res Vet Sci 58:67–69

Homer B L, Li C, Berry K H et al 2001 Soluble scute proteins of healthy and ill desert tortoises *(Gopherus agassizii)*. Am J Vet Res 62(1):104–110

Hulbert A J 2000 Thyroid hormones and their effects: A new perspective. Biol Rev 75:519–631

Innis C J, Garner M, Tabaka C et al 2003 Clinical and histopathology findings in Sulawesi tortoises *(Indotestudo forstenni)* with necrotizing sinusitis and rhinitis. Proc Assoc Reptil Amphib Vet, Reno, NV 96–100

Jacobson E R, Schumacher J, TelfordJr S R et al 1994 Intranuclear coccidiosis in radiated tortoises *(Geochelone radiata)*. J Zoo Wildl Med 25(1):95–102

Kelly T R, Walton W, Nadelstein B et al 2005 Phacoemulsification of bilateral cataracts in a loggerhead sea turtle *(Caretta caretta)*. Vet Rec 156:774–777

Koelle P, Hoffman R 2002 Urinalysis in European tortoises. Part II. Proc Assoc Rept Amphib Vet 115–117

Knotek Z 2014 Alfaxalone as an induction agent for anaesthesia in terrapins and tortoises. Vet Rec 175:327

Lafortune M, Wellehan J F X, Terrell S P et al 2005 Shell and systemic hyalohyphomycosis in fly river turtles, *Carettochelys insculpta*, caused by *Paecilomyces lilacinus*. J Herp Med Surg 15(2):15–19

Marshang R E, Ruemenapf T H 2002 Virus "X"; characterizing a new viral pathogen in tortoises. Proc Assoc Reptil Amphib Vet, Reno, NV 101–102

Mehlhorn H, Schmahl G, Frese M et al 2005 Effects of a combination of emodepside and praziquantel on parasites of reptiles and rodents. Parasitol Res 97:S64S69

Meyer J 1998 Gastrografin as a gastrointestinal contrast agent in the Greek tortoise *(Testudo hermanni)*. J Zoo Wildl Med 29(2):183–189

Neiffer D L, Lydick D, Burks K et al 2005 Hematologic and plasma biochemical changes associated with fenbendazole administration in Hermann's tortoises *(Testudo hermanni)*. J Zoo Wildl Med 36(4):661–672

Nicasio J, Campillo B, Frye F L 2002 Preliminary report of subepidermal mite infestation in an African spurred tortoise, *Geochelone sulcata*. Proc ARAV 17

Philbey A W 2006 Amoebic enterocolitis and acute myonecrosis in leopard tortoises *(Geochelone pardalis)*. Vet Rec 158:567–569

Philbey A W, Lawrie A M, Taylor D J et al 2006 Lower urinary tract obstruction in a Mediterranean spur-thighed tortoise *(Testudo graeca)* with coxofemoral arthritis. Vet Rec 159:492–495

Pizzi R, Goodman G, Gunn-Moore D et al 2005 *Pieris japonica* intoxication in an African spurred tortoise *(Geochelone sulcata)*. Vet Rec 156:487–488

Redrobe S P, Scudamore C L 2000 Ultrasonographic diagnosis of pericardial effusion and atrial dilation in a spur-thighed tortoise *(Testudo graeca)*. Vet Rec 146:183–185

Rose F L, Koke J, Koehn R 2001 Identification of the aetiological agent for necrotizing scute disease in the Texas tortoise. J Wildl Dis 37:223–228

Sales M J, Ferrer D, Castellà J et al 2003 Myiasis in two Hermann's tortoises *(Testudo hermanni)*. Vet Rec 153:600–601

Sengupta A, Ray P P, Chaudri-Sengupta S et al 2003 Thyroidal modulation following hypo- and hyperthermia in the soft-shelled turtle *Lissemys punctata punctata Bonnoterre*. Eur J Morphol 41(5):149–154

Soldati G, Lu Z H, Vaughan L et al 2004 Detection of mycobacteria and chlamydiae in granulomatous inflammation of reptiles: A retrospective study. Vet Pathol 41:388–397

Taylor S K, Citino S B, Zdziarski J M et al 1996 Radiographic anatomy and barium sulphate transit time of the gastrointestinal tract of the leopard tortoise *(Testudo pardalis)*. J Zoo Wildl Med 27(2):180–186

Werner R E 2003 Parasites in the diamondback terrapin, *Malaclemys terrapin*: A review. J Herp Med and Surg 13(4):5–9

Willer C J, Lewbart G A, Lemons C 2003 Aural abscesses in wild eastern box turtles, *(Terrapene carolina carolina)*, from North Carolina: Aerobic bacterial isolates and distribution of lesions. J Herp Med Surg 13(2):4–9

Chapter 13

Bicknese E J, Cranfield M J 1995 Cyanoacrylate treatment for corneal ulcers in Kokoe-Pa poison dart frogs *(Dendrobates histrionicus)*. Proc Assoc Reptil Amphib Vet 67–73

Crawshaw G J 1998 Amphibian emergency and critical care. Vet Clin North Am Exot Anim Pract 1(1):207–231

D'Agostino J J, West G, Booth D M 2007 Plasma pharmacokinetics of selamectin after a single topical administration in the American bullfrog *(Rana catesbeiana)*. J Zoo Wildl Med 38:51–54

Green S L, Moorhead R C, Bouley D M 2003 Thermal shock in a colony of South African clawed frogs *(Xenopus laevis)*. Vet Rec 152:336–337

Jacobson E R, Robertson D R, Lafortune M et al 2004 Renal failure and bilateral thymoma in an American bullfrog *Rana catesbiana*. J Herpetol Med Surg 14(2):6–11

Mayer J, Martin J C, Garner M M et al 2000 Chromoblastomycosis due to a synanamorph of *Veronaea botryosa* in a colony of White's tree frogs *(Litoria caerula)*. Br Vet Zoo Soc Proc Spring Meeting 11

Minter L J, Clarke E O, Gjeltema J L 2011 Effects of intramuscular meloxicam administration of prostaglandin E2 synthesis in the North American bullfrog *(Rana catesbeiana)*. J Zoo Wildl Med 42:680–685

Pessier A P, Roberts D R, Linn M et al 2002 "Short tongue syndrome," Lingual squamous metaplasia and suspected hypovitaminosis A in captive Wyoming toads, *Bufo baxteri*. Proc Assoc Reptil Amphib Vet 151–153

Shaw S D, Bishop P J, Harvey C et al 2012 Fluorosis as a probable factor in metabolic bone disease in captive New Zealand native frogs *(Leiopelma* species). J Zoo Wildl Med 43(3):549–565

Stevens C W 2011 Analgesia in amphibians: Preclinical studies and clinical applications. Vet Clin North Am Exot Anim Pract 14:33–44

Williams D L, Whitaker B R 1994 The amphibian eye: a clinical review. J Zoo Wildl Med 25(1):18–28

Wright K M 1995 Amphibian medicine. Proc Assoc Reptil Amphib Vet 1995:59–64

Chapter 14

Britt T, Weisse C, Weber S et al 2002 Use of pneumocystoplasty for overinflation of the swim bladder in a goldfish. J Am Vet Med Assoc 221(5):690–693

Bunnajirakul S, Steinhagen D, Hetzel U et al 2000 A study of histopathology of *Trypanoplasma borreli* (Protozoa: Kinetoplastida) in susceptible common carp *Cyprinus carpio*. Dis Aquat Organ 39(3):221–229

Burghdorf-Moisuk A, Mitchel M A, Watson M 2011 Clinical and physiological effects of sodium chloride baths in goldfish *(Carassius auratus)*. J Zoo Wildl Med 42(4):586–592

Conroy G, Conroy D A 1999 Acid-fast bacterial infection and its control in guppies *(Lebistes reticulatus)* reared on an ornamental fish farm in Venezuela. Vet Rec 144:177–178

Dezfuli B S, Simoni E, Rossi R et al 2000 Rodlet cells and other inflammatory cells of *Phoxinus phoxinus* infected with *Raphidascaris acus* (Nematoda). Dis Aquat Organ 43(1):61–69

Govett P D, Olby N J, Marcellin-Little D J et al 2004 Stabilisation of scoliosis in two koi *(Cyprinus carpio)*. Vet Rec 155:115–119

Jepson L 2001 Koi medicine. Kingdom Books, Havant

Meyer C, Ganter M, Korting W et al 2002 Effects of a parasite-induced nephritis on osmoregulation in the common carp *Cyprinus carpio*. Dis Aquat Organ 8(50):127–135

Molnar K 2002 Differences between the European carp *(Cyprinus carpio carpio)* and the coloured carp *(Cyprinus carpio haematopterus)* in susceptibility to *Thelohanellus nikolskii* (Myxosporea) infection. Acta Vet Hung 50(1):51–57

Pasnik D J, Smith S A, Wolf J C 2003 Accidental electroshock of fish in a recirculation facility. Veterinary Record 153:562–564

Patino R 1997 Manipulations of the reproductive system of fishes by means of exogenous chemicals. Prog Fish Cult 59(1):18–128

Sano T, Morita N, Shima N et al 1991 Herpesvirus cyprini: Lethality and oncogenicity. J Fish Dis 14:533–543

Yokohama H, Liyanage Y S, Sugai A et al 1999 Efficacy of fumagillin against haemorrhagic thelohanellosis caused by *Thelohanellus hovorkai* (Myxosporea: Myyxozoa) in coloured carp, *Cyprinus carpio L.* J Fish Dis 22:243–245

Chapter 15

Aloo P A 2002 A comparative study of helminth parasites from the fish *Tilapia zillii* and *Oreochromis leucostictus* in Lake Naivasha and Oloidien Bay, Kenya. J Helminthol 76(2):95–104

Britt T, Weisse C, Weber S et al 2002 Use of pneumocystoplasty for overinflation of the swim bladder in a goldfish. J Am Vet Med Assoc 221(5):690–693

Conroy G, Conroy D A 1999 Acid-fast bacterial infection and its control in guppies *(Lebistes reticulatus)* reared on an ornamental fish farm in Venezuela. Vet Rec 144:177–178

Francis-Floyd R, Bolon B, Frase W et al 1993 Lip fibromas associated with retrovirus-like particles in angelfish. J Am Vet Med Assoc 202(10):1547–1548

Gonzalez-Solis D, Moravec F 2002 A new atractid nematode, *Atractis vidali* sp. *n.* (Nematoda: Atractidae), from cichlid fishes in southern Mexico. Folia Parasitol (Praha) 49(3):227–230

Lewbart G A, Stone E A, Love N E 1995 Pneumocystectomy in a Midas cichlid. J Am Vet Med Assoc 207:319–321

Miles D J, Kanchanakhan S, Lilley J H et al 2001 Effect of macrophages and serum of fish susceptible or resistant to epizootic ulcerative syndrome (EUS) on the EUS pathogen, *Aphanomyces invadans*. Fish Shellfish Immunol 11(7):569–584

Negm-Eldin M M, Davies R W 1999 Simultaneous transmission of *Trypanosoma mukasai, Babesiosoma mariae* and *Cyrilia nili* to fish by the leech *Batracobdelloides tricarinata*. Dtsch Tierarztl Wochenschr 106(12):526–527

Noga E J, Flowers J R 1995 Invasion of *Tilapia mossambica* (cichlidae) viscera by the monogenean *Enterogyrus cichlidarum*. J Parasitol 81(5):815–817

Noga E J, Wright J F, Pasarell L 1990 Some unusual features of mycobacteriosis in the cichlid fish *Oreochromis mossambicus*. J Comp Pathol 102(3):335–344

Pasnik D J, Smith S A, Wolf J C 2003 Accidental electroshock of fish in a recirculation facility. Vet Rec 153:562–564

Pimenta Leibowitz M, Ariav R, Zilberg D 2005 Environmental and physiological conditions affecting *Tetrahymena* sp. infection in guppies, *Poecilia reticulata* Peters. J Fish Dis 28:539–547

Silva-Souza A T, Eiras J C 2002 The histopathology of the infection of *Tilapia rendalli and Hypostomus regani (Osteichthyes)* by lasidium larvae of *Anodontites trapesialis* (Mollusca, Bivalvia). Mem Inst Oswaldo Cruz 97(3):431–433

Vidal-Martinez V M, Kennedy C R 2000 Potential interactions between the intestinal helminths of the cichlid fish *Cichlasoma synspilum* from southeastern Mexico. J Parasitol 86(4):691–695

Wildgoose W 1998 Skin disease in ornamental fish: Identifying common problems. In Pract 20:226–243

Yanong R P, Curtis E, Russo R et al 2004 *Cryptobia iubilans* infection in juvenile discus. J Am Vet Med Assoc 224(10):1644–1650

Chapter 16

Beier M, Anken R H, Rahmann H 2002 Susceptibility to abnormal (kinetotic) swimming fish correlates with inner ear carbonic anhydrase-reactivity. Neurosci Lett 335(1):17–20

Blasiola G C, Turnier J C, Hurst E E 1981 Metastatic thyroid adenocarcinomas in a captive population of kelp bass, *Paralabrax clanthatus*. J Nat Cancer Inst 66:51–59

Bullard S A, FrascaJr S, Benz G W 2000 Skin lesions caused by *Dermophthirius penneri* (Monogenea Microbothriidae) on wild-caught blacktip sharks *(Carcharinus limbatus)*. J Parasitol 86(3):618–622

Carrillo J, Martinez J, Divanach P et al 1999 Unilateral eye abnormalities in reared Mediterranean gilthead sea bream. Vet Rec 145:494–497

Conroy G, Conroy D A 1999 Acid-fast bacterial infection and its control in guppies *(Lebistes reticulatus)* reared on an ornamental fish farm in Venezuela. Vet Rec 144:177–178

Fairbanks M B, Hoffert J R, Fromm P O 1974 Short circuiting of the ocular oxygen concentrating mechanism in the Teleost *Salmo gairdneri* using carbonic anhydrase inhibitors. J Gen Physiol 64:263–273

Greenwell M G, Vainisi S J 1994 Surgical management of lipid keratopathy in green moray eels *(Gynothorax funebris)*. Proc Am Assoc Zoo Vet 179–181

LePage V, Dutton C J, Crawshaw G et al 2014 A study of diseases in captive yellow seahorse *Hippocampus kuda*, pot-bellied seahorse *Hippocampus abdominalis* and weedy seadragon *Phyllopteryx taeniolatus*. J Fish Dis 2014 May 13; [Epub 2014 May 13]

Lin Q, Lin J, Huang L 2010 Effects of light intensity, stocking density and temperature on the air-bubble disease, survivorship and growth of early juvenile seahorse *Hippocampus erectus* Perry, 1810. Aquaculture Research 42:91–98

Oestmann D J 1985 Environmental and disease problems in ornamental marine aquariums. Comp Cont Ed Pract Vet 7(8):656–667

Pasnik D J, Smith S A, Wolf J C 2003 Accidental electroshock of fish in a recirculation facility. Vet Rec 153:562–564

Shields R P, Popp J A 1979 Intracardial mesotheliomas and a gastric papilloma in a giant grouper, *Epinephelus itajara*. Vet Pathol 16:191–198

Stoskopf M K 1993 Clinical pathology of sharks, skates and rays. Fish medicine. Saunders, Philadelphia

Varner P W, Lewis D H 1991 Characterization of a virus associated with head and lateral line erosion syndrome in marine angelfish. J Aquat Health 3:198–205

Vincent A C J, Clifton-Hadley R S 1989 Parasitic infection of the seahorse *(Hippocampus erectus)*. A case report. J Wildl Dis 25(3):404–406

Index

Page numbers followed by "*f*" indicate figures, "*t*" indicate tables, and "*b*" indicate boxes.